Tissue and Organ Regeneration

Tissue and Organ Regeneration

Advances in Micro- and Nanotechnology

edited by
Lijie Grace Zhang
Ali Khademhosseini
Thomas J. Webster

PAN STANFORD PUBLISHING

Published by

Pan Stanford Publishing Pte. Ltd.
Penthouse Level, Suntec Tower 3
8 Temasek Boulevard
Singapore 038988

Email: editorial@panstanford.com
Web: www.panstanford.com

British Library Cataloguing-in-Publication Data
A catalogue record for this book is available from the British Library.

Tissue and Organ Regeneration: Advances in Micro- and Nanotechnology

Copyright © 2014 Pan Stanford Publishing Pte. Ltd.

All rights reserved. This book, or parts thereof, may not be reproduced in any form or by any means, electronic or mechanical, including photocopying, recording or any information storage and retrieval system now known or to be invented, without written permission from the publisher.

For photocopying of material in this volume, please pay a copying fee through the Copyright Clearance Center, Inc., 222 Rosewood Drive, Danvers, MA 01923, USA. In this case permission to photocopy is not required from the publisher.

Cover image: Courtesy of Juan Carlos Izpisua Belmonte, Salk Institute for Biological Studies. Neural differentiation in an embryoid body derived from human iPS cells (beta-III tubulin in green and DAPI in blue).

ISBN 978-981-4411-67-7 (Hardcover)
ISBN 978-981-4411-68-4 (eBook)

Printed in the USA

Contents

Preface   xxi

Part I: Micro and Nanotechnology

1. **Nano/Microfabrication Techniques for Tissue and Organ Regeneration**   3
   Benjamin Holmes, Thomas J. Webster, and Lijie Grace Zhang

   1.1 Introduction   3
        1.1.1 Introduction and Clinical Challenges   3
        1.1.2 Tissue Engineering   4
        1.1.3 Scaffold-Based Approaches and Scaffold Roles   4
   1.2 Electrospinning   5
        1.2.1 Introduction   5
        1.2.2 Basic Principles, Materials and Practices   5
        1.2.3 Modification of Scaffold Porosity   7
        1.2.4 Electrospun Composite Scaffolds   8
        1.2.5 Novel Methodology   10
            1.2.5.1 Co-spun scaffolds and co-deposited materials   10
            1.2.5.2 Wet-electrospinning   13
            1.2.5.3 Novel nanocomposites   14
   1.3 3D Printing   16
        1.3.1 Introduction to 3D Printing and Medical Applications   16
        1.3.2 Methods   17
            1.3.2.1 Fused deposition modeling   17
            1.3.2.2 Selective laser sintering and stereolithography   19
            1.3.2.3 Laminated object manufacturing   21

		1.3.2.4	Inkjet 3D printing	22
		1.3.2.5	Novel methodology and applications	23
	1.4	Other Current Methodology		25
		1.4.1	Solvent Casting	25
		1.4.2	Gas Foaming	26
		1.4.3	Phase Separation	27
	1.5	Summary		27

2. Three-Dimensional Micropatterning of Biomaterial Scaffolds for Tissue Engineering — 37

Joseph C. Hoffmann and Jennifer L. West

	2.1	Need for 3D Micropatterning in Tissue Engineering		37
	2.2	3D Printing		39
		2.2.1	Direct-Write Bioprinting	40
		2.2.2	Inkjet Bioprinting	43
		2.2.3	Biological Laser Printing	46
	2.3	Photolithography		49
		2.3.1	Post-Gelation Photopatterning	50
		2.3.2	Stereolithography	61
	2.4	The Future of Micropatterning in Tissue Engineering		66

3. Nanobiotechnology and Biomaterials for Regenerative Medicine — 75

Nupura S. Bhise and Jordan J. Green

	3.1	Introduction		76
	3.2	Polymeric 3-D Systems for Tissue Regeneration		79
		3.2.1	Hydrogel Systems	79
		3.2.2	Nano/Micro-Fabricated Systems	80
			3.2.2.1 Photolithography	81
			3.2.2.2 Electrospinning	83
	3.3	Nanoparticle-Based Delivery Systems for Programming and Reprogramming Cell Fate		89
	3.4	High-Throughput Combinatorial Strategies for Biomaterial Development		93
	3.5	Conclusions		97

4. Micro- and Nanotechnology Engineering Strategies for Tissue Interface Regeneration and Repair — 105
Torri E. Rinker and Johnna S. Temenoff

- 4.1 Introduction — 106
- 4.2 Co-Culture Systems for in vitro Analysis of Tissue Interfaces — 108
  - 4.2.1 Two-Dimensional Systems — 108
    - 4.2.1.1 Physically separated cell populations — 109
    - 4.2.1.2 Direct-contact cell populations — 111
  - 4.2.2 Three-Dimensional Systems — 115
    - 4.2.2.1 Physically separated cell populations — 115
    - 4.2.2.2 Direct-contact cell populations — 118
- 4.3 Scaffold Types for in vivo Applications in Interface Tissue Engineering — 121
  - 4.3.1 Gradiated Scaffolds — 122
    - 4.3.1.1 Composition gradients — 123
    - 4.3.1.2 Structure gradients — 124
    - 4.3.1.3 Biomolecular gradients — 127
  - 4.3.2 Braided Scaffolds — 129
  - 4.3.3 Microsphere-Containing Scaffolds — 130
  - 4.3.4 Natural Scaffolds — 131
- 4.4 Scaffold Fabrication — 133
  - 4.4.1 Nanofibrous Scaffold Fabrication — 133
    - 4.4.1.1 Self-assembly — 133
    - 4.4.1.2 Phase separation — 134
    - 4.4.1.3 Electrospinning — 135
  - 4.4.2 Gradiated Scaffolds — 136
    - 4.4.2.1 Flow-based systems — 136
    - 4.4.2.2 Diffusion — 137
    - 4.4.2.3 Time-dependent exposure — 138
  - 4.4.3 Rapid Prototyping — 139
    - 4.4.3.1 Inkjet printing — 140
    - 4.4.3.2 Multinozzle low-temperature deposition — 141
- 4.5 Future Directions — 141

5. Spatiotemporal Genetic Control of Cellular Systems   157
Lauren R. Polstein and Charles A. Gersbach

  5.1 Introduction   157
  5.2 Time-Independent Gene Regulation Systems   158
      5.2.1 Constitutive Gene Expression Systems   158
      5.2.2 Constitutive Gene Silencing   163
  5.3 Systems for Temporal Control of Gene Regulation   164
      5.3.1 Chemically Induced Gene Regulation Systems   165
            5.3.1.1 Tetracycline-inducible system   165
            5.3.1.2 Small molecule–induced dimerizers   171
      5.3.2 Hormone-Induced Systems   174
  5.4 Spatiotemporal Gene Regulation Systems   177
      5.4.1 Heat-Inducible Gene Regulation   177
      5.4.2 Ultraviolet Radiation-Induced Gene Expression   178
      5.4.3 Light-Induced Gene Regulation Systems   181
      5.4.4 Spatiotemporal Genetic Control Using Scaffolds   186
  5.5 Conclusion   188

6. Biomimetic Design of Extracellular Matrix-Like Substrate for Tissue Regeneration   199
Chao Jia, Seyed Babak Mahjour, Lawrence Chan, Da-wei Hou, and Hongjun Wang

  6.1 Introduction   200
  6.2 Electrospinning and Electrospun Fibers   201
  6.3 Incorporation of Various Biomolecules (Like ECM Molecules, Growth Factors) into Nanofibers   205
  6.4 Control of Fiber Spatial Arrangement   211
  6.5 Formation of Multifunctional Hierarchical Structures Enabled by Nanofibers   214
      6.5.1 Formation of Acellular Sandwiched Structures   214
      6.5.2 Formation of Cell/Fiber Multilayered Structure   217

		6.5.3	Three-Dimensional Tissue Formation from the Assembled Cell/Fiber Structure	219
	6.6	Future Perspectives		220
	6.7	Conclusion		221

7. Degradable Elastomers for Tissue Regeneration — 231

G. Rajesh Krishnan, Michael J. Hill, and Debanjan Sarkar

	7.1	Introduction		231
	7.2	Characteristics of Elastomers		232
	7.3	Design of Biodegradable Elastomers		234
		7.3.1	Polyesters	234
		7.3.2	Polyamides/Peptides	240
		7.3.3	Polyurethanes	242
		7.3.4	Hydrogels	245
	7.4	Applications of Biodegradable Elastomers in Tissue Regeneration		248
		7.4.1	Blood Vessels	248
		7.4.2	Bladder	250
		7.4.3	Cardiac Tissue Engineering	251
		7.4.4	Tracheal, Neural, and Retinal	253
	7.5	Conclusion		255

8. Protein Engineering Strategies for Modular, Responsive, and Spatially Organized Biomaterials — 265

Ian Wheeldon

	8.1	Introduction	266
	8.2	Modular Design of Multi-Functional and Bioactive Hydrogels	268
	8.3	Protein Engineering of Stimuli-Responsive Hydrogels	273
	8.4	Nanoscale Spatial Organization of Bioactive Signals in Protein Hydrogels	278
	8.5	Future Direction of Protein and Peptide Biomaterials	283

Part II: Tissue and Organ Regeneration

9. Design and Fabrication of Biomimetic Microvascular Architecture — 295
Thomas M. Cervantes and Joseph P. Vacanti

- 9.1 Introduction — 295
  - 9.1.1 Clinical Need for Whole Organ Fabrication — 295
  - 9.1.2 Mass Transport and Manufacturing Limitations — 296
- 9.2 Biomimetic Vascular Design Principles — 298
  - 9.2.1 Functional Motif — 299
  - 9.2.2 Pressure and Flow Conditions — 300
  - 9.2.3 Shear Stress — 302
  - 9.2.4 Aspect Ratio — 305
  - 9.2.5 Vessel Length — 307
  - 9.2.6 Diameter Relationships — 308
  - 9.2.7 Branching Angle — 309
  - 9.2.8 Boundary Layer Profile at Intersections — 311
  - 9.2.9 Computational Design Tools — 312
- 9.3 Microfabrication Technologies — 313
  - 9.3.1 Micromolding — 314
  - 9.3.2 Direct Fabrication — 318
  - 9.3.3 Sacrificial Molding — 319
  - 9.3.4 Self-assembly and Bioprinting — 322

10. Tissue Engineering of Human Bladder — 335
Anthony Atala

- 10.1 Introduction — 336
- 10.2 Basics of Tissue Engineering — 336
  - 10.2.1 Biomaterials Used in Genitourinary Tissue Construction — 337
  - 10.2.2 Design and Selection of Biomaterials — 338
  - 10.2.3 Types of Biomaterials — 339
  - 10.2.4 Cells for Urogenital Tissue Engineering Applications — 342

		10.2.5	Stem Cells and Other Pluripotent Cell Types	344
	10.3		Tissue Engineering Strategies for Bladder Replacement	348
		10.3.1	Biomaterial Matrices for Bladder Regeneration	348
		10.3.2	Regenerative Medicine for Bladder Using Cell Transplantation	350
	10.4		Conclusions	354
11.	The Self-Assembling Process of Articular Cartilage and Self-Organization in Tissue Engineering			369

Pasha Hadidi, Rajalakshmanan Eswaramoorthy, Jerry C. Hu, and Kyriacos A. Athanasiou

	11.1	Introduction		369
		11.1.1	Scaffoldless versus Scaffold-Based Engineered Tissue	370
		11.1.2	Scaffoldless Methods of Generating Tissue	372
		11.1.3	Self-Organization and the Self-Assembling Process in Tissue Engineering	375
	11.2	Examples of Self-Organization in Tissue Engineering		377
		11.2.1	Tendon and Ligament	378
		11.2.2	Liver	379
		11.2.3	Vascular	380
		11.2.4	Bone	381
		11.2.5	Optic and Nerve Tissues	382
	11.3	Biological Mechanisms Underlying the Self-Assembling Process		383
		11.3.1	The Differential Adhesion Hypothesis and the Self-Assembling Process as an Energy-Driven Process	383
		11.3.2	Cell Contraction and the Cytoskeleton in Cell Sorting	385
	11.4	The Self-Assembling Process in Tissue Engineering: Articular Cartilage and Fibrocartilage		387

  11.4.1 Distinct Phases of Self-Assembling
     Cartilage Reminiscent of Morphogenesis   387
  11.4.2 Native Tissue Dimensions and Morphology
     in Self-Assembling Cartilage   389
  11.4.3 Near-Native Biomechanical Properties of
     Self-Assembling Cartilage   390
 11.5 Signals Used to Engineer Self-Organizing and
   Self-Assembling Tissues   391
  11.5.1 Soluble Signals   391
  11.5.2 Mechanical Signals   392
  11.5.3 Coordinated Soluble and Mechanical
     Signaling   393
 11.6 Conclusion and Future Directions   393

12. Environmental Factors in Cartilage Tissue Engineering   409
Yueh-Hsun Yang and Gilda A. Barabino

 12.1 Articular Cartilage   410
  12.1.1 Structure and Function   410
  12.1.2 Degeneration and Repair   411
  12.1.3 Cartilage Tissue Engineering   412
 12.2 Environmental Stimuli   414
  12.2.1 Mechanical Forces   415
    12.2.1.1 Deformational loading   415
    12.2.1.2 Hydrostatic pressure   417
    12.2.1.3 Laminar flow   418
    12.2.1.4 Turbulent flow   419
  12.2.3 Biochemical Signals   421
    12.2.3.1 Fetal bovine serum   422
    12.2.3.2 Growth factors: insulin-like growth
        factor-1 and transforming growth
        factor-β   423
 12.3 Interplay between Mechanical and Biochemical
   Stimuli   425
  12.3.1 Low Serum Effects on Cultivation of
     Neocartilage   425

		12.3.2	Continuous versus Transient Exposure of Engineered Cartilage to Growth Factors	428

	12.4	Multipotent Mesenchymal Stem Cells	431
		12.4.1 Driving Forces of MSC Chondrogenic Differentiation	432
		12.4.2 Coculture-Enabled MSC Chondrogenesis	434
	12.5	Conclusions and Future Directions	437

13. Bone Regenerative Engineering: The Influence of Micro- and Nano-Dimension — 455

Roshan James, Meng Deng, Sangamesh G. Kumbar, and Cato T. Laurencin

13.1	Introduction	455
13.2	Understanding Native Bone	457
	13.2.1 Hierarchical Organization of Bone	458
	13.2.2 Biology of Bone	461
13.3	Bone Grafts	463
	13.3.1 Autografts	463
	13.3.2 Allografts	463
	13.3.3 Bone Graft Substitutes	464
13.4	Design Considerations for Bone Graft Substitutes	464
13.5	Regeneration Using Surface Topography and Scaffold Architecture	467
13.6	Stem Cells	475
13.7	Conclusions	482

14. Stem Cells and Bone Regeneration — 495

Martin L. Decaris, Kaitlin C. Murphy, and J. Kent Leach

14.1	Introduction	495
14.2	Sources of Stem Cells for Bone Regeneration	497
	14.2.1 Pluripotent Stem Cells	498
	14.2.2 Adult Stem Cells	499
14.3	Osteogenic Induction of Stem Cells	503
	14.3.1 Soluble Osteogenic Factors	504
	14.3.2 Bulk Material Properties	506

14.3.3	Material Surface Properties	509
14.3.4	Cell–Cell Interactions	512
14.3.5	Genetic Modification of Stem Cells	513
14.4	Stem Cell–Based Approaches to Bone Formation	515
14.4.1	Ex vivo Bone Formation	515
14.4.2	Bone Formation in vivo	517
14.5	Conclusions	520

15. Notch Signaling Biomaterials and Tissue Regeneration — **535**

Thanaphum Osathanon, Prasit Pavasant, and Cecilia Giachelli

15.1	Introduction	535
15.2	The Notch Signaling Pathway	536
15.2.1	Notch Family of Receptors and Their Ligands	537
15.2.2	Notch Signaling	538
15.2.2.1	Canonical Notch signaling pathway	539
15.2.2.2	Non-canonical Notch signaling pathway	540
15.3	Role of Notch Signaling in Stem Cells	541
15.3.1	Notch Signaling in Hematopoietic Stem Cells	541
15.3.2	Notch Signaling in Adipose-Derived Mesenchymal Stem Cells	542
15.3.3	Notch Signaling in Dental Tissue-Derived Mesenchymal Stem Cells	542
15.3.4	Notch Signaling in Epithelial Stem Cells	544
15.4	Notch Signaling Biomaterials	545
15.4.1	Notch Signaling Surfaces	545
15.4.1.1	Indirect affinity immobilization of Notch ligands	545
15.4.1.2	Site-specific binding via Fc domain	546
15.4.1.3	An antigen–antibody reaction combined with biotin-streptavidin chemistry	547

		15.4.2	Potential Use of Notch Signaling Biomaterials in Regenerative Medicine	548
			15.4.2.1 Notch signaling biomaterials and HSC expansion and differentiation	548
			15.4.2.2 Notch signaling biomaterials and bone regeneration	548
			15.4.2.3 Notch signaling biomaterials and periodontal tissue regeneration	549
			15.4.2.4 Notch signaling biomaterials and cardiac regeneration	550
	15.5	Conclusions		551

16. Stem Cell-Based Dental, Oral, and Craniofacial Tissue Engineering — 565

Sahng G. Kim, Chang Hun Lee, Jian Zhou, Mo Chen, Ying Zheng, Mildred C. Embree, Kimi Kong, Karen Song, Susan Y. Fu, Shoko Cho, Nan Jiang, and Jeremy J. Mao

	16.1	Introduction		565
	16.2	Challenges of Orofacial Tissue Regeneration		565
	16.3	Orofacial Stem/Progenitor Cells		566
		16.3.1	Dental Epithelial Stem Cells	567
		16.3.2	Dental Mesenchyme Stem/Progenitor Cells	567
			16.3.2.1 Periodontal ligament	567
			16.3.2.2 Dental pulp	568
			16.3.2.3 Dental follicle	568
	16.4	Tooth Regeneration		569
	16.5	Dental Pulp and Dentin Regeneration		571
	16.6	Periodontal Regeneration		573
	16.7	Calvarial Bone Regeneration		575
	16.8	Clinical Engagement and Training for Regenerative Therapies		577
	16.9	Summary		578

17. Engineering Functional Bone Grafts for Craniofacial Regeneration   589

Pinar Yilgor Huri and Warren L. Grayson

  17.1 Introduction   589
      17.1.1 Overview of Bone Tissue Engineering for Craniofacial Applications   590
  17.2 Principles of Craniofacial Graft Design   591
      17.2.1 Cell Sources for Craniofacial Bone Tissue Engineering   591
      17.2.2 Scaffold Biomaterials   595
      17.2.3 Engineering Anatomically Shaped Craniofacial Grafts   600
      17.2.4 Growth Factors and Delivery Strategies   601
      17.2.5 Bone Bioreactor   605
  17.3 Impact of Micro- and Nano-Technologies in Craniofacial Bone Tissue Engineering   607
      17.3.1 Biomimetic Nanofibrous Scaffolds   607
      17.3.2 Topographical Cues   608
  17.4 Summary   609

18. Nanotechnology in Osteochondral Regeneration   621

Nathan J. Castro, Joseph R. O'Brien, and Lijie Grace Zhang

  18.1 Introduction   622
  18.2 Osteochondral Anatomy and Physiology   623
  18.3 Osteochondral Tissue Regeneration   625
      18.3.1 Introduction   625
      18.3.2 Nanobiomaterials for Osteochondral Regeneration   627
            18.3.2.1 Self-assembling nanobiomaterials   627
            18.3.2.2 Carbon-based nanobiomaterials   630
            18.3.2.3 Other therapeutic encapsulated nanobiomaterials   631
      18.3.3 Three-Dimensional Nanocomposite Scaffolds For Osteochondral Regeneration   634

		18.3.3.1	3D stratified/graded nano osteochondral scaffolds	634
		18.3.3.2	Emerging 3D printed nanocomposite osteochondral scaffolds	635
18.4	Conclusions			637

19. Aortic Heart Valve Tissue Regeneration — 645

Bin Duan, Laura A. Hockaday, Kevin H. Kang, and Jonathan T. Butcher

19.1	Introduction			646
19.2	Heart Valve Function, Structure, and Physiology			647
	19.2.1	Heart Valve Function and Structure		647
	19.2.2	Aortic Valve Cellular Composition		649
		19.2.2.1	Valvular endothelial cells	650
		19.2.2.2	Valve interstitial cells	650
	19.2.3	Interaction between Valve Interstitial Cells and Microenvironment		651
19.3	Tissue-Engineered Aortic Heart Valve			652
	19.3.1	Principles and Criteria		652
		19.3.1.1	Decellularized valves	653
		19.3.1.2	Natural biomaterials for TEHV	656
		19.3.1.3	Biodegradable synthetic polymers	657
		19.3.1.4	In vivo–engineered valve-shaped tissues	658
	19.3.2	Strategies for TEHV Scaffold Fabrication		659
	19.3.3	Cell Sources		660
	19.3.4	Heart Valve Tissue Bioreactors		662
		19.3.4.1	Component bioreactors	663
		19.3.4.2	Whole valve scale bioreactors	667
	19.3.5	In vivo Animal Models and Approaches for Heart Valve Regeneration		674
19.4	Future Direction			675
19.5	Conclusions			676

20. Micro and Nanotechnology in Vascular Regeneration — 695
Vivian Lee and Guohao Dai

- 20.1 Overview of Angiogenesis and Vasculogenesis — 696
- 20.2 Biomaterial Scaffold to Promote Vascularization — 697
  - 20.2.1 Biomaterials for Controlled Release of Angiogenic Factors — 697
  - 20.2.2 Immobilization of Bioactive Molecules to Enhance Angiogenesis — 700
  - 20.2.3 Engineering Biomaterial Architecture to Promote Infiltration of Vascular Cells — 701
- 20.3 Micro- and Nanotechnologies to Create Precise Vascular Patterns — 702
  - 20.3.1 Microfabrication-Based Approaches — 702
  - 20.3.2 Multiphoton Polymerization of Hydrogels for Vascular Patterns — 704
  - 20.3.3 Rapid Prototyping and Solid Free form Techniques — 705
  - 20.3.4 Bottom-Up Approach: Self-Assembling of Cell-Laden Hydrogels — 708
  - 20.3.5 Cell Sheet Technology — 709
- 20.4 Summary — 712

21. Micro- and Nanofabrication Approaches to Cardiac Tissue Engineering — 725
Nicole Trosper, Petra Kerscher, Jesse Macadangdang, Daniel Carson, Elizabeth Lipke, and Deok-Ho Kim

- 21.1 Introduction — 726
- 21.2 Multiscale Features of Cardiac Tissue Environments — 727
- 21.3 Current Challenges in Cardiac Tissue Engineering — 729
- 21.4 Micro- and Nanofabrication Techniques — 733
  - 21.4.1 Electron Beam Lithography — 733
  - 21.4.2 Template Molding — 734
  - 21.4.3 Microcontact Printing — 735
  - 21.4.4 Electrospun Nanofibers — 736
- 21.5 Applications of Micro- and Nanofabrication in Cardiac Tissue Engineering — 737

	21.5.1 Cell Sheet Engineering	740
	21.5.2 Cell-Laden Scaffolds	741
	21.5.3 Nanoparticles	744
21.6	Conclusion	746

22. Engineering of Skeletal Muscle Regeneration: Principles, Current State, and Challenges — 755

Weining Bian, Mark Juhas, and Nenad Bursac

22.1	Biology of Skeletal Muscle Regeneration	755
	22.1.1 Overview of Skeletal Myogenesis	756
	22.1.2 Muscle Regeneration in Acute Trauma and Chronic Degenerative Diseases	759
	22.1.3 Role of Satellite Cells in Muscle Regeneration	761
	22.1.4 Role of Non-Myogenic Cells in Muscle Regeneration	762
	22.1.5 Role of Extracellular Matrix in Muscle Regeneration	763
22.2	Current Advances toward Therapeutic Muscle Regeneration	765
	22.2.1 Artificial Stem Cell Niches for Cell Expansion	766
	22.2.2 In situ Tissue Regeneration	767
	22.2.3 In vitro Generation of Functional Skeletal Muscle Tissues	768
22.3	Existing Challenges and Future Work	770
	22.3.1 Optimal Cell Source	771
	22.3.2 Optimal Biomaterial	774
	22.3.3 Neurovascular Integration	776
22.4	Concluding Remarks	778

Index — 791

Preface

This premier edition of *Tissue and Organ Regeneration: Advances in Micro- and Nanotechnology* provides an extensive overview of micro- and nanoscale technological advancements for a variety of tissue/organ regeneration such as bone, cartilage, craniofacial, osteochondral, muscle, bladder, cardiac, and vascular tissues. Specifically, it emphasizes state-of-the-art biomimetic spatio-temporally controlled scaffold fabrication as well as directed stem-cell behavior and fate by micro- and nanoscale cues. Owing to the rapid progression of micro- and nanotechnology for tissue and organ regeneration and the extensive amount of resources available, it is at times difficult to ascertain a solid understanding of cutting-edge research. Therefore, the current text aims to provide an up-to-date survey of this fast-developing research focus.

This current edition is divided into two main areas: (1) an overview of current advances in micro- and nanotechnology and (2) micro- and nanotechnology for tissue and organ applications. As our collective understanding of the interactions between tissue/organ extracellular matrix components and native cells increases, novel strategies for the seamless integration of micro- and nanoscale features, biochemical signaling, and stem cell biology have become ever more important for tissue engineers and scientists. This text will serve as a comprehensive resource for students and experts alike and is intended to be used as an excellent teaching tool for advanced undergraduate and graduate courses. In addition, contributions from many world leaders in tissue and organ regeneration with respect to specific tissue/organ systems that have been shown to be of greatest clinical value provide researchers and scientists a unique perspective of micro/nanotechnology, biomaterials, stem cell biology, and tissue engineering.

In addition, we have given particular attention to stem cells, including adult stem cells and progenitor populations that may soon lead to new tissue-engineering therapies for various tissue regenerations and a wide variety of other clinically relevant diseases. This up-to-date coverage of stem cell and biological cues and other emerging technologies is complemented by a series of chapters applying micro- and nanotechnology for tissue engineering. The result is a valuable book that we believe not only will be useful in understanding recent breakthroughs and ongoing challenges in this dynamic research area but also will spur the cultivation of new strategies that may foster future and developing research.

Lijie Grace Zhang
Ali Khademhosseini
Thomas J. Webster

Part 1

Micro- and Nanotechnology

Chapter 1

Nano/Microfabrication Techniques for Tissue and Organ Regeneration

Benjamin Holmes,[a] Thomas J. Webster,[b] and Lijie Grace Zhang[a]

[a]*Department of Mechanical and Aerospace Engineering and Department of Medicine, The George Washington University, 801 22nd Street NW, 726 Phillips Hall, Washington, DC 20052, USA*
[b]*Department of Chemical Engineering, Northeastern University, 360 Huntington Avenue, 313 Snell Engineering Center, Boston, MA 02115, USA*

lgzhang@gwu.edu

1.1 Introduction

1.1.1 Introduction and Clinical Challenges

Current medical treatment methods have shifted toward more customizable, patient-specific options through the evolution of technology in modern medicine. Nowhere is this more evident than in tissue repair and organ regeneration [3,33]. Currently, the treatment of defects and injury to tissues with limited regenerative capacity, such as cartilage, vasculature, cardiac tissue, and nerves involve highly invasive and painful procedures, such as a total hip or knee replacement. In many of the cases listed, there are inadequate alternative treatment methods available other than traditional organ/tissue transplants, which contain their own inherent complications. In recent years, a great deal of research has focused

---

Tissue and Organ Regeneration: Advances in Micro- and Nanotechnology
Edited by Lijie Grace Zhang, Ali Khademhosseini, and Thomas J. Webster
Copyright © 2014 Pan Stanford Publishing Pte. Ltd.
ISBN 978-981-4411-67-7 (Hardcover), 978-981-4411-68-4 (eBook)
www.panstanford.com

on the treatment of traumatic and congenital injuries via stem cell therapy [25,79,97]. Although stem cells hold great promise in regenerative medicine, long-term success has been difficult to achieve when they are used alone.

1.1.2 Tissue Engineering

Tissue engineering (TE) may hold the key to unlocking the potential of stem cell-based organ repair and tissue regeneration, and lead to better treatments which were previously only available at a great expense, if at all. Drs. Langer and Vacanti defined TE as "an interdisciplinary field that applies the principles of engineering and life sciences toward the development of biological substitutes that restore, maintain, or improve tissue function or a whole organ" [40,82]. In the ensuing years, this discipline quickly developed to encompass a variety of cell types (e.g., stem cells, chondrocytes, osteoblasts, endothelial cells, fibroblasts, and smooth muscle cells), scaffolds (e.g., biodegradable, natural or synthetic materials, polymers, and nanocomposites), bioactive factors (e.g., various growth factors and cytokines), and physical stimuli (mechanical, electrical, etc.) to form biomimetic tissues and organs. Specifically, scaffolds play a critical role in providing a 3D environment to support cell growth, control cell differentiation, improve matrix deposition, and tissue/organ regeneration.

1.1.3 Scaffold-Based Approaches and Scaffold Roles

In scaffold-based TE, a micro/nanoscale biocompatible and biodegradable material is designed with biomimetic features for enhanced and directed cell behavior. Stem cell behavior can be controlled not only by changing the physical dimensions of biomimetic scaffolds, but also by modulating the composition, surface chemistry, and mechanical properties [1,14,65].

An ideal scaffold should fulfill four key characteristics. It should provide (1) adequate structural support with a suitable degradation rate; (2) modulate the cellular microenvironment; (3) encourage cellular attachment, ingrowth and tissue formation, and (4) easily exchange nutrients and waste to and from cells within the construct [40,82,91]. Researchers in TE have been making great strides in designing and fabricating TE scaffolds to satisfy these design constraints via various nano- and microtechniques. This chapter will focus on two promising fabrication methods for micro- and nanofeatured TE scaffolds: electrospinning [101] and three-dimensional (3D) printing [12,18]. Both methods offer a high degree of control over scaffold architecture and composition to include the incorporation of morphogenetic constituent materials. In addition to these two methods, several other scaffold fabrication techniques for the manufacture of TE scaffolds will be discussed.

1.2 Electrospinning

1.2.1 Introduction

Novel methodologies for TE scaffold fabrication have been explored and developed in order to solve and improve current medical problems. For many years, creating polymer scaffolds as a substrate for tissue growth has been one of the most popular and most promising approaches for various tissue regeneration applications [29]. A very common and well-established method for creating these scaffolds is a process known as electrospinning. Electrospinning has been considered favorable because of the ability of researchers to create fibrous porous polymer scaffolds with features ranging from the micro- to the nanoscale mimicking the extracellular matrix (ECM) of native tissue and creating an environment for improved cell behavior [74]. While the system parameters needed to obtain desired fiber dimensions have been thoroughly investigated, a great deal of research is currently focused on means to fabricate polymeric scaffolds with modified physical and compositional complexities. In order to elucidate the current state of electrospinning for TE and its future directions, the clinical challenges facing tissue engineers and an explanation of electrospinning/its application to TE will be discussed in the following sections.

1.2.2 Basic Principles, Materials and Practices

Electrospun polymer scaffolds may provide an advantageous new approach to organ/tissue defect treatment. Because of the ease by which one can create a scaffold of desired physical and mechanical dimensions with incorporated nano- and microcomposite materials, there is great potential to influence and promote cell differentiation and proliferation [27].

Electrospinning is a process for creating inherently porous materials composed of micro- and/or nanoscale polymer fibers. Briefly, a solid polymer is dissolved in an organic solvent to produce a viscous solution, which is then loaded into a syringe with a blunt point needle or capillary and syringe pump. The expelled mixture is subjected to a high voltage potential over a specific working distance used to charge the polymer chains drawing a long fiber to a grounded collector plate [55,74,91]. The solvent evaporates, due to either the voltage potential or natural evaporation in air, and a mesh of solid polymer fibers is created [49,55,80]. There are currently a number of different synthetic and natural polymers used in electrospinning. Synthetic polymers are chosen for their biodegradability and biocompatibility, as well as their ability to match characteristics of the target tissue [14,27,101]. Some popular polymers include poly-L-lactic acid (PLLA) and poly-caprolactone (PCL) for electrospinning in bone, cartilage and neural regeneration applications [15,60,66], while other materials such as polyaniline (PAN) and polypyrrole (PPy) are used for cardiac and other neural applications due to their inherent electrical conductivity [62]. In the case of natural polymers, materials such as collagen and chitosan are very often used [6,7,42,60,99] for various tissue regeneration constructs because of their biocompatibility properties. However, when electrospun, these materials are weak and require structural support, so they are often electrospun into coatings or in conjunction with a stronger, synthetic polymer [6,27]. It is important to know that the number of polymers, both synthetic and natural, that are used for electrospinning are numerous, and chosen based on whatever specific application the scaffold will be used for [62,92,101].

The variation of parameters in electrospinning, such as voltage, working distance, and polymer-solvent solution concentration, in correlation to scaffold characteristics have been well established and understood. This being the case, electrospinning has already been used in a wide variety of practical and experimental applications. One of the simplest applications is for surface coatings and membranes [62,80]. Because of the ability of electrospinning to produce physical properties that mimic the ECM, it is often used to create coatings on implants and devices in order to promote cell adhesion [62]. Electrospinning can also be used to deposit natural polymers, proteins, and peptides onto surfaces, as well as onto electrospun polymer scaffolds for enhanced cell growth [15,62,80]. The same principles that make electrospun surface coatings on materials useful for promoting tissue regeneration also make electrospinning advantageous for scaffold design. Unlike coating an implant, where the goal is to induce existing cells and tissue to adhere on a biocompatible material, artificial tissue can be grown and incorporated into a target area in the body [29,88,91]. There are two different approaches to scaffold design: 2D and 3D scaffolds. An electrospun 2D scaffold is typically only several layers of fibers thick, and is intended to grow only one layer of cells [70]. While 2D scaffolds have been shown to promote cell growth, 3D scaffolds provide much better results, and are considered the most promising approach [6,42].

An electrospun 3D scaffold is many fiber layers thick and is intended to fully mimic the ECM of the natural tissue. 3D scaffolds have been shown to promote much better cell adhesion and growth as compared to 2D scaffolds, and are potentially very powerful for their ability to grow larger amounts of bulk tissue at a time, as well as having the promise of being able to grow whole organs and systems [29,40,82].

As discussed, the ultimate goal of a scaffold is to provide a framework that provides structural support for growing cells, as well as promoting cell growth and directed cell differentiation. Cells are seeded onto a pre-fabricated, electrospun scaffold and are promoted to grow for an extended period of time, usually around one month in an experimental setting. Typically, cells in native tissues/organs are seeded into an electrospun scaffold for specific tissue/organ regeneration such as chondrocytes for cartilage, osteoblasts for bone regeneration [46,58,68,80]. In more recent years research has been moving towards seeding electrospun scaffolds with various stem cells and attempting to direct their differentiation and proliferation to a desired tissue type [66,68].

1.2.3 Modification of Scaffold Porosity

Enhancing porosity of TE scaffolds for tissue regeneration has been another important way to modify electrospun polymer scaffolds. In native tissue, the ECM forms naturally porous, nanostructured environments, which promote cell adhesion, proliferation, and differentiation [29,88]. Therefore, it is important to construct a scaffold that mimics the scale and structure of the native ECM [60]. However, it is difficult to obtain purely electrospun polymers on the true nanoscale due to the inherent limitations of the technology as well as the loss of structural and mechanical integrity of a scaffold with small fiber dimensions. Because of these considerations, more and more research has sought to modify the surface characteristics of microscale and sub-micron scaffold fibers. One potential approach is to co-spin finer fibers onto thicker fibers in order to achieve nano-texturization of micro scale fibers [80]. This creates appropriate nanostructures on microscaled fibers, which have been shown to promote better cell adhesion, proliferation, and differentiation [80]. Another novel method for creating porous scaffolds is through a technique known as wet electrospinning. In wet electrospinning, fibers are collected in a coagulation bath of methanol or some other liquid, as opposed to on a collector plate in open air [73] yielding a highly porous structure that greatly improves cell adhesion. It was reported that cellular growth was four times greater than a control group after a 28-day growth period [35]. Yet another method for generating highly porous scaffolds is to fabricate a composite scaffold combining a chosen electrospun polymer as the matrix and an inherently porous material as a constituent. In one instance, a PCL scaffold was co-spun with mesoporous bioactive glass (MBG), which is a commonly used material in bone regeneration because of its high bioactivity [93]. This scaffold was then coated with hydroxyapatite (HA) and collagen to further enhance cell adhesion and tissue formation. The initial incorporation of MBG into the scaffold not only greatly enhanced osteoconductivity, biocompatibility, and cell affinity, but allowed for a reduced coating time and a more effective HA and collagen coating [93].

1.2.4 Electrospun Composite Scaffolds

One of the most widely investigated methods to modify electrospun scaffolds for TE is the fabrication of composite scaffolds. Like other methods discussed, composite TE scaffolds contain constituent materials blended into a fibrous polymer matrix for enhanced structural and mechanical characteristics, modified surface chemistry, additional porosity and surface roughness or enhanced cellular properties. For osteogenic modification, for instance, one of the most frequently investigated materials for electrospun composite scaffolds is HA crystals [62]. Often, HA is simply blended with the polymer solution at a desired concentration and then electrospun into a scaffold per normal fabrication procedures [63]. HA is attractive because it fortifies and enhances several important scaffold parameters at once [17,41,63]. The incorporation of HA into a scaffold has shown to stimulate the proliferation of osteoblasts and osteoblast-like cells and the differentiation and proliferation of bone marrow mesenchymal stem cells (MSCs) [54,55,60]. In several cases, MSCs have been seeded onto composite scaffolds containing nano-HA (nHA), and in all have shown improved results with regard to proliferation and osteogenic differentiation [56,60]. Besides stimulated cellular growth, nHA also greatly enhances the surface roughness of electrospun fibers, specifically at the nanoscale [15,41]. Cells preferentially adhere to rough surfaces with nanoscaled features and surface modifications provided by the addition of nHA greatly facilitates cellular adhesion and growth [17,36,60,73]. Another important aspect for the inclusion of HA on electrospun scaffolds is an enhancement of mechanical properties [41,54]. It has been shown that the inclusion of HA in a scaffold matrix increases scaffold yield strength, as well as Young's modulus, which not only creates a more robust and functional scaffold but also may help to direct the differentiation of stem cells [54].

In addition to HA, many other constituent materials have been used to enhance cell behavior for bone application. One such material is tricalcium phosphate (TCP). Tricalcium phosphate is a bioceramic found in both bone and in geological environments [89]. It is commonly used for hard tissue regeneration due to its beneficial effect on improving cell activity, but it lacks toughness [15,89]. Hence, its combination with an electrospun scaffold is advantageous because TCP scaffolds require structural support [89]. Another material with similar bioactive applications is collagen. Collagen is a natural polymer that is a critical component of the native ECM in a variety of native tissues [6,10,55].

As previously discussed, there are a wide variety of ways that collagen can be incorporated into a polymeric scaffold. Typically, collagen is used as a surface treatment to render a scaffold more cell-adherent as in the deposition of nanofibrous collagen on electrospun scaffolds [30,42,80]. However, collagen lacks significant structural and mechanical integrity and must be used with a robust polymer or other composite materials for functional TE scaffolds [89]. In lieu of these materials that naturally occur in human tissues, xeno-derived, natural, or synthetic materials have also been explored for bone tissue engineering applications. One common material is chitosan, a natural component found in the exoskeleton of crustaceans [6]. Chitosan has been shown to enhance cellular adhesion and growth, but needs to be structurally supported [6]. Other materials that have been investigated to increase porosity and surface roughness for bone regeneration include bioactive glass, gelatin, and the blending of different polymers [15,17,46,56,60]. One particularly interesting application of a blended polymer was the inclusion of a "sacrificial" PEO fibrous element to a PCL/collagen scaffold. In an aqueous and/or cellular active environment, the PEO fibers degraded much more rapidly, leaving a highly porous, complex PCL/collagen scaffold that greatly enhanced the osteogenesis of MSCs [60]. This is an especially important example because it highlights the novel application of materials to create dynamic scaffolds and systems.

1.2.5 Novel Methodology

As has been shown, there are many newly developed approaches to electrospin scaffolds for TE and regenerative medicine applications. Such new methods improve the functionality of scaffolds. This ranges from fiber dimensions to yield strength to directing the phenotypic expression of stem cells. While the direct correlation of these modifications on cellular growth has yet to be fully understood, enough information has been accumulated that researchers are already looking at more novel ways to control the properties of electrospun tissue engineering scaffolds. These methods largely consist of creative new modifications and the manipulation of the electrospinning fabrication process, or the use of novel and highly experimental materials.

1.2.5.1 Co-spun scaffolds and co-deposited materials

One of the most heavily researched experimental methods for electrospun scaffolds has been co-electrospinning scaffolds.

Co-spinning refers to the simultaneous deposition of two or more different materials onto a single collection agent in order to achieve a novel combination, distribution, or structure (see Fig. 1.1). As has already been discussed, this method has been applied to achieve a desired distribution of chemicals, constituents, and drugs, to create novel core-shell fiber structures for drug delivery, and to deposit materials in such a way as to create surface features of a desired size on larger, structural elements [64,65,80,81,90]. This method is also being investigated in relation to combining electrospinning and electrospraying, a process similar to electrospinning where the material is deposited in micro- or nano-sized beads, as opposed to fibers (see Fig. 1.2) [21,58,62]. This unique combination of electrospinning and electrospraying has just begun to be investigated by researchers, but has already been utilized in some creative ways [22,58].

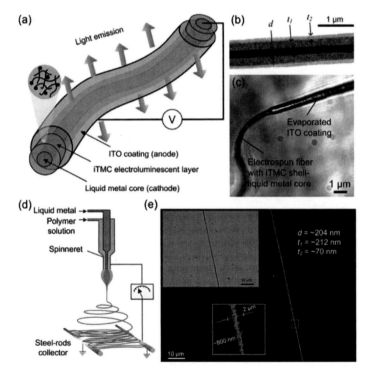

Figure 1.1 Diagram, TEM image and Raman spectroscopic image of novel core-sheath electrospun fibers for optical fabric [16].

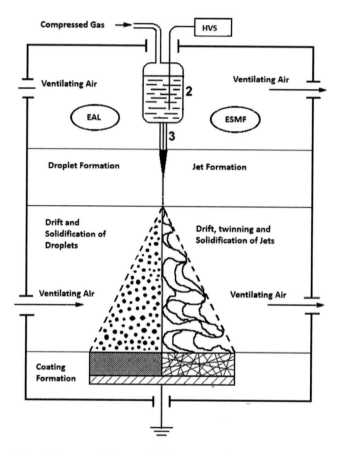

Figure 1.2 Diagram of electrospinning versus electrospraying [20].

The combination of electrospinning/electrospraying has been used to create composite materials. For example, Francis et al. used the process to create composite scaffolds consisting of electrospun gelatin (gel) and electrosprayed nHA. Scaffolds were fabricated in a 4:1 and 2:1 Gel/nHA compositional ratio and were then evaluated for surface topography, material distribution and mechanical properties. The scaffolds were also analyzed for biocompatibility in vitro by seeding human fetal osteoblasts on the fabricated scaffolds. The studies showed that these composite scaffolds yielded better cell proliferation and enhanced biomineralization [21].

The novel application of combining electrospinning/electrospraying has not been limited to composite scaffolding. For example, Paletta et al. published a recent study where osteoblasts suspended in medium were electrosprayed onto scaffolds composed of PLLA and PLLA/collagen. This method was not shown to inhibit cellular growth or scaffold degradation, and it was concluded by the researcher to be a suitable method for cell seeding of electrospun TE scaffolds [58].

1.2.5.2 Wet-electrospinning

Another example of novel modifications to the electrospinning process is that of "wet electrospinning." The process of wet electrospinning entails a standard electrospinning setup augmented with the collector plate submerged in a liquid bath (see Fig. 1.3). Shin et al. used wet electrospinning to create a 3D poly(trimethyle necarbonate-co-epsilon-caprolactone)-block-co-poly(p-dioxanone) scaffold for bone regeneration that was 90% porous and exhibited interconnected pores. This highly porous scaffold showed good cellular adhesion of osteoblasts at the center of the scaffold after only four days of in vitro cell seeding. The cells also proliferated 1.5 times faster than the control after seven days.

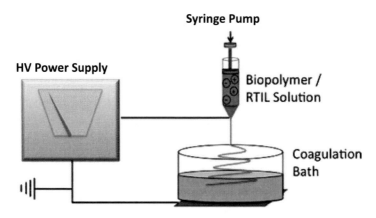

Figure 1.3 Diagram of wet electrospinning [50].

In addition, alkaline phosphate (a marker of bone formation) was four times higher than the control after 28 days [73]. These results showed that wet electrospun scaffolds can be a promising approach to creating scaffolds that are advantageous for bone growth.

1.2.5.3 Novel nanocomposites

With the amount of investigation into using natural materials native to bone and cartilage tissue, a novel area of research has been to incorporate non-natural or unconventional materials into scaffolds. One such material is octadecylamine-functionalized nanodiamonds (ND-OCT) [98]. Nanodiamonds (ND) are 5 nm diamond particles surrounded by amorphous and graphitic carbon, which has a large number of different functional groups on its surface. Because of this, NDs have chemically complex surfaces with the potential for combination with a variety of chemicals [53]. In a recent study, Zhang et al. created ND-OCT for use as a mechanically enhancing constituent for electrospun PLLA scaffolds. OCT was chosen as a functional group because it causes the NDs to be immiscible in water and hydrophilic organic solvents, but to have a high affinity toward hydrophobic solvents, making them ideal for uniform dispersion in a polymer while also being resilient in a biological environment [53,98]. At 10 wt%, PLLA-ND-OCT scaffolds exhibited a 200% increase in Young's modulus and an 800% increase in hardness thus enhancing the mechanical properties of the ND-OCT-PLLA scaffold and rendering them very close to that of natural bone [98]. ND-OCTs also exhibited autofluorescence, giving off a very bright blue light when excited [53,98]. However, unlike other fluorophores, ND-OCTs are non-toxic and very stable, which could make them a potentially powerful tool for in vivo analysis [53,98].

Increasingly, nanotubes and nanotube/nanofibrous structures are being explored as a novel nanocomposite for electrospun scaffolds. Rosette nanotubes (RNTs) are an example of novel tubular structures currently being used. Rosette nanotubes are self-assembling tubes consisting of stacked disk shaped rings, or rosettes, made of the DNA base pairs guanine and cytosine [76]. Due to their unique biological and physiochemical properties, RNTs provide significant potential to enhance and promote cellular growth and development [9,76,96]. For example, Chen et al. used a novel electrospinning technique to fabricate hydrogel, rosette nanotube, and fibroblast-like cells into novel 3D scaffold for cartilage implantation. The results of their study showed that electrospun RNT/hydrogel composites improved both fibroblast and chondrocyte functions. RNT/hydrogel composites promoted fibroblast cell chondrogenic differentiation in two-week culture experiments. Furthermore, studies demonstrated that RNTs enhanced the hydrogel adhesive strength to that of severed collagen. These results, thus, provided a nanostructured scaffold that enhanced fibroblast cell adhesion, viability, and chondrogenic differentiation [9].

In addition to RNTs, both single-walled and multiwalled carbon nanotubes (CNTs and MWCNTs) have been used to enhance the mechanical and physiochemical characteristics of electrospun scaffolds [51,59]. CNTs and MWCNTs have a radius of around 10 to 20 nm and 50 to 60 nm, respectively, and are thus very biomimetic [95]. They are also electrically conductive, which can be conducive for certain types of tissue regeneration such as neural or cardiac applications, and they are also easily functionalized with biological molecules and/or proteins [83,86,95]. Pan et al. fabricated microcomposite fibers of regenerated silk fibroin (RSF) and MWCNTs by electrospinning. A quiescent blended solution and a three-dimensional Raman image of the composite fibers showed that functionalized MWCNTs (F-MWCNTs) were well dispersed in the solution and the RSF fibers, respectively. The mechanical properties of the RSF electrospun fibers were improved drastically by incorporating F-MWCNTs. Compared with the pure RSF electrospun fibers, a 2.8-fold increase in breaking strength, a 4.4-fold increase in Young's modulus, and a 2.1-fold increase in breaking energy was observed for the composite fibers with 1.0 wt% F-MWCNTs. Cytotoxicity tests preliminarily demons-trated that the electrospun fiber mats have good biocompatibility for tissue engineering scaffolds [59].

Sharma et al. used electrospinning to fabricate polyaniline-carbon nanotube/poly(N-isopropyl acrylamide-co-methacrylic acid) (PANI-CNT/PNIPAm-co-MAA) composite nanofibers and PNIPAm-co-MAA nanofibers as a three-dimensional conducting smart tissue scaffold. Cellular responses on the nanofibers were studied with mice L929 fibroblasts, and the PANI-CNT/PNIPAm-co-MAA composite nanofibers were shown to have the highest cell growth and cell viability as compared to PNIPAm-co-MAA nanofibers. Cell viability in the composite nanofibers was 98% higher, indicating that the composite nanofibers provided a better environment as a 3D scaffold for cell proliferation and attachment and are suitable for tissue engineering applications [69].

1.3   3D Printing

1.3.1   Introduction to 3D Printing and Medical Applications

While electrospinning has been established as one of the most widely and thoroughly investigated methods for scaffold fabrication, it still presents a number of limitations such as having weak or poor mechanical properties, having non-uniform pore distribution, random pore interconnectivity and void space, and limited control over the size, and distribution of fibers within the micro and nanoarchitecture of the scaffold [28,62]. Recently, 3D printing and rapid prototyping processes have been used to create scaffolds that are 3D with user defined microstructures and microscaled architectures [12,13]. This ensures that the scaffold is fully unoccluded with uniformly interconnected pores and has a more complex, controlled architecture.

Hard tissue is one of the most readily researched and treated defect and injury sites for TE scaffold-based solutions. One of the critical 3D scaffold design criteria for hard tissues is that they must have suitable mechanical properties. In addition, interconnected pores, specifically pore structures at the microscale, interconnected by smaller pores on a nano-scale are also indicative of the ECM of hard tissues, and are very important for hard tissue scaffold design [85,89,98]. This sort of complicated, hierarchical structure is one that is difficult to recapitulate, if at all, and then more difficult to control in even very advanced electrospinning setups and other common scaffold fabrication techniques. With the application of 3D printing, there is an allowance not only for the creation of delicate and intricate structures from the advanced working of strong and robust materials, but the potential to create highly ordered structures that could conceivably match any desired architecture [44]. This later advantage is one that also makes 3D printing attractive for other types of targeted tissue 3D scaffolds.

Theoretically, the versatility and precision of 3D printing could be used to print not only small scaffolds and patches for defect repair, but could eventually be used to print whole organs. Currently, 3D printing as applied to TE uses a layered manufacturing method of printing thin depositions of material in a given pattern on top of previously printed and cured material [13,44]. This could allow for large, macro-scale objects that have complex, user-defined internal features, mimicking the architecture a given organ. This could also allow for materials to be printed that encapsulate living cells into the artificial organ construct, creating a complex network of cells, advantageous architecture and structure conducive to organ function and cell/tissue growth [87]. Examples and discussion of this will be presented later in the chapter.

Moreover, one of the most important challenges facing 3D TE construct design is vascularization. Scaffolds seeded with cells that begin to mature and form tissue have problems with the transportation of nutrients and essential signaling chemicals and growth factors, as well as removal of waste products within the internal structure of the scaffold [11,18,60]. In the body, vascular networks accomplish this task, but new and under-formed vasculature presents a daunting limitation to scaffold-based tissue repairs. However, if a scaffold can be fabricated with designed transport channels and structures that mimic vascularized tissue, then it could be possible to alleviate this issue [84]. 3D printing presents a potential ability to accomplish this because, as stated previously, it is possible to create structures with predesigned complex, microscale internal architectures.

1.3.2 Methods

There are currently a number of methods for 3D printing and rapid prototyping that have been directly applied to the manufacture of 3D TE constructs. These methods provide fast and affordable design prototypes that have been applied in novel ways and modified to use and create unique materials and structures for TE purposes.

1.3.2.1 Fused deposition modeling

Fused deposition modeling (FDM) is one of the simplest forms of 3D fabrication. In FDM, a computer-aided design (CAD) drawing is used in conjunction with a 3D printer to create polymeric 3D structures. A FDM machine consists of a slightly heated printing bed, a printing head capable of 3D axial movement and a computer/controller. The printing head draws a solid polymeric filament and forces it through a heated extruder head, which heats up the material and deposits it, in a molten form, on the printing surface in a thin layer. The machine then prints multiple thin layers on top of the previously deposited layer. In the end, one is left with a 3D construct of pre-determined design (see Fig. 1.4) [37,67]. Fused deposition modeling is very rudimentary compared to other 3D fabrication methods, but it is important because it establishes an overarching methodology in all 3D fabrication techniques, where a fully 3D-designed structure is disassembled into very thin, successive slices and then physically recreated layer-by-layer. Fused deposition modeling itself has strong potential as a 3D fabrication method for 3D TE scaffolds because of its ability to employ a number of different polymers, but is not often utilized because it lacks a low enough resolution to create complex and biomimetic nano/microstructures [5].

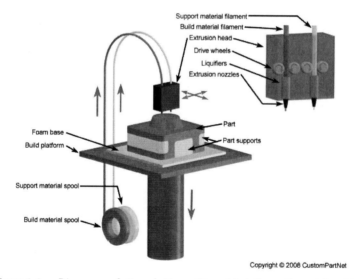

Figure 1.4 Diagram of Fused Deposition Modeling. Copyright 2008 CustomPartNet.

Shim et al. used a deposition system similar to FDM called solid freeform fabrication (see Fig. 1.5). A 3D scaffold was printed from a deposited, structurally sound polymer, while a cell-laden hydrogel was infused into the void spaces The printed hard scaffold served as a structural support while the printed soft hydrogel served to encapsulate cells and ensure their even distribution throughout the construct [72].

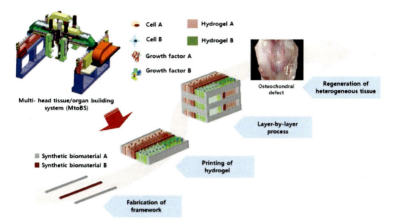

Figure 1.5 Fabrication diagram of a composite solid freeform fabrication of a hydrogel/polymer scaffold [71].

1.3.2.2 Selective laser sintering and stereolithography

Selective laser sintering (SLS) uses a construction method similar to FDM (see Fig. 1.6). In SLS, a printing surface on a movable piston is loaded with a material in powder form. A high-power pulsed laser is then used to cure a layer of the material in a defined pattern based on a user-designed CAD drawing. Once the layer is cured, the piston lowers the printing platform by one layer thickness. The powdered printing material is replenished and the laser cures the next layer of the structure [34,35,39]. Kolan et al. used SLS to fabricate porous constructs made of 13–93 bioactive glass, using stearic acid as a polymeric binder. The effect of particle size distribution, binder content, processing parameters, and sintering schedule on the microstructure and mechanical properties of porous constructs was investigated, and importantly improved mechanical properties were reported [39]. Lohfeld et al. created SLS scaffolds of PCL and PCL/TCP for bone tissue regeneration. Different scaffold designs were generated, and assessed for manufacturability, porosity, and mechanical performance. Furthermore, scaffolds were generated with increasing TCP content, and scaffold fabrication from PCL and PCL/TCP mixtures with up to a 50 mass% TCP was shown to be possible. With increasing macroporosity, the stiffness of the scaffolds dropped. However, the stiffness increased by minor geometrical changes, such as the addition of a cage around the scaffold [47].

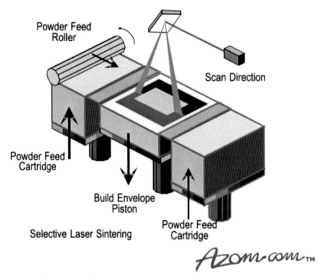

Figure 1.6 Diagram of selective laser sintering. Copyright azom.

Stereolithography (SL) is another laser-based printing method (see Fig. 1.7). SL also employs a moveable build platform and prints materials layer-by-layer. The platform and piston are immersed in a photocurable resin, which uses an ultraviolet wavelength laser

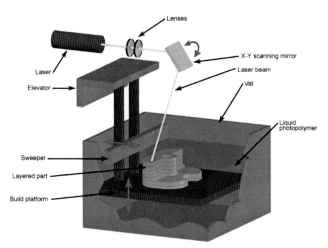

Figure 1.7 Diagram of traditional Stereolithography. Copyright 2008 CustomPartNet.

to cure the polymer resin [32,48,94]. That is to say, that it is a liquid polymer that cross-links and forms a solid structure when exposed to certain wavelengths of light, as opposed to a polymer material that is sintered together at high energies as with SLS.

Increasingly, modified SLS, SL and other laser-based printing methods have become very popular for the manufacture of 3D TE constructs, due to the versatility of materials that can be printed and the high resolutions achievable. SL has also been especially popular due to the fact that there are a number of photocurable polymers that have ideal properties for biological applications and cell encapsulation. Catros et al. used a combination of a laser-based curing process called laser assisted bioprinting and electrospinning. Thin PCL membranes were spun and then patterned with a laser-cured bioink comprising MG63 cells and alginate in dispersion patterns. The finished 2D scaffold layers were then stacked to form a 3D construct. Circular patterns were maintained in vitro during the first week but they were no longer observable after 2 weeks, due to cell proliferation. The layer-by-layer printed construct provided an appropriate 3D environment for cell survival and enhanced cell proliferation in vitro and in vivo [4]. Koch et al. also used laser-assisted bioprinting to create 3D structured scaffolds for skin grafts. Fibroblasts and keratinocytes suspended in collagen were used as the print medium. It was demonstrated that the printed constructs incited cells to have enhanced adhesion and an affinity for the formation of gap junctions [38].

1.3.2.3 Laminated object manufacturing

Laminated object manufacturing (LOM) uses a large sheet of the printing material, coated with an adhesive, and a cutting tool or laser to cut out a given layer of a designed 3D shape and deposit it on top of the preexisting printed form (see Fig. 1.8). Laminated object manufacturing does not demonstrate the level of resolution of SLS or SL, but because of increased work into developing methods for 2D tissue engineering scaffolds and films, it could be a potential tool for processing such 2D constructs easily into a functional 3D scaffold [57]. Pirlo et al. created a series of formed and molded 2D biopapers, which were then stacked. 2D biopapers were created by pouring polymer dissolved in solvent into molds patterned with NaCl crystals. When hardened, the salt was washed off, leaving a robust pattered film.

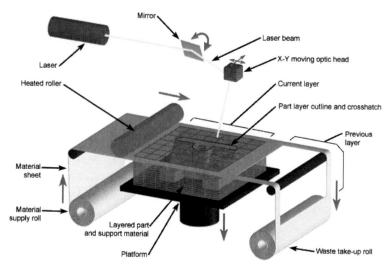

Figure 1.8 Diagram of laminated object manufacturing. Copyright 2008 CustomPartNet.

Laser Assisted Bioprinting was then used to deposit human umbilical vein endothelial cells onto the bioapaper, which was then stacked. The purpose was to create a pre-vascularized scaffold environment for future TE applications [61].

1.3.2.4 Inkjet 3D printing

Inkjet 3D Printing (3DP), like many other methods discussed, uses CAD or a computer generated drawing to create a 3D shape that is subsequently fabricated layer-by-layer (see Fig. 1.9). In 3DP, a printing head similar to that found in an inkjet printer moves across a bed of powdered printing material and selectively deposits a binding agent in the cross section of that layer. The construct is then coated in a new layer of powder and the process is continued. 3DP is popular because of the ease and cost effectiveness of the equipment and setup [12,24]. Recently, it has become popular for 3D TE scaffold fabrication because it can use a wide variety of materials, and its inert fabrication method is not damaging to biological materials, growth factors, chemicals and even living cells that might be printed in a scaffold or construct.

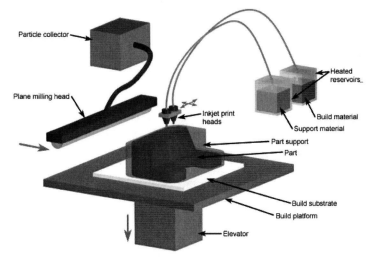

Figure 1.9 Diagram of inkjet 3D printing. Copyright 2008 CustomPartNet.

Gaetani et al. utilized a deposition process similar to inkjet printing called tissue printing. Human cardiac-derived cardiomyocyte progenitor cells were printed into an alginate matrix where they experienced enhanced proliferation and cardiac differentiation. The printed scaffold was also put into contact with and showed migration into a matrigel layer, which served as a simulation of targeted cell delivery into native tissue at the defect site [23].

Xu et al. took a unique approach to 3D TE construct fabrication by fabricating a construct without the scaffold materials. Inkjet printing was utilized to print cells into a network of zigzagging tubes mimicking the size and shape of native tissue vascularization. The lack of a base scaffold material and the ability to achieve appropriately sized and shaped vasculature-like tubes made this a potential first step toward full organ printing [87].

1.3.2.5 Novel methodology and applications

In addition to the pre-established 3D printing fabrication methods discussed thus far, several unique fabrication methods for controlled, 3D TE scaffolds have been recently investigated. One such method that has been gaining popularity is 3D fiber deposition. 3D fiber deposition is similar to FDM, where a heated nozzle is used to deposit a melted polymer, but the outlet used is on the order of several hundred microns in diameter. The process yields micro-fiber arrays, with controllable fiber spacing and deposition angle. Fedorovich et al. used 3D Fiber Deposition to create alginate hydrogel matrices containing chondrocytes and osteogenic progenitors, as well as separate printed layers for osteoblasts and osteoblast growth for osteochondral defects. Good cellular growth results were reported and a high degree of effect was demonstrated on the scaffold architecture by modulation of the above mentioned process parameters [19]. Sun et al. also used 3D fiber deposition to create and compare porous PCL scaffolds containing osteoblasts, which were fabricated at 45 degree and 90° deposition angles. The 3D printed scaffolds were compared to traditional salt-leeched scaffolds. The cell distribution on the 3D scaffolds was more homogeneous than the salt-leached scaffolds, demonstrating that 3D scaffolds are more effective for tissue engineering. The results also showed that it is possible to design and optimize the properties of amorphous polymer scaffolds by 3D fiber deposition [77].

Other novel demonstrations have been recently investigated that show the versatility and adaptability of 3D fabrication methods. Tarafder et al. recently used microwave sintering to create a 3D, porous TCP scaffold for bone tissue engineering. Tricalcium phosphate was printed into a microscale scaffold using 3D printing, but was then sintered in a microwave furnace. A significant increase in compressive strength, between 46% and 69% was achieved by this process, as compared to conventional sintering due to more efficient densification. In vitro cell studies exhibited an increase in cell density with a decrease in macropore size using human osteoblast cells. Histomorphological analysis also revealed that the presence of both micro- and macropores facilitated osteoid-like new bone formation [78].

Lu et al. also utilized projection printing, which works similarly to photolithography, in which a photo-mask is used to cure layers of photosensitive material in designed patterns when exposed to light. In projection printing, a UV light source is used in conjunction with a micro-mirror array, a digital masking device, imaging optics and a photocurable resin to photopolymerize the resin into complex, biomimetic shapes. Lu et al. was able to use this process to print precise closed channels and cavities that mimicked native vasculature [48].

1.4 Other Current Methodology

Electrospinning and 3D printing are currently the two most promising and most widely investigated methods for 3D scaffold fabrication. There are, however, a number of other preexisting methods that have been in use as 3D scaffold fabrication methods. Traditional methods do not offer the same level of control, biomimetic structure formation, or improved material, chemical and cellular incorporation into the construct, but there are several methodologies that are still being applied to TE scaffold fabrication in novel and relevant ways. In the following, we will briefly discuss several well-established methods.

1.4.1 Solvent Casting

Solvent casting is a process in which a polymer is dissolved in an organic solvent, after which particles of a specific or desired dimension are added to the solution. The solution is then added to a mold, where the solvent evaporates off, leaving a solid structure. The evaporation of the solvent in and of itself is not remarkable, but solvent-polymer solutions can be cast in molds of virtually any shape or size. This means that molds with complex micro-architectures can be fabricated and used to create highly ordered and biomimetic polymer scaffolds [2,45,92]. In some cases, the pre-cast solvent-polymer mixture is incorporated with some micro- or nano-sized porogen material. Once the solution is cast, the solid structure is put into a water bath, which dissolves the incorporated porogen leaving behind a rigid, porous structure. Yu et al. used a solvent casting method to create stackable poly(3-hydroxybutyrate-co-3-hydroxyhexanoate) films, which were then seeded with mesenchymal stem cells leading to enhanced adhesion, cellular aggregate formation, proliferation, and cellular migration within the scaffold [92]. Azami et al. devised a nanostructured scaffold for bone repair using hydroxyapatite and gelatin as its main components.

The scaffold was prepared via layer solvent casting combined with freeze-drying and lamination techniques. Engineering analyses show that the scaffold possessed a three dimensional interconnected homogenous porous structure with a porosity of about 82% and pore sizes ranging from 300 to 500 µm. The mechanical properties measured also matched those of spongy bone. The results obtained from biological assessment show that this scaffold did not negatively affect osteoblast proliferation rate and actually improved osteoblast function as shown by increasing the alkaline phosphate (ALP) activity and calcium deposition and formation of mineralized bone nodules. In addition, the scaffold promoted healing of critical sized calvarial bone defect in rats [2].

1.4.2 Gas Foaming

Gas foaming is a process for scaffold fabrication similar to solvent casting where a foam-forming agent, such as ammonium bicarbonate, is added to a polymer solvent solution. The polymer-solvent foam is then dried, and the solvent evaporates, leaving a rigid and porous structure. Gas foaming is very simple, in that one cannot create highly ordered or controllable porous materials. However, because of the inert nature of the pore formation process, a variety of materials and composite materials can be utilized to create tissue-engineered scaffolds. Ji et al. used gas foaming to create highly porous poly-DL-lactide and poly(ethylene glycol) co-polymer scaffolds foamed with CO_2 [31]. In addition to composite materials, gas foaming has the potential to create pre-seeded scaffolds, and to utilize material mixtures that have incorporated living cells and biological material into them. Chen et al. used a novel method to seed a calcium phosphate cement with human umbilical cord cells encapsulated in hydrogel spheres. The calcium phosphate/hydrogel sphere mixture was then foamed with a porogen to achieve high porosity and good cellular dispersion [7, 8]. Zhou et al. employed a new technique where "solid-state" foaming (SSF) was combined with immiscible polymer blends to achieve a variety of different pore sizes and distributions within the same structure. That is to say, highly interconnected micro- and nanopores were observed [100]. Gas foaming, due to the relative ease of preparation, also has great potential as a mass-production fabrication method for TE scaffolds and TE biomaterials. Henke et al. conducted a study into the effectiveness of oligo(poly(ethylene glycol)fumarate) (OPF) gas foamed hydrogel scaffolds for cell culture. Ready to use OPF-hydrogel scaffolds were prepared by gas foaming, freeze drying, individual packing into bags and subsequent gamma-sterilization. The scaffolds could be stored and used "off-the-shelf" without any need for further processing prior to cell culture. Thus, the handling was simplified and the sterility of the cell carrier was assured [26].

1.4.3 Phase Separation

In phase separation, a polymer in liquid form is polymerized into a block co-polymer of different block morphologies that separate homogenously throughout the structure to form uniform, ordered, nanoscale structures. Chemical and molecular incompatibilities in the polymer blocks cause this phenomenon to occur, and the same principle can be applied to different materials as well. Zhao et al. used phase separation to create highly porous poly(propylene carbonate) scaffolds for bone regeneration with nanofibrous chitosan interconnecting the macropores. It was reported that these scaffolds were able to achieve as high as 91.9% porosity [99]. Sun et al. used a combination of injection molding and phase separation to create multi-channeled PLLA scaffolds intended for neuronal and tendon regeneration. These highly complex and porous scaffolds showed greatly enhanced protein adsorption and cellular adhesion [75]. Moawad et al. were able to employ sintered heat transfer to induce phase separation in glass–ceramic mixtures to form highly porous TE scaffolds with pores on the nanoscale [52]. Lee et al. was also able to employ a novel phase separation technique by using room-temperature ionic liquid to induce pore formation in poly(lactic acid) (PLA) scaffolds [43].

1.5 Summary

Today's clinical challenges provide great opportunity for the development of highly customizable methodologies for the treatment and repair of diseased, damaged, and injured tissue and organs. Stem cells provide a great deal of promise, but require chemical and physical cues for adequate differentiation and tissue formation. Scaffold-based TE approaches achieve this by using highly designed, biodegradable and biocompatible constructs with biomimetic micro/nano-featured architecture, modified surface chemistries and incorporated biological and chemical factors for enhanced cellular adhesion, proliferation and differentiation. Electrospinning is one popular method for scaffold fabrication that creates micro and nano fibrous materials. It can be used with a variety of polymers, constituent materials, and can be augmented to work in tandem other fabrication processes, but it has begun to reach limitations. 3D printing does not have the ability to create biomimetic features as small as electrospinning, but it can create much more controlled and well-designed structures, and could potentially be used to rapidly produce constructs of complex micro and macro architecture. Several other popular methods exist, including solvent casting, gas foaming and phase separation that rely on more rudimentary chemical reactions and phenomena to create porous, biomimetic scaffolds. Still, they can be used with a variety of materials and continue to be applied in valid and novel ways.

References

1. Ahn, S. H., Lee, H. J., Kim, G. H. (2011). Polycaprolactone scaffolds fabricated with an advanced electrohydrodynamic direct-printing method for bone tissue regeneration, *Biomacromolecules*, **12**, 4256–4263.
2. Azami, M., Tavakol, S., Samadikuchaksaraei, A., et al. (2012). A porous hydroxyapatite/gelatin nanocomposite scaffold for bone tissue repair: in vitro and in vivo evaluation, *J Biomater Sci Polym Ed*, DOI:10.1163/156856211X617713.
3. Berthiaume, F., Maguire, T. J., Yarmush, M. L. (2011). Tissue engineering and regenerative medicine: history, progress, and challenges, *Annu Rev Chem Biomol Eng*, **2**, 403–430.
4. Catros, S., Guillemot, F., Nandakumar, A., et al. (2012). Layer-by-layer tissue microfabrication supports cell proliferation in vitro and in vivo, *Tissue Eng Part C Methods*, **18**, 62–70.
5. Centola, M., Rainer, A., Spadaccio, C., et al. (2010). Combining electrospinning and fused deposition modeling for the fabrication of a hybrid vascular graft, *Biofabrication*, **2**, 014102.

6. Chen, L., Zhu, C., Fan, D., et al. (2011). A human-like collagen/chitosan electrospun nanofibrous scaffold from aqueous solution: Electrospun mechanism and biocompatibility, *J Biomed Mater Res Part A*, **99A**, 395–409.
7. Chen, W., Zhou, H., Tang, M., et al. (2012). Gas-foaming calcium phosphate cement scaffold encapsulating human umbilical cord stem cells, *Tissue Eng Part A*, **18**, 816–827.
8. Chen, W., Zhou, H., Weir, M. D., et al. (2012). Umbilical cord stem cells released from alginate-fibrin microbeads inside macroporous and biofunctionalized calcium phosphate cement for bone regeneration, *Acta Biomater*, **8**, 2297–2306.
9. Chen, Y., Bilgen, B., Pareta, R. A., et al. (2010). Self-assembled rosette nanotube/hydrogel composites for cartilage tissue engineering, *Tissue Eng Part C Methods*, **16**, 1233–1243.
10. Chen, Z. C., Ekaputra, A. K., Gauthaman, K., et al. (2008). In vitro and in vivo analysis of co-electrospun scaffolds made of medical grade poly(epsilon-caprolactone) and porcine collagen, *J Biomater Sci Polym Ed*, **19**, 693–707.
11. Chung, E. J., Sugimoto, M., Koh, J. L., et al. (2012). Low-pressure foaming: a novel method for the fabrication of porous scaffolds for tissue engineering, *Tissue Eng Part C Methods*, **18**, 113–121.
12. Cui, X., Boland, T., D'Lima, D. D., et al. (2012). Thermal inkjet printing in tissue engineering and regenerative medicine, *Recent Part Drug Deliv Formul*, **6**, 149–155.
13. Cui, X., Breitenkamp, K., Finn, M. G., et al. (2012). Direct human cartilage repair using three-dimensional bioprinting technology, *Tissue Eng Part A*, **18**, 1304–1312.
14. de Valence, S., Tille, J. C., Mugnai, D., et al. (2012). Long term performance of polycaprolactone vascular grafts in a rat abdominal aorta replacement model, *Biomaterials*, **33**, 38–47.
15. Dinarvand, P., Seyedjafari, E., Shafiee, A., et al. (2011). New approach to bone tissue engineering: simultaneous application of hydroxyapatite and bioactive glass coated on a poly(L-lactic acid) scaffold, *ACS Appl Mater Interfaces*, **3**, 4518–4524.
16. Dong, L. (2012). Coaxial electrospinning produces a self-supporting micro/nanofiber electronic light source: SPIE Newsroom; Contract No.: Document Number.
17. Fang, R., Zhang, E., Xu, L., et al. (2010). Electrospun PCL/PLA/HA based nanofibers as scaffold for osteoblast-like cells, *J Nanosci Nanotechnol*, **10**, 7747–7751.

18. Fedorovich, N. E., Alblas, J., Hennink, W. E., et al. (2011). Organ printing: the future of bone regeneration?, *Trends Biotechnol*, **29**, 601–606.
19. Fedorovich, N. E., Schuurman, W., Wijnberg, H. M., et al. (2012). Biofabrication of osteochondral tissue equivalents by printing topologically defined, cell-laden hydrogel scaffolds, *Tissue Eng Part C Methods*, **18**, 33–44.
20. Filatov, Y., Budyka, A., Kirichenko, V. (eds.) (2007). *Electrospinning of Micro- and Nanofibers: Fundamentals in Separation and Filtration Processes*. Redding: Begell House Inc publisher.
21. Francis, L., Venugopal, J., Prabhakaran, M. P., et al. (2010). Simultaneous electrospin-electrosprayed biocomposite nanofibrous scaffolds for bone tissue regeneration, *Acta Biomater*, **6**, 4100–4109.
22. Francis, L., Venugopal, J., Prabhakaran, M. P., et al. (2010). Simultaneous electrospin-electrosprayed biocomposite nanofibrous scaffolds for bone tissue regeneration, *Acta Biomater*, **6**, 4100–4109.
23. Gaetani, R., Doevendans, P. A., Metz, C. H., et al. (2012). Cardiac tissue engineering using tissue printing technology and human cardiac progenitor cells, *Biomaterials*, **33**, 1782–1790.
24. Godino, N., Gorkin, R., Bourke, K., et al. (2012). Fabricating electrodes for amperometric detection in hybrid paper/polymer lab-on-a-chip devices, *Lab Chip*, **12**, 3281–3284.
25. Gupta, P. K., Das, A. K., Chullikana, A., et al. (2012). Mesenchymal stem cells for cartilage repair in osteoarthritis, *Stem Cell Res Ther*, **3**, 25.
26. Henke, M., Baumer, J., Blunk, T., et al. (2012). Foamed oligo(poly(ethylene glycol)fumarate) hydrogels as versatile prefabricated scaffolds for tissue engineering, *J Tissue Eng Regen Med*, doi: 10.1002/term.1517.
27. Holmes, B., Castro, N. J., Zhang, L. G., et al. (2012). Electrospun fibrous scaffolds for bone and cartilage tissue generation: recent progress and future developments, *Tissue engineering Part B, Reviews*, **18**, 478–486.
28. Holzwarth, J. M., Ma, P. X. (2011). Biomimetic nanofibrous scaffolds for bone tissue engineering, *Biomaterials*, **32**, 9622–9629.
29. Hutmacher, D. W. (2000). Scaffolds in tissue engineering bone and cartilage, *Biomaterials*, **21**, 2529–2543.
30. Shabani, I., Haddai, V.-A., Soleimani, M., Seyedjafari, E., Babaeijandaghi, F., Ahmadbeigi, N. (2011). Enhanced infiltration and biomineralization of stem cells on collagen-grafted three-dimensional nanofibers, *Tissue Eng Part A*, **17**, 1209–1218.

31. Ji, C., Annabi, N., Hosseinkhani, M., et al. (2012). Fabrication of poly-DL-lactide/polyethylene glycol scaffolds using the gas foaming technique, *Acta Biomater*, **8**, 570–578.
32. Jolly, S. W., He, Z., McGuffey, C., et al. (2012). Stereolithography based method of creating custom gas density profile targets for high intensity laser-plasma experiments, *Rev Sci Instrum*, **83**, 073503.
33. Jones, A. C., Arns, C. H., Sheppard, A. P., et al. (2007). Assessment of bone ingrowth into porous biomaterials using MICRO-CT, *Biomaterials*, **28**, 2491–2504.
34. Kang, H., Long, J. P., Urbiel Goldner, G. D., et al. (2012). A paradigm for the development and evaluation of novel implant topologies for bone fixation: implant design and fabrication, *J Biomech*, **45**, 2241–2247.
35. Kettner, M., Schmidt, P., Potente, S., et al. (2011). Reverse engineering–rapid prototyping of the skull in forensic trauma analysis, *J Forensic Sci*, **56**, 1015–1017.
36. Ki, C. S., Park, S. Y., Kim, H. J., et al. (2008). Development of 3-D nanofibrous fibroin scaffold with high porosity by electrospinning: implications for bone regeneration, *Biotechnol Lett*, **30**, 405–410.
37. Kim, J., McBride, S., Tellis, B., et al. (2012). Rapid-prototyped PLGA/beta-TCP/hydroxyapatite nanocomposite scaffolds in a rabbit femoral defect model, *Biofabrication*, **4**, 025003.
38. Koch, L., Deiwick, A., Schlie, S., et al. (2012). Skin tissue generation by laser cell printing, *Biotechnol Bioeng*, **109**, 1855–1863.
39. Kolan, K. C., Leu, M. C., Hilmas, G. E., et al. (2012). Effect of material, process parameters, and simulated body fluids on mechanical properties of 13–93 bioactive glass porous constructs made by selective laser sintering, *J Mech Behav Biomed Mater*, **13C**, 14–24.
40. Langer, R., Vacanti, J. P. (1993). Tissue engineering, *Science*, **260**, 920–926.
41. Lao, L., Wang, Y., Zhu, Y., et al. (2011). Poly(lactide-co-glycolide)/hydroxyapatite nanofibrous scaffolds fabricated by electrospinning for bone tissue engineering, *J Mater Sci Mater Med*, **22**, 1873–1884.
42. Lee, H., Yeo, M., Ahn, S., et al. (2011). Designed hybrid scaffolds consisting of polycaprolactone microstrands and electrospun collagen-nanofibers for bone tissue regeneration, *J Biomed Mater Res Part B: Appl Biomater*, **97B**, 263–270.
43. Lee, H. Y., Jin, G. Z., Shin, U. S., et al. (2012). Novel porous scaffolds of poly(lactic acid) produced by phase-separation using room

temperature ionic liquid and the assessments of biocompatibility, *J Mater Sci Mater Med*, **23**, 1271–1279.

44. Lee, M., Wu, B. M. (2012). Recent Advances in 3D printing of tissue engineering scaffolds, *Methods Mol Biol*, **868**, 257–267.

45. Li, X., Nan, K., Shi, S., et al. (2012). Preparation and characterization of nano-hydroxyapatite/chitosan cross-linking composite membrane intended for tissue engineering, *Int J Biol Macromol*, **50**, 43–49.

46. Linh, N. T., Lee, B. T. (2011). Electrospinning of polyvinyl alcohol/gelatin nanofiber composites and cross-linking for bone tissue engineering application, *J Biomater Applications*, **27**, 255–266.

47. Lohfeld, S., Cahill, S., Barron, V., et al. (2012). Fabrication, mechanical and in vivo performance of polycaprolactone/tricalcium phosphate composite scaffolds, *Acta Biomater*, **8**, 3446–3456.

48. Lu, Y., Chen, S. (2012). Projection printing of 3-dimensional tissue scaffolds, *Methods Mol Biol*, **868**, 289–302.

49. Ma, Z., Kotaki, M., Inai, R., et al. (2005). Potential of nanofiber matrix as tissue-engineering scaffolds, *Tissue Eng*, **11**, 101–109.

50. Meli, L., Miao, J., Dordick, J. S., et al. (2010). Electrospinning from room temperature ionic liquids for biopolymer fiber formation *Green Chem*, **12**, 1883–1892.

51. Miao, J., Miyauchi, M., Dordick, J. S., et al. (2012). Preparation and characterization of electrospun core sheath nanofibers from multi-walled carbon nanotubes and poly(vinyl pyrrolidone), *J Nanosci Nanotechnol*, **12**, 2387–2393.

52. Moawad, H. M., Jain, H. (2012). Fabrication of nano-macroporous glass-ceramic bioscaffold with a water soluble pore former, *J Mater Sci Mater Med*, **23**, 307–314.

53. Mochalin, V. N. (2010). *Nanodiamond*, AJ Drexel Nanotechnology Institute.

54. Mouthuy, P. A., Y. H., Triffitt, J., Oommen, G., Cui, Z. (2010). Physico-chemical characterization of functional electrospun scaffolds for bone and cartilage tissue engineering, *Proc. Inst Mechan Eng*, **224**, 1401–1414.

55. Nair, L. S., Bhattacharyya, S., Laurencin, C. T. (2004). Development of novel tissue engineering scaffolds via electrospinning, *Expert Opin Biol Ther*, **4**, 659–668.

56. Nandakumar, A., Fernandes, H., de Boer, J., et al. (2010). Fabrication of bioactive composite scaffolds by electrospinning for bone regeneration, *Macromol Biosci*, **10**, 1365–1373.

57. Nie, W., Zhang, J., Wang, Z., et al. (2008). [Rapid-prototyping manufacture of human scoliosis based on laminated object technology], Sheng Wu Yi Xue Gong Cheng Xue Za Zhi, **25**, 1260–1263.
58. Paletta, J. R., Mack, F., Schenderlein, H., et al. (2011). Incorporation of osteoblasts (MG63) into 3D nanofibre matrices by simultaneous electrospinning and spraying in bone tissue engineering, *Eur Cell Mater*, **21**, 384–395.
59. Pan, H., Zhang, Y., Hang, Y., et al. (2012). Significantly reinforced composite fibers electrospun from silk fibroin/carbon nanotube aqueous solutions, *Biomacromolecules*, **13**, 2859–2867.
60. Phipps, M. C., Clem, W. C., Grunda, J. M., et al. (2012). Increasing the pore sizes of bone-mimetic electrospun scaffolds comprised of polycaprolactone, collagen I and hydroxyapatite to enhance cell infiltration, *Biomaterials*, **33**, 524–534.
61. Pirlo, R. K., Wu, P., Liu, J., et al. (2012). PLGA/hydrogel biopapers as a stackable substrate for printing HUVEC networks via BioLP, *Biotechnol Bioeng*, **109**, 262–273.
62. Prabhakaran, M. P., Ghasemi-Mobarakeh, L., Ramakrishna, S. (2011). Electrospun Composite Nanofibers for Tissue Regeneration, *J Nanosci Nanotechnol*, **11**, 3039–3057.
63. Rainer, A., Spadaccio, C., Sedati, P., et al. (2011). Electrospun hydroxyapatite-functionalized PLLA scaffold: potential applications in sternal bone healing, *Ann biomed Eng*, **39**, 1882–1890.
64. Samavedi, S., Olsen Horton, C., Guelcher, S. A., et al. (2011). Fabrication of a model continuously graded co-electrospun mesh for regeneration of the ligament–bone interface, *Acta Biomater*, **7**, 4131–4138.
65. Samer Srouji, D. B.-D., Rona Lotan, Erella Livne, Ron Avrahami, Eyal Zussman. (2011). Slow-release human recombinant bone morphogenetic protein-2 embedded within electrospun scaffolds for regeneration of bone defect: in vitro and in vivo evaluation, *Tissue Eng Part A*, **17**, 269–277.
66. Schofer, M. D., Roessler, P. P., Schaefer, J., et al. (2011). Electrospun PLLA nanofiber scaffolds and their use in combination with BMP-2 for reconstruction of bone defects, *PLoS ONE*, **6**, e25462.
67. Schumann, D., Ekaputra, A. K., Lam, C. X., et al. (2007). Biomaterials/scaffolds. Design of bioactive, multiphasic PCL/collagen type I and type II-PCL-TCP/collagen composite scaffolds for functional tissue engineering of osteochondral repair tissue by using electrospinning and FDM techniques, *Methods Mol Med*, **140**, 101–124.

68. Shafiee, A., Soleimani, M., Chamheidari, G. A., et al. (2011). Electrospun nanofiber-based regeneration of cartilage enhanced by mesenchymal stem cells, *J Biomed Mater Res Part A*, **99A**, 467–478.
69. Sharma, Y., Tiwari, A., Hattori, S., et al. (2012). Fabrication of conducting electrospun nanofibers scaffold for three-dimensional cells culture, *Int J Biol Macromol*, **51**, 627–631.
70. Shim, I. K., Jung, M. R., Kim, K. H., et al. (2010). Novel three-dimensional scaffolds of poly(L-lactic acid) microfibers using electrospinning and mechanical expansion: Fabrication and bone regeneration, *J Biomed Mater Res Part B: Appl Biomater*, **95B**, 150–160.
71. Shim, J.-H., Lee, J.-S., Kim, J. Y., et al. (2012). Bioprinting of a mechanically enhanced three-dimensional dual cell-laden construct for osteochondral tissue engineering using a multi-head tissue/organ building system. *J Micromechan Microeng*, **22**, 085014.
72. Shim, J. H., Kim, J. Y., Park, M., et al. (2011). Development of a hybrid scaffold with synthetic biomaterials and hydrogel using solid freeform fabrication technology, *Biofabrication*, **3**, 034102.
73. Shin, T. J., Park, S. Y., Kim, H. J., et al. (2010). Development of 3-D poly(trimethylenecarbonate-co-epsilon-caprolactone)-block-poly (p-dioxanone) scaffold for bone regeneration with high porosity using a wet electrospinning method, *Biotechnol Lett*, **32**, 877–882.
74. Smith, L. A., Ma, P. X. (2004). Nano-fibrous scaffolds for tissue engineering, *Colloids Surf B Biointerf*, **39**, 125–131.
75. Sun, C., Jin, X., Holzwarth, J. M., et al. (2012). Development of channeled nanofibrous scaffolds for oriented tissue engineering, *Macromol Biosci*, **12**, 761–769.
76. Sun, L., Zhang, L., Hemraz, U. D., et al. (2012). Bioactive rosette nanotube-hydroxyapatite nanocomposites improve osteoblast functions, *Tissue Eng Part A*, **18**, 1741–1750.
77. Sun, Y., Finne-Wistrand, A., Albertsson, A. C., et al. (2012). Degradable amorphous scaffolds with enhanced mechanical properties and homogeneous cell distribution produced by a three-dimensional fiber deposition method, *J Biomed Mater Res A*, **100**, 2739–2749.
78. Tarafder, S., Balla, V. K., Davies, N. M., et al. (2012). Microwave-sintered 3D printed tricalcium phosphate scaffolds for bone tissue engineering, *J Tissue Eng Regen Med*, **7**, 631–641.
79. Tel-Vered, R., Yehezkeli, O., Willner, I. (2012). Biomolecule/nanomaterial hybrid systems for nanobiotechnology, *Adv Exp Med Biol*, **733**, 1–16.

80. Thorvaldsson, A., Stenhamre, H., Gatenholm, P., et al. (2008). Electrospinning of highly porous scaffolds for cartilage regeneration, *Biomacromolecules*, **9**, 1044–1049.
81. Toyokawa, N., Fujioka, H., Kokubu, T., et al. (2010). Electrospun synthetic polymer scaffold for cartilage repair without cultured cells in an animal model, arthroscopy: *J Arthroscopic Amp Relat Surg*, **26**, 375–383.
82. Vacanti, J. P., Langer, R. (1999). Tissue engineering: the design and fabrication of living replacement devices for surgical reconstruction and transplantation, *Lancet*, **354**, Suppl. 1, SI32–34.
83. van der Zande, M., Walboomers, X. F., Olalde, B., et al. (2011). Effect of nanotubes and apatite on growth factor release from PLLA scaffolds, *J Tissue Eng Regen Med*, **5**, 476–482.
84. Visconti, R. P., Kasyanov, V., Gentile, C., et al. (2010). Towards organ printing: engineering an intra-organ branched vascular tree, *Expert Opin Biol Ther*, **10**, 409–420.
85. Wang, Q., McGoron, A. J., Pinchuk, L., et al. (2010). A novel small animal model for biocompatibility assessment of polymeric materials for use in prosthetic heart valves, *J Biomed Mater Res A*, **93**, 442–453.
86. Xie, F., Weiss, P., Chauvet, O., et al. (2010). Kinetic studies of a composite carbon nanotube-hydrogel for tissue engineering by rheological methods, *J Mater Sci Mater Med*, **21**, 1163–1168.
87. Xu, C., Chai, W., Huang, Y., et al. (2012). Scaffold-free inkjet printing of three-dimensional zigzag cellular tubes, *Biotechnol Bioeng*, **109**, 3152–3160.
88. Yaszemski, M. J., Payne, R. G., Hayes, W. C., et al. (1995). The ingrowth of new bone tissue and initial mechanical properties of a degrading polymeric composite scaffold, *Tissue Eng*, **1**, 41–52.
89. Yeo, M., Lee, H., Kim, G. (2010). Three-dimensional hierarchical composite scaffolds consisting of polycaprolactone, β-tricalcium phosphate, and collagen nanofibers: fabrication, physical properties, and in vitro cell activity for bone tissue regeneration, *Biomacromolecules*, **12**, 502–510.
90. Yoon, H., Kim, G. (2011). A three-dimensional polycaprolactone scaffold combined with a drug delivery system consisting of electrospun nanofibers, *J Pharm Sci-Us*, **100**, 424–430.
91. Yoshimoto, H., Shin, Y. M., Terai, H., et al. (2003). A biodegradable nanofiber scaffold by electrospinning and its potential for bone tissue engineering, *Biomaterials*, **24**, 2077–2082.

92. Yu, B. Y., Chen, P. Y., Sun, Y. M., et al. (2012). Response of human mesenchymal stem cells (hMSCs) to the topographic variation of poly(3-hydroxybutyrate-co-3-hydroxyhexanoate) (PHBHHx) films, *J Biomater Sci Polym Ed*, **23**, 1–26.

93. Yun H. S., K. S., Khang D. W., Choi J. I., Kim H. H., Kang M. J. (2011). Biomimetic component coating on 3D scaffolds using high bioactivity of mesoporous bioactive ceramics *Intl J Nanomed*, **6**, 2521–2531.

94. Zhang, A. P., Qu, X., Soman, P., et al. (2012). Rapid fabrication of complex 3D extracellular microenvironments by dynamic optical projection stereolithography, *Adv Mater*, **24**, 4266–4270.

95. Zhang, K., Choi, H. J., Kim, J. H. (2011). Preparation and characteristics of electrospun multiwalled carbon nanotube/polyvinylpyrrolidone nanocomposite nanofiber, *J Nanosci Nanotechnol*, **11**, 5446–5449.

96. Zhang, L., Hemraz, U. D., Fenniri, H., et al. (2010). Tuning cell adhesion on titanium with osteogenic rosette nanotubes, *J Biomed Mater Res A*, **95**, 550–563.

97. Zhang, L., Zhou, Y., Zhu, J., et al. (2012). An updated view on stem cell differentiation into smooth muscle cells, *Vascul Pharmacol*, **56**, 280–287.

98. Zhang, Q., Mochalin, V. N., Neitzel, I., et al. (2011). Fluorescent PLLA-nanodiamond composites for bone tissue engineering, *Biomaterials*, **32**, 87–94.

99. Zhao, J., Han, W., Chen, H., et al. (2012). Fabrication and in vivo osteogenesis of biomimetic poly(propylene carbonate) scaffold with nanofibrous chitosan network in macropores for bone tissue engineering, *J Mater Sci Mater Med*, **23**, 517–525.

100. Zhou, C., Ma, L., Li, W., et al. (2011). Fabrication of tissue engineering scaffolds through solid-state foaming of immiscible polymer blends, *Biofabrication*, **3**, 045003.

101. Zhou, H., Lawrence, J. G., Bhaduri, S. B. (2012). Fabrication aspects of PLA-CaP/PLGA-CaP composites for orthopedic applications: a review, *Acta Biomater*, **8**, 1999–2016.

Chapter 2

Three-Dimensional Micropatterning of Biomaterial Scaffolds for Tissue Engineering

Joseph C. Hoffmann and Jennifer L. West

Department of Biomedical Engineering, Duke University, 2138 Campus Drive, Box 90281, Durham, NC 27708, USA

jennifer.l.west@duke.edu

2.1 Need for 3D Micropatterning in Tissue Engineering

The broad-scale clinical success of tissue engineering applications has thus far been limited to simple tissues with few complex microstructures. Notably, all of the tissue engineering products currently on the market have focused on thin, avascular tissues in which oxygen and nutrients diffuse throughout the tissue constructs to sustain cellular viability. When attempting to construct thicker, more complex tissues such as those in the heart, lungs, kidney, and liver, cells more than several hundred microns from the nearest capillary have been shown to suffer from hypoxia and subsequent cell death [48]. In order to engineer more complex tissues and organs, it will be necessary, therefore, to form a microvasculature that allows for sufficient gas exchange and nutrient supply to sustain high cell viability within the tissues. Further, since the specific

---

Tissue and Organ Regeneration: Advances in Micro- and Nanotechnology
Edited by Lijie Grace Zhang, Ali Khademhosseini, and Thomas J. Webster
Copyright © 2014 Pan Stanford Publishing Pte. Ltd.
ISBN 978-981-4411-67-7 (Hardcover), 978-981-4411-68-4 (eBook)
www.panstanford.com

microstructure of endogenous vascular networks relates directly to the ability of a tissue to function properly [24], it will be necessary to precisely control the density and spatial orientation of capillaries within biomaterial scaffolds.

Hydrogels have emerged as a leading material candidate in which to engineer tissue microenvironments since they possess the innate advantages of mimicking the mechanical properties of soft tissues, possessing a high level of biological compatibility, and offering opportunities for biofunctionalization and cell encapsulation [39]. The porous and aqueous nature of hydrogels also allows for diffusion of cellular metabolites, such as nutrients and wastes, which is a condition critical to high cellular viability. In recent years, hydrogels have been selected and modified with a variety of growth factors and cell adhesive ligands to produce cellular effects ranging from endothelial cell tubule formation [47], to guided neurite extension [62], to osteoblast differentiation and mineralization [61].

While tissue engineering in hydrogels has seen fundamental success, precise spatial control of cellularized hydrogel structures on the micron scale, such as that required to spatially dictate the position of individual capillaries, has long stood as a particularly technical challenge in tissue engineering. Researchers have made progress toward this goal through the development of micropatterning technologies that facilitate physical and biochemical manipulation of scaffolds, and ultimately, control of cellular behavior; however, techniques to manipulate biomaterials have traditionally been highly two-dimensional in scope. For example, micro-contact printing has utilized elastomeric stamps to immobilize distinct patterns of adhesive molecules, such as fibronectin, onto the surface of biomaterial substrates [11]. Further, techniques have also been developed to pattern self-assembled monolayers [45] or to control the formation of wrinkles on hydrogel surfaces [28] in order to probe cell behavior. These methods have proved to be useful in the study of complex cellular interactions as they allow for the dictation of cell morphology and the organization of cells into complex, pre-designed microstructures. However, they are less directly applicable to tissue engineering as they fail to allow for the fabrication of three-dimensional (3D) physical and biochemical structures that are necessary to mimic the physiological microenvironment and ultimately develop complex tissues. To this point, recent findings have shown that nearly all cell types require three-dimensional

(3D) cues to produce a physiologically relevant cellular response [25]. For example, researchers have observed drastic differences in attachment, morphology, migration, and proliferation between cells in 2D versus 3D environments [17,22,75].

As a consequence, tissue engineers have turned their attention to the development of 3D technologies capable of hydrogel scaffold manipulation on the micron scale [35]. In this chapter, we review the most recent advances of 3D micropatterning technologies and discuss their application in the field of tissue engineering and regenerative medicine. Specifically, we discuss the continued development of 3D printing and photolithography as a means to three-dimensionally dictate biomaterial properties and cell behavior, and examine the progress thus far toward the development of more complex tissues and organs.

2.2 3D Printing

Early 3D printing systems for tissue engineering were borrowed from the field of materials manufacturing and were composed of a print head mounted on X–Y rails, a building platform with an axial elevator, and a powder dispensing roller. Scaffolds were fabricated by laying down a powder across the building platform, and then directing the print head to dispense a liquid binder in designed two-dimensional patterns. After axial adjustment, another layer of powder was applied and bound in the areas where the binding liquid was deposited [13]. Using computer automated design software, a series of two-dimensional images were thereby translated into a 3D tissue engineering scaffold. In 2002, this type of 3D printing patterned a scaffold with controlled properties to better mimic the characteristics of both bone and cartilage [60]. Specifically, the top section of a scaffold was printed using poly(D,L,-lactide-co-glycolide) (PLGA) and L-poly lactic acid (PLA) at 90% porosity with staggered macroscopic channels to facilitate chrondrocyte seeding and cartilage formation. The bottom portion of the same scaffold was printed into a cloverleaf shape using PLGA and calcium phosphate at 55% porosity to achieve strong mechanical properties and initiate bone growth. This 3D printing technology demonstrated control of porosity, material composition, physical structure, and mechanical properties within a 3D biomaterial scaffold, with the goal of fabricating multifaceted materials for total joint replacement [60]. Excited by early success, engineers have since moved to 3D printing of hydrogel structures on the micron scale. Further, over the last 10 years the term 3D printing has evolved and split to encompass at least three valuable yet distinct technologies now being utilized in the tissue engineering community. These technologies, known as direct-write bioprinting, inkjet bioprinting, and biological laser printing will now each be discussed in turn, with an emphasis on recent successes in tissue engineering applications.

2.2.1 Direct-Write Bioprinting

Direct-write bioprinting involves the use of a three-dimensionally controlled actuator to extrude a liquid material, or bioink, through a dispensing pen in the form of a designed pattern (Figs. 2.1a,b) [10,43]. The pattern is subsequently cross-linked or gelled using chemical reagents or environmental factors. 3D structures are then built through an additive layer-by-layer process (Fig. 2.1c). Direct-write bioprinting generally prints a continuous line of material extruded from the dispensing pen and the resolution is highly dependent on the printing material, including its viscosity, as well as cross-linking or gelling conditions [10]. Some direct-write bioprinters are capable of printing 3D structures as small as 5 µm and as large as many millimeters [10,66]. Direct-write bioprinting was recently utilized to print 3D collagen scaffolds containing microfluidic channels [41].

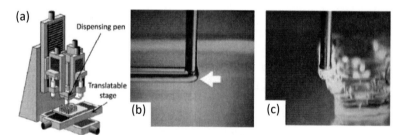

Figure 2.1 Direct-Write Bioprinting. (a) A schematic of a direct-write bioprinting apparatus. Biomaterials are dispensed by a pen onto a translatable stage to form a scaffold. Adapted from Lewis et al. [43]. (b) Close up image of a dispensing pen extruding the first layer of a hydrogel biomaterial onto a surface (arrow is leading edge). (c) After curing the first layer, additional layers are deposited to form 3D structures. Adapted from Chang et al. [10].

In this example, a scaffold was fabricated by first printing collagen into a designed pattern and then cross-linking it with nebulized sodium bicarbonate using a custom designed 3D bioprinter (Fig. 2.2a) [41]. Heated gelatin was then printed into the regions of the scaffold where collagen was not present and cross-linked via temperature cooling. Using a layer-by-layer method, 400 μm wide 3D channels of gelatin were patterned within the collagen scaffold (Fig. 2.2b) [41]. The scaffold was heated to liquefy and then rinse away the gelatin, leaving hollow channels behind (Fig. 2.2c) [41]. To demonstrate mechanical integrity of the scaffold, a complex rotary pattern of hollow channels was fabricated and perfused with blue microspheres in phosphate buffered saline (PBS) (Fig. 2.2d) [41].

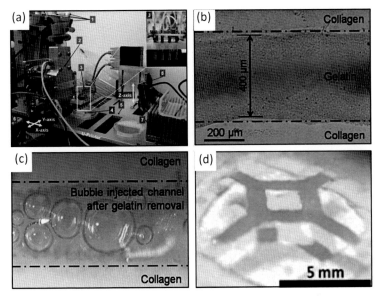

Figure 2.2 Direct-Write Bioprinting Collagen Scaffolds with Microfluidic Channels. (a) A photograph of the custom designed 3D bioprinter, including (1) a four-channel syringe unit, (2) a heating and cooling element, (3) a four-channel dispensing unit, (4) a target substrate, and (5) a vertical, and (6) horizontal stage. (b) This bioprinter was utilized to fabricate 3D collagen scaffolds containing 400 μm wide 3D channels of gelatin. (c) The channels became hollow when heated and washed, thus allowing for air bubbles to be injected into them. (d) Perfusion of blue microspheres in PBS was demonstrated in a rotary pattern of hollow channels within a collagen scaffold. Adapted from Lee et al. [41].

Finally, when dermal fibroblasts were seeded on this material, the micropatterned channels allowed for better nutrient transport and increased cell viability as opposed to scaffolds without channels [41]. In addition to collagen and gelatin, direct-write bioprinting has been demonstrated using a wide variety of hydrogel biomaterials, including agarose [50], alginate [15], pluronic F127 [66], Matrigel [23], a hyaluronan-gelatin copolymer [64], and a synthetic copolymer containing poly(ethylene glycol) [8]. This bioprinting technique has the ability to encapsulate highly viable cells [10], thus allowing for spatially controlled formation of 3D cellularized scaffolds. As example, rat microvascular cells were incorporated into a collagen bioink, and a multilayer 3D structure was printed with cell viability over 90 percent [65].

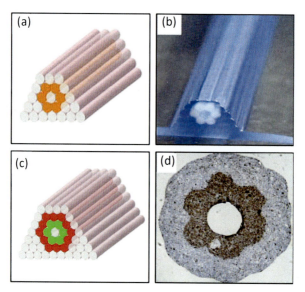

Figure 2.3 Direct-write bioprinting of cellularized spheroids. (a) Design template to form hollow tubules from cylindrical fused cell spheroids (orange) and non-adhesive agarose rods. (b) Printed construct with non-adhesive agarose rods in blue and cell spheroids in white. (c) Design to form double layered vascular wall with vascular smooth muscle cell cylinders (green) and fibroblast cells (red). (d) Histological examination of double layered vascular wall. The brown staining (smooth muscle α-actin) and blue staining (hematoxylin) are used to clearly differentiate the two cellular layers. Adapted from Norotte et al. [50].

Researchers have even utilized direct-write bioprinting in a scaffoldless approach in which cylinders composed only of fused cell spheroids were three-dimensionally positioned between non-adhesive agarose rods to form vessel-like tubules of various geometries (Figs. 2.3a,b) [50]. The same group was then able to combine both vascular smooth muscle cell cylinders and fibroblast cylinders in order to fabricate a multiwalled structure that mimicked the multilayer structures that occur naturally in blood vessels as shown in Figs. 2.3c,d [50].

Most recently, direct-write bioprinting has combined multiple cell types to form different tissues when implanted in vivo [23]. Endothelial progenitor cells encapsulated in Matrigel in one section of a printed scaffold were formed vessels containing red blood cells after a 6-week implantation in immunodeficient mice. A different section of the same scaffold was printed with mesenchymal stem cells and calcium phosphate micro particles in Matrigel and demonstrated significant bone formation after a six week implantation [23]. The capability of direct-write bioprinting to pattern 3D structures of multiple cells types within various biomaterials should have an important future impact on tissue engineering as we move closer to fabricating complex organs.

2.2.2 Inkjet Bioprinting

Another newly developed 3D printing technique, known as inkjet bioprinting, involves the use of modified commercial printers to dispense cells or cell-biomaterial mixtures in a precise, micropatterned manner [58]. In this technique commercial print heads are modified with needles or nozzles and commercial printer ink is replaced with bioink consisting of living cells in solution (Fig. 2.4a) [73].

Printers are exposed to UV light and modified cartridges are wiped down with ethanol in order to provide cells with a sterile environment. Desktop thermal printers are most common in inkjet bioprinting and operate by using a heating element to induce a small liquid bubble that then forces a precise amount of liquid through a series of nozzles [58], each of which is about 50 µm in diameter [56] (Fig. 2.4b). When the heat pulse is removed, the bubble collapses, and the subsequent loss of volume draws more fluid into the chamber. The inkjet bioprinting process proceeds via repeated generation of microdroplets of bioink that are subsequently deposited onto a biomaterial substrate, or biopaper, in computer-specified patterns. In one of the first examples of inkjet printing of mammalian cells, Chinese hamster ovary (CHO) cells were deposited onto collagen or agarose hydrogels into distinct patterns with less than 10% loss of cell viability [74]. Researchers have also used inkjet printers to simultaneously deposit both viable cells and a biomaterial scaffold. For example, in one recent study, a solution containing thrombin and human microvascular endothelial cells (HMECs) served as bioink that was printed onto a fibrinogen-coated coverslip [16]. With incubation at 37°C for 20 min, a mechanically stable fibrin scaffold with 100 μm diameter fibers formed. After 21 days in culture, the HMECs coalesced to form high integrity microvascular tubules aligned along the fibrin scaffolds [16].

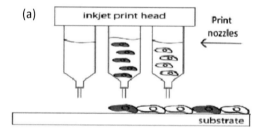

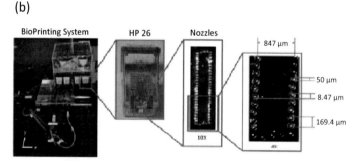

Figure 2.4 Inkjet bioprinting. (a) Schematic of inkjet bioprinting in which an inkjet print head containing nozzles dispenses cells onto a biomaterial substrate. Adapted from Wust et al. [73]. (b) An inkjet bioprinting system is pictured. This system uses an HP26 ink cartridge with 50 nozzles, each of which is 50 μm in width. Adapted from Pepper et al. [56].

Three-dimensionality in most inkjet bioprinting systems has been achieved through the stacking of multiple biomaterial substrates. For example, in one study, five sequential layers of fibrin were printed in a layer-by-layer manner, with each layer containing neuronal cells and possessing a thickness of about 50 µm [74]. While promising for some applications, automated and precise 3D control of hydrogel scaffolds using inkjet bioprinting has been limited because printing a liquid material on a hydrogel substrate causes the liquid to spread out, thus diminishing axial thickness and limiting lateral pattern resolution to hundreds of micrometers. Researchers have recently overcome this obstacle using modified inkjet printers to pattern quick gelling alginate droplets [55]. Alginate forms a hydrogel almost immediately when exposed to calcium, and therefore, droplets can be cross-linked before spreading occurs, thus greatly increasing resolution and 3D patterning capabilities.

As example, alginate microdroplets were recently printed onto a gelatin substrate that contained calcium chloride [55]. As the alginate droplets were printed, calcium ions diffused into them, triggering gelation. Each gelled calcium droplet then acted as a building block for 3D structures (Fig. 2.5a). Researchers in this study achieved excellent cell viability within the alginate droplets and a maximum resolution of under 3 µm. Using this technique, a bifurcating hollow microchannel, reminiscent of those seen in the microvasculature, was patterned (Figs. 2.5b,c) and subsequently supported physiologic flow conditions without leaking [55]. Finally, this research group demonstrated that this inkjet printing platform could be used to provide 3D structure to slower gelling, more biologically active materials by combing them with alginate. To accomplish this advancement, alginate and collagen were mixed and structures were first formed using the fast- gelling alginate process. The collagen was then allowed to slowly gel when heated. After collagen gelation, the alginate was removed via chelation, leaving behind a 3D collagen structure [55]. With its ability to control the placement of both cells and bioactive materials on the micron scale, inkjet bioprinting will likely be a critical micropatterning technology as the tissue engineering field progresses.

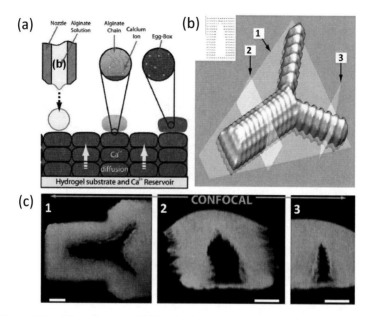

Figure 2.5 Microdrop scaffold fabrication using an inkjet bioprinter. (a) Alginate microdroplets are printed onto a gelatin hydrogel permeated with calcium chloride. Calcium ions diffuse upwards and rapidly cross-link the droplets allowing for the formation of 3D structures. (b) Model of a bifurcating channel to be printed with indicated slices corresponding to confocal images below. Inset: model of droplets needed to form larger channel. (c) Confocal images of the cross-linked alginate channel with each image corresponding to the indicated plane in the model above. All scale bars = 200 μm. Adapted from Pataky et al. [55].

2.2.3 Biological Laser Printing

Biological laser printing (BioLP) has emerged as a parallel process to dictate the microstructure of cells on hydrogel biomaterials. BioLP is a modified laser-induced forward transfer technique that involves the use of a high pulsed laser to transfer cells onto a biomaterial substrate in a highly controlled manner. With this technology, a laser is focused on a target material consisting of a transparent mechanical support layer (glass or quartz), an energy conversion layer (gold or titanium), and a liquid transfer layer containing the cells to be printed (Fig. 2.6) [58]. The laser is specifically focused on the energy conversion layer, which absorbs the laser light and transmits it to the cell containing transfer material. This results in a jet of cell-containing material being transferred to a biomaterial substrate in the exact location of the laser pulse [58].

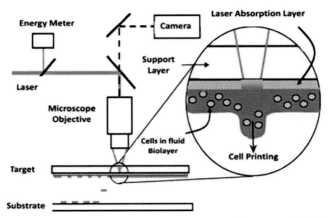

Figure 2.6   Biological laser printing setup. A schematic of biological laser printing is depicted. The laser is focused on the laser absorption layer (also known as the energy conversion layer). Energy is transmitted to the cell-laden transfer layer, which results in a jet of material being transferred to the biomaterial substrate [58].

The amount of material transferred per laser pulse is generally about 500 femtoliter [4], and the resulting resolution has been reported to be less than 5 µm [3]. The biomaterial substrate receiving surface is normally controlled by a CAD/CAM interface that allows for translation of the printed substrate and therefore the fabrication of patterned hydrogels.

Numerous cell types have been shown to survive this process with cell viability near 100 percent [2,4,32,58], and different kinds of cells have been deposited adjacent to one another [3] and in single cell arrays on biomaterial surfaces [2]. Recently, high-throughput BioLP systems have been designed that allow for the rapid printing of different kinds of cells or biological materials. For example, a "multicolor" BioLP system was utilized to rapidly print alginate droplets, hydroxyapatite nanocrystals, and endothelial cells with high precision using the same automated printing system [26]. This was achieved using a single infrared laser and a rotating carousel that could quickly change between printing materials [26]. Multiple populations of endothelial cells were later printed into juxtaposed concentric patterns with high resolution between the cell types (Fig. 2.7) [27].

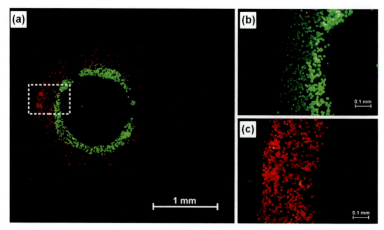

Figure 2.7 Multicolor biological laser printing. (a) Human endothelial cells were labeled with green or red fluorescent dyes and printed into a pattern of concentric circles using BioLP. (b, c) Higher magnification of the patterned cellular structures. The two cellular circles partially overlap at their interface [27].

In moving toward a 3D constructs, a 500 µm thick fibrin scaffold was fabricated with BioLP by printing thrombin onto a fibrinogen biopaper [27]. Using a 200 mm/s scan speed, a 4 cm^2 patterned array of fibrin fibers containing endothelial cells was printed in just a few seconds [27].

BioLP has also been applied in a layer-by-layer method to fabricate thicker constructs closer to the size scale of naturally occurring tissues and organs. For example in one study, human osteosarcoma cells were printed into a distinct pattern on a thin layer of basement membrane hydrogel (Matrigel) [3,58]. A second Matrigel layer was then applied on top of the cells, and a different pattern of osteosarcoma cells was printed. Interestingly, the cells were printed onto the soft hydrogel with enough force to be encapsulated in a 3D manner, rather than simply adhering to the surface. Using this layer-by-layer method, three cell patterns were incorporated into a 3D hydrogel, with each layer comprising approximately 50–75 µm in thickness [3,58]. In a different study, salt leached PLGA impregnated with collagen or Matrigel was utilized with BioLP to print endothelial cells into distinct patterns of microscopic lines [57]. The endothelial cells were seen to form vessel-like networks and maintain their pattern configurations. Further, the PLGA-based biopapers were sturdy enough to be physically stacked together to form a 3D construct, which served as a proof of concept for fabricating 3D vascularized scaffolds [57]. When used in this manner, BioLP holds great promise for fabricating more complex tissues and organs.

2.3 Photolithography

In parallel with the development of 3D printing, photolithography for bioengineering applications has evolved into an array of techniques capable of precise patterning of polymers on the micron scale. Originally developed and long used in the microelectronics industry, photolithography involves spatial and temporal control of light-based chemical reactions using a photomask to facilitate or alter the cross-linking of polymers. Photolithography in tissue engineering has developed with the introduction of macromolecular precursors that can be polymerized via a free radical induced cross-linking reaction in order to form photopolymerized hydrogels [49]. The propagation of free radicals to induce cross-linking is generally created by the photocleavage of an initiator upon light activation at the appropriate wavelength. Specifically, photoinitiators such as benzoin derivatives, benziketals, acetophenone derivatives, and hydroxyalkylphenones achieve free radical polymerization via the photocleavage of carbon–carbon, carbon–chlorine, carbon–oxygen, or carbon–sulfur bonds when exposed to light [49]. When selecting an initiator, one must consider the biocompatibility, water solubility, cytotoxicity, and excitation wavelength of the chosen molecule so that the initiator best fits the needs of a particular application. The molecules 2,2-dimethoxy-2-phenylacetophenone, 4-(2-hydroxyethoxy) phenyl-(2-propyl) ketone, eosin Y and camphorquinone are all commonly utilized to induce cross-linking of macromolecular precursors into polymerized hydrogel networks. Such hydrogel fabrication schemes offer several important advantages for tissue engineering. Specifically, photopolymerized hydrogels offer both a high level of spatial and temporal control during fabrication as well as opportunities to incorporate biomolecules for increased functionality [49]. It has also been shown that cells may be encapsulated in photopolymerizable hydrogels and retain high viability after macromolecular cross-linking. For example, minimal cell death was demonstrated for both osteoblasts photoencapsulated in 10% poly(ethylene glycol) diacrylate (PEG-DA) hydrogel networks [7] and endothelial cells encapsulated in poly(propylene fumarate-co-ethylene glycol) networks [68]. Certain photoinitiators, such as 4-(2-hydroxyethoxy) phenyl-(2-propyl) ketone (Irgacure 2959) and eosin Y, are particularly well suited for use in cell encapsulations as they allow lower cytotoxicity and higher cell viability throughout the photopolymerization process [6].

Photolithographic techniques have allowed for the fabrication of hydrogel scaffolds with detailed features by employing photomasks to dictate controlled photo-initiated cross-linking of synthetic and natural prepolymer materials. The current approaches to micropattern scaffolds using controlled light exposure in 3D hydrogels can be classified into 2 distinct approaches, namely post-gelation photopatterning and stereolithography [36]. Recent progress with these approaches will now be discussed in detail, with an emphasis on advancement toward engineering functional tissues.

2.3.1 Post-Gelation Photopatterning

Post-gelation photopatterning involves the cross-linking of a preformed hydrogel and the subsequent micropatterning of physical or biochemical structures within that hydrogel by exposing portions of the gel to light of a particular wavelength [36]. Post-gelation patterning is often achieved by permeating the pre-formed hydrogel with photoinitiator molecules as well as biomolecules to be patterned into the gel. At other times, however, simple light exposure is enough to alter the physical or chemical structure of the hydrogel. In either case, cells may be encapsulated within the hydrogel prior to patterning or may be seeded onto the hydrogel subsequently. Early techniques utilized transparency masks to control photochemical reactions within preformed hydrogels. For example, researchers utilized basic transparency photomasks to micropattern the cell adhesive peptide Arg-Gly-Asp-Ser (RGDS) onto the surface of non-adhesive poly(ethylene glycol) diacrylate (PEG-DA) hydrogels [46]. In these experiments, a PEG-DA hydrogel was first photopolymerized with UV light and an acrylate-poly(ethylene glycol)-RGDS molecule (PEG-RGDS) was applied to the surface of the hydrogel along with a photoinitiator. Using a photomask, UV light was then selectively applied to the hydrogel and distinct patterns of PEG-RGDS were cross-linked onto the hydrogel surface. With this technique, researchers were able to pattern 50 μm lines of PEG-RGDS, and upon seeding with endothelial cells, cellular cord-like tubules formed along the lines in an organized manner [46]. Others have used post-gelation photopatterning to manipulate the degradability of hydrogel scaffolds. In one such case, a naturally degradable hyaluronan-based scaffold was designed such that when the scaffold was exposed to UV light, additional bonds were formed that rendered the scaffold impervious to degradation [37]. By exposing UV light through a photomask, patterned regions of non-degradable material could be fabricated within these scaffolds. In validation of the technique, encapsulated mesenchymal stem cells spread out and remodeled the non-patterned hydrogel matrix but were unable to elongate within the patterned hydrogel, with this result ultimately influencing stem cell differentiation [37].

An advance in post-gelation photopatterning has come with the use of lasers to control photochemical reactions in hydrogels. In early work, researchers developed a degradable agarose hydrogel modified with a cysteine-based sulphydryl protecting group that was cleavable with UV light [44]. By application of a UV laser, these protecting groups were cleaved into the shape of a channel, and the free sulphydryl groups were then chemically reacted with the biomolecule malemide-GRGDS. This scheme created channels of adhesive GRGDS into which neural cells migrated, demonstrating the guidance of cells in a micropatterned 3D biomaterial [44]. The application of lasers for photopatterning became even more prevalent with the advent of laser scanning lithography (LSL) with confocal microscopes [29]. These instruments scan precisely focused laser light over a specified area and use an adjustable light collection pinhole to eliminate out of focus light and allow for optical sectioning with low axial resolution [63]. In LSL, the laser light from a confocal laser scanning microscope excites a photoinitiator and cross-links biomolecules within a hydrogel to subsequently guide cellular organization. For example, researchers soaked PEG-RGDS and the photoinitiator eosin y into PEG-based hydrogels and then patterned the materials using a 514 nm argon laser attached to a confocal microscope [29]. To achieve high spatial resolution, computerized virtual masks were implemented that directed the precise spatial location of the laser. This type of control allowed for the fabrication of microscopic patterns of bioactivity on the otherwise non-adherent PEG hydrogel surface [29]. LSL has been utilized to pattern vascular endothelial growth factor and RGDS onto the surface of PEG-based hydrogels in the form of 10 μm lines [42]. Endothelial cells seeded on these surfaces aligned along the patterns and rapidly formed vessel-like tubes [42].

While surface studies remain excellent methods to study cell behavior, scientists have increasingly focused on controlling the cellular microenvironment in three dimensions. Recently, laser scanning lithography has been transformed into a more powerful 3D technology by the increased availability of two-photon microscopes. In order to recognize the significance of this advance, however, one must first understand the basic principles of a two- photon excitation event. In normal photonic excitation, a fluorophore is excited with light of the appropriate wavelength, and an electron is allowed to reach an excited energy state. Upon relaxation of this electron, energy is released in the form of a photon, producing the fluorescent effect. In two-photon excitation, the simultaneous excitation of two photons of a lower energy is used to excite a fluorophore, which may then release a photon at a higher energy than either of the two excitatory photons. Two-photon excitation using light at 720 nm, for example, will allow for fluorophore excitation at 360 nm. The probability of two-photon excitation is very low, and thus a high-frequency pulsed laser, such as a titanium sapphire laser, is traditionally required to achieve the effect. A Ti:Sapphire laser is capable of producing light pulses faster than 100 fs at a frequency of 75 Mhz [67]. The pulse nature of such a laser allows peak excitation power to be very high (1–10 kW), while the average power is sufficiently low as to not cause damage to materials and even allow for cell viability.

Two-photon excitation has several innate advantages over one-photon excitation. First, the probability of simultaneous excitation of two photons is proportional to the square of the light intensity, and thus excitation decays away rapidly with the fourth power of distance from the focal point [21]. Functionally, this allows for the excitation to be limited to a microscopic, three-dimensional volume at the focal point of excitation light; therefore, while one photon excitation would excite a fluorophore throughout the axial direction of a sample, two-photon excitation allows for innate three-dimensionality in which the fluorophore is only excited where the light is precisely focused [67]. Another advantage of two-photon excitation is that long wavelength infrared light (between 720–1200 nm) normally passes through biological water-based materials with significantly less scattering than visible or ultraviolet light, thereby allowing for high-resolution excitation at greater axial depths. While traditionally applied to optical imaging, two-photon excitation has now been utilized in combination with laser scanning lithography to confine photo-reactive processes to three-dimensional focal volumes with high resolution [30].

The use of a two-photon excitation process to directly modify photosensitive hydrogel scaffolds offers a novel method for the fabrication of 3D microenvironments. This technique, known as two-photon laser scanning lithography (TP-LSL), was utilized in photosensitive acrylate-based PEG hydrogels to confine photo-reactive processes to focused, 3D micro-volumes, leaving all other points along the laser's optical path unaltered [31,40]. Specifically, fluorescent PEG-RGDS was soaked into a preformed PEG-DA hydrogel, and through the utilization of a laser scanning microscope, a focused, two-photon laser excited photoinitiator molecules, thereby inducing free-radical based chemical cross-linking of the PEG-RGDS at the microscopic, three-dimensional volume of the laser focal point. Un-cross-linked molecules were then washed away, leaving behind precisely designed three-dimensional regions of bioactivity within the preformed hydrogel scaffolds (Fig. 2.8). TP-LSL has been utilized to pattern biomolecules in precisely designed 3D volumes in several different hydrogel systems via various photochemical mechanisms [19,30,31,72]. In all systems, 3D micropatterning was achieved by designating regions of interest for patterning in the X–Y lateral direction and controlling the focus of the laser beam for patterning in the Z direction.

The capabilities and parameters of TP-LSL systems have been explored extensively in recent years. PEG-RGDS micropatterns as small as 1 μm in the lateral direction and 5 μm in the axial direction have been fabricated in PEG-based hydrogels, demonstrating the superior resolution of the technique [31]. Variation of laser power and scan speed have also shown to directly correlate with the concentration of cross-linked biomolecules, with higher powers and slower scan speeds inducing higher PEG-RGDS concentrations within PEG-based hydrogels [30,31,71]. Further, different kinds of biomolecules have been three-dimensionally patterned into the same microenvironment [31,71]. For example, PEG-RGDS was first micropatterned into a hydrogel using a designed virtual mask. After soaking out non-patterned PEG-RGDS, a different acrylate-PEG-peptide, PEG- QILDVPST, was soaked into the hydrogel and patterned using a different virtual mask in either a juxtaposed or overlapping manner to the original RGDS peptide (Fig. 2.9a) [31]. In another example, high affinity binding proteins streptavidin/biotin and barstar/barnase were utilized with TP-LSL to facilitate the 3D patterning of multiple bioactive proteins [71]. To do this, streptavidin and barnase were sequentially immobilized in unique micropatterns via two-photon chemistry within an agarose hydrogel. The fusion proteins barstar-sonic hedgehog (SHH) and biotin-ciliary neurotrophic factor (CNTF) were then synthesized.

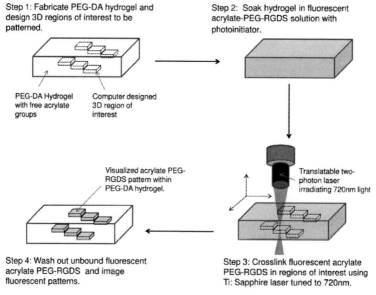

Figure 2.8 Post-gelation photopatterning via two-photon laser scanning lithography. Acrylate-based PEG hydrogels were fabricated and 3D regions of interest were designed on a computer. Fluorescent acrylate-PEG-RGDS with photoinitiator was then soaked into the hydrogel and a translatable two-photon laser irradiating at 720 nm was used to cross-link the fluorescent PEG-RGDS molecules into the desired 3D micropatterns. The gels were then washed to yield only the designed 3D regions of patterned biomolecules [31].

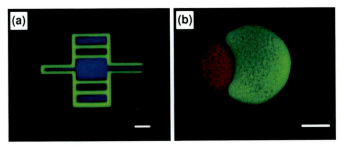

Figure 2.9 Photopatterning multiple biomolecules within a hydrogel microenvironment. (a) Two-photon laser scanning lithography (TP-LSL) was used to pattern PEG-RGDS (green) and PEG-QILDVPST (blue) into a complicated channel pattern within a PEG-based hydrogel. Scale bar = 25 μm. Adapted from Hoffmann et al. [31]. (b) TP-LSL was used to pattern streptavidin and barnase into an agarose hydrogel via two photon chemistry. The fusion proteins barstar-sonic hedgehog (green) and biotin-ciliary neurotrophic factor (red) were then washed into the gel and bound by their micropatterned binding partner. Adapted from Wylie et al. [71].

The fusion proteins were simply soaked into the gel and were immediately bound by their micropatterned binding partners, thus facilitating the control of bioactive proteins in 3D (Fig. 2.9b) [71]. These micropatterning capabilities can serve as important tools to manipulate and recapitulate complex cellular microstructures within hydrogels.

Bioengineers have recently introduced cells into TP-LSL micropatterned hydrogels with the goal of controlling cellular behavior on the microscale for tissue engineering applications. In one example, human dermal fibroblasts in a fibrin clot were first encapsulated in an enzymatically degradable PEG hydrogel [40]. A branching micropattern of PEG-RGDS, approximately 100 μm in width, was then fabricated using TP-LSL. Subsequent fibroblast migration was observed to be directly guided along the micropattern as the cells extended processes and invaded only into regions of RGDS within the gel (Fig. 2.10a) [40].

TP-LSL has also been demonstrated to three-dimensionally direct endothelial cells [1] and neurons [59]. To guide endothelial cells, TP-LSL was used to pattern a 3D gradient of vascular endothelial growth factor (VEGF) in agarose hydrogels [1]. This was achieved using a macro program that continually increased laser power as patterning progressed in the Z dimension. When seeded on the surface of the hydrogels, primary brain microvascular endothelial cells formed tubule-like structures and migrated over 200 µm down an optimal VEGF gradient (Fig. 2.10b) [1]. In order to guide neural cells, a scanning two-photon laser and a digital micromirror device were utilized to cross-link biotinylated protein structures within hyaluroninc acid hydrogels [59]. An avidin-biotin bridge was then formed by washing in avidin and biotinylated biomolecules such as a biotin-modified IKVAV peptide. A set of four helixes decorated with the IKVAV peptide was fabricated in this manner and dorsal root ganglia cells were guided down the helix with 5 µm resolution (Fig. 2.10c). This ability to control complex scaffold architectures in a 3D cellular environment will undoubtedly have an important impact on future tissue engineering constructs.

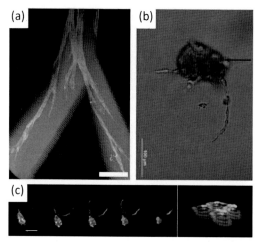

Figure 2.10 Guiding 3D cell migration in photopatterned hydrogels. (a) A branching micropattern of fluorescent PEG-RGDS (green) guides the migration of fibroblast cells (DAPI-blue, phalloidin-red) within a PEG based hydrogel. Scale bar = 100 µm. Adapted from Lee et al. [40]. (b) Primary endothelial cells migrated into an agarose hydrogel down a patterned VEGF gradient. The arrow indicates the hydrogel surface. Scale bar = 100 µm. Adapted from Aizawa et al. [1]. (c) Dorsal root ganglia cells migrating down a helix pattern. The left image is the hydrogel surface and images to the right are at increasing depth, indicating guided 3D migration. The far right image is a projection of the 4 helix pattern before cell seeding. Scale bar = 50 µm. Adapted from Seidlits et al. [59].

TP-LSL can also physically remove microstructures from preformed hydrogels to manipulate cell behavior. For example, three-dimensional channels were ablated within collagen gels using a two-photon laser tuned to 830 nm with 400 mW focal power [34]. These channels, which ranged in size from 3 µm × 3 µm × 150 µm to 30 µm × 30 µm × 150 µm, were then able to guide collective cell migration from an encapsulated cell spheroid [34]. In another example, photodegradable, synthetic hydrogels were fabricated to control the 3D microenvironment of biomaterial scaffolds [38]. Poly(ethylene glycol) hydrogels were rendered photodegradable through the inclusion of a nitrobenzyl ether-derived moiety in the polymer backbone [38]. TP-LSL micropatterning was then utilized to generate a variety of hollow 3D volumes within these PEG-based hydrogels. Using this technique, the relative spreading and differentiation of human mesenchymal stem cells was regulated via controlled photodegradation of hydrogel matrices [38,69]. In follow up work, hydrogels were formulated that could be modified via orthogonal photoconjugation and photocleavage reactions [20]. Specifically, hydrogels with polymer backbones containing both a nitrobenzyl ether derived moiety for photodegradation as well as a vinyl group for facile linking to thiol containing peptide and protein structures were created by means of copper free alkine-azide reactions [20]. Functionally, this allowed for 3D photodegradation of PEG hydrogels with two-photon laser light at 720 nm and 3D photocoupling of biomolecules to the same hydrogel using the eosin Y photointiator and two-photon laser light at 860 nm. Researchers were then able to control 3D cellular migration by patterning both hollow channels as well as the RGD adhesive ligand (Fig. 2.11) [20].

Such multifunctional materials offer bioengineers unprecedented regulation of the cellular microenvironment, but researchers have only just begun to fully apply this control in a manner more directly related to tissue engineering applications. For instance, while many researchers have reported micropatterning of hydrogels and subsequent cellular control with TP-LSL, almost all of these studies have utilized simple geometric shapes when defining virtual masks to spatially dictate the location of the laser. Recently, however, scientists have significantly advanced 3D patterning into a technology directly applicable to tissue engineering with the advent of Image-Guided TP-LSL. In this technique, 3D microscopic tissue images are directly translated to 3D biomolecule micropatterns within preformed hydrogels (Fig. 2.12a) [18]. In one example of Image-Guided TP-LSL, a series of X–Y cross-sectional images of the endogenous microvasculature was obtained as the focus was translated in the Z direction [18].

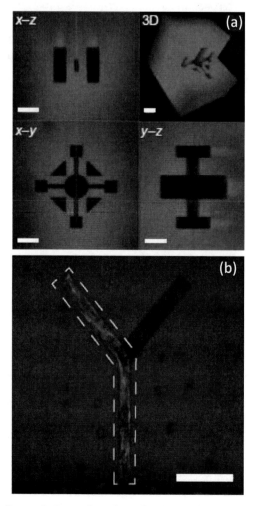

Figure 2.11 Post-gelation photodegradation and photopatterning of hydrogels. (a) Two-photon laser scanning lithography (TP-LSL) was utilized to degrade a complex 3D structure within a PEG hydrogel. Scale bar = 100 μm. (b) A photodegraded channel was patterned with RGD and shown to direct the migration of fibroblast cells. Scale bar = 100 μm. Adapted from DeForest et al. [20].

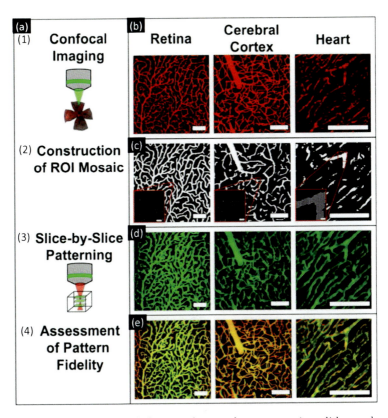

Figure 2.12 Image guided two-photon laser scanning lithography. (a) Tissue structures are imaged on a confocal microscope and converted to a region of interest mosaic (aka virtual mask). Biomolecules are then patterned into a hydrogel slice by slice to three-dimensionally mimic original tissue structures. (b) 3D image projections of vasculature from the retina, cerebral cortex, and heart. (c) Virtual masks consisting of a series of regions of interest. (d) 3D projections of fluorescent PEG-RGDS patterned within a PEG based hydrogel. (e) A merge of the imaged vasculature and patterned hydrogels, with yellow indicating excellent overlap. Scale bars = 100 μm (5 μm for inserts) [18].

Each image of the microvessels was computationally converted to a virtual mask that then directed a two-photon laser to pattern biomolecules in a hydrogel into the exact structure of the vessels in the original image. All of the virtual masks within the series were sequentially micropatterned with the appropriate axial spacing between each slice so that a biomolecule micropattern was formed that exactly mimicked the natural microvessels in all three dimensions. Using this technique, PEG-RGDS was biomimetically patterned within a degradable PEG-based hydrogel in the exact shape of murine microvessels from the heart, brain, and eye as shown in Figs. 2.12b–e [18].

Image-guided TP-LSL has also been utilized to micropattern multiple aspects of a complex microenvironment [18]. Specifically, the architecture of the murine neural stem cell niche was first elucidated by fluorescent immunohistochemistry with a Ki67 antibody to neural stem cells and anti-PECAM for the endothelial cells of microvessels. Images of the two different niche components were next converted to virtual masks to direct the two-photon laser. PEG-RGDS was patterned into a PEG-based hydrogel in the shape of the microvessels, while a different peptide, PEG-IKVAV, was patterned into the structure of the neural stem cells. Each of these patterns precisely mimicked the two endogenous structures from the neural stem cell niche [18]. The capability to pattern multiple biological molecules into distinct biomimetic structures within hydrogel scaffolds will be directly applicable to tissue engineering as scientists look to control the organization and function of multiple cell types on the microscale. Most recently, and perhaps most exciting for the tissue engineering field, bioengineers have utilized Image-Guided TP-LSL to guide the cellular organization of engineered vessel structures within a hydrogel to directly mimic the microvasculature of the brain [18].

This was achieved through micropatterning PEG-RGDS into the structure of the cerebral cortex microvessels within a PEG-based hydrogel containing endothelial cells and pericyte precursor cells. As the cells assembled into vessels, their architecture was guided by the patterned RGDS molecules, thus resulting in the biomimetic vessels that precisely mimicked the vasculature of the cerebral cortex (Fig. 2.13) [18]. Since the spatial arrangement of vessels is directly related to tissue function [24], the ability to engineer tissue specific vessel morphologies will be critical as the field moves toward the fabrication of complex tissues and organs. Tissue engineering applications of post-gelation photopatterning techniques, such as those involving image-guided TP-LSL, are expected to increase exponentially in the near future.

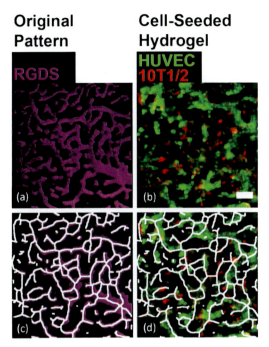

Figure 2.13 Engineered biomimetic microvasculature. (a) A degradable PEG-based hydrogel with a PEG-RGDS pattern (purple) in the shape of the vessels in the cerebral cortex. (b) Endothelial cells (green) and pericyte cells (red) formed vessel tubules that align with the RGDS pattern of the vessels in the cerebral cortex. (c) Tracing of RGDS pattern to highlight structure. (d) Pattern tracing overlaid on organized vessels to show alignment of vessels to pattern. Scale bar = 50 µm [18].

2.3.2 Stereolithography

In parallel with the development of post-gelation photopatterning, stereolithography (SLA) has developed into an important patterning technology for the fabrication of tissue engineering scaffolds. SLA employs a layer-by-layer strategy in which a thin, spatially defined layer of hydrogel is first photopolymerized from a precursor solution [36]. The hydrogel precursor solution normally contains a photo-cross-linkable polymer, a photoinitiator, and, at times, living cells. After cross-linking the first hydrogel layer, excess solution is washed away, and a second layer of precursor solution is deposited and subsequently polymerized. This process is then repeated until hydrogel scaffolds with the desired 3D architecture have been achieved.

As in the case of post-gelation patterning, several different methods have been developed to control the features of photopolymerized hydrogel scaffolds using SLA. Early researchers employed molds and transparency photomasks to control the structure of each layer. For example, with energy from a UV light source, Teflon spacers and a photomask depicting a series of uniform spheres and channels were utilized to photopolymerize a poly(2-hydroxyethyl methacrylate) (polyHEMA) hydrogel micropatterned with a controlled porosity and gel thickness [5]. Specifically, 62 μm pores and 200 μm channels were fabricated. After collagen deposition, these poly(HEMA) scaffolds supported the spreading and differentiation of myoblasts into fibrilliar structures that aligned along the micropatterned porosity [5]. In a different study, PEG-DA hydrogels were polymerized in an interfacial manner to facilitate layer-by-layer patterning [54]. Specifically, PEG-DA mixed with poly(ethylene glycol)-amino acrylate (PEG-AA) was photopolymerized onto an eosin y functionalized surface. After the photopolymerization of the first layer, the initiator was soaked into the hydrogel to react with free amines of the PEG-AA, thus providing a newly functionalized surface onto which the next hydrogel layer was polymerized. Using this technique, a series of complex transparency photomasks allowed fabrication of hydrogels into a high-resolution (50 μm) structure that resembled a complex vascular architecture [54]. Hydrogels created with transparency photomasks have also been shown to facilitate high cell viability during cross-linking and even increased nutrient transport and cell function compared with bulk, non-patterned hydrogels [70].

The use of laser light sources and virtual masks in the fabrication of photopolymerized hydrogel structures has become increasingly common in SLA to achieve both high resolution and increased automation.

In one example, a UV laser was utilized in combination with a platform that translates in the Z direction in order to polymerize multilayer, cellularized PEG-DA hydrogels (Fig. 2.14a) [9,36]. CAD software directed the UV laser to photopolymerize a cell-laden hydrogel into a cross-hatch structure (Fig. 2.14b). The platform was moved axially after the initial polymerization and a second layer was photopolymerized onto the first layer. Unique populations of fibroblasts were also incorporated into different layer sets of the hydrogel to successfully fabricate a complex, multilayer tissue engineering scaffold (Fig. 2.14c) [9].

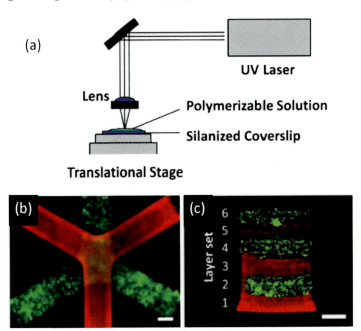

Figure 2.14 Stereolithographic scaffold fabrication. (a) Stereolithography experimental setup where a UV laser is used to polymerize a monomer solution into distinct shapes using a translational stage. To form each new layer, the stage moves axially. Adapted from Khetan et al. [36]. (b) A multi-layer PEG-based hydrogel forming a complex cross hatch structure. The first layer set of the scaffold contains green fluorescent fibroblasts while the second layer set contains red fluorescent fibroblasts. Scale bar = 1 mm. (c) A cross-sectional view of a multilayer PEG-based hydrogel with each layer containing red or green labeled fibroblasts. Six sets of layers are shown, with each layer set approximately 500 μm. Scale bar = 1 mm. Adapted from Chan et al. [9].

A microfluidic system was also recently developed in which multiple types of photopolymerizable materials could be rapidly polymerized into 3D structures on the microscale in a highly automated way [12]. This system involved flowing a hydrogel precursor solution into a chamber, polymerizing it with a 532 nm laser, and then washing away un-cross-linked material (Fig. 2.15a). The process was repeated with various hydrogel precursor solutions to form complex, multi-component hydrogel structures with 3 µm resolution as shown in Fig. 2.15b [12]. These types of high-throughput techniques will likely prove essential to fabricating multifaceted scaffolds for biomimetic tissue engineering.

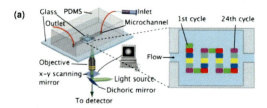

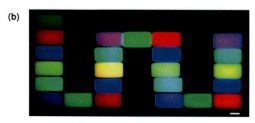

Figure 2.15 Microfluidic stereolithographic patterning. (a) Microfluidic patterning setup. A microfluidic device was placed on the stage of a confocal microscope. Photocurable agents were injected via the inlet. Structures were then polymerized and washed before the next cycle began. (b) PEG-based hydrogels fabricated within a microfluidic system. 24 compositionally unique microscopic PEG-based hydrogels were fabricated using 24 cycles of this process. Scale bar = 200 µm. Adapted from Cheung et al. [12].

As with post-gelation photopatterning, the recent increased availability of high-frequency pulsed lasers allows SLA to incorporate two-photon polymerization of hydrogel structures.

Two-photon SLA involves polymerizing polymer structures through an exact 3D control of the laser focal spot, which can be achieved using a laser scanning microscope or various alterative setups that allow for three axis control. Using this technique, 3D structures were polymerized via a layer-by-layer method until the desired architecture was achieved. In one reported system, a copolymer with both poly(caprolactone) and poly(ethylene glycol) was used in combination with a two-photon laser to fabricate complex 3D biomaterial structures with 4 µm resolution [14]. Fibroblasts seeded onto the microstructured material were both highly viable and proliferative [14]. In a different set of experiments, methacylamide-modified gelatin was photo-cross-linked into a biocompatible scaffold on a larger scale with similar microscopic resolution [51]. Specifically, a computer designed scaffold was photopolymerized as an array of 50 µm thick struts. To fabricate each strut, the two-photon laser was adjusted 2 µm axially between each layer. The struts were patterned together to form a series of pores with each pore having dimensions of 250 µm × 250 µm × 300 µm Four layers of a 10 × 10 array of pores were fabricated in this manner resulting in final scaffold dimensions of 2.5 mm × 2.5 mm × 1.2 mm as shown in Fig. 2.16a. Importantly, upon treatment with collagenase, ridges in the scaffold were observed to correspond to the 2 µm spaced patterned layers of each strut, indicating high resolution despite the relatively large overall scaffold size (Fig. 2.16b) [51].

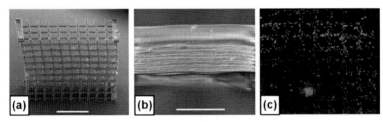

Figure 2.16 Two-photon stereolithography. (a) Methacylamide-modified gelatin was photo-cross-linked using a two-photon laser into a series of pores. Four layers of a 10 × 10 array of pores were fabricated. Scale bar = 1 mm. (b) After collagenase treatment, ridges in the scaffold were observed that corresponded to the 2 µm spaced patterned layers of each ridge. Scale bar = 50 µm. (c) Porcine mesenchymal stem cells (green) were seeded on scaffold and observed to proliferate after 11 days in culture. Adapted from Ovsianikov et al. [51].

Mesenchymal stem cells seeded onto this scaffold were shown to adhere, proliferate, and differentiate successfully (Fig. 2.16c) [51]. In another example of the versatility of TP-LSL, 2.5 mm^3 scaffolds of biocompatible photoresist polymers were fabricated with sub-micrometer resolution in only 2 h [33]. Others yet have fabricated bioactive PEG-DA scaffolds with feature resolution as low as 200 nm [53]. With such exquisite control of biomaterial scaffold design, photolithography has become an exciting tool for tissue engineers as they look to bridge length scales and move toward the micropatterning of more complex, functional tissues.

2.4 The Future of Micropatterning in Tissue Engineering

Over the last decade, 3D printing and photolithography technologies have advanced rapidly, with these techniques readily adapted to the field of tissue engineering. While much progress has been made toward the common goal of generating functional tissue replacements, it is prudent to note that each technique still possesses distinct advantages and disadvantages (Table 2.1). For example, direct-write bioprinting and stereolithography are best suited for fabricating 3D structures, but in many cases lack the resolution necessary to manipulate individual cells into complex tissue microstructures. Biological laser printing has become a fine way to manipulate cell position, but has limited ability to fabricate spatially complex 3D structures.

Table 2.1 Pros and cons of 3D microfabrication technologies

	Pros	**Cons**
Direct-write bioprinting	– Fabricates large structures – Fabricates 3D structures	– Lacks 3D resolution – Difficult to pattern multiple bioactive molecules
Inkjet bioprinting	– Accessible and economical – Incorporation of multiple cell types	– Difficult to achieve 3D structures – Difficult to pattern multiple bioactive molecules
Biological laser printing	– Allows for precise placement of cells – Incorporation of multiple cell types	– Difficult to achieve 3D structures – Difficult to pattern multiple bioactive molecules
Post-gelation photo-patterning	– High-resolution 3D patterning – Incorporation of multiple materials/cell types	– Difficult to fabricate large structures
Stereolithography	– Fabricates large 3D structures – Incorporation of multiple materials/cell types	– Lacks 3D resolution

Inkjet printing is promising in terms of accessibility and economics, but fabrication of larger 3D structures with precise resolution is in its nascent stages. Additionally, difficulties in photopatterning large structures with very fine 3D resolution are only just beginning to be addressed. Incremental improvements in the shortcomings of these technologies will significantly impact the ability of researchers to organize cells into complex microstructures on the path toward developing functional tissue engineering therapeutics.

While a variety of micropatterning techniques have been separately discussed in this chapter, they are not necessarily mutually exclusive. For example, two-photon stereolithography has been combined with biological laser printing in order to first fabricate high-resolution 3D scaffolds and then print different cell types onto this scaffold in a controlled manner [52]. Future research will similarly focus on the development and application of combination micropatterning technologies to address multiple needs in tissue engineering scaffold fabrication. In fact, it is likely that some combination of layer-by-layer fabrication and post-gelation or cellular patterning will be necessary to give tissue engineering constructs a physical 3D microstructure as well as intricately patterned biology. Future micropatterning tissue engineering research must also address issues surrounding the achievement of functional tissue engineering outcomes. For example, can the engineered microvasculature support gas exchange and nutrient transport to sustain increased cell viability? Will the tissue constructs assume specific functions such as blood detoxification in the liver or sufficient mechanical support for bone? These and other questions will be the central focus as bioengineers look to continually optimize micropatterning technologies toward the ultimate goal of engineering functional organs to improve patient outcomes.

References

1. Aizawa, Y., Wylie, R., and Shoichet, M., Endothelial Cell Guidance in 3D Patterned Scaffolds, *Advanced Materials*, **22** (2010), 4831–4835.
2. Barron, J. A., Krizman, D. B., and Ringeisen, B. R., Laser printing of single cells: Statistical analysis, cell viability, and stress, *Annals of Biomedical Engineering*, **33** (2005), 121–130.

3. Barron, J. A., Wu, P., Ladouceur, H. D., and Ringeisen, B. R., Biological laser printing: A novel technique for creating heterogeneous 3-dimensional cell patterns, *Biomedical Microdevices*, **6** (2004), 139–147.

4. Barron, J. A., Young, H. D., Dlott, D. D., Darfler, M. M., Krizman, D. B., and Ringeisen, B. R., Printing of protein microarrays via a capillary-free fluid jetting mechanism, *Proteomics*, **5** (2005), 4138–4144.

5. Bryant, S. J., Cuy, J. L., Hauch, K. D., and Ratner, B. D., Photo-patterning of porous hydrogels for tissue engineering, *Biomaterials*, **28** (2007), 2978–2986.

6. Bryant, S. J., and Anseth, K. S., Photopolymerization of hydrogel scaffolds, in *Scaffolding in Tissue Engineering* (Ma, P. M., and Elisseeff, J., eds.), Taylor and Francis Group, Boca Raton, 2006, pp. 71–91.

7. Burdick, J. A., and Anseth, K. S., Photoencapsulation of osteoblasts in injectable RGD-modified PEG hydrogels for bone tissue engineering, *Biomaterials*, **23** (2002), 4315–4323.

8. Censi, R., Schuurman, W., Malda, J., di Dato, G., Burgisser, P. E., Dhert, W. J. A., et al., A printable photopolymerizable thermosensitive p(HPMAm-lactate)-PEG hydrogel for tissue engineering, *Advanced Functional Materials*, **21** (2011), 1833–1842.

9. Chan, V., Zorlutuna, P., Jeong, J. H., Kong, H., and Bashir, R., Three-dimensional photopatterning of hydrogels using stereolithography for long-term cell encapsulation, *Lab on a Chip*, **10** (2010), 2062–2070.

10. Chang, C. C., Boland, E. D., Williams, S. K., and Hoying, J. B., Direct-write bioprinting three-dimensional biohybrid systems for future regenerative therapies, *Journal of Biomedical Materials Research Part B—Applied Biomaterials*, **98B** (2011), 160–170.

11. Chen, C. S., Alonso, J. L., Ostuni, E., Whitesides, G. M., and Ingber, D. E., Cell shape provides global control of focal adhesion assembly, *Biochemical and Biophysical Research Communications*, **307** (2003), 355–361.

12. Cheung, Y. K., Gillette, B. M., Zhong, M., Ramcharan, S., and Sia, S. K., Direct patterning of composite biocompatible microstructures using microfluidics, *Lab on a Chip*, **7** (2007), 574–579.

13. Chu, T.-M. G., Solid freeform fabrication of tissue engineering scaffolds, in *Scaffolds in Tissue Engineering* (Ma, P. M., and Elisseeff, J., eds.), Taylor and Francis, Boca Raton (2006), pp. 139–155.

14. Claeyssens, F., Hasan, E. A., Gaidukeviciute, A., Achilleos, D. S., Ranella, A., Reinhardt, C., et al., Three-dimensional biodegradable structures fabricated by two-photon polymerization, *Langmuir*, **25** (2009), 3219–3223.
15. Cohen, D. L., Malone, E., Lipson, H., and Bonassar, L. J., Direct freeform fabrication of seeded hydrogels in arbitrary geometries, *Tissue Engineering*, **12** (2006), 1325–1335.
16. Cui, X., and Boland, T., Human microvasculature fabrication using thermal inkjet printing technology, *Biomaterials*, **30** (2009), 6221–6227.
17. Cukierman, E., Pankov, R., Stevens, D. R., and Yamada, K. M., Taking cell-matrix adhesions to the third dimension, *Science*, **294** (2001), 1708–1712.
18. Culver, J. C., Hoffmann, J. C., Poche, R. A., Slater, J. H., West, J. L., and Dickinson, M. E., Three-dimensional biomimetic patterning in hydrogels to guide cellular organization, *Advanced Materials*, **24** (2012), 2344–2348.
19. DeForest, C. A., Polizzotti, B. D., and Anseth, K. S., Sequential click reactions for synthesizing and patterning three-dimensional cell microenvironments, *Nature Materials*, **8** (2009), 659–664.
20. DeForest, C. A., and Anseth, K. S., Cytocompatible click-based hydrogels with dynamically tunable properties through orthogonal photoconjugation and photocleavage reactions, *Nature Chemistry*, **3** (2011), 925–931.
21. Denk, W., Strickler, J. H., and Webb, W. W., Two-photon laser scanning fluorescence microscopy, *Science*, **248** (1990), 73–76.
22. Dikovsky, D., Bianco-Peled, H., and Seliktar, D., Defining the Role of Matrix compliance and proteolysis in three-dimensional cell spreading and remodeling, *Biophysical Journal*, **94** (2008), 2914–2925.
23. Fedorovich, N. E., Wijnberg, H. M., Dhert, W. J. A., and Alblas, J., Distinct tissue formation by heterogeneous printing of osteo-and endothelial progenitor cells, *Tissue Engineering—Part A*, **17** (2011), 2113–2121.
24. Gerhardt, H., and Betsholtz, C., How do endothelial cells orientate?, in *Mechanisms of Angiogenesis* (Clauss, M., and Breier, G., eds.), Birkhauser Verlag, Basel (2005).
25. Griffith, L. G., and Swartz, M. A., Capturing complex 3D tissue physiology in vitro, *Nature Reviews Molecular Cell Biology*, **7** (2006), 211–224.

26. Guillemot, F., Souquet, A., Catros, S., Guillotin, B., Lopez, J., Faucon, M., et al., High-throughput laser printing of cells and biomaterials for tissue engineering, *Acta Biomaterialia*, **6** (2009), 2494–2500.
27. Guillotin, B., Souquet, A., Catros, S., Duocastella, M., Pippenger, B., Bellance, S., et al., Laser assisted bioprinting of engineered tissue with high cell density and microscale organization, *Biomaterials*, **31** (2010), 7250–7256.
28. Guvendiren, M., and Burdick, J. A., The control of stem cell morphology and differentiation by hydrogel surface wrinkles, *Biomaterials*, **31** (2010), 6511–6518.
29. Hahn, M. S., Miller, J. S., and West, J. L., Laser scanning lithography for surface micropatterning on hydrogels, *Advanced Materials*, **17** (2005), 2939–2942.
30. Hahn, M. S., Miller, J. S., and West, J. L., Three-dimensional biochemical and biomechanical patterning of hydrogels for guiding cell behavior, *Advanced Materials*, **18** (2006), 2679–2684.
31. Hoffmann, J. C., and West, J. L., Three-dimensional photolithographic patterning of multiple bioactive ligands in poly(ethylene glycol) hydrogels, *Soft Matter*, **6** (2010), 5056–5063.
32. Hopp, B., Smausz, T., Kresz, N., Barna, N., Bor, Z., Kolozsvari, L., et al., Survival and proliferative ability of various living cell types after laser-induced forward transfer, *Tissue Engineering*, **11** (2005), 1817–1823.
33. Hsieh, T. M., Ng, C. W. B., Narayanan, K., Wan, A. C. A., and Ying, J. Y., Three-dimensional microstructured tissue scaffolds fabricated by two-photon laser scanning photolithography, *Biomaterials*, **31** (2010), 7648–7652.
34. Ilina, O., Bakker, G. J., Vasaturo, A., Hofmann, R. M., and Friedl, P., Two-photon laser-generated microtracks in 3D collagen lattices: principles of MMP-dependent and -independent collective cancer cell invasion, *Physical Biology*, **8** (2011), 1–8.
35. Khademhosseini, A., Langer, R., Borenstein, J., and Vacanti, J. P., Microscale technologies for tissue engineering and biology, *Proceedings of the National Academy of Sciences*, **103** (2006), 2480–2487.
36. Khetan, S., and Burdick, J. A., Patterning hydrogels in three dimensions towards controlling cellular interactions, *Soft Matter*, **7** (2010), 830–838.
37. Khetan, S., and Burdick, J. A., Patterning network structure to spatially control cellular remodeling and stem cell fate within 3-dimensional hydrogels, *Biomaterials*, **31** (2010), 8228–8234.

38. Kloxin, A. M., Kasko, A. M., Salinas, C. N., and Anseth, K. S., Photodegradable hydrogels for dynamic tuning of physical and chemical properties, *Science*, **324** (2009), 59–63.
39. Lavik, E., and Langer, R., Tissue engineering: current state and perspectives, *Applied Microbiology and Biotechnology*, **65** (2004), 1–8.
40. Lee, S.-H., Moon, J. J., and West, J. L., Three-dimensional micropatterning of bioactive hydrogels via two-photon laser scanning photolithography for guided 3D cell migration, *Biomaterials*, **29** (2008), 2962–2968.
41. Lee, W., Lee, V., Polio, S., Keegan, P., Lee, J.-H., Fischer, K., et al., On-demand three-dimensional freeform fabrication of multi-layered hydrogel scaffold with fluidic channels, *Biotechnology and Bioengineering*, **105** (2010), 1178–1186.
42. Leslie-Barbick, J. E., Shen, C., Chen, C., and West, J. L., Micron-scale spatially patterned, covalently immobilized vascular endothelial growth factor on hydrogels accelerates endothelial tubulogenesis and increases cellular angiogenic responses, *Tissue Engineering Part A*, **17** (2010), 221–229.
43. Lewis, J. A., and Gratson, G. M., Direct writing in three dimensions, *Materials Today*, **7** (2004), 32–39.
44. Luo, Y., and Shoichet, M. S., A photolabile hydrogel for guided three-dimensional cell growth and migration., *Nature Materials*, **3** (2004), 249–253.
45. Miller, J. S., Béthencourt, M. I., Hahn, M., Lee, T. R., and West, J. L., Laser-scanning lithography (LSL) for the soft lithographic patterning of cell-adhesive self-assembled monolayers, *Biotechnology and Bioengineering*, **93** (2006), 1060–1068.
46. Moon, J. J., Hahn, M. S., Kim, I., Nsiah, B. A., and West, J. L., Micropatterning of poly(ethylene glycol) diacrylate hydrogels with biomolecules to regulate and guide endothelial morphogenesis, *Tissue Engineering Part A*, **15** (2009), 579–585.
47. Moon, J. J., Lee, S. H., and West, J. L., Synthetic biomimetic hydrogels incorporated with Ephrin-A1 for therapeutic angiogenesis, *Biomacromolecules*, **8** (2007), 42–49.
48. Moon, J. J., and West, J. L., Vascularization of engineered tissues: Approaches to promote angiogenesis in biomaterials, *Current Topics in Medicinal Chemistry*, **8** (2008), 300–310.
49. Nguyen, K. T., and West, J. L., Photopolymerizable hydrogels for tissue engineering applications, *Biomaterials*, **23** (2002), 4307–4314.

50. Norotte, C., Marga, F. S., Niklason, L. E., and Forgacs, G., Scaffold-free vascular tissue engineering using bioprinting, *Biomaterials*, **30** (2009), 5910–5917.
51. Ovsianikov, A., Deiwick, A., Van Vlierberghe, S., Dubruel, P., Moller, L., Drager, G., et al., Laser fabrication of three-dimensional CAD scaffolds from photosensitive gelatin for applications in tissue engineering, *Biomacromolecules*, **12** (2011), 851–858.
52. Ovsianikov, A., Gruene, M., Pflaum, M., Koch, L., Maiorana, F., Wilhelmi, M., et al., Laser printing of cells into 3D scaffolds, *Biofabrication*, **2** (2010), 1–7.
53. Ovsianikov, A., Malinauskas, M., Schlie, S., Chichkov, B., Gittard, S., Narayan, R., et al., Three-dimensional laser micro- and nano-structuring of acrylated poly(ethylene glycol) materials and evaluation of their cytoxicity for tissue engineering applications, *Acta Biomaterialia*, **7** (2011), 967–974.
54. Papavasiliou, G., Songprawat, P., Perez-Luna, V., Hammes, E., Morris, M., Chiu, Y. C., et al., Three-dimensional patterning of poly(ethylene glycol) hydrogels through surface-initiated photopolymerization, *Tissue Engineering Part C-Methods*, **14** (2008), 129–140.
55. Pataky, K., Braschler, T., Negro, A., Renaud, P., Lutolf, M. P., and Brugger, J., Microdrop printing of hydrogel bioinks into 3D tissue-like geometries, *Advanced Materials*, **24** (2012), 391–396.
56. Pepper, M. E., Parzel, C. A., Burg, T., Boland, T., Burg, K. J. L., and Groff, R. E., Design and implementation of a two-dimensional inkjet bioprinter, in *2009 Annual International Conference of the IEEE Engineering in Medicine and Biology Society* (IEEE, 2009), pp. 6001–6005.
57. Pirlo, R. K., Wu, P., Liu, J., and Ringeisen, B., PLGA/hydrogel biopapers as a stackable substrate for printing HUVEC networks via BioLP (TM), *Biotechnology and Bioengineering*, **109** (2011), 262–273.
58. Ringeisen, B. R., Othon, C. M., Barron, J. A., Young, D., and Spargo, B. J., Jet-based methods to print living cells, *Biotechnology Journal*, **1** (2006), 930–948.
59. Seidlits, S. K., Schmidt, C. E., and Shear, J. B., High-resolution patterning of hydrogels in three dimensions using direct-write photofabrication for cell guidance, *Advanced Functional Materials*, **19** (2009), 3543–3551.
60. Sherwood, J. K., Riley, S. L., Palazzolo, R., Brown, S. C., Monkhouse, D. C., Coates, M., et al., A three-dimensional osteochondral composite scaffold for articular cartilage repair, *Biomaterials*, **23** (2002), 4739–4751.

61. Shin, H., Zygourakis, K., Farach-Carson, M., Yaszemski, M. J., and Mikos, A. G., Modulation of differentiation and mineralization of marrow stromal cells cultured on biomimetic hydrogels modified with Arg-Gly-Asp containing peptides, *Journal of Biomedical Materials Research Part A*, **69A** (2004), 535–543.
62. Shoichet, M. S., and Kapur, T. A., Immobilized concentration gradients of nerve growth factor guide neurite outgrowth, *Journal of Biomedical Materials Research Part A*, **68A** (2004), 235–243.
63. Shotton, D. M., Confocal scanning optical microscopy and its applications for biological specimens, *Journal of Cell Science*, **94** (1989), 175–206.
64. Skardal, A., Zhang, J. X., McCoard, L., Xu, X. Y., Oottamasathien, S., and Prestwich, G. D., Photocrosslinkable hyaluronan-gelatin hydrogels for two-step bioprinting, *Tissue Engineering Part A*, **16** (2010), 2675–2685.
65. Smith, C. M., Christian, J. J., Warren, W. L., and Williams, S. K., Characterizing environmental factors that impact the viability of tissue-engineered constructs fabricated by a direct-write bioassembly tool, *Tissue Engineering*, **13** (2007), 373–383.
66. Smith, C. M., Stone, A. L., Parkhill, R. L., Stewart, R. L., Simpkins, M. W., Kachurin, A. M., et al., Three-dimensional bioassembly tool for generating viable tissue-engineered constructs, *Tissue Engineering*, **10** (2004), 1566–1576.
67. Soeller, C., and Cannell, M. B., Two-photon microscopy: imaging in scattering samples and three-dimensionally resolved flash photolysis, *Microscopy Research and Technique*, **47** (1999), 182–195.
68. Suggs, L. J., and Mikos, A. G., Development of poly(propylene fumarate-co-ethylene glycol) as an injectable carrier for endothelial cells, *Cell Transplantation*, **8** (1999), 345–350.
69. Tibbitt, M. W., Kloxin, A. M., Dyamenahalli, K. U., and Anseth, K. S., Controlled two-photon photodegradation of PEG hydrogels to study and manipulate subcellular interactions on soft materials, *Soft Matter*, **6** (2010), 5100–5108.
70. Tsang, V. L., Chen, A. A., Cho, L. M., Jadin, K. D., Sah, R. L., DeLong, S., et al., Fabrication of 3D hepatic tissues by additive photopatterning of cellular hydrogels, *The FASEB Journal*, **21** (2007), 790–801.
71. Wylie, R. G., Ahsan, S., Aizawa, Y., Maxwell, K. L., Morshead, C. M., and Shoichet, M. S., Spatially controlled simultaneous patterning of multiple growth factors in three-dimensional hydrogels, *Nature Materials*, **10** (2011), 799–806.

72. Wylie, R. G., and Shoichet, M. S., Two-photon micropatterning of amines within an agarose hydrogel, *Journal of Materials Chemistry*, **18** (2008), 2716–2721.
73. Wüst, S., Müller, R., and Hofmann, S., Controlled positioning of cells in biomaterials—approaches towards 3D tissue printing, *Journal of Functional Biomaterials*, **2** (2011), 119–154.
74. Xu, T., Jin, J., Gregory, C., Hickman, J. J., and Boland, T., Inkjet printing of viable mammalian cells, *Biomaterials*, **26** (2005), 93–99.
75. Zaman, M. H., Trapani, L. M., Siemeski, A., MacKellar, D., Gong, H. Y., Kamm, R. D., et al., Migration of tumor cells in 3D matrices is governed by matrix stiffness along with cell-matrix adhesion and proteolysis, *Proceedings of the National Academy of Sciences of the United States of America*, **103** (2006), 10889–10894.

Chapter 3

Nanobiotechnology and Biomaterials for Regenerative Medicine

Nupura S. Bhise and Jordan J. Green

Department of Biomedical Engineering,
Johns Hopkins University School of Medicine,
400 North Broadway, Wilmer Smith Building, Room 5017,
Baltimore, MD 21231, USA

green@jhu.edu

The field of nanobiotechnology holds great promise to develop multiscale fabrication techniques that benefit regenerative medicine. The combination of nano/micro-fabrication techniques with novel biomaterials provides a unique opportunity to create extracellular matrices that mimic native three-dimensional tissue microstructure. This chapter presents advances in nanobiotechnology techniques to develop biomaterial-based matrices and drug delivery systems for regenerative medicine applications. The discussion focuses on systems using hydrogel matrices, nano/micro-fabrication platforms, electrospun nanofibrous matrices, and nano/micro-particles for drug and biomacromolecule delivery. Each technique is discussed from a biomaterials perspective and specific examples are cited to explain their application in tissue repair and regeneration.

Tissue and Organ Regeneration: Advances in Micro- and Nanotechnology
Edited by Lijie Grace Zhang, Ali Khademhosseini, and Thomas J. Webster
Copyright © 2014 Pan Stanford Publishing Pte. Ltd.
ISBN 978-981-4411-67-7 (Hardcover), 978-981-4411-68-4 (eBook)
www.panstanford.com

3.1 Introduction

Tissues are composed of a complex arrangement of cells within a surrounding three-dimensional (3-D) extracellular matrix (ECM). Their physiological function depends on the complexity that results from the tissue-specific arrangement of different cell types, ECM molecules and their interactions (cell–cell and cell–ECM). A pathological dysfunction of any of these components results in degeneration of the supporting tissue architecture, cell death, and eventual loss of function in the damaged tissue. The discipline of tissue engineering emerged to allow the re-creation of this complex 3-D architecture that mimics a tissue in vitro, with the ultimate goal of using these fabricated constructs to regenerate a damaged, degenerated, or lost tissue [44]. The key components of a tissue-engineered construct are cells, scaffold/matrix and biomolecules (for example, growth factors, cytokines and genes). Since the seminal paper by Langer and Vacanti in 1993 [44], this interdisciplinary field has propelled forward based on principles adapted from engineering, material science and life sciences.

Nanobiotechnology and biomaterials can benefit the field of regenerative medicine in numerous ways. One critical aspect is in scaffold design. Biomaterial selection is critical for scaffold design as it determines the physical, chemical, and biological properties of the scaffold, including its biocompatibility and degradation rate, and can modulate cell differentiation and proliferation. Cells interact with and respond to topographical features on the surrounding matrix at all length scales, including nanoscale features such as pores, ridges, and fibers [21,77] (Fig. 3.1). Nanobiotechnologies allow scaffold fabrication, incorporation of biomolecules, and tailoring of topology on a nanoscale. Another critical area of regenerative medicine that benefits from biomaterials and nanobiotechnology is drug delivery. Choice of biomaterial in this instance is especially important to control degradation rate and drug release rate, in addition to also controlling biocompatibility and structural properties of a controlled release device. Nanobiotechnology is crucial to enabling intracellular delivery, where a sensitive cargo is not just released extracellularly, but ferried into a target cell for delivery to a specific compartment within the cell as shown in Fig. 3.2 [25]. Nanobiotechnology is particularly important for the delivery of sensitive biological molecules, including DNA,

RNA, peptides, and proteins that can modulate cell function for regenerative medicine.

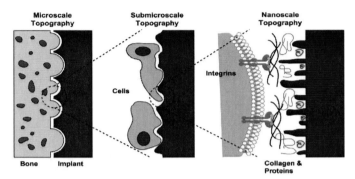

Figure 3.1 Cells interact with and respond to different length-scale topographical features on the scaffold/implant. Reprinted from *Biomaterials*, 32/13, Gittens, R. A., McLachlan, T., Olivares-Navarrete, R., Cai, Y., Berner, S., Tannenbaum, R., Schwartz, Z., Sandhage, K. H., and Boyan, B. D. The effects of combined micron-/submicron-scale surface roughness and nanoscale features on cell proliferation and differentiation, 3395–3403, Copyright 2011, with permission from Elsevier.

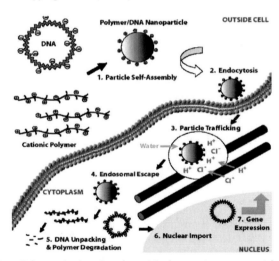

Figure 3.2 Schematic showing the critical steps in nanoparticle mediated intracellular gene delivery. Reprinted with permission from Green, J. J., Langer, R., and Anderson, D. G. (2008). A combinatorial polymer library approach yields insight into nonviral gene delivery. *Accounts Chem Res*, **41**, 749–759. Copyright 2008, American Chemical Society.

A variety of stem cells and adult progenitor cells have been investigated as candidates for cell transplantation therapies due to their capacity to regenerate and differentiate into multiple cell types. Unfortunately, regenerative strategies based on cell transplantation alone are challenged by setbacks, including rapid clearance of transplanted cells, the failure of cell homing and retention at the damaged site, and the shortage of accessible and ethical sources of genetically matched transplantable cells. The recent development of induced pluripotent stem cell (iPSC)–based regenerative techno-logies hold the potential to revolutionize the field of regenerative medicine as it provides a source of ethically derived, inexhaustible and genetically matched source of pluripotent cells [75]. However, for a successful regenerative strategy the cells need to be guided by a supporting matrix that provides physical and chemical cues for the cells to repair the damaged tissue.

Two types of scaffold-based approaches for tissue repair have been widely investigated [41]: in the first approach, a synthetic scaffold, pre-seeded ex vivo with cells isolated from host tissue, is implanted in the damaged area to promote regeneration. The scaffold acts as a 3-D ECM to guide the cell growth and differentiation in vivo. The scaffold material properties are tuned to allow biodegradability at a rate similar to tissue regeneration and are bio-inert to avoid rejection by the host immune system. In the second approach, acellular scaffolds are implanted in the damaged area and act as a depot of biomolecules. The biomolecules are released from the implant at a controlled rate for a sustained period to allow recruitment and homing of cells to the damaged area. Different proliferation and differentiation signals can also be delivered to aid regeneration. Delivery can be directly from a scaffold or from nano/micro-particles embedded within the scaffold. Such composite scaffolds acting as depots for biomolecule delivery may be ideal for stem cell applications such as the generation or programming of induced pluripotent stem cells (iPSCs) that require sustained expression of factors for a period of several weeks.

The delivery of biomolecules in their protein form is inefficient and costly due to rapid clearance in vivo, the expense of recombinant proteins and the need for repeated administration [32]. The sustained delivery of genes encoding these factors is a potentially promising alternative approach. A new paradigm in bioactive scaffold engineering is to deliver therapeutic protein-encoding genes from an implanted scaffold to the target cells [10,60,64]. Recently, "bioactive scaffold" strategies combining the above two approaches have been developed to allow controlled release of biomolecules from pre-seeded scaffolds to promote growth of progenitor cells during ex vivo culture and the biomolecules delivery is sustained post-implantation for enhanced tissue regeneration in vivo [38,58].

3.2 Polymeric 3-D Systems for Tissue Regeneration

Successfully engineered constructs for tissue regeneration have been mostly limited to skin epidermal wounds, cartilage injuries and corneal implants. Tissue-engineered constructs for treating degeneration of complex organ systems such as cardiovascular, nervous, hepatic, and orthopedic remain a challenge. To re-create a functional tissue, the engineered constructs need to recapitulate the complex nano- and micro-scale features of the native ECM as well as control the spatial and temporal organization of cells. The field of nanotechnology holds great promise to develop multiscale fabrication techniques that benefit regenerative medicine. The spatial and temporal control facilitated by these techniques further enhances the ability to generate functional biomaterials and platforms for evaluating regenerative capacity. Fabrication patterns range from a few hundred nanometers to micrometers. Fabricating scaffolds with two-dimensional (2-D) topographical patterns allows manipulation of cellular behaviors, including cell attachment, proliferation migration, and differentiation. Recent developments have focused on extending topology control to 3-D to more precisely recapitulate the complexity of tissues.

3.2.1 Hydrogel Systems

Hydrogel systems are excellent scaffold materials for mimicking the native 3-D extracellular environment [35]. They are networks of cross-linked hydrophilic polymers that swell in aqueous environment by holding water in their porous structure [8]. A variety of natural polymers (for example, collagen, alginate, hyaluronic acid, elastin, and fibrin) and synthetic polymers (for example, polyethylene glycol, poly(hydroxyethyl methacrylate) and polyacrylamide) have been used to mimic the physical properties, including elasticity, of the native tissue (ranging from <1 kPa for brain tissue to ~45 kPa for osteoblasts) as well as to encapsulate cells for creating pre-seeded scaffolds for tissue regeneration [33].

Natural polymers may inherently be well suited from the standpoint of biocompatibility and native tissue-like elasticity, but synthetic polymers often have superior mechanical properties, allow regulation of biophysical properties and are perhaps better suited for controlling microenvironmental factors and cellular behavior. Moreover, "intelligent" synthetic polymer systems designed to undergo conformational changes in response to an external stimuli are important for temporal and spatial regulation during tissue regeneration and constitute an important class of drug delivery platforms [34]. The external stimuli include pH, temperature, ions, electric fields and light or ultra-violet (UV) radiation. Hydrogels with degradable moieties susceptible to cellular enzymes such as matrix metalloproteinases (MMPs) allow simulation of the native degradation rate during tissue regeneration or repair [49]. Hydrogels have been used in various biomedical applications, such as contact lenses in ophthalmology, absorbable adjuncts to sutures in surgery, wound dressings, barriers to prevent post-operative adhesion formation, injectable decellularized matrices for in vivo tissue repair, scaffolds for tissue engineering, cell encapsulation systems and as drug delivery platforms [13,15,30,59,63]. In many cases, nanoscale features of these hydrogels are key for their chemical and biological function. For a more comprehensive review of hydrogel systems, which is beyond the scope of this chapter, readers are referred to recent reviews [63].

3.2.2 Nano/Micro-Fabricated Systems

Many fabrication techniques used for engineering 3-D biologics have been adapted from the traditional engineering fields. These include photolithographic micropatterning from electrical engineering, robotic printing and rapid prototyping from mechanical engineering and, electrospinning and emulsification techniques from chemical engineering [79]. Biomaterial selection is important for each of these fabrication approaches.

3.2.2.1 Photolithography

Photomask-based lithography is a technique where a photocurable polymer is patterned using a photoresist mask. A photoinitiator decomposes when exposed to light of a particular wavelength to produce free radicals that initiate the cross-linking reaction in the portion of the polymer left exposed by the mask. Hydrogels and acrylated polymer-based systems are widely used with this technique. Care must be taken to reduce cytotoxicity by optimizing the reaction parameters such as prepolymer and photoinitiator concentrations, wavelength of the exposed light (mostly UV wavelengths) as well as the length and intensity of light exposure, and the reaction solvent. Polyethylene glycol (PEG)–based hydrogels have been extensively used for cell-based applications since the hydrophilic backbone enhances nutrient diffusion and improves cell viability. The polymers commonly used for photolithography include diacrylated PEG (PEGDA) and methacrylated hyaluronic acid (meHA). Functional hepatic tissues have been fabricated using PEGDA photolithography approach [48,69]. A three step photolithographic approach was used to generate honeycomb structures to surround individual hepatic microtissues. RGD, the cell-binding motif of ECM proteins, -functionalized PEGDA was mixed with primary hepatic cells and the mixture was placed in chambers to control the height by removable spacers. 3-D structures were created by exposure to UV light using different photomasks in a layered fashion and 500 μm features were photopatterned to facilitate nutrient and oxygen transport. The cells remained viable in the 3-D constructs and were able to produce urea and albumin demonstrating their hepatic functionality in the macroscale constructs.

Mold-based lithography involves the use of an elastomeric polymer that can be casted to form molds. The pattern of the mold confers the shape to the cross-linked gel formed from UV cross-linking a prepolymer solution in the areas exposed by the mold. Polymers used for micromolding include polydimethylsiloxane (PDMS), polyurethanes, polyamines, and Teflon. Polydimethylsiloxane-based molds created using a silicon master is the most common method used to create 3-D tissue constructs by mold-lithography. The PDMS molds are coated with polymers that promote cell attachment and growth. In one study by Tekin et al., NIH-3T3 cells were cultured for three days on poly(*N*-isopropylacrylamide) (PNIPAAm)-coated PDMS molds with microgrooves to form tissue fibers and these fibers were retrieved by inverting the mold on a glass slide at room temperature and allowing the NIPAAm to expand [67]. These tissue parts were then combined to form larger constructs for tissue engineering. Subsequently the same group used the temperature dependent shrinkage and expansion of PNIPAAm to create multicomponent coculture hydrogels [68]. PNIPAAm patterned micromolds were created by UV cross-linking and equilibration at 24°C to obtain the mold shape. Cells were encapsulated in agarose gel precursor, poured on the PNIPAAm molds and the mixture was micropatterned by incubation at 25°C to cross-link the agarose gel. Since PNIPAAm shrinks at 37°C, the cell/agarose microgels were retrieved from the molds by incubating at 37°C. A second cell type was encapsulated in agarose and was allowed to fill the spaces created by the shrunken PNIPAAm mold to achieve patterned coculture in the same gel as shown in Fig. 3.3. Such multicomponent microfabricated systems allow the investigation of unique cell–cell interactions that cannot be achieved by conventional culture systems. Mold features can be designed at the microscale and at the nanoscale.

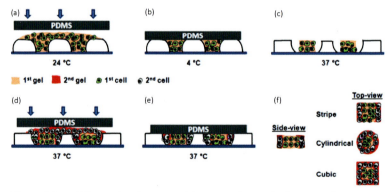

Figure 3.3 Schematic of sequential patterning technique used to create coculture hydrogel microstructures with temperature responsive micromolds. Reprinted with permission from Tekin, H., Tsinman, T., Sanchez, J. G., Jones, B. J., Camci-Unal, G., Nichol, J. W., Langer, R., and Khademhosseini, A. Responsive micromolds for sequential patterning of hydrogel microstructures. *J Am Chem Soc*, **133**, 12944–12947. Copyright 2011 American Chemical Society.

3.2.2.2 Electrospinning

Bioactive scaffolds are ideal as they present both biological and physical cues for cells to grow. Electrospun scaffolds have gained popularity due to their ease in manufacture, ability to control nanoscale fiber diameters, and high surface to volume ratio useful for biomolecule delivery [28]. Electrospinning is a technique in which a polymer solution is spun or melted into whipped jets using electrostatic force to generate continuous ultrathin fibers with nano- and submicron-scale diameters. The grounded collector can be in a static or dynamic state to generate random or aligned fibers respectively. The variables that influence the electrospinning process are polymer solution properties (type of solvent, polymer structure, concentration and molecular weight), environmental factors (humidity and temperature) and setup parameters (applied voltage, collecting distance, solution flow rate). It is important to optimize these variables for successful generation of continuous fibers and to avoid undue effects like bead/droplet formation.

These fibers, as with other biomaterials used for regenerative medicine, should be designed to mimic the native tissue environment. Biomaterials used for electrospinning can be divided into two types: natural polymers and synthetic polymers. Considerable success has been achieved with natural polymers such as collagen, gelatin, chitin, and fibrin [18,28]; however, poor mechanical and thermal properties limit the application of these biopolymers. On the other hand, synthetic polymers enable fine-tuning of chemical properties and are also better suited for processing. The most commonly used synthetic polymers are poly(alpha-hydroxy esters), specifically polycaprolactone (PCL), polylactic acid (PLA), polyglycolic acid (PGA) and poly(lactic-co-glycolic acid) (PLGA), since these have been approved by FDA as biodegradable and biocompatible polymers [46] (Fig. 3.4). Recently, polymer composites have been used to enhance the properties of spun fibers. Polymer composites enable tuning of hydrophilicity, optimal porosity to allow diffusion of nutrients, controllable biodegradability, increased control of mechanical properties, reduced potential cytotoxicity, and improved cell attachment for proliferation and differentiation [40].

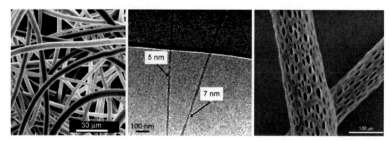

Figure 3.4 Scanning electron microscopy images of electrospun polyamide (left) and polylactic acid (right) nanofibers. Transmission electron microscopy image of electrospun polylactide nanofibers (middle). Reprinted with permission of John Wiley & Sons, Copyright 2007 from Greiner, A., and Wendorff, J. H. (2007). Electrospinning: a fascinating method for the preparation of ultrathin fibers. *Angew Chem*, **46**, 5670–5703.

It is important that cell-biomaterial interactions are enhanced and to promote these interactions biomolecules can be integrated into electrospun scaffolds by one of the following approaches: physical adsorption, blend or coaxial electropspinning, and covalent immobilization. The simplest way to load a biomolecule onto an electrospun scaffold is by dipping the scaffold in an aqueous solution containing the biomolecule post-electrospinning. The biomolecules are physically adsorbed on the scaffold surface via electrostatic forces. Although this approach preserves the native form of the protein or gene, the biggest disadvantage is the uncontrolled release profile. In this method, the biomolecule release is fast (within days to a couple of weeks), whereas other biomolecule methods enable sustained release lasting for months. Nie et al. have shown that when bone morphogenetic protein 2 (BMP2) was adsorbed onto a PLGA scaffold more than 75% of the total loaded amount was released within 5 days with almost 100% release reached in 20 days during a bone regeneration study. This rate was much faster when compared to rate of BMP2 released from scaffolds prepared by blend electrospinning [57].

The technique of blend electrospinning involves mixing biomolecules within a polymer solution and electrospinning this pre-mixed solution to form hybrid scaffolds. Alternatively, in a modified version of blend electrospinning termed emulsion electrospinning, the biomolecule can be suspended in an organic solvent and emulsified with the polymer solution via ultrasonication or homogenization. Scaffolds fabricated using either of these methods can achieve sustained release profiles lasting for as long as 3 months [16]. However, the biomolecule activity can be affected by the mechanical forces involved in the fabrication steps and the conformational changes in the protein caused by the organic solvent. Various strategies have been used to avoid these issues. To avoid harsh processing steps (ultrasonication or homogenization), salt complexation is used instead of emulsification to enhance protein solubility [74]. Addition of hydrophilic polymers such as PEG and PEO in the aqueous biomolecule solution improves protein stability [45] and increases the viscosity of biomolecule solution to prevent formation of beads [72]. These hydrophilic additives and others such as hydroxyapetite crystals also enhance water uptake by the scaffolds and help accelerate the protein released by passive diffusion [57].

Scaffolds fabricated by blend electrospinning typically have an initial burst release in the span of hours, followed by a sustained release profile that is almost linear. The release profiles can be tuned by varying the polymer composition, which affects the degradation rate of the scaffold. In an early gene delivery study, Luu et al. showed a burst release of β-galactosidase within a couple of hours followed by a sustained release for 20 days using PLA-PEG block copolymer blended with varying compositions of PLGA, whereas others have reported a linear release profile sustaining several months from composite PLGA spun scaffolds [50]. This technique has been widely used for delivering a range of biomolecules, including growth factors such as BMP2, basic fibroblast growth factor and epidermal growth factor, bovine serum albumin, enzymes such as lysozyme and genes such as β-galactosidase and BMP2 plasmid [40]. For 3-D cell tissue regeneration applications, it is important to adjust the porosity of the nanofibrous scaffolds to allow sufficient cell infiltration into the scaffolds. The pore size in a random mesh elecctrospun scaffold can be tuned by using these dual composition electrospinning strategies and by varying the relative composition of the two polymers [31].

Recently, coaxial electrospinning has emerged as an attractive strategy in the field for delivery of biomolecules highly susceptible to denaturation during processing [47]. In this method, the biomolecule and polymer solution are simultaneously fed through different capillary channels into a single needle in a coaxial manner that results in the formation of nanofibrous scaffolds with an organized core-shell structure. The core solution consists of a hydrophilic polymer that enables loading and preservation of protein bioactivity, while the hydrophobic shell solution facilitates fiber formation. The fabrication process is affected by various parameters such as feeding rates of the two solutions and their interfacial tension and viscosity. Because of the processing complexity, this method is less common than blend electrospinning, however, the core-shell structure provides an added advantage for biomolecule delivery as it can potentially protect the native structure during fabrication. The biomolecule release profile is similar to blend electrospinning, however much less protein releases in the initial burst release stage and thereby the release can be sustained for a longer time period [39]. This behavior is attributed to the encapsulation of biomolecules in the inner core fibers as the outer shell fibers act as a membrane-barrier for diffusion.

Coaxial electrospinning has been used to encapsulate various proteins for tissue regeneration studies, including fibroblast growth factor, platelet-derived growth factor, and nerve growth factor (NGF). An interesting study conducted by Wang et al. reported the use of aligned core-shell nanofibers to deliver NGF to aid sciatic nerve regeneration [72]. The nanofiber shell solution consisted of PLGA dissolved in hexafluoroisopropanol (HFIP) organic solution and the core solution consisted of NGF dissolved in an aqueous PEG solution. Aligned nanofibers were fabricated by rotating the collector wheel at a fixed speed to control fiber orientation and the nanofibrous scaffolds were reeled into aligned nerve guidance conduits (PLGA/NGF NGC). In a rat sciatic nerve model, the PLGA/NGF NGC group performed significantly better (approximately 1.5-fold higher nerve conduction velocity and compound motor action potential) than the PLGA alone group for promoting nerve regeneration [72].

Saraf et al. reported the use of coaxial electrospun scaffolds for gene delivery [61]. Their coaxial nanofibrous system consisted of EGFP-DNA plasmid dissolved in an aqueous PEG solution to form the core component and the shell component was formed from a solution of hyaluronic acid (HA) modified polyethylenimine (PEI) used as the delivery biomaterial dissolved in an organic polymer solution of poly(e-capralactone) (PCL). They showed that the plasmid diffusing out from the core successfully formed gene delivery particles by complexing with the cationic PEI-HA released from the shell. The particles were able to transfect cells present on the scaffold for a sustained period of 60 days at an average transfection efficiency of 15%. The efficiency was found to correlate with the concentration and molecular weight of the core PEG polymer.

The covalent immobilization strategy involves tethering the biomolecule onto the fiber surface via formation of a chemical bond. Many surface chemistries have been exploited, but the most common method is formation of peptide bonds between amino and carboxyl groups. Incorporation of bonds susceptible to enzyme cleavage allows controlling the release profile of biomolecules by adjusting the cleavage rate. Kim et al. incorporated matrix metalloproteinases (MMPs) cleavable linkers to tether gene delivery nanoparticles to electrospun scaffolds that allowed tuning the release profile by controlling MMP mediated bond cleavage [42]. Specifically, linear polyethyleneimine (LPEI) was covalently immobilized to amine groups on the surface of the nanofibrous matrix via an MMP-cleavable peptide linker, followed by electrostatic incorporation of DNA on the scaffold (Fig. 3.5). In vivo transfection efficiency with the LPEI-immobilized nanofibrous matrix was approximately 50-fold higher when compared to transfection efficiency with naked DNA or 10-fold higher when compared to DNA-incorporated in the absence of LPEI immobilized with MMP-cleavable peptides (Fig. 3.6).

Although considerable progress has been achieved in preserving the bioactivity of biomolecules in electrospun scaffolds fabricated by the above methods, the requirement for suspension of biomolecules in polymeric solutions instead of their natural aqueous environment is an unresolved liability. To address this, sophisticated scaffolds have been designed that combine nanoparticle-based delivery with polymeric fibrous scaffolds as multicomponent drug delivery systems. While the scaffolds act as reservoirs for the carriers to improve their in vivo half-life and stability, the embedded carriers encapsulate therapeutic biomolecules (hydrophobic or hydrophilic) and preserve their bioactivity before releasing it at the target site [55].

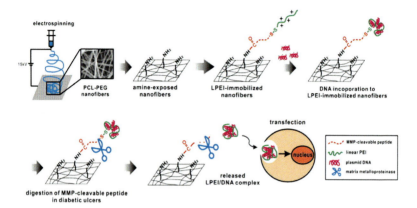

Figure 3.5 Schematic representation of therapeutic gene delivery from MMP-responsive electrospun LPEI immobilized nanofibrous scaffold. Reprinted from *J Control Release*, 145/3, Kim, H. S., and Yoo, H. S., MMPs-responsive release of DNA from electrospun nanofibrous matrix for local gene therapy: in vitro and in vivo evaluation, 264–271, Copyright 2010, with permission from Elsevier.

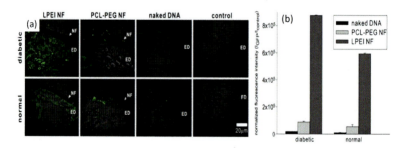

Figure 3.6 In vivo transfection efficiency data of green fluorescent protein (GFP) DNA delivered from DNA/LPEI immobilized nanofibrous matrix with MMP-susceptible linker (LPEI NF), DNA/PCL-PEG nanofibrous matrix without LPEI (PCL-PEG NF) or without any matrix (naked DNA). Reprinted from *J Control Release*, 145/3, Kim, H. S., and Yoo, H. S., MMPs-responsive release of DNA from electrospun nanofibrous matrix for local gene therapy: in vitro and in vivo evaluation, 264–271, Copyright 2010, with permission from Elsevier.

3.3 Nanoparticle-Based Delivery Systems for Programming and Reprogramming Cell Fate

Engineering complex tissues requires simultaneous development of multiple cell types in a spatially and temporally controlled manner within the scaffold. Conventional global presentation of differentiation factors through culture media fails to recapitulate the controlled presentation of cues found in vivo; therefore spatiotemporal differentiation of stem cells into various cell types cannot be achieved. To overcome this challenge, stem cell fate can be controlled by functionalizing scaffolds with drug delivery nanoparticles carrying differentiation cues. Nanoparticle-based drug delivery systems have been used to achieve controlled release of differentiation cues in the form of plasmids (genes), proteins (growth factors) and siRNA (gene silencing). The release of appropriate signals can be controlled by modulating the biophysical properties of these nano-reservoirs, including degradation rate and size range. Examples of nano-reservoirs used as drug delivery systems include polymeric nanoparticles, liposomes, polymeric micelles, quantum dots, carbon nanotubes, gold nanoparticles, and dendrimers [19] (Fig. 3.7). For a more comprehensive review of the different types of nanoparticles, readers are referred to recent reviews [17,19,23].

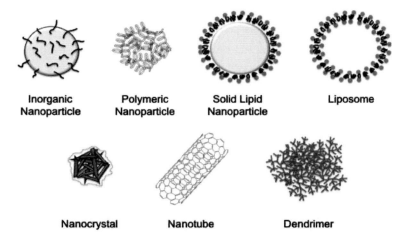

Figure 3.7 Types of nanoparticle-based drug delivery systems. Reprinted from *Bioorg Med Chem*, 17/8, Faraji, A. H., and Wipf, P., Nanoparticles in cellular drug delivery, 2950–2962, Copyright 2009, with permission from Elsevier.

Andersen et al. achieved spatially controlled differentiation of MSCs into two different cell lineages, osteogenic and chondrogenic, by functionalizing nanostructured PCL scaffolds with nanoparticles containing siRNA targeted for differentiation toward specific cell lineages [2]. Scanning electron microscopy (SEM) data indicated two different pore size distributions within the scaffold that greatly enhanced the surface area available for seeding cells and loading nanoparticles. Larger pores with diameters >50 μm provided a site for cells to migrate and attach, while the smaller pores <15 nm were filled with siRNA nanoparticles with a size of approximately 200 nm. The siRNA nanoparticle loaded scaffolds were able to achieve dual differentiation in vivo by loading different siRNAs in specific locations within the implanted scaffold.

In a study involving plasmid delivery, Yang et al. used nonviral biodegradable poly-β-amino ester (PBAE)–based nanoparticles to engineer MSCs and MSC-like cells derived from ESCs to express vascular endothelial growth factor (VEGF) to promote angiogenesis in a graft implanted in mouse ischemic hindlimbs [76]. The scaffolds seeded with modified MSCs helped vascularization of the tissue construct and reduced degeneration of the ischemic limb. PBAEs are a newer class of polycations with a hydrolytically degradable backbone developed by Langer and coworkers for drug delivery applications [27,51,52,65]. They self-assemble with negatively charged nucleic acids due to their positive backbone to form nanoparticles of approximately 100 nm. Researchers demonstrated the use of PBAE-based nanoparticles to deliver genes to human ESC colonies while stably maintaining the pluripotent state [26]. The efficacy of gene transfer was shown to be higher than that of the commonly used commercial agent Lipofectamine 2000. Human umbilical vein endothelial cells (HUVECs), as primary human endothelial cells, are an important cell model for studying angiogenesis and the promotion of angiogenesis is important for increasing nutrient and gas transfer in tissue-engineered constructs. Researchers have recently described the use of biodegradable poly(ester amine)-based and poly(amido amine)-based nanoparticles to deliver siRNA as well as DNA effectively to HUVECs [70]. Biomaterial and nanoparticle properties are key to identify which material is most effective for delivery for each type of cargo [24]. For example, the design of a biomaterial's or nanoparticle's mechanism of degradation was found to be particularly important for the delivery of siRNA compared to DNA. Polymers terminated with a newly described cystamine end-group, consisting of disulfide bonds, had improved efficacy for delivering siRNA compared with DNA as the reductive environment of the cytoplasm enabled a quick, triggered release of nucleic acid cargo via reduction of the disulfide linkages. In contrast, nonreducible, hydrolytic degradable linkages facilitated enhanced DNA delivery to the nucleus, where biodegradation occurred over a longer period of time. Bhise et al. used 10 different PBAE nanoparticle formulations to transfect mammary epithelial cells in both traditional 2-D monolayer and in 3-D organotypic cultures [11]. This study elucidated the differences in gene delivery efficacy between 2-D monolayer models and 3-D models, and indicated that small differences in the chemical structure of a biomaterial can tune gene delivery efficacy (Fig. 3.8).

The combined approach of codelivering siRNA and DNA to simultaneously inhibit the expression of inhibitory factors (siRNA) and enhance the expression of differentiation factors (DNA) has the potential to act synergistically for stem cell fate control. Jeon et al. codelivered a SOX9 expressing gene and an anti-Cbfa-1 siRNA by coating them on PLGA nanoparticles in order to differentiate MSCs into chondrocytes [37]. In addition to stem cell differentiation, codelivery of multiple nucleic acids to the same target is often a requirement for factor-based stem cell reprogramming [78]. Biomaterial and nanoparticle-based strategies for safely and effectively reprogramming human somatic cells to human induced pluripotent stem cells (hiPSCs) are very promising to the field of regenerative medicine. To improve the design of nanoparticle-based codelivery systems for reprogramming and codelivery of therapeutic genes, Bhise et al. developed a novel nanoparticle assay to quantify the number of plasmids encapsulated in a single polymeric nanoparticle [12]. They reported a range of 30 to 100 plasmids per particle depending on the polymer structure and evaluated PBAE-based nanoparticles for codelivery of reporter plasmids in human fibroblasts (Fig. 3.9). The nanoparticles with the higher plasmid per particle count had greater codelivery efficiency than the nanoparticles with the lower plasmid per particle count. Montserrat et al. have successfully reprogrammed human fibroblasts to hiPSCs using PBAE-based nanoparticles for delivering reprogramming factors; however they failed to generate transgene-free hiPSCs, which is a critical requirement for clinical application of these cells [56]. Future research in nanobiotechnology may enable the generation of hiPSCs in a highly safe and efficient manner, and such cells would be good candidates for tissue engineering applications.

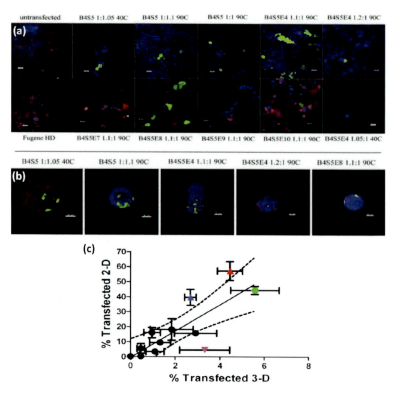

Figure 3.8 20× confocal stacks (8 μM) showing transfection efficiency of different versions of PBAE polymers 2 days post-transfection in (a) 2-D EPH4 cells and (b) mammary epithelial fragments cultured in a 3-D matrigel. Cells were fixed with 4% PFA and stained with Phalliodin-Alexa 568 (actin) and DAPI (nuclei). (c) Scatter-plot comparing the transfection efficacy (% positive) of polymeric nanoparticles in 2-D culture and 3-D organotypic culture. Reprinted from *Biomaterials*, 13, Bhise, N. S., Gray, R. S., Sunshine, J. C., Htet, S., Ewald, A. J., and Green, J. J. The relationship between terminal functionalization and molecular weight of a gene delivery polymer and transfection efficacy in mammary epithelial 2-D cultures and 3-D organotypic cultures, 8088–8096, Copyright 2010, with permission from Elsevier.

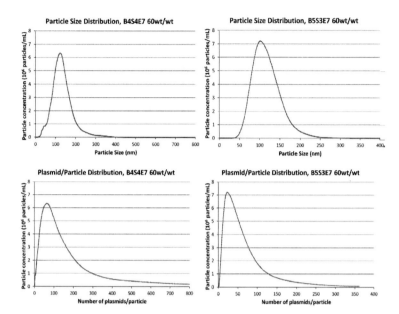

Figure 3.9 Size distribution (top) and plasmid per particle distribution (bottom) data of PBAE (B4S4E7 and B5S3E7, both 60:1 polymer to DNA wt/wt) based nanoparticles. Reprinted from *Small*, 8, Bhise, N. S., Shmueli, R. B., Gonzalez, J., and Green, J. J. A novel assay for quantifying the number of plasmids encapsulated by polymer nanoparticles, 367–373, Copyright 2012, with permission from Wiley-VCH.

3.4 High-Throughput Combinatorial Strategies for Biomaterial Development

The in vivo fate of stem cells is controlled by the complex microenvironment surrounding them, often referred to as a niche. The niche provides biochemical and biophysical cues to stem cell to remain in a quiescent state, differentiate to a specific cell type, or self-renew. This biological response depends on not just a single signal, but on a multitude of cues from the extracellular microenvironment. The development of bioactive degradable matrices that locally control cellular behavior holds immense potential in the field of regenerative medicine [29]. A variety of biomaterials have been explored for providing biophysical and biochemical instructive cues to the cells, however the traditional methods employed to investigate cell and biomaterial interactions are often low throughput. In an effort to address this issue and accelerate the development of effective biomaterials for regenerative medicine applications, combinatorial and high-throughput approaches to synthesize and screen biomaterials and cellular microenvironments to probe cell behavior have been reported [14,36,54] (Fig. 3.10).

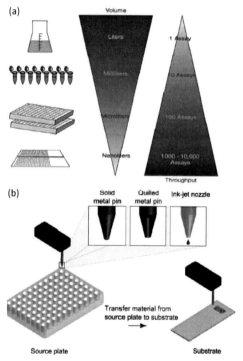

Figure 3.10 High-throughput technologies allow rapid synthesis and screening of biomaterials, enable miniaturization of cell assays and reduce costs. (a) Schematic demonstrating a continuous increase in throughput with a parallel decrease in sample/reagent volume. Reprinted from *Drug Discov Today*, 11/13–14, Castel, D., Pitaval, A., Debily, M. A., and Gidrol, X., Cell microarrays in drug discovery, 616–622, Copyright 2006, with permission from Elsevier. (b) Robotic printing techniques used to create materials microarrays. Reprinted from *Biomaterials*, 31/2, Hook, A. L., Anderson, D. G., Langer, R., Williams, P., Davies, M. C., and Alexander, M. R., High throughput methods applied in biomaterial development and discovery, 187–198, Copyright 2010, with permission from Elsevier.

Langer, Anderson, Green, and others have developed large libraries of synthetic polymers using high-throughput, miniaturized systems to evaluate diverse arrays of biomaterials for their use as cellular substrates, bioactive depots for drug delivery and nanoparticle systems [1,3–5,25,52,62] (Fig. 3.11). In one of these studies, Anderson et al. reported nanoliter-scale synthesis of a library of photopolymerizable biomaterials to screen more than 1700 diverse human embryonic stem cell (hESC)-material interactions [4]. This study was followed by a more exhaustive screening of about 3500 combinations of biodegradable polymers with neural stem cells, human mesenchymal stem cells and neural stem cells [6]. These approaches have also been used to develop degradable photo-cross-linkable materials [7] and degradable polymers for nucleic acid delivery [62,65,70].

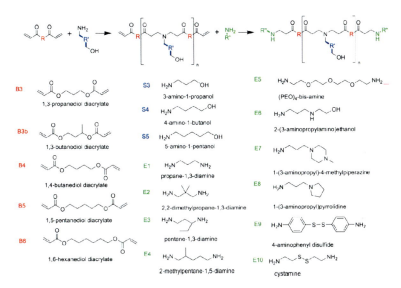

Figure 3.11 Reaction scheme and chemical structures of monomers used to synthesize a combinatorial PBAE library.

High-throughput artificial niche microarrays allow for a rapid and quantitative investigation of the interaction of microenvironmental factors and cell fate [20]. In a recent work by Gobaa et al., topographically structured soft hydrogel microwell arrays were used to modulate substrate stiffness, cell density, and micropatterned signaling proteins that enabled studying the effect of artificial niches on the differentiation ability of MSCs at a single cell level [22]. Robotic protein spotting was used to create printed stamps and subsequently these stamps were used for microcontact printing on the PEG hydrogels, thus allowing precise control of the protein type, amount, and combination printed on the microwells. The proteins used for probing included those involved in cell-ECM signaling such as fibronectin and cell-cell signaling such as cadherins [53]. Signaling cues in the local niche may also be provided in the form of nanoscale topographies, small molecules, siRNA and DNA [9,14,43,54,71] (Fig. 3.12).

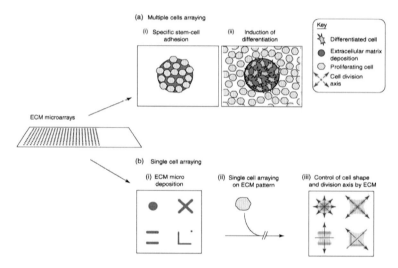

Figure 3.12 Applications of ECM microarrays for high-throughput screening of combinations of ECM components used to control stem cell fate. Reprinted from *Drug Discov Today*, 11/13–14, Castel, D., Pitaval, A., Debily, M. A., and Gidrol, X., Cell microarrays in drug discovery, 616–622, Copyright 2006, with permission from Elsevier.

High-throughput nanotopography screening has helped elucidate the role of physical cues in the microenvironment on cellular behavior. Washburn et al. investigated the effect of nanoscale surface roughness on osteoblast proliferation by modulating polymer crystallinity [73]. Taqvi and Roy studied the effect of scaffold's compression modulus, controlled by changing scaffold pore size and polymer concentration, on differentiation of mouse ESCs toward hematopoietic lineage [66]. Such combinatorial methods in nanotechnology and microfabrication are ideal tools for developing high-throughput and automated platforms to study 3-D microenvironments and enable rapid translation of regenerative medicine therapies to the clinic.

3.5 Conclusions

This chapter describes recent advances in biomaterials and nanobiotechnology for regenerative medicine. Two key uses for biomaterials are as tissue engineering scaffolds and as drug and biomolecule delivery systems. Nanobiotechnology enables fine-tuning of the physical, chemical, and biological characteristics of these biomaterials, devices, and delivery systems. Multiscale fabrication techniques allow the design of scaffolds with nano/micro-scale topographies to control stem cell fate and the creation of complex 3-D tissue constructs. New high-throughput strategies are allowing the synthesis, characterization, and evaluation of many new biodegradable materials and systems for regenerative medicine. When combined with the appropriate human stem cell source, which these biomaterials can themselves also help directly to generate, these cell-biomaterial systems are promising to recapitulate critical aspects of in vivo tissue function and may enable future translational utilization.

References

1. Akinc, A., Zumbuehl, A., Goldberg, M., Leshchiner, E. S., Busini, V., Hossain, N., Bacallado, S. A., Nguyen, D. N., Fuller, J., Alvarez, R., et al. (2008). A combinatorial library of lipid-like materials for delivery of RNAi therapeutics. *Nat Biotechnol*, **26**, 561–569.

2. Andersen, M. O., Nygaard, J. V., Burns, J. S., Raarup, M. K., Nyengaard, J. R., Bunger, C., Besenbacher, F., Howard, K. A., Kassem, M., and Kjems, J. (2010). siRNA nanoparticle functionalization of nanostructured scaffolds enables controlled multilineage differentiation of stem cells. *Mol Ther*, **18**, 2018–2027.

3. Anderson, D. G., Lynn, D. M., and Langer, R. (2003). Semi-automated synthesis and screening of a large library of degradable cationic polymers for gene delivery. *Angew Chem Int Edit*, **42**, 3153–3158.

4. Anderson, D. G., Levenberg, S., and Langer, R. (2004). Nanoliter-scale synthesis of arrayed biomaterials and application to human embryonic stem cells. *Nat Biotechnol*, **22**, 863–866.
5. Anderson, D. G., Akinc, A., Hossain, N., and Langer, R. (2005). Structure/property studies of polymeric gene delivery using a library of poly (beta-amino esters). *Mol Ther*, **11**, 426–434.
6. Anderson, D. G., Putnam, D., Lavik, E. B., Mahmood, T. A., and Langer, R. (2005). Biomaterial microarrays: rapid, microscale screening of polymer-cell interaction. *Biomaterials*, **26**, 4892–4897.
7. Anderson, D. G., Tweedie, C. A., Hossain, N., Navarro, S. M., Brey, D. M., Van Vliet, K. J., Langer, R., and Burdick, J. A. (2006). A combinatorial library of photocrosslinkable and degradable materials. *Adv Mater*, **18**, 2614–2618.
8. Anseth, K. S., Bowman, C. N., and Brannon-Peppas, L. (1996). Mechanical properties of hydrogels and their experimental determination. *Biomaterials*, **17**, 1647–1657.
9. Bailey, S. N., Sabatini, D. M., and Stockwell, B. R. (2004). Microarrays of small molecules embedded in biodegradable polymers for use in mammalian cell-based screens. *Proc Natl Acad Sci USA*, **101**, 16144–16149.
10. Bhise, N. S., Shmueli, R. B., Sunshine, J. C., Tzeng, S. Y., and Green, J. J. Drug delivery strategies for therapeutic angiogenesis and antiangiogenesis. *Exp Opin Drug Deliv*, **8**, 485–504.
11. Bhise, N. S., Gray, R. S., Sunshine, J. C., Htet, S., Ewald, A. J., and Green, J. J. (2010). The relationship between terminal functionalization and molecular weight of a gene delivery polymer and transfection efficacy in mammary epithelial 2-D cultures and 3-D organotypic cultures. *Biomaterials*, **31**, 8088–8096.
12. Bhise, N. S., Shmueli, R. B., Gonzalez, J., and Green, J. J. (2012). A novel assay for quantifying the number of plasmids encapsulated by polymer nanoparticles. *Small*, **8**, 367–373.
13. Burdick, J. A. (2012). Injectable gels for tissue/organ repair. *Biomedical materials*, **7**, 020201–020201.
14. Castel, D., Pitaval, A., Debily, M. A., and Gidrol, X. (2006). Cell microarrays in drug discovery. *Drug Discov Today*, **11**, 616–622.
15. Cellesi, F., Tirelli, N., and Hubbell, J. A. (2002). Materials for cell encapsulation via a new tandem approach combining reverse thermal gelation and covalent crosslinking. *Macromol Chem Phys*, **203**, 1466–1472.

16. Chew, S. Y., Wen, J., Yim, E. K., and Leong, K. W. (2005). Sustained release of proteins from electrospun biodegradable fibers. *Biomacromolecules*, **6**, 2017–2024.

17. Cho, K. J., Wang, X., Nie, S. M., Chen, Z., and Shin, D. M. (2008). Therapeutic nanoparticles for drug delivery in cancer. *Clin Cancer Res*, **14**, 1310–1316.

18. Cui, W. G., Zhou, Y., and Chang, J. (2010). Electrospun nanofibrous materials for tissue engineering and drug delivery. *Sci Technol Adv Mater*, **11**, 014108.

19. Faraji, A. H., and Wipf, P. (2009). Nanoparticles in cellular drug delivery. *Bioorg Med Chem*, **17**, 2950–2962.

20. Flaim, C. J., Teng, D., Chien, S., and Bhatia, S. N. (2008). Combinatorial signaling microenvironments for studying stem cell fate. *Stem Cells Dev*, **17**, 29–39.

21. Gittens, R. A., McLachlan, T., Olivares-Navarrete, R., Cai, Y., Berner, S., Tannenbaum, R., Schwartz, Z., Sandhage, K. H., and Boyan, B. D. (2011). The effects of combined micron-/submicron-scale surface roughness and nanoscale features on cell proliferation and differentiation. *Biomaterials*, **32**, 3395–3403.

22. Gobaa, S., Hoehnel, S., Roccio, M., Negro, A., Kobel, S., and Lutolf, M. P. (2011). Artificial niche microarrays for probing single stem cell fate in high throughput. *Nat Methods*, **8**, 949–955.

23. Goldberg, M., Langer, R., and Jia, X. Q. (2007). Nanostructured materials for applications in drug delivery and tissue engineering. *J Biomat Sci-Polym E*, **18**, 241–268.

24. Green, J. J. (2011). Rita schaffer lecture: nanoparticles for intracellular nucleic acid delivery. *Ann Biomed Eng*, **40**, 1408–1418.

25. Green, J. J., Langer, R., and Anderson, D. G. (2008). A combinatorial polymer library approach yields insight into nonviral gene delivery. *Acc Chem Res*, **41**, 749–759.

26. Green, J. J., Zhou, B. Y., Mitalipova, M. M., Beard, C., Langer, R., Jaenisch, R., and Anderson, D. G. (2008). Nanoparticles for gene transfer to human embryonic stem cell colonies. *Nano Lett*, **8**, 3126–3130.

27. Green, J. J., Zugates, G. T., Langer, R., and Anderson, D. G. (2009). Poly(beta-amino esters): procedures for synthesis and gene delivery. *Methods Mol Bio*, **480**, 53–63.

28. Greiner, A., and Wendorff, J. H. (2007). Electrospinning: a fascinating method for the preparation of ultrathin fibers. *Angew Chem*, **46**, 5670–5703.

29. Griffith, L. G., and Naughton, G. (2002). Tissue engineering--current challenges and expanding opportunities. *Science*, **295**, 1009–1014.
30. Grinstaff, M. W. (2007). Designing hydrogel adhesives for corneal wound repair. *Biomaterials*, **28**, 5205–5214.
31. Guimaraes, A., Martins, A., Pinho, E. D., Faria, S., Reis, R. L., and Neves, N. M. Solving cell infiltration limitations of electrospun nanofiber meshes for tissue engineering applications. *Nanomedicine (Lond)*, **5**, 539–554.
32. Gupta, R., Tongers, J., and Losordo, D. W. (2009). Human studies of angiogenic gene therapy. *Circ Res*, **105**, 724–736.
33. Guvendiren, M., and Burdick, J. A. (2012). Stiffening hydrogels to probe short- and long-term cellular responses to dynamic mechanics. *Nat Commun*, **3**, 792.
34. Hoffman, A. S. (1995). "Intelligent" polymers in medicine and biotechnology. *Artif organs*, **19**, 458–467.
35. Hoffman, A. S. (2001). Hydrogels for biomedical applications. *Ann New York Acad Sci*, **944**, 62–73.
36. Hook, A. L., Anderson, D. G., Langer, R., Williams, P., Davies, M. C., and Alexander, M. R. (2010). High throughput methods applied in biomaterial development and discovery. *Biomaterials*, **31**, 187–198.
37. Jeon, S. Y., Park, J. S., Yang, H. N., Woo, D. G., and Park, K. H. (2012). Co-delivery of SOX9 genes and anti-Cbfa-1 siRNA coated onto PLGA nanoparticles for chondrogenesis of human MSCs. *Biomaterials*, **33**, 4413–4423.
38. Ji, W., Sun, Y., Yang, F., van den Beucken, J. J., Fan, M., Chen, Z., and Jansen, J. A. Bioactive electrospun scaffolds delivering growth factors and genes for tissue engineering applications. *Pharm Res*, **28**, 1259–1272.
39. Ji, W., Yang, F., van den Beucken, J. J., Bian, Z., Fan, M., Chen, Z., and Jansen, J. A. Fibrous scaffolds loaded with protein prepared by blend or coaxial electrospinning. *Acta Biomater*, **6**, 4199–4207.
40. Ji, W., Sun, Y., Yang, F., van den Beucken, J. J. J. P., Fan, M. W., Chen, Z., and Jansen, J. A. (2011). Bioactive Electrospun Scaffolds Delivering Growth Factors and Genes for Tissue Engineering Applications. *Pharm Res*, **28**, 1259–1272.
41. Khademhosseini, A., Langer, R., Borenstein, J., and Vacanti, J. P. (2006). Microscale technologies for tissue engineering and biology. *Proc Natl Acad Sci USA*, **103**, 2480–2487.
42. Kim, H. S., and Yoo, H. S. MMPs-responsive release of DNA from electrospun nanofibrous matrix for local gene therapy: in vitro and in vivo evaluation. *J Control Release*, **145**, 264–271.

43. Lamers, E., van Horssen, R., te Riet, J., van Delft, F. C. M. J. M., Luttge, R., Walboomers, X. F., and Jansen, J. A. (2010). The Influence of Nanoscale Topographical Cues on Initial Osteoblast Morphology and Migration. *Eur Cells Mater*, **20**, 329–343.
44. Langer, R., and Vacanti, J. P. (1993). Tissue engineering. *Science*, **260**, 920–926.
45. Li, C. M., Vepari, C., Jin, H. J., Kim, H. J., and Kaplan, D. L. (2006). Electrospun silk-BMP-2 scaffolds for bone tissue engineering. *Biomaterials*, **27**, 3115–3124.
46. Li, W. J., Cooper, J. A., Mauck, R. L., and Tuan, R. S. (2006). Fabrication and characterization of six electrospun poly(alpha-hydroxy ester)-based fibrous scaffolds for tissue engineering applications. *Acta Biomater*, **2**, 377–385.
47. Liao, I. C., Chew, S. Y., and Leong, K. W. (2006). Aligned core-shell nanofibers delivering bioactive proteins. *Nanomedicine (Lond)*, **1**, 465–471.
48. Liu Tsang, V., Chen, A. A., Cho, L. M., Jadin, K. D., Sah, R. L., DeLong, S., West, J. L., and Bhatia, S. N. (2007). Fabrication of 3D hepatic tissues by additive photopatterning of cellular hydrogels. *FASEB J*, **21**, 790–801.
49. Lutolf, M. P., Raeber, G. P., Zisch, A. H., Tirelli, N., and Hubbell, J. A. (2003). Cell-responsive synthetic hydrogels. *Adv Mater*, **15**, 888–892.
50. Luu, Y. K., Kim, K., Hsiao, B. S., Chu, B., and Hadjiargyrou, M. (2003). Development of a nanostructured DNA delivery scaffold via electrospinning of PLGA and PLA-PEG block copolymers. *J Control Release*, **89**, 341–353.
51. Lynn, D. M., and Langer, R. (2000). Degradable poly(beta-amino esters): Synthesis, characterization, and self-assembly with plasmid DNA. *J Am Chem Soc*, **122**, 10761–10768.
52. Lynn, D. M., Anderson, D. G., Putnam, D., and Langer, R. (2001). Accelerated discovery of synthetic transfection vectors: Parallel synthesis and screening of degradable polymer library. *J Am Chem Soc*, **123**, 8155–8156.
53. MacBeath, G., and Schreiber, S. L. (2000). Printing proteins as microarrays for high-throughput function determination. *Science*, **289**, 1760–1763.
54. Mei, Y., Goldberg, M., and Anderson, D. (2007). The development of high-throughput screening approaches for stem cell engineering. *Curr Opin Chem Biol*, **11**, 388–393.

55. Mickova, A., Buzgo, M., Benada, O., Rampichova, M., Fisar, Z., Filova, E., Tesarova, M., Lukas, D., and Amler, E. Core/Shell Nanofibers with Embedded Liposomes as a Drug Delivery System. *Biomacromolecules*, 952–962.

56. Montserrat, N., Garreta, E., Gonzalez, F., Gutierrez, J., Eguizabal, C., Ramos, V., Borros, S., and Izpisua Belmonte, J. C. (2011). Simple generation of human induced pluripotent stem cells using poly-beta-amino esters as the non-viral gene delivery system. *J Bio Chem*, **286**, 12417–12428.

57. Nie, H., Soh, B. W., Fu, Y. C., and Wang, C. H. (2008). Three-dimensional fibrous PLGA/HAp composite scaffold for BMP-2 delivery. *Biotechnol Bioeng*, **99**, 223–234.

58. Prabhakaran, M. P., Ghasemi-Mobarakeh, L., and Ramakrishna, S. Electrospun composite nanofibers for tissue regeneration. *J Nanosci Nanotechnol*, **11**, 3039–3057.

59. Rich, W. J., Condon, P. I., and Percival, S. P. B. (1988). Hydrogel Intraocular-Lens Experience with Endocapsular Implantation. *Eye*, **2**, 523–528.

60. Roy, K., Wang, D., Hedley, M. L., and Barman, S. P. (2003). Gene delivery with in-situ crosslinking polymer networks generates long-term systemic protein expression. *Mol Ther*, **7**, 401–408.

61. Saraf, A., Baggett, L. S., Raphael, R. M., Kasper, F. K., and Mikos, A. G. Regulated non-viral gene delivery from coaxial electrospun fiber mesh scaffolds. *J Control Release*, **143**, 95–103.

62. Shmueli, R. B., Sunshine, J. C., Xu, Z., Duh, E. J., and Green, J. J. (2012). Gene delivery nanoparticles specific for human microvasculature and macrovasculature. *Nanomed nanotechnology, Bio, Med*, **8**, 1200–1207.

63. Slaughter, B. V., Khurshid, S. S., Fisher, O. Z., Khademhosseini, A., and Peppas, N. A. (2009). Hydrogels in Regenerative Medicine. *Adv Mater*, **21**, 3307–3329.

64. Storrie, H., and Mooney, D. J. (2006). Sustained delivery of plasmid DNA from polymeric scaffolds for tissue engineering. *Adv Drug Deliv Rev*, **58**, 500–514.

65. Sunshine, J., Bhise, N., and Green, J. J. (2009). Degradable polymers for gene delivery. Conference proceedings: *Annual International Conference of the IEEE Engineering in Medicine and Biology Society IEEE Engineering in Medicine and Biology Society Conference*, **2009**, pp. 2412–2415.

66. Taqvi, S., and Roy, K. (2006). Influence of scaffold physical properties and stromal cell coculture on hematopoietic differentiation of mouse embryonic stem cells. *Biomaterials*, **27**, 6024–6031.

67. Tekin, H., Ozaydin-Ince, G., Tsinman, T., Gleason, K. K., Langer, R., Khademhosseini, A., and Demirel, M. C. Responsive microgrooves for the formation of harvestable tissue constructs. *Langmuir*, **27**, 5671–5679.

68. Tekin, H., Tsinman, T., Sanchez, J. G., Jones, B. J., Camci-Unal, G., Nichol, J. W., Langer, R., and Khademhosseini, A. Responsive micromolds for sequential patterning of hydrogel microstructures. *J Am Chem Soc*, **133**, 12944–12947.

69. Tsang, V. L., and Bhatia, S. N. (2007). Fabrication of three-dimensional tissues. *Adv Biochem Eng Biotechnol*, **103**, 189–205.

70. Tzeng, S. Y., Yang, P. H., Grayson, W. L., and Green, J. J. (2011). Synthetic poly(ester amine) and poly(amido amine) nanoparticles for efficient DNA and siRNA delivery to human endothelial cells. *Intl J Nanomed*, **6**, 3309–3322.

71. Unadkat, H. V., Hulsman, M., Cornelissen, K., Papenburg, B. J., Truckenmuller, R. K., Carpenter, A. E., Wessling, M., Post, G. F., Uetz, M., Reinders, M. J., et al. (2011). An algorithm-based topographical biomaterials library to instruct cell fate. *Proc Natl Acad Sci USA*, **108**, 16565–16570.

72. Wang, C. Y., Liu, J. J., Fan, C. Y., Mo, X. M., Ruan, H. J., and Li, F. F. (2012). The Effect of Aligned Core-Shell Nanofibres Delivering NGF on the Promotion of Sciatic Nerve Regeneration. *J Biomater Sci-Polymer Ed*, **23**, 167–184.

73. Washburn, N. R., Yamada, K. M., Simon, C. G., Jr., Kennedy, S. B., and Amis, E. J. (2004). High-throughput investigation of osteoblast response to polymer crystallinity: influence of nanometer-scale roughness on proliferation. *Biomaterials*, **25**, 1215–1224.

74. Wernig, M., Zhao, J. P., Pruszak, J., Hedlund, E., Fu, D., Soldner, F., Broccoli, V., Constantine-Paton, M., Isacson, O., and Jaenisch, R. (2008). Neurons derived from reprogrammed fibroblasts functionally integrate into the fetal brain and improve symptoms of rats with Parkinson's disease. *Proc Natl Acad Sci United States Am*, **105**, 5856–5861.

75. Wu, S. M., and Hochedlinger, K. Harnessing the potential of induced pluripotent stem cells for regenerative medicine. *Nat Cell Biol*, **13**, 497–505.

76. Yang, F., Cho, S. W., Son, S. M., Bogatyrev, S. R., Singh, D., Green, J. J., Mei, Y., Park, S., Bhang, S. H., Kim, B. S., et al. (2010). Genetic engineering of human stem cells for enhanced angiogenesis using biodegradable polymeric nanoparticles. *Proc Natl Acad Sci USA,* **107**, 3317–3322.

77. Yang, Y., and Leong, K. W. (2010). Nanoscale surfacing for regenerative medicine. *Wiley Interdisciplinary Rev Nanomed Nanobiotechnol,* **2**, 478–495.

78. Yu, J., Hu, K., Smuga-Otto, K., Tian, S., Stewart, R., Slukvin, II, and Thomson, J. A. (2009). Human induced pluripotent stem cells free of vector and transgene sequences. *Science,* **324**, 797–801.

79. Zorlutuna, P., Annabi, N., Camci-Unal, G., Nikkhah, M., Cha, J. M., Nichol, J. W., Manbachi, A., Bae, H., Chen, S., and Khademhosseini, A. Microfabricated Biomaterials for Engineering 3D Tissues. *Adv Mater,* **24**, 1782–1804.

Chapter 4

Micro- and Nanotechnology Engineering Strategies for Tissue Interface Regeneration and Repair

Torri E. Rinker and Johnna S. Temenoff

The Wallace H. Coulter Department of Biomedical Engineering,
Georgia Institute of Technology, 313 Ferst Drive, Atlanta, GA 30332, USA

trinker3@gatech.edu, johnna.temenoff@bme.gatech.edu

Tissue interfaces are the regions between two divergent tissues that act as a transition point in structure, function, and composition. They are required for proper tissue function, but when injured, can be very difficult to regenerate. Recently, interface tissue engineering has emerged as a new focus for researchers in the field of regenerative medicine. In interface tissue engineering, many traditional tissue engineering strategies have been employed, while other strategies incorporating micro- and nanotechnologies have been modified or newly developed to meet the specific needs of interface development. This chapter will begin by discussing the use of in vitro two- and three-dimensional co-culture to study cellular communication mediated by both soluble factor exchange and cell–cell contacts. Then, current types and fabrication methods of scaffolds/constructs for interface tissue engineering will be

---

Tissue and Organ Regeneration: Advances in Micro- and Nanotechnology
Edited by Lijie Grace Zhang, Ali Khademhosseini, and Thomas J. Webster
Copyright © 2014 Pan Stanford Publishing Pte. Ltd.
ISBN 978-981-4411-67-7 (Hardcover), 978-981-4411-68-4 (eBook)
www.panstanford.com

described. With rapidly developing innovative platforms for both in vitro and in vivo study, interface tissue engineering strategies promise to offer both researchers and clinicians excellent resources for interface reconstruction and repair.

4.1 Introduction

Tissue interfaces are prevalent in the body and are necessary for proper tissue function [79]. These interfaces can occur between organ systems, such as between neural and vascular interfaces and other tissues, or between two disparate tissue types of the same organ, such as within orthopaedic interfaces. Critical to almost all tissues, the vascular interface provides the required blood supply to support tissue function, and in its absence, tissues suffer hypoxia, nutrient deficiency, waste product accumulation, and signaling disruption [2]. Another interface between organs is the neural interface, the regeneration of which has been an area of intense study with the aim of regenerating function over large nerve gaps, currently difficult to achieve [22]. Finally, interfaces between two tissues, such as orthopedic interfaces, involve two tissue types with drastically different biological and mechanical properties. Examples include bone–ligament/tendon, muscle–tendon, and the osteochondral interface, all of which are difficult to repair (Fig. 4.1) [79]. In common to all of these interfaces is the difficulty in their regeneration, due to the multiple cell types and dissimilar extracellular matrix (ECM) [79].

Researchers working on interface tissue engineering (ITE) aim to regenerate and repair both interface function and structure between different tissue types [110]. This has proven challenging, and tissue interfaces are often not successfully regenerated due to the complexities involved in creating an appropriate environment for multiple cell types. Because the tissues on either side of the interface have distinct cellular populations, mechanical properties, composition, and ECM organization, there is a requirement for compositional gradients, subcompartments, and spatial control within systems engineered to mimic the interface [79,86]. Also, as cellular behavior is directed by structures on micro- and nanoscale, it is critical to utilize micro- and nanotechnologies to control material properties [153]. Currently, many strategies employing these technologies are prevalent in ITE and many more are rapidly developing.

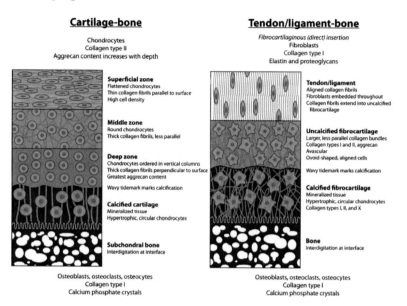

Figure 4.1 A diagram depicting the cartilage–bone and tendon/ligament-bone interfaces and their compositions. Orange indicates levels of aggrecan concentration, light blue indicates collagen fibers, and dark blue indicates mineralized tissue. Reprinted from Yang, P. J. and Temenoff, J. S. (2009). Engineering orthopedic tissue interfaces, *Tissue Eng. Pt. B-Rev.*, **15**, 127–41.

In this review, we will begin by highlighting the two- and three-dimensional (2D and 3D, respectively) co-culture systems that are used to study interface-relevant cellular communication in vitro. These systems include physically separated cell populations, which allows for analysis of secreted factors and their effects on other cells, as well as cell populations in direct contact, which provides a platform on which to analyze effects of both soluble factors and cell–cell contacts. Then, we will provide an overview of the types of scaffolds used for ITE, including those that are gradiated, braided, formed from microspheres, and derived from natural sources. Finally, we will end our discussion by giving a brief overview of current scaffold fabrication techniques, including those used to fabricate gradiated scaffolds, nanofibrous matrices, and computer-assisted designs.

4.2 Co-Culture Systems for in vitro Analysis of Tissue Interfaces

In interface tissue engineering, knowledge of how cells communicate is critical, as cell organization, boundaries, fate, function, and communication are implicated in interfacial tissue development [59,86,87,140]. Many studies have demonstrated the utility of using in vitro co-culture systems to study these interactions, as they can provide a platform to analyze the mechanisms governing interface regeneration through understanding heterotypic cellular interactions (communication between two different cell types) [86,87]. Thus, in vitro co-culture systems have and will continue to increase our understanding of cellular communication in ITE [78].

Not only do in vitro systems provide insight into cellular communication, but they also provide information about how cells respond to biomimetic materials and how materials can be engineered to direct cell behavior [87,110]. Biomaterial scaffolds are often critical for creating organized tissue structures to understand mechanisms of cell communication at millimeter and centimeter scales [86]. By understanding these interactions in vitro, tissue formation rates in vivo may be enhanced through scaffold optimization prior to implantation [78,86,87]. Thus, in vitro co-culture can also provide a platform on which to analyze the simultaneous interaction between two different cell types as dictated by a selected biomaterial. To this end, both 2D and 3D environments have been used to study cellular communication with strict control over both spatial and temporal presentation of each cell type.

4.2.1 Two-Dimensional Systems

Two-dimensional cell culture systems involve the analysis of the heterotypic cellular communication of cells adhered to a 2D surface. In general, 2D cell culture has been traditionally employed due to ease of use, convenience, and high cell viability [67]. While 2D systems have some significant limitations over 3D systems [1,19,67,131,137] (discussed in Section 4.2.2), they still can provide a useful platform for studying basic questions relating to cellular communication. 2D systems can be fabricated to achieve cell populations that are physically separated or in direct contact.

4.2.1.1 Physically separated cell populations

Physical separation can be achieved through physical constraints placed on the culture system. Benefits of this technique include the ability to separate cell populations for further analysis, as well as limiting communication to that only mediated by secreted paracrine factors. One limitation of the technique is the lack of cell–cell contacts, an interaction that acts as a common avenue of communication in tissues [75]. Physically separated cell populations can be achieved through transwell systems, selective surface cell seeding, and cell patterning.

Commonly employed, transwell systems involve two chambers separated by a flexible membrane that prevents the passage of cells but allows transport of soluble factors [50]. These systems have been used to study the interactions at the interface of many cell types, with a primary function of elucidating the contribution of soluble factor secretion compared to that of cell–cell or cell–matrix contacts on cellular behavior. This is exemplified in a study of the developing growth plate, which involved rat osteoblast and bovine articular chondrocyte co-culture in a transwell system. [93]. Comparing the transwell co-culture to direct co-culture that allowed for cell–cell contact, it was found that osteoblastic differentiation, determined by alizarin red and alkaline phosphatase (ALP) staining, was suppressed in direct culture but not in transwell culture with chondrocytes after two weeks [93]. Furthermore, suppression of proteoglycan deposition by chondrocytes was observed in the transwell system but not in the direct cell-contact culture [93]. Thus, it was realized that understanding both direct and indirect cellular communication would be essential for effective growth plate regeneration [93].

In the previous example, the soluble factors that influenced cell behavior remained undefined, but it is possible to identify such factors using transwell systems. For example, a co-culture with rat neurons and mouse endothelial cells (ECs) via a transwell system showed that EC soluble factors were neuroprotective and reduced neuronal cell death under hypoxic conditions [34]. To further elucidate this neuroprotective behavior, it was possible to test the hypothesis that the EC-released soluble factor responsible for this protection was brain-derived neurotrophic factor (BDNF) by removing it from EC conditioned media by filtering against a soluble antagonist (TrkB-Fc) [34]. Again using a transwell system, it was found that the neuroprotective nature of EC conditioned media was lost upon removal of BDNF, implicating it as an important means of communication between ECs and neurons [34]. In another example, a transwell system was used to co-culture Sprague–Dawley rat pup osteoblasts and dural cells to study the mechanisms behind reossification in infant large calvarial defects [121]. Osteoblasts were seen to proliferate more rapidly when co-cultured with rat dural cells and showed greater levels of differentiation, as determined by increased gene expression of collagen IαI, ALP, osteopontin, and osteocalcin [121]. Transforming growth factor (TGF)-β1 and Fibroblast Growth Factor (FGF)-2, both osteoinductive cytokines, were suspected be likely players in this cellular communication [121]. This was supported by the fact that relative expression of both were seen to be high in dural cells while low in osteoblasts [121]. Thus, transwell systems can both establish that cellular communication is occurring between given cell types and then can be further employed for study of specific soluble factor secretion and its influences on cellular behavior.

In selective surface cell seeding, cells are cultured in spatially segregated regions that are in contact with the same media source. This technique has been used to study the anterior cruciate ligament (ACL)-to-bone interface, which consists of a transition from a non-mineralized to mineralized fibrocartilage region (Fig. 4.1) [139]. Thus, the mechanisms that govern regeneration of this tissue interface were examined by culturing interface-relevant cell types [139]. Bovine osteoblasts (bone) and fibroblasts (tendon) were cultured on coverslips in a culture dish separated by agarose-encapsulated fibroblasts, chondrocytes, or bone marrow stromal cells [139]. From the study, it was observed that all differentiated cells maintained their phenotype, while stem cells showed increased ALP activity and type II collagen and glycosaminoglycan (GAG) production, indicating possible differentiation down (fibro)chondrogenic and osteogenic lineages [139]. This technique is advantageous as it requires few materials and no special patterning techniques, and in general, much information can be gained through the soluble factor exchange and its influence on cellular behavior. However, spatial control is limited, as cell populations cannot be as precisely patterned as they can be in more sophisticated patterning techniques.

In cell-signaling studies, exact placement of cells is often critical, as cellular response is determined by the concentration and spatiotemporal characteristics of the soluble factors they are exposed to [61]. Therefore, advanced two-dimensional cell-patterning techniques have been developed and provide excellent spatial control over cell populations. In one example, a cell-patterning technique consisted of a dual patterned surface on which cells preferentially adhered in response to temperature [135]. This thermoresponsive surface consisted of an initial layer of poly(*N*-isopropylacrylamide) (PIPAAm) and was patterned with P(IPAAm-*n*-butyl methacrylate) (PIPAAm-BMA) by using masks during electron beam polymerization [134,135]. At 27°C, the bottom layer of PIPAAm repelled cells, but the patterned PIPAAm-BMA promoted cell adhesion, allowing culture of one cell type on the precisely patterned surface [134,135]. Then, by changing the temperature to 37°C, a second cell type could also adhere to the PIPAAm, creating patterned co-cultures of both cell types [134,135]. By regulating temperature, it was possible to obtain co-cultures of bovine hepatocytes and rat ECs seeded in desired geometries [135]. Results showed gradiated differences in hepatocyte phenotypic albumin synthesis based on their proximity to ECs, with those nearest ECs producing more protein than those further away [134,135]. This suggests that diffusion of soluble factors to hepatocytes from the vascular system may be essential for optimal cell function, providing further insight into the vascularization requirements for liver tissue regeneration [134,135]. Thus, cell-patterning techniques provide platforms on which to study how spatial orientation influences cell behavior. Furthermore, cell patterning can provide excellent control of cell–cell contacts, which will be discussed in the next section.

4.2.1.2 Direct-contact cell populations

Controlling cell–cell contact is important for development of in vitro systems that mimic normal tissue architecture [62,75]. Cell contact-based communication can occur via adherens junctions, desmosomes, tight junctions, or gap junctions [75]. One disadvantage to direct-contact cell populations is the inability to retrieve and isolate different cell types within the co-culture. However, direct-contact studies are valuable as it is possible to observe phenomenon like cell migration, cell morphology, and gene expression [2,76,140].

Direct cell contact can be established through seeding multiple cells types on the same surface, cell patterning, or microfluidic manipulation.

When seeding cells on the same surface, cells are labeled or specifically stained and can be studied using imaging technologies [2,76,140]. For example, in one study of ligament-bone interface formation, bovine fibroblasts and osteoblasts were seeded on opposite sides of the same tissue culture well surface and both migration and gene expression were analyzed [140]. Cells migration was tracked by using different dyes for each cell type and subsequent imaging with light microscopy, which indicated that both cell types migrated to the interface [140]. Gene expression of interface relevant markers collagen type I and aggrecan were elevated in co-culture as compared to monoculture controls, suggesting that osteoblast–fibroblast interactions may initiate formation of fibrocartilage, found within this tissue interface [140]. Similar analysis techniques have also been used to study interactions between MSCs and ECs and their progenitors when seeded on the same surface [2,76]. While this technique is fast and requires little to no specialized equipment to obtain direct-contact co-cultures, it cannot achieve the spatial or temporal control that is possible with patterned co-culture systems.

In contrast to random seeding, patterned co-culture systems provide more exact control over homotypic and heterotypic communication (communication between the same and different cell types, respectively), spatial localization, and cell contact [59,62,125,145]. This is often accomplished by using an elastomeric stamp to localize a desired substrate to specific geometric patterns on a cell culture surface [9,58,145]. To create stamps with specific patterns of raised surface areas, poly(dimethylsiloxane) (PDMS) or a similar polymer solution is poured over machined master molds, resulting in stamps with precise geometrical configuration. For example, a PDMS stamp was used to create a surface of alternating 40 μm-wide strips of laminin and perlecan domain IV peptide by coating the stamp with laminin and applying it to a perlecan-coated cell culture surface [9]. Then, as murine long bone osteocytes preferentially adhered to perlecan and murine dorsal root ganglia neurons to laminin, co-culture with specific geometric patterning of each cell type was established [9]. This type of system provides a platform for the study of direct cell contact between osteocytes and neurons, and the concept of preferential adherence could be applied to other cell types for co-culture experiments [9]. In another study utilizing molds, HeLa cells were cultured with human umbilical vein ECs on a concave polystyrene sheet filled with a convex layer of PDMS [58]. This was manufactured by machining the polystyrene plate as a mold and pouring PDMS around it, resulting in a precise fit between the two materials [58]. Faster migration was seen with cells in co-culture than in monoculture, suggesting that cellular interactions influence migration in this model of tumor vasculogenesis [58]. Both of these techniques show how molds can provide precise patterns for 2D co-culture to investigate cellular interactions.

2D patterning is also achieved by using stimuli responsive materials that can be switched from cell/protein repulsive to cell/protein adherent [62,99,150]. Surface-switching can be employed to temporally and spatially control cell adhesion, exemplified in a study of human neuroblastoma and rat glial cell co-culture [150]. From a silicon master, PDMS stamps with 60 μm-wide grooves were fabricated and then used to stamp cell culture surfaces with a cell-resistant polyelectrolyte [150]. Neuroblastoma cells were then cultured on the polyelectrolyte-free portions of the patterned surface, resulting in alternating strips of cells and polyelectrolyte coating [150]. Then, glial cells were added to the culture with chitosan, reversing the cell-resistant properties of the patterned strips and allowing adhesion of the glial cells to the polyelectrolyte-coated surface, which resulted in a final alternating pattern of neuroblastoma and glial cells [150]. This technique provides a valuable tool for future study of neurons and glial cells, especially toward the regeneration of damaged neurons [150]. Another example of switchable surfaces involves a similar technique in which an initially cell-repulsive surface was modified to become cell-adherent in a temporally controlled manner [62]. In this system, a glass surface was patterned with alternating hyaluronic acid (HA) (less cell adherent) and fibronectin (highly cell adherent) [62]. The first cell type was added to the surface and bound only to the regions patterned with fibronectin [62]. Then, the HA surface was switched to cell adherent by applying poly-L-lysine (PLL), which interacts electrostatically with HA and allowed for a second cell type to adhere to regions of HA/PLL complexes [62]. Successful co-cultures of both murine hepatocytes and embryonic stem cells (ESCs) with fibroblasts was achieved for at least 5 days in this system, and future studies will seek to identify the biochemical interactions between the two populations [62]. In general, switchable surfaces can be used to achieve precise patterning up to the spatial resolution permitted by substrate coating techniques, and provide excellent platforms for co-culture studies.

Microfluidic techniques provide control of the local cellular environment and can be used for 2D cell patterning [83,152]. By employing fluid flow through materials such as silicon or silicone elastomer (PDMS), microfluidics can provide physically and biochemically controlled microenvironments by using guiding structures or specially designed channels [98]. In one study that employed fluid flow to precisely localize cells within a microfluidic channel, PDMS cured on a silicon master was used to form capillary channels when placed on a cell culture dish [127]. Three separate inlets converged into a single channel, allowing for up to three different cell types to be co-cultured simultaneously [127]. Both chicken erythrocytes and bovine ECs could be patterned in this device, and further applications could include more complicated channel design to achieve different geometrically configured co-cultures as well as culture of different cell types [127]. Microfluidics can provide spatial patterning on a small scale and have endless applications due to the many possible configurations of channels, channel dimensions, and fluid flow parameters.

Besides using microfluidic devices to precisely pattern cells, it is also possible to use fluid flow as a factor within the co-culture system to better mimic the in vivo environment. For example, in one study, two PDMS layers sandwiched a thin, porous polyester membrane to form a microfluidic device [118]. In the top PDMS layer, a thin channel carrying human MDA-MB-231 breast cancer cells ran parallel to the porous membrane, on which human dermal ECs were cultured [118]. In the bottom layer, two distinct cavities held chemokines, which could diffuse through the endothelium layer in the porous polyester membrane and interact with the human MDA-MB-231 breast cancer cells [118]. In effect, this system is similar to transwell systems but adds a flow component that is necessary to better model endothelial cell culture [118]. This model was advantageous to study how localization of chemokines influences endothelial stimulation to promote cancer cell adhesion and can be used for further studies of endothelial cell interaction with other cell types and stimuli [118]. Thus, microfluidic devices can be used to incorporate fluid flow in a co-culture system as well as precisely pattern cells or growth factors.

4.2.2 Three-Dimensional Systems

While useful for certain studies, the culture of cells in 2D limits the inclusion of parameters known to be important in the 3D in vivo environment, where cells have an ECM meshwork on which to communicate [1,19,42,49,67,131,137]. These parameters include mechanical cues, communication between cells and matrix, and communication between adjacent cells [42]. Thus, 3D co-culture systems provide an opportunity to study cellular interaction with both heterotypic cell types and biomaterials that more closely mimic the 3D tissue environment. These studies can be used to understand mechanisms of interface development and can act as preliminary studies for future in vivo applications.

4.2.2.1 Physically separated cell populations

The soluble factors released from cells cultured in a 3D environment can be studied through physically separated cell populations. A variety of systems, utilizing hydrogels and microfluidics, have been used to achieve 3D systems that allow for physical cell separation yet maintain the potential for cell signaling. Hydrogels can be used to study cellular communication that occurs at a distance, which is often applicable in ITE. Hydrogels are versatile, porous 3D constructs consisting primarily of water [24,80,131]. Synthetic and natural polymers can be used to form gels, either of which can be modified to achieve desired bioactivity [24,80,131]. Because of their aqueous nature, hydrogels provide a low barrier to soluble factor diffusion between cells. Also key to their utility in interface tissue engineering is the ability to manipulate hydrogel properties for optimal culture of many different cell types [36,37,56,57]. Furthermore, different hydrogel materials can be joined together to form co-culture systems that best mimic interfaces [36,37,56,57].

While hydrogels have been applied to study many different tissue interfaces, one study that revolves around osteochondral interface regeneration highlights how the diverse properties of hydrogels can be used to mimic biological tissues [57]. In this study, hydrogels of divergent composition were employed to study the osteochondral interface, the region between articular cartilage and the bone, comprised of mineralized cartilage and a tidemark that demarcates the hyaline articular cartilage from the calcified cartilage region (Fig. 4.1) [56,57]. It has been hypothesized that cellular communication within the osteochondral interface plays a part in tissue regeneration [56,57]. To test this hypothesis, a co-culture of bovine osteoblasts and chondrocytes was achieved by fabricating a multiphase scaffold of agarose hydrogel (for chondrocytes) and sintered microspheres of polylactide-*co*-glycolide (PLGA) and 45S5 bioactive glass (BG) composite (for osteoblasts), materials chosen to mimic the diverging mechanical properties at the interface [57]. Between these two phases, a hybrid agarose-PLGA-BG interface was used promote a calcified-cartilage region [57]. In the co-culture system, total collagen and GAG content increased with time and compared to a culture system without BG, a mineralized matrix was produced [57]. These results indicate that both cellular communication and scaffold composition, which can be easily tuned when using hydrogels as the scaffold, are necessary for osteochondral regeneration.

Not only are material properties of hydrogels diverse, but there are also a variety of ways in which they can be manipulated. For example, rather than connecting hydrogels together, one study developed a co-culture system by culturing bovine chondrocytes from different zones of articular cartilage in separate agarose hydrogels in the same cell-culture well [56]. In this system, a decrease in mineralization was observed in the deep zone chondrocytes when cultured with articular surface chondrocytes [56]. Another study that also focused on zonal organization of cartilage assessed bilayered photopolymerizable hydrogels seeded with bovine chondrocytes [111]. Deep zone and superficial chondrocytes were again observed to communicate, as co-cultured deep zone chondrocytes were seen to have increased total collagen and GAG production as compared to controls [111]. Thus, through two co-culture models involving either connected or disconnected cell-laden hydrogels, it was ascertained that chondrocytes from different cartilage layers communicate, providing further insight into how the zonal structure of cartilage is maintained [56,111]. Hydrogel manipulation was also employed to analyze communication between the cell types present in the bone marrow niche [37]. Photopatterning of poly(ethylene glycol) (PEG)-based hydrogels was used to fabricate a 3D co-culture system of human osteoblasts, adipocytes, and MSCs, which could be subsequently separated after co-culture to obtain distinct cell populations for gene expression analysis [36,37]. For culture systems of one, two, or three cell types, distinct expression dynamics for osteogenic, adipogenic, chondrogenic, and myogenic transcriptional regulators were observed, indicating cellular communication within the construct [37]. This study demonstrates that hydrogel platforms allowing both co-culture and subsequent separation of cell populations may allow for examination of a host of biological questions [37]. Due to their diversity and ease of manipulation, hydrogels provide an excellent 3D scaffold for studying cellular communication for a variety of tissue interfaces and have been reviewed thoroughly [10,33,41,63,67,106,151].

In other patterning methodologies, microfluidics can be used to achieve excellent spatial control in 3D. In a 3D environment, microfluidic flow can be used to pattern materials or cells. To pattern both matrix material and cells simultaneously in a controlled spatial configuration, a layered co-culture between human ECs, smooth muscle cells (SMCs), and fibroblasts was created [129]. One by one, cell-laden matrices were loaded into the channel and allowed to settle and solidify before the next layer was added, maintaining separation between each cell population [129]. Cell viability was maintained in the culture system and it was found that matrix material could be used to control the rate of SMC migration [129]. Collagen and collagen-chitosan matrices promoted SMC migration into fibroblast layers within one and two days, respectively, while matrigel matrices showed limited SMC migration over the culture time [129]. This type of system could be used to pattern other cell types and matrices for further co-culture analysis [129]. In another system, microfluidic cell patterning was achieved by utilizing three channels made of PDMS, each coated with collagen to promote cell adhesion and also separated by collagen scaffolds to allow for cell migration between the channels [15]. Co-culture of human ECs and mouse smooth muscle precursor cells was established by putting cells in two different channels, allowing for adherence, growth, and communication of two separated cell populations [15]. It was observed that smooth muscle cells suppressed the migration of ECs, and further studies with this system could elucidate the role of smooth muscle cell recruitment in newly formed capillary stabilization [15]. Overall, microfluidics can be utilized both in the fabrication of 3D systems and as a variable parameter in 3D co-culture.

4.2.2.2 Direct-contact cell populations

In-contact 3D co-culture provides cells with the ability to communicate through soluble factors, cell–cell contact, and cell–matrix contacts. Micromass culture, ECM-like matrices, cell-patterning, and microfluidics are commonly used to achieve direct cell contact in 3D co-culture. Purely cell-based systems, such as cell spheroids and micromasses, utilize the tendency of cells to self-aggregate [42]. These cell-based 3D systems are valuable because scaffold materials do not interfere with cell–cell contacts [132]. Cell spheroids are one type of multicellular aggregates that has been used to study cell adhesion, migration, and differentiation, especially during tissue formation [132]. Often, imaging techniques are employed to study cellular behavior within the spheroid [42]. Similar to the examples in 2D culture, 3D culture systems with cell-contact can be used to elucidate which effects arise from cell–cell contact and which from soluble factors. For example, to study angiogenesis and its function in bone formation and repair, spheroid co-culture between human ECs and osteoblasts was generated by culturing equal amounts of suspended osteoblasts and ECs in non-adhesive tissue culture plates [122,142]. From these experiments, it was observed that over time, cells organize so that a core of osteoblasts was surrounded by a layer of ECs [122]. Changes in gene expression (downregulation of vascular endothelial growth factor (VEGF) and upregulation of ALP in osteoblasts; upregulation of VEGF receptor-2 in ECs) were seen to be cell-contact dependent, as conditioned media did not cause the same gene expression changes as the co-culture system [122]. Such systems could be used to study other interfaces in the future.

Micromass culture has been used to study cellular interactions between specific tissue types [5,38,55,130]. An example of this was demonstrated in a study of the interactions between bovine osteoblasts and chondrocytes for osteochondral interface regeneration applications [55]. Osteoblasts were allowed to adhere directly to a chondrocyte micromass, creating a scaffold on which to study cell–cell interactions [55]. Co-culture seemed to modulate cell phenotype, as chondrocyte GAG production and osteoblasts mineral deposition were both decreased [55]. Future studies will involve studying the possible formation of an interfacial region similar to that found in vivo [55]. Although individual cell populations cannot be studied with this technique, micromass co-culture is a valuable technique to study communication mediated by cell–cell contact and has been implemented in many other biomedical applications [38,64,69].

Besides purely cell-based systems, scaffolds similar to the native tissue environment have been employed and include decellularized ECM and tissue explants. Especially critical for cell types with complex ECM, naturally derived scaffolds can allow cells to be studied in a scaffold that closely mimics the in vivo environment while still allowing the study of specific factors [12]. For example, to ensure proper nutrient supply to provide a more physiological tissue environment, a 3D bioartificial vascularized scaffold (BioVaSc®) was developed, based upon a decellularized porcine small bowl segment [109]. The vascular structures within the cell-free collagen matrix were seeded with multiple cell types, such as human hepatocytes and ECs, and promoted heterotypic cellular communication, ascertained through VEGF expression [109].

Tissue explants can be partially decellularized and utilized for co-culture systems [12]. To maintain the native complexity of bone, bovine bone explants with in situ osteocytes were developed by removing surface cells through a PBS water jet and a Trypsin-EDTA wash [12]. In order to study the mechanisms in which osteocytes and osteoblasts communicate, primary bovine osteoblasts were seeded on the explant [12]. The system allowed for the study of intercellular communication through gap junctions and permitted mechanical load testing, showing that prostaglandin E_2 release and bone formation increased with dynamic deformational loading [12]. When utilized for in vitro culture, natural scaffolds can provide a biomimetic environment for cell communication studies. In ITE, this could be particularly beneficial, as precisely mimicking interface regions with artificial biomaterials can prove challenging due to diverging mechanical and compositional properties.

Cell patterning, as seen in 2D systems, provides excellent spatial control of cell populations. In 3D cell culture with cell–cell contact, cell patterning can be used to build 3D tissue that mimics the native environment in the body, as layered tissues are interconnected to form a continuous 3D tissue lattice [39]. Often, thermoresponsive surfaces are used to pattern cells because they provide user-defined control over cell adherence to a surface. In one study, the PIPAAm thermoresponsive surfaces discussed earlier were used to culture human ECs and rat hepatocytes in 2D cell sheets, which were stacked to form 3D constructs [39]. Cell viability was maintained for at least 41 days and hepatocytes in contact with ECs took on a more rounded cell shape and had increased albumin expression compared to surrounding hepatocytes that were not in contact with the ECs, suggesting that contact with ECs promoted maintenance of differentiated function [39]. Another technique for tissue layering also involved the thermoresponsive properties of PIPAAm [136]. PIPAAm and polyacrylamide (PAAm), a non-adhesive material, were patterned in alternating strips onto silanized coverslips [136]. Human ECs were then cultured on the cell-adherent PIPAAm lanes, allowing detachment at 20°C [136]. On separate PIPAAm surface, human fibroblasts were cultured to confluency [136]. Then, a gelatin stamp was applied to the fibroblast layer at 20°C, causing fibroblasts to be repelled from the PIPAAm and adhere to the gelatin stamp [136]. The gelatin-fibroblast stamp was next applied to the patterned ECs at 20°C, and in a similar manner, ECs were repelled from the PIPAAm surface and adhered to the fibroblasts [136]. Finally, the gelatin-fibroblast-EC stamp was applied to another confluent fibroblast layer under the same conditions, creating a fibroblast-EC-fibroblast co-culture [136]. Cells proved viable after 5 days and the system can be used in future studies of angiogenesis and cellular communication [136]. A plethora of cell-patterning techniques have been used for 3D co-culture and provide excellent spatial and temporal control of cells within 3D scaffolds [59]. For ITE, cell-patterning is especially useful as it can be used to mimic the distribution of various cell types within the interface.

Microfluidic techniques can be used to generate 3D scaffolds with cell contacts and have been recently employed in spheroid co-culture. In spheroid formation, commonly used formation techniques often lack efficiency, ability to generate long-term culture, control of spheroid size, and ability to uniformly distribute cells [48]. Researchers have started to overcome these problems by using microfluidic fabrication techniques. For example, a microfluidic cell patterning method was developed to allow for the pre-positioning of multiple cell types before and during spheroid formation [132].

Hydrodynamic forces focused cells on geometric features in the bottom layer of a microfluidic device, so when two types of cells were introduced to separate inlets that merged to a larger channel, they were simultaneously seeded in defined spatial arrangements [132]. By altering the geometry of the channels, the size and shape of the cellular patterning could be controlled, and a co-culture of mouse hepatocytes and embryonic stem cells remained in their defined locations for at least 14 days [132]. Spatially varied stem cell pluripotency, as determined by levels of OCT4 promoter expression, was observed based on the orientation of hepatocytes around the embryonic stem cells, suggesting cellular communication between the two cell types [132]. Microfluidics strategies have also been successfully implemented in hepatocyte, endothelial, osteoblast, monocyte, macrophage, and cancer cell co-culture [48,124,143]. These techniques are used for diverse applications and have proven successful in generating co-culture systems with great precision and repeatability.

Two and three-dimensional co-culture models provide excellent platforms on which cellular communication can be studied. Often, the information learned from such model systems can be applied to fabricate scaffolds used for in vivo applications. Also, the biological information gained regarding the effects of cellular communication and biomaterials on cell behavior in vitro may help formulate the questions that direct in vivo studies of interface tissues.

4.3 Scaffold Types for in vivo Applications in Interface Tissue Engineering

Currently, one of the most promising approaches in interface tissue engineering involves seeding donor cells onto porous 3D scaffolds, which provide an environment for cells and developing tissues [4,86]. Besides heterogeneity, scaffolds can provide cells with nano-, micro-, and macro-scale topological features, an appropriate biomechanical environment, and key surface ligands [4]. In general, scaffolds should be biocompatible to reduce the risk of an uncontrolled inflammatory response, be biodegradable into non-toxic products, have appropriate topological features to encourage ideal cell behavior and scaffold integration, have mechanical strength to withstand relevant stresses and strains, and be easily manufactured and sterilized [4]. Specifically challenging in

ITE applications is the requirement to engineer an environment that supports development of multiple tissues, as well as the interfaces in between. Thus, an ideal scaffold for ITE must support growth and differentiation of multiple cell populations, direct homotypic and heterotypic cellular communication, and promote the formation and maintenance of matrix heterogeneity [79,87]. With these requirements in mind, significant strides in ITE have been made through use of biomimetic scaffold that are gradiated, braided, generated from microspheres, and derived from natural sources (Fig. 4.2).

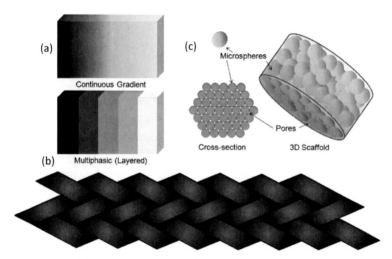

Figure 4.2 Schematic diagrams of scaffold types, including gradient scaffolds (a), braided scaffolds (b), and microsphere-based scaffolds (c).

4.3.1 Gradiated Scaffolds

Tissue interfaces, especially those in the musculoskeletal system, are anisotropic and exhibit gradients of structural properties, mechanics, biomolecules, and types of cells (Fig. 4.1) [79,110]. Due to these heterogeneous properties and cell populations, homogenous biomaterials may not be successful in regenerating musculoskeletal tissue interfaces [110]. Thus, many musculoskeletal ITE scaffolds exhibit a gradient of structural and mechanical properties that mimic those of the native insertion site [78,87]. This gradiated structure offers the possibility of continuous, multitissue generation on a single scaffold system as well as improved biological fixation at the point of injury [78,79].

Gradients can be multiphasic or continuous (Fig. 4.2a) [79]. In multiphasic scaffolds, several distinct sections have unique structural and biomolecular properties that promote growth for specific cell types [110]. Continuously gradiated scaffolds have a continuous transition in compositional and/or mechanical properties, and may better recapitulate the native transition within the interface region [79]. Both types of scaffolds will be considered in our discussion of gradients in composition, structure, and biomolecules.

4.3.1.1 Composition gradients

Anisotropy in the cellular microenvironment occurs when a heterogeneous distribution of cells and molecules exists within spatially varying ECM [25]. As these gradients play important roles in biological function [25], composition gradients in materials have been fabricated to better mimic native tissue interfaces, so that one scaffold can have various biological and mechanical functions designed for either a specific cell type or a specific mix of cell types. For example, collagen matrices have been continuously gradiated with minerals through diffusive techniques for osteochondral regeneration [72], hydrogels have been continuously gradiated using microfluidics [25], continuous organic to inorganic gradients have been developed using PEG and PDMS composite scaffolds for bone to fibrocartilage transition [89], multiphasic composites of calcium phosphate and HA sponge have been used for articular cartilage repair [31], and PLGA with additions of polyglycolic acid (PGA) fibers, BG, or calcium sulfate have been developed as multiphasic composite scaffolds for osteochondral defects [94]. Comprehensive reviews detail other strategies involving compositional gradients [2,79,84,87,110,151].

Gradiated scaffolds are often employed in bone–soft tissue interfaces to mimic compositional differences in each tissue type, as well as the transition zone in the middle. Mineral deposition and as a consequence, mechanical strength, are often the gradiated components of these systems [72,119,120,128]. In one study of biphasic scaffolds for bone–soft tissue interface, a tri-phasic scaffold system was fabricated and utilized for co-culture of bovine osteoblasts and fibroblasts [119]. Phase A was developed for soft tissue, formed from polyglactide knitted mesh sheets; phase B for fibrocartilage, consisting of sintered PLGA-based microspheres; and phase C for bone, comprised of sintered PLGA-based microspheres and 45S5 bioactive glass [119]. Upon seeding bovine fibroblasts in phase A and osteoblasts in phase C, migration of both cell types was seen into the middle phase B [119]. When expanded to a tri-culture system by adding chondrocytes to the middle layer and subcutaneously implanting the scaffold into a rat model, tissue ingrowth was observed in all three scaffold phases [120]. Phase A consisted of high levels of collagen I and III, ascertained through immunostaining, and phase C was highly mineralized, while phase B was moderately mineralized and contained collagen I and II [120]. As the scaffold resulted in distinct yet continuous cellular and matrix regions, it demonstrates the possibility of multitissue regeneration on a single scaffold [120]. Another study utilized a multiphasic scaffold with layers of PLGA-tricalcium phosphate (TCP) and PLGA to obtain a mineral composition gradient [72]. Six weeks after implantation of the rabbit bone-marrow derived cell-seeded scaffold into a cartilage defect of a rabbit model, spatially segregated cartilage-like and bone-like tissue growth were seen, as compared to the fibrous tissue growth seen in controls with no scaffold implantation [72]. Continuously gradiated scaffolds are also employed to mimic the gradients present at tissue interfaces. In one study for bone regeneration, a nanofibrous poly(ε-caprolactone) (PCL) scaffold with continuously gradiated calcium phosphate nanoparticles (nACP) was used to study murine osteoblast response to mineralization [105]. Osteoblast adhesion and proliferation were enhanced on nACP-rich region [105].

These three studies provide examples of a commonly encountered phenomenon in gradiated scaffold engineering: In scaffolds with composition gradients, cell behavior responds in a similarly gradiated fashion. Thus, such scaffolds are useful in ITE because they can support multiple cell types and matrix formation as well as direct cell behavior.

4.3.1.2 Structure gradients

Scaffolds, acting often as a temporary support for tissues during regeneration, must be able to withstand forces exerted upon them during and after implantation, requiring specific mechanical properties for each tissue engineering application [138]. In ITE, gradiated mechanical properties are often required due to the heterogeneous cell populations and ECM content at the interface. The osteochondral interface provides an example of divergent mechanical properties (Fig. 4.1). The modulus of bone, with its extensively mineralized matrix, is much higher than that of cartilage, where collagen, proteoglycans, and osmotic pressure contribute to the mechanical strength of the tissue [151]. Thus, to support multiple tissue types on one scaffold, anisotropic mechanical properties are often employed and are achieved through structural gradients of porosity, stiffness, and fiber orientation.

Porosity and stiffness gradients are often integrated into hydrogel, ceramic, and nanofibrous scaffolds. Porosity gradients can be achieved by using a porogen, which is a solute, often a salt, dispersed throughout a solvent containing a polymer solution. The solution is cast into a mold so that the polymer creates a scaffold around the porogen while the solvent evaporates. The porogen can be removed from the final scaffold by placing the salt-laden composite in water to remove the salt (or by other techniques appropriate for the specific porogen). These porogens can be integrated into the scaffold in a gradiated matter (the gradient formation techniques discussed in Section 4.4.2 apply to porogens as well), creating porosity gradients. Such gradients influence cell behavior, as seen in PLGA scaffolds and agarose-gelatin-based hydrogels, in which cell growth was reduced as porosity decreased, resulting in gradiated cell density [112,133].

Stiffness gradients can be developed in hydrogels by manipulating the cross-linking density, which can be thought of as the distance between polymer chains within the hydrogel. For example, higher cross-linking density, created by increasing the stimulus for polymerization (cross-linking initiator concentration, UV light intensity, or temperature), creates a smaller pore size and thus a stiffer gel [110]. In both hydrogels and nanofibrous matrices, cellular migration toward regions of increased stiffness has been observed [68,73,144]. Mechanical properties can be controlled through mineral content, as exemplified in a study in which TCP nanoparticles were incorporated into PCL nanofibers at continuously varied concentrations [28]. This resulted in a 3D scaffold with gradiated concentrations of TCP nanoparticles and mechanical properties [28]. As TCP concentrations increased from 0% to 12%, elongation break values decreased from 259% to 171% while modulus values increased from 18.5 to 27.5 kPa [28]. After four weeks of murine osteoblast culture on this scaffold, it was found that tissue constructs resembled the bone-cartilage interface in regards to calcium type I and ECM distribution, observed by histological analysis, as well as in the spatial variation of mechanical properties [28]. TCP gradients have also been used in the bone layer of a scaffold for osteochondral regeneration in a porcine animal model [44]. The tri-phasic implant had a PCL phase (cartilage), a PCL-TCP phase (bone), and an additional mesh phase, comprised of PCL and collagen, incorporated at the end of the cartilage scaffold to achieve integration with host tissue [44]. When seeded with porcine MSCs and inserted into a defect at the medial condyle and the patellar groove in a porcine model, more GAG content and mineralization was found at the cartilage and bone interfaces, respectively, as compared to controls in which only cells or only the scaffold was implanted [44]. From this, it was determined that this cell-seeded gradiated scaffold enhanced healing of the osteochondral interface [44].

Fiber organization is a commonly observed property that is gradiated within tissue interfaces and can direct cell behavior both in vivo and in vitro. One biological example of dissimilar fiber organization is the tendon–bone interface, in which fibers are organized along the axis of loading in the tendon, whereas this is not the case in bone. As repaired tendons can be re-injured due to the lack of regeneration of the transitional interface that exists in uninjured tissue, this organizational transition is an area of study in ITE [44]. By developing a nanofibrous scaffold that mimicked the aligned collagen fibers of normal tissue and the more randomly aligned fibers in the bone, one study showed that it was possible to promote different orientation in rat tendon fibroblasts in each region [147]. Specifically, it was shown that cells aligned with fibers when organized and oriented randomly when fibers were unorganized [147]. Mechanical testing showed increased toughness, modulus, and ultimate stress in aligned fibers in comparison to randomly oriented fibers, consistent with the hypothesis that mechanical properties depend on fiber alignment [147]. Thus, for musculoskeletal interfaces that involve two tissues with different mechanical properties, there is evidence that structurally gradiated scaffolds can promote tissue-specific ECM deposition. Developing biomimetic structural scaffolds is a worthwhile avenue to pursue in ITE, especially for musculoskeletal applications.

4.3.1.3 Biomolecular gradients

Biomolecular gradients of growth factors, ECM components, and genetic material have been fabricated for ITE applications [61,107,114]. In many biomolecular gradient studies, cells have been observed to migrate toward higher concentrations of growth factors. Human smooth muscle cells (SMCs) have been see to migrate toward basic fibroblast growth factor (bFGF) [20], Sprague–Dawley rat neural stem cells (NSCs) demonstrated increasing levels of astrocytic markers with increasing levels of ciliary neurotrophic factor (CNTF) [53], and rat pheochromocytoma cell neurites were guided up concentration gradients of nerve growth factor (NGF) in poly(2-hydroxyethyl-methacrylate) (p(HEMA)) scaffolds [60]. In a slightly different type of study, patterns of bone morphogenetic protein-2 (BMP-2) were printed on fibrin-coated glass slides [102]. Interestingly, researchers used different numbers of overprints to generate spatially defined amounts of BMP-2 [102]. Murine muscle-derived stem cells were cultured on the slides and it was observed that markers of osteogenic differentiation, evidenced by ALP expression, increased with increasing number of overprints, even in myogenic culture conditions, while control cell populations on non-printed substrate underwent myogenic differentiation, observed through myotube formation and myosin heavy chain (fast) gene expression [102].

The influence of multiple growth factors on cellular behavior within a single scaffold has also been studied [23,53]. By creating a gradient of growth factors, a single scaffold has the potential to direct one cell type down several different lineages or behavioral pathways. In one example, growth factor gradients were created by printing different portions of a hydrogel with FGF-2 and CNTF [53]. As FGF-2 has been shown previously to maintain a proliferative state while CNTF to induce differentiation, this gradient was employed to further understand Sprague–Dawley rat NSC differentiation [53]. In areas of CNTF, NSCs expressed differentiation markers such as smooth muscle gene SMA and glial fibrillary acidic protein (GFAP), while NSCs on areas printed with FGF-2 did not [53]. From these examples, it is clear that growth factor gradients have the potential to direct cell migration and differentiation in ITE, providing a means of developing anisotropic cell populations to mimic different tissues.

Similar to that of growth factors, gradients of ECM proteins have resulted in directed cellular behavior. In a poly(methylglutarimide) nanofiber mat, murine fibroblast density and adherence was increased at the region where fibronectin was most concentrated [113]. Similarly, human ECs were observed to show increased attachment and spreading with increased concentrations of RGDS in PEG-diacrylate (DA) hydrogels [43]. Interestingly, neurite extension rate of chicken dorsal root ganglia were significantly higher in anisotropic scaffolds of ECM protein laminin-1 (LN-1) as compared to isotropic scaffolds [22]. Clearly, local concentration of growth factors and ECM has a strong influence on cell migration, adhesion, and differentiation, and through manipulating these concentrations, cell behavior can be more tightly controlled within a scaffold. While the scaffolds presented above were not developed toward interface tissue applications, this tight control of cell behavior provides rationale for using ECM gradients to develop anisotropic scaffolds for ITE scaffold formation.

Finally, gradients of genetic materials have been established. Genetic approaches to gradient formation might be beneficial as they overcome the short half-life inherent to other cell-signaling molecules used to create gradients, such as proteins [103]. To study the ability for retroviral gradients to engineer gradients of differential cell function, gradients of immobilized retrovirus encoding osteogenic transcription factor Runx were established via deposition of controlled PLL densities [103]. Zonal organization of osteoblastic and fibroblastic phenotypes were achieved both in vitro and in vivo after seeding Wistar rat fibroblasts on the gradiated scaffold, with increased osteogenic phenotype in areas of highly concentrated retrovirus [103]. This specific scaffold has applications toward musculoskeletal interface regeneration, especially for the bone–ligament/tendon interface. In general, genetic gradients have the potential to provide a more persistent signal to cells for cases in which cell-signaling molecules can only achieve a transient response.

4.3.2 Braided Scaffolds

Fibrous scaffolds can be fabricated using braiding techniques (Fig. 4.2b) and are beneficial for two main reasons. First, the braiding process permits control of pore diameter, porosity, mechanical properties, and geometry [16]. Second, they can be composed of nanofibers, which mimic ECM in their porous and fibrillar structure as well as provide large surface area and roughness for cell contact [110,153]. With superior control of mechanical properties and porosity, braided scaffolds are a popular scaffold choice for many tissue engineering applications. They have been previously investigated for tendon/ligament regeneration [16,17,77], cartilage regeneration [88], nerve regeneration [8], rotator cuff regeneration [30], ACL regeneration [29], and many other applications [32,66]. Notably, none of these applications involve tissue interfaces; rather, they involve many of the tissues that are found on one side of important interfaces. It may be interesting to join these braided scaffolds with other fibrous scaffolds to create biphasic scaffolds for ITE. Also, it may be desirable to develop methods that allow for gradiated fabrication of braided scaffolds for heterogeneous cell type culture. A few examples of braided scaffolds and their applications are given below.

With the application of mimicking the native ACL, polylactide-*co*-glycolide (PLAGA) fibers were braided to obtain a similar architecture to that of the native collagen fiber matrix [16]. On either end of the scaffold, high angle fiber orientation was used to mimic the bony attachment sites, while the middle of the scaffold consisted of lower angle fiber orientation to mimic the intra-articular zone [16]. Initial studies indicated proliferation, attachment, and growth of white rabbit primary ACL fibroblasts and mouse fibroblasts, demonstrating good biocompatibility of the scaffold [16]. Employing similar techniques, PLLA braided scaffolds with fibronectin coating were fabricated and seeded with rabbit primary ACL fibroblasts [17]. Then, scaffolds were fixed by sutures at the femoral and tibial tunnels in a rabbit model for in vivo studies to regenerate the ACL [17]. After twelve weeks, histological sections of the cell-seeded scaffold showed more tissue ingrowth and aligned collagen fibers as compared to the unseeded control, demonstrating possible healing of the rabbit ACL [17]. This example, while still designed to mimic only one tissue, provides a clear example of how anisotropic properties can be developed in a braided scaffold. Thus, it would be possible to expand this technology to use braided scaffolds for ITE applications in the future.

4.3.3 Microsphere-Containing Scaffolds

Microparticles have gained attention in scaffold-design, as they can be used as supporting matrices for cell adhesion (Fig. 4.2c) or carriers of bioactive agents for controlled delivery of exogenous signals [115]. As building blocks, microspheres are beneficial due to ease of fabrication, as well as good control over morphology and physicochemical characteristics [116]. Microparticle scaffolds can be composite in structure, meaning that only portions of the scaffold are made of microparticles, or continuous, meaning that the entire scaffold is composed of microparticles (Fig. 4.2c). As supporting matrices, microparticles are often employed to provide mechanical characteristics that mimic native tissue. For example, microspheres have been used in two composite scaffolds to mimic bone and fibrocartilagenous ECM [57,119,120]. In a tri-phasic scaffold to promote ACL-to-bone interface regeneration, sintered microspheres were used for the fibrocartilagenous and bone mimicking regions, as these regions required long-term integrity and supported cell growth [119,120]. Similarly, another scaffold that was used to mimic the osteochondral interface employed microspheres for the bone-like region and a microsphere-hydrogel composite for the fibrocartilagenous region [57]. The microsphere composite was shown to improve bovine osteoblast calcium phosphate deposition and to mimic the mechanical properties of the interface [57]. Thus, microspheres allow for control of mechanical properties and consequent cell behavior within a scaffold, providing another tool to generate ITE scaffolds that have specific structural requirements.

As carriers for bioactive agents, microparticles provide much versatility in release of a variety of encapsulated factors [116]. A study for osteochondral repair provides an example of microparticle delivery of TGF-β1, seen to enhance chondrocyte differentiation, proliferation, and ECM deposition [47]. A composite of an oligo(poly(ethylene glycol) fumarate) (OPF) hydrogel and growth factor-loaded gelatin microparticles was shown to accelerate host cell infiltration when implanted in a condyle defect in a rabbit model [47]. Fourteen weeks after implantation, scaffolds with TGF-β1-loaded microparticles in the chondral portion of the scaffold showed slight improvement in histological evaluation of cell infiltration, matrix deposition, and degradation of the scaffold, indicating that growth factor release could be beneficial to the osteochondral defect repair [47]. In scaffolds for ITE, microparticles provide another means to allow for controlled material properties. Microparticles can be gradiated within the scaffold as well, allowing desired anisotropic mechanical properties or growth factor release to be obtained.

4.3.4 Natural Scaffolds

Natural scaffolds include those that utilize autologous tissue grafts or ECM and scaffold-less approaches. Autologous scaffolds are advantageous because they reduce the risk of host rejection, but still the autologous tissue must be obtained from the host, which often results in invasive procedures that can cause harm in the region of explant. Generally, once autologous tissue is obtained, it is treated with growth factors, cells, or other chemicals intrinsic to the healing process prior to reimplantation [82,85,92]. Many ITE-relevant decellularized scaffolds have proven successful and include cartilage, bone, tendon/ligament, nerves, and blood vessels [26,104]. More extensive reviews on decellurization provide ample examples and overview common techniques used to obtain decellularized matrices [3,11,46].

The possibilities in autologous explant manipulation for ITE applications were explored in the following two studies. In a rabbit model, adenovirus-BMP-2, shown to improve tendon graft insertion into native bone, or the BMP-2 gene was injected into autologous tendon grafts prior to implantation [85]. In this approach, the BMP-2-treated grafts showed similar tendon–bone interface in the osseous tunnel to that of normal ACL insertion, determined through histological and mechanical analysis [85]. Another similar study also sought to improve tendon–bone attachment and used tendon grafts in which both ends were soaked in calcium phosphate for regeneration in a rabbit model [92]. The calcium phosphate was hypothesized to promote bone tissue formation at the ends of the graft, and the soaked graft did show enhanced healing at the bone–tendon interface when implanted into a rabbit model, indicated by cartilage formation between the tendon and bone as compared to the fibrous interface formed in control groups [92]. Both of these approaches highlight the possibility of obtaining better scaffold-native tissue integration by modifying native tissue explants prior to implantation, which is beneficial to ITE as many musculoskeletal interfaces have poor scaffold–host integration after surgical repair.

Similar to co-culture with spheroids and micromasses, scaffold-less approaches rely on cell–cell adhesions and ECM deposition and not on cell interactions with traditional biomaterials [42,132]. For in vivo applications, scaffold-less approaches are attractive because they may reduce the risk of an inflammatory response to non-biological scaffolds in the host after implantation [4]. While not for the specific application of ITE, examples that have utilized scaffold-less technologies include MSCs that have been cued to form hyaline cartilage [27], bone-marrow stromal cells that have been shown to successfully self-assemble into ligament [35], and fibrochondrocytes and chondrocytes that have self-assembled to form cartilage-like tissue for possible knee meniscus applications [45]. Toward an ITE application, 3D bone-like tissue structures composed solely of rat bone marrow stromal cells (BMSCs) were generated [126]. BMSCs were cultured on a laminin-coated silicone elastomer and after sufficient ECM production occurred, the tissue monolayer lifted from the substrate and self-assembled into a cylindroid tissue [126]. Both osteogenic and fibroblastic differentiation, as determine by ALP activity, collagen type I deposition, and mineralization, were seen within the construct, which may indicate that the mechanical cues that occurred during tissue development influenced stem cell differentiation [126]. As a continuation to this study, bone–ligament–bone (BLB) constructs were generated by culturing a monolayer of BMSCs in ligament-differentiation media and then securing a bone construct on top of the monolayer [81]. The ligament-like BMSCs monolayer rolled up around the bone construct, forming a BLB construct that was tested in vivo by suturing it to the points of insertion of the femur and tibia in a rat model [81]. The explanted BLB construct stained positively for type I collagen and elastin one month after implantation and was well vascularized after two months [81]. Explants also demonstrated a functionally graded response similar to native tissue inhomogeneity [81]. Scaffold-less tissue engineering is intriguing, because rather than engineering cues to direct tissue development, it utilizes the native developmental cues inherent to each cell type to form new tissue.

4.4 Scaffold Fabrication

The complexity and intricacies required for ITE scaffold fabrication have necessitated the development of innovative, reliable, and reproducible fabrication methods for a new generation of tissue scaffolds. The scaffolds previously discussed can be generally categorized as nanofibrous scaffolds, gradiated scaffolds, and computer generated scaffolds. Scaffold formation methods are often used in combination and are constantly modified for specific applications, so here we will provide a general overview of several techniques, as well as ITE-specific scaffold fabrication methods, if examples are available.

4.4.1 Nanofibrous Scaffold Fabrication

Nanofibrous scaffolds are beneficial, as they can mimic the porosity and fibrillar nature of the native ECM and provide large surface area for cell attachment [110,153]. Once fabricated, some nanofibrous matrices are easily tunable to provide the biological and chemical cues offered by the native ECM [110]. Currently, self-assembly, phase separation, and electrospinning are the principle methods employed to create nanofibrous scaffolds [91].

4.4.1.1 Self-assembly

Self-assembly is a process in which individual, preexisting components organize themselves into an ordered structure without human intervention [91,117]. During self-assembly, non-covalent bonds produce stable structures that can closely match biological systems [51,91,96,97,123,154]. One disadvantage of this technique is the limited number of polymers that can achieve self-assembly, as well as the lack of control over fiber orientation [91]. However, this technique is advantageous as it requires no harmful organic solvents that reduce biocompatibility [91]. For example, in one study, self-assembled 3D nanofiber networks were achieved upon adding peptide amphiphile (PA) molecules to fluids containing polyvalent metal ions [6,40]. In fluids containing mouse osteoblasts, cells were trapped during self-assembly and survived in the fibrous matrix for at least three weeks [6].

An example of self-assembly for an ITE application involves a study in which a hybrid bone implant material of Titanium-6Al-4V foam and self-assembling PA nanofiber matrix was fabricated in order to eliminate the need for the cement fixation often required for orthopedic and dental implants [108]. In this system, the pores of the titanium scaffold were filled with self-assembling PA nanofibers, creating a biocompatible matrix [108]. When laden with pre-osteoblastic mouse cells and implanted in a defect on the diaphysis of the femur in a rat model, bone formation was seen around and inside the scaffold through histological analysis [108]. As shown in this example, integrating self-assembly with other ITE techniques, such as porosity gradiated scaffolds, could potentially provide anisotropic distribution of matrix that might be hard to obtain otherwise.

4.4.1.2 Phase separation

Phase separation can be used to produce nano-fibrous structures without use of sophisticated equipment [91]. In the general procedure, polymers are first dissolved in a solvent, which can include porogens to obtain increased scaffold porosity, and then the temperature is decreased to promote the initially homogenous solution to separate into a polymer-rich and a polymer-poor phase [14]. The solvent in the phase of low polymer concentration is later removed through extraction, evaporation, or sublimation, leaving behind open pores surrounded by the solidified polymer-rich phase [14]. While some control of structural properties, such as shape, pore size, interfiber distance, and fiber diameter can be controlled, control of fiber orientation has not been obtained [91]. In one study, poly(L-lactic acid) (PLLA) solutions were cast over paraffin spheres and were then thermally phase-separated to form fibrous matrices with nano structures [13]. This technique allowed for control of the macroscopic shape of the scaffold, the spherical pore size, interfiber distance, and fiber diameter [13]. In another study, a PLLA scaffold generated by phase separation was utilized for neonatal mouse cerebellum C17-2 stem cell culture [149]. Within the matrix, nerve stem cells proliferated, migrated, and showed signs of differentiation, ascertained through morphological analysis via scanning electron microscopy and actin content using confocal microscopy [149]. This is only one example of how phase separation can be used to produce nano-structured scaffolds that allow for cell adhesion and differentiation in vitro [149]. Many reviews and reports detailing strategies for phase separation are available [91,117].

4.4.1.3 Electrospinning

Electrospinning employs electrostatic forces to produce polymer fibers with diameters between 10 and 1000 nm, which can subsequently be surface-modified to increase cellular compatibility (Fig. 4.3) [110]. By using electrospinning as a fabrication technique, it is possible to control fiber orientation, a critical parameter in fibrous scaffold formation that can influence cellular growth and orientation [91,147]. Mechanistically, electrospinning employs electrostatic forces to produce ultra-thin polymer fibers with defined spatial orientation, high aspect ratio, high surface area, and good control over pore geometry [91]. Briefly, a spinneret is connected to a syringe that acts as a reservoir for the polymer solution, and polymer droplets get electrified at the tip of the spinneret [91]. Once the electrostatic force exceeds the viscoelastic force and surface tension of the droplet, a charged fine polymer jet ejects from the tip of the droplet [91]. The jet moves toward the counter electrode, also known as the collector, and while in transit, solvent evaporates and the different polymer strands separate due to mutual repulsion [91]. Various fiber orientations are achieved by modifying the collector (Fig. 4.3) [91].

Recently, gradations in nanofibrous scaffolds have been achieved during the electrospinning process. In one example, extrusion has been combined with electrospinning in order to incorporate different chemical or growth factors into the mesh with temporal control, allowing for spatially gradiated meshes [110]. In another study, a 2-spinnerette method was developed and involved a fabrication setup in which two spinnerettes are placed side by side and each dispense different types of nanofibers simultaneously, producing an overlapping pattern (Fig. 4.3b) [105]. Random-to-aligned gradients in structure have also been achieved through electric field manipulation [147]. Finally, porosity can also be controlled in electrospun scaffolds. Nano- and micro-scale porous structures can be obtained by incorporating micro- and nano-sized salt particles into the initial polymer solutions before electrospinning [141]. After electrospinning, salts can be leached out, leaving secondary porous structures [141]. Numerous reviews provide a more comprehensive description of the electrospinning process and cellular interactions to electrospun scaffolds [7,90,91,95,117,146].

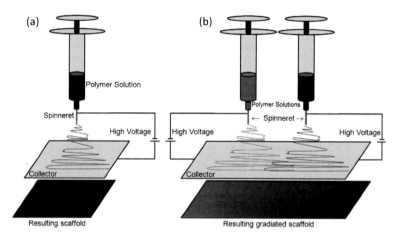

Figure 4.3 Schematic of electrospinning process. (a) A polymer solution held in a syringe is pushed through a spinneret, creating a droplet. A fine polymer jet is ejected from the tip of the spinneret when the electrostatic forces exceed viscoelastic forces, and the jets move to the collector and create a fibrous scaffold. (b) To make a gradient nanofibrous scaffold, two spinnerets are placed side by side and electrospin two different polymer solutions onto the same collector.

4.4.2 Gradiated Scaffolds

By employing micro- and nanotechnologies, it is possible to create gradients both in composition and properties within a single scaffold while still achieving interconnected and integrated phases [87,110]. Gradiated scaffolds can be formed using flow-based systems, diffusion, and time-dependent exposure.

4.4.2.1 Flow-based systems

Flow-based systems include both microfluidics and gradient makers, which utilize controlled pumping of materials to achieve spatial variations within a scaffold. Microfluidic techniques control fluid flow in micrometer-scale channels and can produce concentration gradients with both spatial and temporal control [20,21,54,60, 107,110,114,115]. Often, PDMS molds and controlled pumps are employed to move fluids and molecules at desired rates [25,43]. In one study, PDMS molds were used to create a microfluidic channel, which was pre-filled with low concentration of PEG-DA [43]. A solution with high concentrations of PEG-DA and cell adhesion ligand RGDS was then introduced into the channel, creating a gradient that could be stabilized with photopolymerization [43]. In another study, programmable pumps were employed to generate a gradient of osteogenic- and chondrogenic-growth factor-loaded microspheres [23]. The flow rates for each microsphere solution was controlled so that the final scaffold consisted of top and bottom quarters of solely osteogenic or chondrogenic microspheres, while the middle half contained a linear gradient of each [23]. As is the case with most of their applications, microfluidics provide control of scaffold structure at the micro-scale that may be hard to achieve using other techniques.

On a larger scale, gradient makers are commercially available and can produce concentration gradients in hydrogels. Gradient makers employ multiple syringe pumps in tandem to pump different solutions at controllable flow rates into a mixer [107]. Then, the mixed solution is pumped out into a mold for further use and stabilization [107]. Gradient makers can be modified and manipulated for a particular application. In one study employing PEG-based hydrogels, bFGF concentration gradients were created using a gradient maker [20]. Two solutions, one of PEG-DA and the other of acryloyl-PEG-bFGF, were contained in two chambers separated by a Teflon valve, allowing for a mixed solution flow [20]. Gradient makers and controlled pumping are commonly employed in tissue engineering and have been used in a plethora of studies involving culture of interface-relevant cell types, including rat neuronal cells, porcine chondrocytes, human smooth muscle cells, and mouse fibroblasts [20,60,74,114].

4.4.2.2 Diffusion

Gradient scaffolds can be created through diffusion [110]. In this method, pre-fabricated scaffolds (hydrogels, nanofibrous matrices, etc.) are exposed to highly concentrated solution of some type of molecule [110]. The molecules then diffuse from a region of high concentration to a region of lower concentration, creating a gradient across the scaffold [110]. Pre-fabricated nanofibrous scaffolds can be subjected to diffusion-based approaches to achieve spatial gradations, illustrated in one study where a nanofibrous collagen scaffold was sandwiched between two nylon meshes [70]. A chamber filled with phosphate solution was positioned above the collagen scaffold while a calcium filled chamber rested below [70]. As the solution diffused into the collagen scaffold, nano-hydroxyapatite crystallites precipitated within the scaffold, resulting in less precipitate on the calcium side of the scaffold [70].

Diffusive strategies can also be used in hydrogels to obtain gradients. Photo- or chemical immobilization can be combined with diffusion-mediated gradient formation to make gradients of growth factors [22,52,101]. In one study, a combination of diffusion and photoimmobilization was used to generate LN-1 gradients in agarose gels [22]. The agarose gel was placed in a chamber with a LN-1 solution on one side and a buffer on the other side [22]. Diffusion down the concentration gradient resulted in a gradient of LN-1 throughout the gel [22]. Photoimmobilization of LN-1 in the agarose gel was achieved through exposure to UV light [22]. With this setup, it was also possible to create gradients with different slopes, enabling generation of steep or gentle gradients [22]. In another technique, diffusion was used to create gradient composites of hydrogel and microparticles. A gradient of loaded microparticles was created within a hydrogel, and upon microparticle degradation, diffusion of soluble factors out of the particle created gradients across the hydrogel [101]. Diffusion-based techniques are valuable in ITE for gradiated scaffold creation.

4.4.2.3 Time-dependent exposure

Scaffolds can be exposed to a solute-containing fluid at a controlled rate in order to obtain spatial gradients of the solute throughout the scaffold. This technique is commonly employed for pre-fabricated nanofibrous scaffolds. In some studies, scaffolds are dipped into the solute-containing fluid at a defined rate. For example, gradients of PLL were created by dipping collagen scaffolds into a PLL solution at controlled rate using a motorized dip coater [103]. Runx2 retrovirus was then immobilized by exploiting the ability of the cationic PLL to charge neutralize and aggregate viral particles [103].

In other studies, the scaffold sits in a chamber that is filled with the solute-containing fluid at a controlled rate [113]. This was employed to generate a fibronectin gradient by filling of a chamber containing a pre-fabricated nanofibrous matrix composed of poly(methylglutarimide) with a fibronectin-containing solution [113]. This resulted in a scaffold of high fibronectin concentration at one end with a gradiated decrease toward the other end [113]. Another study used a similar technique: by filling a vial housing a PLGA-based scaffold at a controlled rate with a calcium phosphate solution, the portion of the matrix in contact with the bottom of the vial had a higher mineral content as compared to the part of the matrix nearest the top of the vial [68]. Time-dependent exposure techniques are limited in that they require a second step after pre-fabrication of the scaffold, thus increasing total manufacture time, but advantageous because they require only relatively simple equipment.

4.4.3 Rapid Prototyping

Rapid prototyping (RP), or solid free-form fabrication (SFF), is a common name for several techniques involving the automatic manufacturing of 3D objects in a layer-by-layer fashion as specified by computer-assisted drawings (CAD) [52,65,100]. RP is an efficient way to reproduce scaffolds with well-defined properties on large scale and in a reproducible manner [52,65]. Recently, solvent-free, aqueous-based RP systems have been developed, allowing for production of biologically based scaffolds [52]. Some RP techniques include stereolithography, selective laser sintering, 3D printing, shape deposition manufacturing, electron beam melting, and extrusion based technologies (fused deposition modeling, 3D plotting, multiphase jet solidification, and precise extrusion manufacturing) [52,65,100]. As these techniques have been thoroughly reviewed elsewhere [52,65,100], here we will focus on 3D bioprinting, which has been employed for ITE applications due to its versatility and ability to accurately pattern materials and cells. Specifically, we will consider inkjet printing and multinozzle low-temperature deposition.

4.4.3.1 Inkjet printing

Inkjet printers have been employed in a process called "bioprinting," which involves the printing of cells, biomolecules, or hydrogels based on a digital pattern [110]. In this 3D printing process, a binding material is deposited into a material stream and onto a powder bed, causing the particles to join together to form the desired object [4]. Then, a new layer of powder is deposited and can be selectively joined to the previous layer, a process that repeats until the entire scaffold is complete [4]. This process has several advantages. As the ink nozzle does not contact the printed surface, risk of cross-contamination is low [53]. Furthermore, inkjet printing is programmable and requires no significant modification of substrates for printing [102]. While promising, inkjet printing has limitations in generating large-scale tissues as well as printing within 3D hydrogels [110].

Inkjet printing has been employed to print ECM, cells, proteins, and DNA at low cost in many biomedical applications [53]. Gradients can be obtained by employing grayscale patterns of different intensities in the CAD [53], or by applying different number of overprints to achieve higher concentration in specified regions [102]. Collagen I scaffolds with defined microchannels and internal structures have been created with jet-printing [138]. Processing did not affect the structural stability of the collagen and this scaffold will be further applied for bone tissue engineering applications [138]. Inkjet printing can also be used to precisely pattern cells. Cellular printing was achieved using a layer-by-layer bioprinting assembly to print PEG mixed with human chondrocytes to fabricate osteochondral plugs [18]. Photopolymerization was simultaneously employed to maintain chondrocyte position [18]. This system achieved specific placement of individual cells, high cell viability, maintenance of chondrogenic phenotype as ascertained through aggrecan and collagen type I and II gene expression, and integration with host tissue, assessed by push-out testing to determine interface failure stress [18]. By further modifying inkjet printers to be more suitable for printing cells and ECM materials, this technique has the potential to create structures with very specific internal structures, soluble factor placement, and cell patterning.

4.4.3.2 Multinozzle low-temperature deposition

Multinozzle low-temperature deposition (MLD) is another computer-based rapid prototype technique that can generate a physical model directly from computer-aided design data [52,65,72,100,148]. Using an MLD approach, several materials can be extruded from different nozzles at the same time, resulting in scaffolds with gradient biomaterials, biomolecules, and pore structures [71]. In one study, it was used to generate osteochondral scaffolds [72]. A computer generated model was divided into three regions, including the subchondral bone, the calcification layer, and the cartilage [72]. Mixtures of PLGA-TCP and PLGA-NaCl were placed in two separate displacement nozzles and individually extruded to fabricate the scaffold as defined by the computer model [72]. The resulting scaffolds had sections differing in materials, pore size, and mechanical structure [72]. MLD is a promising technique, as it can extrude many materials at the same time, and could be specifically modified for the particular demands of a given study.

4.5 Future Directions

As highlighted in this chapter, ITE has employed many common tissue engineering techniques in order to fabricate co-culture systems and scaffolds for implantation. One of the critical differences between ITE and other disciplines in tissue engineering is the requirement for heterogeneous materials and cell types to mimic the transition regions inherent to native biological interfaces. To overcome this challenge, cellular communication within in vitro co-culture of interface-relevant cell types has been studied, and results have been used to further improve current interface regeneration strategies. Importantly, it has been realized that the specific type of cellular communication between cells is critical to interface development, maintenance, and generation. For instance, in many cases, it has been observed that direct cell or matrix contact influences cell behavior differently than that of soluble factor signaling. Significant strides have been made in the realm of biomimetic co-culture, especially in the development of platforms that provide tight control over cellular manipulation, but few studies have focused on much more than rudimentary phenotypic information that can be gained from the established cellular interactions. By using these platforms for studies in signaling pathways and systems biology, for example, it may be possible to further elucidate how cellular communication is implicated in interface development.

To achieve anisotropy, ITE scaffolds have required the creative implementation of well-developed tissue engineering techniques. For instance, innovative combinations of previously developed technologies have resulted in gradiated scaffolds appropriate for ITE. Such combinations include microfluidics with standard hydrogel formation techniques to form biomolecular gradients and electrospinning with extrusion to fabricate gradients in nanofibrous scaffolds. These examples have proven beneficial to ITE, and still many opportunities for combining other techniques exist to make more biomimetic scaffolds. For example, braided, naturally derived, and microsphere-containing scaffolds could be fabricated to include biomolecular gradients. In this way, cells could experience both structural and biochemical stimuli within the same scaffold. While scaffold types are being combined in new ways, some currently established scaffold types and fabrication techniques are not yet used in ITE. One example is braided scaffolds, which offer an excellent surface for cell-seeding. Several braided scaffolds of diverging properties could be combined to create tissue interfaces and moreover, scaffolds in which diverging properties are braided into one scaffold could be beneficial for ITE applications.

Fabrication techniques for tissue engineering are rapidly improving and becoming more efficient, yet for many ITE applications, a compromise between scaffold specificity and ease of fabrication must be made. For example, with the techniques currently available for nanofibrous scaffold fabrication, either extensive equipment is needed to fabricate highly specific scaffolds, such as those obtained by electrospinning, or relatively simple processes can be used to fabricate less complex scaffolds, such as phase separation and self-assembly. This makes electrospinning an attractive option, as it provides a highly precise means of developing nanofibrous scaffolds, but it requires extensive equipment and expertise. By improving upon complicated technologies and making them more readily available and usable, complex scaffold fabrication will become more attainable.

While many preliminary studies on the effects of biomolecular and stiffness gradients have been conducted, they have not yet fully explored gradient influence on cell behavior. It may be possible to pattern cells by manipulating their behavior through gradiated scaffolds. For example, two or more different cell types could be stimulated to migrate opposite directions within the same scaffold due to gradients. Biomolecular gradients and their ability to guide stem cell differentiation on scaffolds have been studied, but further in vivo studies could also be valuable in ITE. For instance, to achieve autologous cell transplantation, stem cells, such as MSCs, could be harvested from a host, seeded on a scaffold engineered to direct cell behavior for tissue interface regeneration, and then implanted into the host for interface repair. While basic studies in this area have already been conducted, further experimentation with stem cell manipulation could result in more biomimetic autologous cell scaffolds.

Traditionally, biomaterials have provided the environment on which artificial tissue interfaces have been developed, but it is possible that cellular interactions may form scaffold-less constructs that even better mimic the native tissue environment. Thus, it still remains a critical challenge to find the balance between manipulating biomaterials and taking advantage of natural cellular interactions to form constructs and scaffolds for ITE.

While ITE has the potential to offer integrative graft solutions that can be translated to the clinical setting, biological fixation of a graft or scaffold to native tissue remains a significant obstacle [79,87]. A more thorough understanding of the structure-function relationship at the native insertion site, as well as a deeper understanding how interface tissue develops, is maintained, and regenerates, is still needed [79,87]. Furthermore, clinical implementation requires identification of optimal cell sources that can be quickly isolated and expanded, as well as sterile methods for implantation and long-term storage [79]. While substantial research on characterizing tissue interfaces has been completed to date, future research will need to focus on these fundamental questions in addition to generating sophisticated cell patterns in a repeatable fashion in order to fully translate this research to regenerative medicine applications in a clinical setting. To this end, ITE requires collaborations among cell biologists to provide insight into cellular signaling and relevant intracellular pathways, material scientists to provide expertise on scaffold design and fabrication, clinicians to relate observations about which techniques promote the best healing, and biomedical engineers to integrate these disciplines in order to develop efficacious co-culture techniques and scaffold designs. ITE is a new but rapidly growing branch of tissue engineering that, with further development, holds great potential to help patients with a plethora of injuries and diseases that are currently deemed untreatable.

References

1. Abbott, A. (2003). Biology's new dimension, *Nature*, **424**, 870–872.
2. Aguirre, A., Planell, J. A., and Engel, E. (2010). Dynamics of bone marrow-derived endothelial progenitor cell/mesenchymal stem cell interaction in co-culture and its implications in angiogenesis, *Biochem. Biophys. Res. Co.*, **400**, 284–291.
3. Badylak, S. F., Taylor, D., and Uygun, K. (2011). Whole-organ tissue engineering: decellularization and recellularization of three-dimensional matrix scaffolds, *Annu. Rev. Biomed. Eng.*, **13**, 27–53.
4. Bártolo, P. J., et al. (2011). *Biofabrication Strategies for Tissue Engineering.* (Springer Netherlands, Dordrecht).
5. Battistelli, M., et al. (2005). Cell and matrix morpho-functional analysis in chondrocyte micromasses, *Microsc. Res. Techniq.*, **67**, 286–295.
6. Beniash, E., et al. (2005). Self-assembling peptide amphiphile nanofiber matrices for cell entrapment, *Acta Biomater.*, **1**, 387–397.
7. Bhardwaj, N., and Kundu, S. C. (2010). Electrospinning: a fascinating fiber fabrication technique, *Biotechnol. Adv.*, **28**, 325–347.
8. Bini, T. B., et al. (2004). Peripheral nerve regeneration by microbraided poly(L-lactide-co-glycolide) biodegradable polymer fibers, *J. Biomed. Mater. Res. A*, **68**, 286–295.
9. Boggs, M. E., et al. (2011). Co-culture of osteocytes and neurons on a unique patterned surface, *Biointerphases*, **6**, 200–209.
10. Carletti, E., Motta, A., and Migliaresi, C. (2011). Scaffolds for tissue engineering and 3D cell culture, in *3D Cell Culture Methods and Protocols*, (Haycock, J. W., eds), Humana Press, c/o Springer Science+Business Media, New York, pp. 17–39.

11. Chan, G., and Mooney, D. J. (2008). New materials for tissue engineering: towards greater control over the biological response, *Trends Biotechnol.*, **26**, 382–392.
12. Chan, M. E., et al. (2009). A trabecular bone explant model of osteocyte–osteoblast co-culture for bone mechanobiology, *Cell Mol. Bioeng.*, **2**, 405–415.
13. Chen, V. J., and Ma, P. X. (2004). Nano-fibrous poly(L-lactic acid) scaffolds with interconnected spherical macropores, *Biomaterials*, **25**, 2065–2073.
14. Chen, V. J., and Ma, P. X. (2006) Polymer Phase Seperation, in *Scaffolding in Tissue Engineering*, (Ma, P. X., and Elisseeff, J. H., eds.), Taylor and Francis Group, London pp. 125–138.
15. Chung, S., et al. (2009). Cell migration into scaffolds under co-culture conditions in a microfluidic platform, *Lab Chip*, **9**, 269–275.
16. Cooper, J. A., et al. (2005). Fiber-based tissue-engineered scaffold for ligament replacement: design considerations and in vitro evaluation, *Biomaterials*, **26**, 1523–1532.
17. Cooper, J. A., et al. (2007). Biomimetic tissue-engineered anterior cruciate ligament replacement, *P. Natl. Acad. Sci. USA*, **104**, 3049–3054.
18. Cui, X., et al. (2012). Direct human cartilage repair using three-dimensional bioprinting technology, *Tissue Eng. Pt. A*, **18**, 1–9.
19. Cukierman, E., Pankov, R., and Yamada, K. M. (2002). Cell interactions with three-dimensional matrices, *Curr. Opin. Cell Biol.*, **14**, 633–639.
20. DeLong, S. A., Moon, J. J., and West, J. L. (2005). Covalently immobilized gradients of bFGF on hydrogel scaffolds for directed cell migration, *Biomaterials*, **26**, 3227–3234.
21. Dertinger, S. K. W., et al. (2001). Generation of gradients having complex shapes using microfluidic networks, *Anal. Chem.*, **73**, 1240–1246.
22. Dodla, M. C., and Bellamkonda, R. V. (2006). Anisotropic scaffolds facilitate enhanced neurite extension in vitro, *J. Biomed. Mater. Res. A*, **78**, 213–221.
23. Dormer, N. H., et al. (2012). Osteochondral interface regeneration of the rabbit knee with macroscopic gradients of bioactive signals, *J. Biomed. Mater. Res. A*, **100**, 162–170.
24. Drury, J. L., and Mooney, D. J. (2003). Hydrogels for tissue engineering: scaffold design variables and applications, *Biomaterials*, **24**, 4337–4351.

25. Du, Y., et al. (2010). Convection driven generation of long-range material gradients, *Biomaterials*, **31**, 1–16.
26. Elder, B. D., Eleswarapu, S. V., and Athanasiou, K. A. (2009). Extraction techniques for the decellularization of tissue engineered articular cartilage constructs, *Biomaterials*, **30**, 3749–3756.
27. Elder, S. H., et al. (2009). Production of hyaline-like cartilage by bone marrow mesenchymal stem cells in a self-assembly model, *Tissue Eng. Pt. A*, **15**, 3025–3036.
28. Erisken, C., Kalyon, D. M., and Wang, H. (2008). Functionally graded electrospun polycaprolactone and beta-tricalcium phosphate nanocomposites for tissue engineering applications, *Biomaterials*, **29**, 4065–4073.
29. Freeman, J. W., Woods, M. D., and Laurencin, C. T. (2007). Tissue engineering of the anterior cruciate ligament using a braid-twist scaffold design, *J. Biomech.*, **40**, 243–252.
30. Funakoshi, T., et al. (2005). Application of tissue engineering techniques for rotator cuff regeneration using a chitosan-based hyaluronan hybrid fiber scaffold, *Am. J. Sport. Med.*, **33**, 1193–1201.
31. Gao, J., et al. (2002). Repair of osteochondral defect with tissue-engineered two-phase composite material of injectable calcium phosphate and hyaluronan sponge, *Tissue Eng.*, **8**, 827–837.
32. Ge, Z., et al. (2004). Biomaterials and scaffolds for ligament tissue engineering, *Med. J. Malaysia*, **59**, 71–72.
33. Ge, Z., et al. (2012). Functional biomaterials for cartilage regeneration, *J. Biomed. Mater. Res. A*, 100, 2526–2536.
34. Guo, S., et al. (2008). Neuroprotection via matrix-trophic coupling between cerebral endothelial cells and neurons, *P. Natl. Acad. Sci. USA*, **105**, 7582–7587.
35. Hairfield-Stein, M., et al. (2007). Development of self-assembled, tissue-engineered ligament from bone marrow stromal cells, *Tissue Eng.*, **13**, 703–710.
36. Hammoudi, T., Lu, H., and Temenoff, J. S. (2010). Long-term spatially defined coculture within, *Tissue Eng. Pt. C-Meth.*, **16**, 1621–1629.
37. Hammoudi, T. M., et al. (2012). 3D in vitro tri-culture platform to investigate effects of crosstalk between mesenchymal stem cells, osteoblasts and adipocytes, *Tissue Eng. Pt. A*, **18**, 1686–1697.
38. Handschel, J. G. K., et al. (2007). Prospects of micromass culture technology in tissue engineering, *Head Face Med.*, **3**, 4.

39. Harimoto, M., et al. (2002). Novel approach for achieving double-layered cell sheets co-culture: overlaying endothelial cell sheets onto monolayer hepatocytes utilizing temperature-responsive culture dishes, *J. Biomed. Mater. Res.*, **62**, 464–470.
40. Hartgerink, J., Beniash, E., and Stupp, S. I. (2001). Self-assembly and mineralization of peptide-amphiphile nanofibers, *Science*, **294**, 1684–1688.
41. Haycock, J. W. (2011). *3D Cell Culture Methods and Protocols*. (Humana Press, c/o Springer Science+Business Media, New York).
42. Haycock, J. W. (2011) 3D cell culture: a review of current approaches and techniques, in *3D Cell Culture Methods and Protocols* (Haycock, J. W., eds) Humana Press, c/o Springer Science+Business Media, New York, pp. 1–15.
43. He, J., et al. (2010). Rapid generation of biologically relevant hydrogels containing long-range chemical gradients, *Adv. Funct. Mater.*, **20**, 131–137.
44. Ho, S. T. B., et al. (2010). The evaluation of a biphasic osteochondral implant coupled with an electrospun membrane in a large animal model, *Tissue Eng. Pt. A*, **16**, 1123–1141.
45. Hoben, G. M., et al. (2007). Self-assembly of fibrochondrocytes and chondrocytes for tissue engineering of the knee meniscus, *Tissue Eng.*, **13**, 939–946.
46. Hodde, J. (2002). Naturally occuring scaffolds for soft tissue repair and regeneration, *Tissue Eng.*, **8**, 295–308.
47. Holland, T. A., et al. (2005). Osteochondral repair in the rabbit model utilizing bilayered, degradable oligo(poly(ethylene glycol) fumarate) hydrogel scaffolds, *J. Biomed. Mater. Res. A*, **75**, 156–167.
48. Hsiao, A. Y., et al. (2009). Microfluidic system for formation of PC-3 prostate cancer co-culture spheroids, *Biomaterials*, **30**, 3020–3027.
49. Huang, C. P., et al. (2009). Engineering microscale cellular niches for three-dimensional multicellular co-cultures, *Lab Chip*, **9**, 1740–1748.
50. Huh, D., et al. (2010). Reconstituting organ-level lung functions on a chip, *Science*, **328**, 1662–1668.
51. Hung, A. M., and Stupp, S. I. (2007). Simultaneous self-assembly, orientation, and patterning of peptide-amphiphile nanofibers by soft lithography, *Nano Lett.*, **7**, 1165–1171.
52. Hutmacher, D. W., Sittinger, M., and Risbud, M. V. (2004). Scaffold-based tissue engineering: rationale for computer-aided design and solid free-form fabrication systems, *Trends Biotechnol.*, **22**, 354–362.

53. Ilkhanizadeh, S., Teixeira, A. I., and Hermanson, O. (2007). Inkjet printing of macromolecules on hydrogels to steer neural stem cell differentiation, *Biomaterials*, **28**, 3936–3943.
54. Jeon, N. L., et al. (2000). Generation of solution and surface gradients using microfluidic systems, *Lagmuir*, **16**, 8311–8316.
55. Jiang, J., Nicoll, S. B., and Lu, H. H. (2005). Co-culture of osteoblasts and chondrocytes modulates cellular differentiation in vitro, *Biochem. Biophys. Res. Co.*, **338**, 762–770.
56. Jiang, J., et al. (2008). Interaction between zonal populations of articular chondrocytes suppresses chondrocyte mineralization and this process is mediated by PTHrP, *Osteoarth. Cartilage*, **16**, 70–82.
57. Jiang, J., et al. (2010). Bioactive stratified polymer ceramic-hydrogel scaffold for integrative osteochondral repair, *Ann. Biomed. Eng.*, **38**, 2183–2196.
58. Kaji, H., et al. (2009). Controlled cocultures of HeLa cells and human umbilical vein endothelial cells on detachable substrates, *Lab Chip*, **9**, 427–432.
59. Kaji, H., et al. (2011). Engineering systems for the generation of patterned co-cultures for controlling cell–cell interactions, *Biochem. Biophys. Acta*, **1810**, 239–250.
60. Kapur, T. A., and Shoichet, M. S. (2004). Immobilized concentration gradients of nerve growth factor guide neurite outgrowth, *J. Biomed. Mater. Res. A*, **68**, 235–243.
61. Keenan, T. M., and Folch, A. (2008). Biomolecular gradients in cell culture systems, *Lab Chip*, **8**, 34–57.
62. Khademhosseini, A., et al. (2004). Layer-by-layer deposition of hyaluronic acid and poly-L-lysine for patterned cell co-cultures, *Biomaterials*, **25**, 3583–3592.
63. Kirkpatrick, C. J., Fuchs, S., and Unger, R. E. (2011). Co-culture systems for vascularization--learning from nature, *Adv. Drug Deliv. Rev.*, **63**, 291–299.
64. Korff, T., et al. (2001). Blood vessel maturation in a 3-dimensional spheroidal coculture model: direct contact with smooth muscle cells regulates endothelial cell quiescence and abrogates VEGF responsiveness, *FASEB J.*, **15**, 447–457.
65. Lacroix, D., Planell, J. A., and Prendergast, P. J. (2009). Computer-aided design and finite-element modelling of biomaterial scaffolds for bone tissue engineering, *Philos. T. R. Soc. A*, **367**, 1993–2009.

66. Laurencin, C. T., and Freeman, J. W. (2005). Ligament tissue engineering: an evolutionary materials science approach, *Biomaterials*, **26**, 7530–7536.
67. Lee, J., Cuddihy, M. J., and Kotov, N. A. (2008). Three-dimensional cell culture matrices: state of the art, *Tissue Eng. Pt. B-Rev.*, **14**, 61–86.
68. Li, X., et al. (2009). Nanofiber scaffolds with gradations in mineral content for mimicking the tendon-to-bone insertion site, *Nano Lett.*, **9**, 2763–2768.
69. Lin, R.-Z., Lin, R.-Z., and Chang, H.-Y. (2008). Recent advances in three-dimensional multicellular spheroid culture for biomedical research, *Biotechnol. J.*, **3**, 1172–1184.
70. Liu, C., Han, Z., and Czernuszka, J. T. (2009). Gradient collagen/nano-hydroxyapatite composite scaffold: development and characterization, *Acta Biomater.*, **5**, 661–669.
71. Liu, L., et al. (2008). Multinozzle low-temperature deposition system for construction of gradient tissue engineering scaffolds, *J. Biomed. Mater. Res. B*, **88**, 254–263.
72. Liu, L., et al. (2009). A novel osteochondral scaffold fabricated via multi-nozzle low-temperature deposition manufacturing, *J. Bioact. Compat. Pol.*, **24**, 18–30.
73. Lo, C. M., et al. (2000). Cell movement is guided by the rigidity of the substrate, *Biophys. J.*, **79**, 144–152.
74. Lo, C. T., et al. (2008). Photopolymerized diffusion-defined polyacrylamide gradient gels for on-chip protein sizing, *Lab Chip*, **8**, 1273–1279.
75. Lodish, H., et al. (2008). *Molecular Cell Biology*. (W. H. Freeman and Company), New York, New York.
76. Lozito, T. P., et al. (2009). Human mesenchymal stem cells express vascular cell phenotypes upon interaction with endothelial cell matrix, *J. Cell Biochem.*, **107**, 714–722.
77. Lu, H. H., et al. (2005). Anterior cruciate ligament regeneration using braided biodegradable scaffolds: in vitro optimization studies, *Biomaterials*, **26**, 4805–4816.
78. Lu, H. H., and Jang, J. (2006). Interface tissue engineering and the formulation of multiple-tissue systems, *Adv. Biochem. Eng. Biotechnol.*, **102**, 91–111.
79. Lu, H. H., et al. (2010). Tissue engineering strategies for the regeneration of orthopedic interfaces, *Ann. Biomed. Eng.*, **38**, 2142–2154.

80. Lutolf, M. P. (2009). Biomaterials: spotlight on hydrogels, *Nat. Mater.*, **8**, 451–453.
81. Ma, J., et al. (2009). Morphological and functional characteristics of three-dimensional engineered bone–ligament–bone constructs following implantation, *J. Biomech. Eng.-T. ASME*, **131**, 101017-1-101017-9.
82. Maier, D., et al. (2007). In vitro analysis of an allogenic scaffold for tissue-engineered meniscus replacement, *J. Orthop. Res.*, **25**, 1598–1608.
83. Marimuthu, M., and Kim, S. (2011). Microfluidic cell coculture methods for understanding cell biology, analyzing bio/pharmaceuticals, and developing tissue constructs, *Anal. Biochem.*, **413**, 81–89.
84. Martin, I., et al. (2007). Osteochondral tissue engineering, *J. Biomech.*, **40**, 750–765.
85. Martinek, V., et al. (2002). Enhancement of tendon–bone integration of anterior cruciate ligament grafts with bone morphogenetic protein-2 gene transfer, *J. Bone Joint Surg.*, **84-A**, 1123–1132.
86. Mikos, A. G., et al. (2006). Engineering complex tissues, *Tissue Eng.*, **12**, 3307–3339.
87. Moffat, K. L., et al. (2009). Orthopaedic interface tissue engineering for the biological fixation of soft tissue grafts, *Clin. Sport Med.*, **28**, 157–176.
88. Moutos, F. T., Freed, L. E., and Guilak, F. (2007). A biomimetic three-dimensional woven composite scaffold for functional tissue engineering of cartilage, *Nat. Mater.*, **6**, 162–167.
89. Munoz-Pinto, D. J., et al. (2010). Inorganic-organic hybrid scaffolds for osteochondral regeneration, *J. Biomed. Mater. Res. A*, **94**, 112–121.
90. Murugan, R., and Ramakrishna, S. (2006). Nano-featured scaffolds for tissue engineering: a review of spinning methodologies, *Tissue Eng.*, **12**, 435–447.
91. Murugan, R., and Ramakrishna, S. (2007). Design strategies of tissue engineering scaffolds with controlled fiber orientation, *Tissue Eng.*, **13**, 1845–1866.
92. Mutsuzaki, H., et al. (2004). Calcium-phosphate-hybridized tendon directly promotes regeneration of tendon–bone insertion, *J. Biomed. Mater. Res. A*, **70**, 319–327.
93. Nakaoka, R., Hsiong, S. X., and Mooney, D. J. (2006). Regulation of chondrocyte differentiation level via co-culture with osteoblasts, *Tissue Eng.*, **12**, 2425–2433.

94. Niederauer, G. G., et al. (2000). Evaluation of multiphase implants for repair of focal osteochondral defects in goats, *Biomaterials*, **21**, 2561–2574.
95. Nisbet, D. R., et al. (2009). Review paper: a review of the cellular response on electrospun nanofibers for tissue engineering, *J. Biomater. Appl.*, **24**, 7–29.
96. Palmer, L. C., and Stupp, S. I. (2009). Molecular self-assembly into one-dimensional nanostructures, *Acc Chem. Res.*, **41**, 1674–1684.
97. Paramonov, S. E., Jun, H.-W., and Hartgerink, J. D. (2006). Self-assembly of peptide-amphiphile nanofibers: the roles of hydrogen bonding and amphiphilic packing, *J. Am. Chem. Soc.*, **128**, 7291–7298.
98. Park, J., et al. (2009). Microfluidic compartmentalized co-culture platform for CNS axon myelination research, *Biomed. Microdev*, **11**, 1145–1153.
99. Paz, A. C., Javaherian, S., and McGuigan, A. P. (2012). Micropatterning co-cultures of epithelial cells on filter insert substrates, *J. Epithelial Biol. Pharmacol.*, **5**, 77–85.
100. Peltola, S. M., et al. (2008). A review of rapid prototyping techniques for tissue engineering purposes, *Ann. Med.*, **40**, 268–280.
101. Peret, B. J., and Murphy, W. L. (2008). Controllable soluble protein concentration gradients in hydrogel networks, *Adv. Funct. Mater.*, **18**, 3410–3417.
102. Phillippi, J. A., et al. (2008). Microenvironments engineered by inkjet bioprinting spatially direct adult stem cells toward muscle- and bone-like subpopulations, *Stem Cells*, **26**, 127–134.
103. Phillips, J. E., et al. (2008). Engineering graded tissue interfaces, *P. Natl. Acad. Sci. USA*, **105**, 12170–12175.
104. Place, E. S., Evans, N. D., and Stevens, M. M. (2009). Complexity in biomaterials for tissue engineering, *Nat. Mater.*, **8**, 457–470.
105. Ramalingam, M., et al. (2012). Nanofiber scaffold gradients for interfacial tissue engineering, *J. Biomater. Appl.*, **0**, 1–11.
106. Reddi, A. H., Becerra, J., and Andrades, J. A. (2011). Nanomaterials and hydrogel scaffolds for articular cartilage regeneration, *Tissue Eng. Pt. B-Rev.*, **17**, 301–305.
107. Sant, S., et al. (2010). Biomimetic gradient hydrogels for tissue engineering, *Can. J. Chem. Eng.*, **88**, 899–911.
108. Sargeant, T. D., et al. (2008). Hybrid bone implants: self-assembly of peptide amphiphile nanofibers within porous titanium, *Biomaterials*, **29**, 161–171.

109. Schanz, J., et al. (2010). Vascularised human tissue models: a new approach for the refinement of biomedical research, *J. Biotechnol.*, **148**, 56–63.

110. Seidi, A., et al. (2011). Gradient biomaterials for soft-to-hard interface tissue engineering, *Acta Biomater.*, **7**, 1441–1451.

111. Sharma, B., et al. (2007). Designing zonal organization into tissue-engineered cartilage, *Tissue Eng.*, **13**, 405–414.

112. Sherwood, J. K., et al. (2002). A three-dimensional osteochondral composite scaffold for articular cartilage repair, *Biomaterials*, **23**, 4739–4751.

113. Shi, J., et al. (2010). Incorporating protein gradient into electrospun nanofibers as scaffolds for tissue engineering, *ACS Appl. Mater. Interfaces*, **2**, 1025–1030.

114. Singh, M., Berkland, C., and Detamore, M. S. (2008). Strategies and applications for incorporating physical and chemical signal gradients in tissue engineering, *Tissue Eng. Pt. B-Rev.*, **14**, 341–366.

115. Singh, M., et al. (2008). Microsphere-based seamless scaffolds containing macroscopic gradients of encapsulated factors for tissue engineering, *Tissue Eng. Pt. C-Meth.*, **14**, 299–309.

116. Singh, M., et al. (2010). Microsphere-based scaffolds for cartilage tissue engineering: using subcritical CO(2) as a sintering agent, *Acta Biomater.*, **6**, 137–143.

117. Smith, L. A., and Ma, P. X. (2004). Nano-fibrous scaffolds for tissue engineering, *Colloid Surf. B*, **39**, 125–131.

118. Song, J. W., et al. (2009). Microfluidic endothelium for studying the intravascular adhesion of metastatic breast cancer cells, *PloS One*, **4**, e5756–e5756.

119. Spalazzi, J. P., et al. (2006). Development of controlled matrix heterogeneity on a triphasic scaffold for orthopedic interface tissue engineering, *Tissue Eng.*, **12**, 3497–3508.

120. Spalazzi, J. P., et al. (2008). In vivo evaluation of a multiphased scaffold designed for orthopaedic interface tissue engineering and soft tissue-to-bone integration, *J. Biomed. Mater. Res. A*, **86**, 1–12.

121. Spector, J. A., et al. (2002). Experimental co-culture of osteoblasts with immature dural cells causes an increased rate and degree of osteoblast differentiation, *Plast. Reconstr. Surg.*, **109**, 631–642.

122. Stahl, A., et al. (2004). Bi-directional cell contact-dependent regulation of gene expression between endothelial cells and osteoblasts in a

three-dimensional spheroidal coculture model, *Biochem. Biophys. Res. Co.*, **322**, 684–692.

123. Stendahl, J. C., et al. (2006). Intermolecular forces in the self-assembly of peptide amphiphile nanofibers, *Adv. Funct. Mater.*, **16**, 499–508.

124. Sudo, R., et al. (2009). Transport-mediated angiogenesis in 3D epithelial coculture, *FASEB J.*, **23**, 2155–2164.

125. Suzuki, M., et al. (2008). Negative dielectrophoretic patterning with different cell types, *Biosens. Bioelectron.*, **24**, 1049–1053.

126. Syed-picard, F. N., et al. (2009). Three-dimensional engineered bone from bone marrow stromal cells and their autogenous extracellular matrix, *Tissue Eng. Pt. A*, **15**, 187–195.

127. Takayama, S., et al. (1999). Patterning cells and their environments using multiple laminar, *P. Natl. Acad. Sci. USA*, **96**, 5545–5548.

128. Tampieri, A., et al. (2008). Design of graded biomimetic osteochondral composite scaffolds, *Biomaterials*, **29**, 3539–3546.

129. Tan, W., and Desai, T. A. (2005). Microscale multilayer cocultures for biomimetic blood vessels, *J. Biomed. Mater. Res. A*, **72**, 146–160.

130. Tare, R. S., et al. (2005). Tissue engineering strategies for cartilage generation--micromass and three dimensional cultures using human chondrocytes and a continuous cell line, *Biochem. Biophys. Res. Co.*, **333**, 609–621.

131. Tibbet, M. W., and Anseth, K. S. (2009). Hydrogels as extracellular matrix mimics for 3D cell culture, *Biotechnol. Bioeng.*, **103**, 655–663.

132. Torisawa, Y.-S., et al. (2009). Microfluidic hydrodynamic cellular patterning for systematic formation of co-culture spheroids, *Integr. Biol.*, **1**, 649–654.

133. Tripathi, A., Kathuria, N., and Kumar, A. (2009). Elastic and macroporous agarose-gelatin cryogels with isotropic and anisotropic porosity for tissue engineering, *J. Biomed. Mater. Res. A*, **90**, 680–694.

134. Tsuda, Y., et al. (2005). The use of patterned dual thermoresponsive surfaces for the collective recovery as co-cultured cell sheets, *Biomaterials*, **26**, 1885–1893.

135. Tsuda, Y., et al. (2006). Heterotypic cell interactions on a dually patterned surface, *Biochem. Biophys. Res. Co.*, **348**, 937–944.

136. Tsuda, Y., et al. (2007). Cellular control of tissue architectures using a three-dimensional tissue fabrication technique, *Biomaterials*, **28**, 4939–4946.

137. Vickerman, V., et al. (2008). Design, fabrication and implementation of a novel multi parameter control microfluidic platform for

three-dimensional cell culture and real-time imaging, *Lab Chip*, **8**, 1468–1477.

138. Wahl, D. A., et al. (2007). Controlling the processing of collagen-hydroxyapatite scaffolds for bone tissue engineering, *J. Mater. Sci.*, **18**, 201–209.

139. Wang, I. N. E., and Lu, H. H. (2006). Role of cell–cell interactions on the regeneration of soft tissue-to-bone interface, *Proc. of the 28th IEEE EMBS Annual International Conference*, pp. 783–786.

140. Wang, I. N. E., et al. (2007). Role of osteoblast—fibroblast interactions in the formation of the ligament-to-bone interface, *J. Orthop. Res.*, **25**, 1609–1609.

141. Wang, Y., et al. (2009). A novel method for preparing electrospun fibers with nano-/micro-scale porous structures, *Polym. Bull.*, **63**, 259–265.

142. Wenger, A., et al. (2004). Modulation of in vitro angiogenesis in a three-dimensional spheroidal coculture model for bone tissue engineering, *Tissue Eng.*, **10**, 1536–1547.

143. Wong, A. P., et al. (2008). Partitioning microfluidic channels with hydrogel to construct tunable 3-D cellular microenvironments, *Biomaterials*, **29**, 1853–1861.

144. Wong, J. Y., et al. (2003). Directed movement of vascular smooth muscle cells on gradient compliant hydrogels, *Lagmuir*, **19**, 1908–1913.

145. Wright, D., et al. (2007). Generation of static and dynamic patterned co-cultures using microfabricated parylene-C stencils, *Lab Chip*, **7**, 1272–1279.

146. Xie, J., Li, X., and Xia, Y. (2008). Putting electrospun nanofibers to work for biomedical research, *Macromol. Rapid Comm.*, **29**, 1775–1792.

147. Xie, J., et al. (2010). "Aligned-to-random" nanofiber scaffolds for mimicking the structure of the tendon-to-bone insertion site, *Nanoscale*, **2**, 923–926.

148. Yan, Y., et al. (2003). Layered manufacturing of tissue engineering scaffolds via multi-nozzle deposition, *Mater. Lett.*, **57**, 2623–2628.

149. Yang, F., et al. (2004). Fabrication of nano-structured porous PLLA scaffold intended for nerve tissue engineering, *Biomaterials*, **25**, 1891–1900.

150. Yang, I. H., Co, C. C., and Ho, C.-C. (2005). Spatially controlled co-culture of neurons and glial cells, *J. Biomed. Mater. Res. A*, **75**, 976–84.

151. Yang, P. J., and Temenoff, J. S. (2009). Engineering orthopedic tissue interfaces, *Tissue Eng. Pt. B-Rev.*, **15**, 127–141.

152. Yeon, J. H., and Park, J.-K. (2007). Microfluidic cell culture systems for cellular analysis, *Biochip J.*, **1**, 17–27.

153. Zhang, L., and Webster, T. J. (2009). Nanotechnology and nanomaterials: Promises for improved tissue regeneration, *Nano Today*, **4**, 66–80.

154. Zhang, S., et al. (2002). Design of nanostructured biological materials through self-assembly of peptides and proteins, *Curr. Opin. Cell Biol.*, **6**, 865–871.

Chapter 5

Spatiotemporal Genetic Control of Cellular Systems

Lauren R. Polstein and Charles A. Gersbach

Department of Biomedical Engineering, Duke University,
2353C CIEMAS, PO Box 90281, 136 Hudson Hall, Durham, NC 27708, USA

charles.gersbach@duke.edu

5.1 Introduction

A major hurdle in tissue and organ regeneration has been the recapitulation of native tissue morphology and function. Most native tissues consist of complex multicellular networks that cannot be recreated by any one specific adult cell type. Although it is possible to mimic native tissue environments in vitro by co-culturing two or more cell types [1–4], the current state of these methods is better suited for studying cell–cell interactions and their role in tissue formation rather than for engineering tissues for therapeutic use. This is because these approaches cannot be easily used to create complex patterns of various cell types within a tissue. Therefore there is a need for controlling cell differentiation in complex spatial patterns in vitro. Because cell differentiation and tissue formation are ultimately governed by gene regulation, systems that facilitate

---

Tissue and Organ Regeneration: Advances in Micro- and Nanotechnology
Edited by Lijie Grace Zhang, Ali Khademhosseini, and Thomas J. Webster
Copyright © 2014 Pan Stanford Publishing Pte. Ltd.
ISBN 978-981-4411-67-7 (Hardcover), 978-981-4411-68-4 (eBook)
www.panstanford.com

external spatial and temporal control of gene expression provide a promising approach to creating functional engineered tissues. This strategy enables directed differentiation of select cells in vitro and in vivo, potentially allowing the patterning of cell types and control of cellular communication in a way that promotes the formation of native-like tissues.

There are various levels of genetic control, each of which provides the opportunity to modulate protein expression in time, space, or both. The least specific level of gene regulation involves the use of constitutive promoters upstream of a transgene; in these systems the gene is always expressed. In contrast, gene regulatory systems that activate genes in both space and time in response to various stimuli, including light, ultraviolet (UV) irradiation, and heat, currently provide the greatest level of control. The type of gene regulatory system that one chooses depends on the requirements of the target engineered tissue. Tissues containing only one cell type may only require the simplest form gene regulation, such as a gene driven by a constitutive promoter; however, complex tissues typically require more sophisticated gene regulatory systems.

5.2 Time-Independent Gene Regulation Systems

5.2.1 Constitutive Gene Expression Systems

Simple engineered tissues, such as functional cartilage, skin, and bladder, can be implanted as monocellular tissues and therefore do not require highly sophisticated gene regulation. Unlike thicker tissues, simple tissue types do not need complex vasculature for survival during in vitro culture or after they are implanted. For example, cartilage is naturally avascular, and skin and bladder tissue are thin and have low metabolic activity, allowing the tissues to rely mainly on diffusion for oxygen and nutrients [5]. As a result, simple tissues are typically engineered using a transgene driven by a constitutive promoter, which does not provide any control over the spatial or temporal expression of the transgene (Fig. 5.1a). In some cases, such as with engineered cartilage and skin tissues, genetic modification is not necessary to form implantable tissue. However, cells are often engineered to express genes that will enhance cell expansion, engraftment, or healing or that will systemically treat an underlying condition or disease.

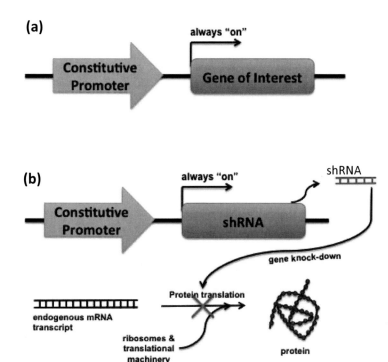

Figure 5.1 Constitutive gene expression systems. (a) Placement of a transgene of interest downstream of a constitutive promoter results in spatially and temporally independent expression of the transgene. (b) Placement of an shRNA construct downstream of a constitutive promoter results in constitutive transcription of the shRNA, which causes silencing of target gene expression through RNA interference.

Cartilage is perhaps the simplest tissue in the human body in that it contains only one cell type (chondrocytes) and is avascular and aneural. However, despite this morphological simplicity, cartilage tissue engineering is complicated by the tissue's role as a low-friction, load-bearing material within the body. For chondrocyte implantation, patient chondrocytes can be isolated and expanded ex vivo [6]. This expansion process provides the opportunity to genetically modify the cells before they are implanted back into the patient. In one study, chondrocytes were transduced with a retroviral vector encoding a constitutively expressed gene for bone morphogenic protein-7 (BMP-7) to expedite the cartilage repair process post-implantation [7]. BMP-7 is normally expressed in articular cartilage [8] and is important for limb and joint formation [9]. Modified or unmodified chondrocytes were suspended in fibrinogen, and this mixture was polymerized in situ in an adult cartilage defect repair horse model. After 4 weeks, implanted BMP-7-expressing chondrocytes exhibited a round, chondrocyte-like morphology and integrated with host subchondral bone, whereas unmodified control chondrocytes were flatter and did not integrate well with host subchondral bone. After 8 months, the appearance, morphology, and integration of treated and control cells were equivalent. Thus, although the end result was the same using genetically modified or unmodified chondrocytes, cells that over-expressed BMP-7 accelerated cartilage tissue repair.

Although it is possible to correct smaller defects in situ and generate cartilage tissue in vitro through expansion of patient-derived chondrocytes, other methods are being explored due to the low availability of chondrocytes and their tendency to dedifferentiate during in vitro culture. These alternative methods are necessary for the repair and replacement of larger defects. There is particular interest in the use of patient-derived adult mesenchymal stem cells (MSCs) for cell-based cartilage repair because they are relatively easy to isolate and expand, and their multipotency enables them to differentiate into multiple connective tissue types [10,11]. There are many factors that govern the differentiation of MSCs into chondrocytes, including transforming growth factor-β (TGF-β) superfamily members, BMPs, Wnt proteins, and fibroblast growth factors (FGFs). Differentiation also depends on the presence of cartilage-specific matrix materials such as type II collagen, aggrecan, and fibronectin [10]. MSCs can be genetically engineered to over-express these factors or deposit these materials to facilitate their differentiation into chondrocytes and improve local cartilage repair [12–14]. For instance, isolated murine muscle-derived stem cells were transduced with retrovirus encoding BMP-4 and LacZ and transplanted into a full thickness articular cartilage defect murine model [15]. Modified cells locally delivered BMP-4, which enhanced chondrocyte differentiation and improved articular cartilage repair as compared to unmodified cells for 24 weeks following cell transplantation.

Genetically modified cells are also being tested for the treatment of debilitating diseases such as rheumatoid arthritis. In a phase I clinical study, autologous synovial fibroblasts were engineered to constitutively express IL-1 receptor antagonist (IL-1Ra), which has been shown to alleviate symptoms of rheumatoid arthritis in mice [13]. These modified cells or control cells were injected into the metacarpophalangeal joints of postmenopausal women suffering from rheumatoid arthritis. After 1 week, joints treated with genetically engineered cells were positive for IL-1Ra mRNA, and the synovial fluid of patients that received intermediate and high doses of treated cells produced high levels of IL-1Ra protein. Future clinical studies are needed to assess the clinical efficacy of the IL-1Ra transgene expression.

In addition to expedited engraftment and healing and treatment of diseases, genetically modified cells can also be used to improve the functionality of implanted constructs and grafts. While simple tissues have been shown to function when implanted as monocellular constructs, functionality can be improved by promoting the recruitment of other cell types once implanted in the body. For example, epidermal keratinocyte skin grafts have been shown to successfully cover wounds, enhance patient survival, and relieve pain due to burns [16], vascular leg ulcers [17], epidermolysis bullosa [18], and other ailments [19], but full, native-like functionality and integration of skin grafts requires the presence of other skin cell types such as mast cells and Langerhans cells. Instead of culturing these cell types along with keratinocytes in vitro before implantation, genetic engineering could be used to release factors that promote migration and infiltration of host cells into the implanted construct. Consequently, improved graft incorporation and functionality may be achieved. This type of modification is short-term such that the treatment lasts only during the wound healing process. Gene expression can be temporarily modified within grafted keratinocytes by immobilizing plasmid DNA or non-integrating virus (i.e., adenovirus) packaged with a desired gene to the scaffold surface. Controlled release of the DNA or virus from the scaffold results in transfection or transduction, respectively, of grafted keratinocytes. Benefits of this approach include local gene delivery only to implanted cells or cells that infiltrate the wound site, protection of the genetic material from proteases present in the healing wound environment, and reduced immunogenicity of the material due to its isolation from host immune cells [20–22].

One study observed the effect of embedded DNA encoding the gene for platelet derived growth factor (PDGF-A or PDGF-B) in a collagen matrix on wound healing [23]. PDGF is a growth factor that been shown to recruit neutrophils, monocytes, fibroblasts, and smooth muscle cells to a healing wound, and reduced expression of PDGF-A had been shown to impair wound healing [24]. Keratinocytes were seeded onto this matrix, and the resulting construct was implanted in an ischemic rabbit ear model. This improved wound healing by reducing wound contraction and increasing host cell infiltration into the wound site.

In some cases, it may be desirable to achieve long-term or permanent gene expression within grafted cells. This is usually done through modification of cells prior to being seeded onto the extracellular matrix scaffold. The most common way to engineer cells for long-term gene expression is via viral transduction using a lentivirus or retrovirus that has been engineered to be replication-incompetent [21,25]. In contrast to adenoviruses and adeno-associated viruses, these viruses are able to integrate a packaged transgene into the cell's genome to achieve sustained gene expression. Long-term gene expression on the order of months to years can also be achieved using adeno-associated viruses, which in nondividing cells persists in an episomal state without integrating into the genome [26–28]. One application of permanent modification of implanted cells is treatment of the underlying disease that caused the patient's need for a graft. For example, diabetic patients often need skin grafts to heal foot and ankle ulcers caused by diabetic neuropathy and ischemia. Keratinocytes have been modified to express and systemically release insulin to reverse hyperglycemia in mice with streptozotocin-induced diabetes [29]. Such keratinocytes could be used to make skin grafts for diabetic patients to help regulate glucose levels.

In vitro viral transduction of cells has also been used to confer anti-microbial properties to grafted keratinocytes. This is highly desirable because infection is the major cause of mortality in burn victims [30]. Furthermore, decreased infection can improve graft integration by reducing host immune response to the graft. Although infection is usually treated using antimicrobial drugs, this management method increases the risk for the emergence of resistant bacteria. In one study, keratinocytes were transduced with retrovirus packaged with the gene encoding human beta-defensin-4 (HBD4) under control of a constitutive promoter [31]. HBD4 has been shown to have bactericidal activity against *Pseudomonas aeruginosa*, a bacteria commonly associated with burn wound infection [30]. The HBD4-expressing keratinocytes showed a significant 29% reduction in bacterial colony formation as compared to control cells.

5.2.2 Constitutive Gene Silencing

Recently, much interest has turned to RNA interference for constitutive knockdown of gene expression (Fig. 5.1b). This has been achieved through delivery of double-stranded RNA molecules conjugated to nanoparticles or by delivery of small-hairpin RNA (shRNA)-encoding DNA vectors [32]. For example, oligonucleotides that are designed to target a gene of interest can be conjugated to gold nanoparticles via thiol groups or electrostatic interactions [33]. Once inside cells, these oligonucleotides have been shown to efficiently scavenge intracellular DNA or RNA to result in knockdown of the targeted gene. Furthermore, one can tune the level of knockdown by changing the density of oligonucleotides on the nanoparticle or by chemically modifying the conjugated oligonucleotides [33,34]. While this technology is still in its infancy, there are many opportunities for its potential use in tissue engineering. For example, it would be beneficial to knockdown genes during in vitro expansion of host cells, such as chondrocytes, to prevent dedifferentiation of cells. Nanoparticles could also be used for gene knock down in implanted cells. For instance, delivery of small interfering RNA (siRNA) that targets inflammatory proteins may mitigate the host's immune response to the tissue construct, improving engraftment.

5.3 Systems for Temporal Control of Gene Regulation

Tissues and organisms naturally develop and regenerate through highly precise temporal control of endogenous genes. When this self-regulation is disrupted, detrimental or fatal effects to individual cells or the entire organism often result. One of the most established examples of this is the process of embryonic and fetal development. Fertilization of an egg initiates a precise order of events involving cell division and differential gene expression that follows an exact temporal schedule. For example, in mouse embryonic heart development, the heart is first recognizable on embryonic day 7.75 as the cardiac crescent. By embryonic day 8.0 the heart tube is visible, and it begins to loop around the lung branchial arches by embryonic day 9.5 [35]. These developments are driven by exactly timed gene expression and cell division; failure of a key gene to be expressed can result in failed development. For instance, *Nanog* null embryos cannot develop beyond implantation [36], suggesting that activation of Nanog at the time of implantation is required for embryonic survival and development.

Precise timing of gene regulation can also be observed in vitro. Because of the promise of stem cells as a cell source for tissue engineering, extensive research has been carried out to determine the key genes and genetic timing of expression in both cells that are coaxed to dedifferentiate into induced pluripotent stem cells (iPSCs) and in multipotent cells that are differentiated into tissue-specific cell types. Discovery of the Yamanaka factors c-Myc, Oct3/4, Klf-4, and Sox2 provided the ability to make iPSCs from differentiated adult human fibroblasts [37]. Further studies have characterized the downstream genetic effects of overexpression of these genes and have discovered that there is distinct sequential activation of pluripotency markers. For instance, mouse somatic cells treated with the four Yamanaka factors via viral transduction show early activation of alkaline phosphatase three days after transduction. This is followed by SSEA1 expression at day 9 and Oct4 and Nanog at day 16 [38]. Clearly, there is a defined timeline of gene activation in induced pluripotency.

In order to recapitulate the morphology and function of native tissues, the effects of temporally defined gene transcription on cellular fate must be understood. As with iPSCs, differentiation of multipotent cells also follows defined timelines of gene activation that are still being elucidated. Differentiation of fibroblasts into myoblasts can be initiated by overexpression of MyoD, which activates the downstream myogenic markers creatine kinase, troponin T, myogenin, and others [39,40]. Expression of these downstream genes induces cell fusion and myotube formation characteristic of muscle tissue.

Temporal gene regulation systems are crucial tools for studying gene induction profiles, and can be valuable for molding engineered tissues from differentiating cells. In order to recapitulate the morphology and function of native tissues, scientists must be able to reproduce temporal patterns of gene expression that occur naturally during development and regeneration. There are several gene regulation systems that enable the temporal regulation of episomal and endogenous genes. Most of these systems can be grouped into two major categories: chemically induced systems and hormonally induced systems. Through various mechanisms, addition of a chemical or hormone in vitro or in vivo elicits a cellular response that activates or represses a target gene. The cellular effect can be easily tuned by changing the concentration of the inducer molecule, enabling control over a wide range of expression levels. This can be used to elucidate the role of a particular gene during tissue development or to construct tissues. Furthermore, the ability to turn a gene "on" or "off" can reduce off-target effects or toxicity of the controlled transgene.

There are also potential applications for temporal gene regulation in the treatment of chronic ailments and diseases, as a therapeutic transgene can be intermittently expressed as needed. For example, temporal control of the expression of growth factors that promote wound healing could be used to treat chronic ulcers [41,42]. Alternatively, chronic inflammation could be treated via expression of anti-inflammatory proteins, such as the peroxisome proliferator-activated receptor γ (PPARγ) for alleviation of intestinal inflammation observed in inflammatory bowel disease [43].

5.3.1 Chemically Induced Gene Regulation Systems

5.3.1.1 Tetracycline-inducible system

One of the most widely used gene regulation systems for temporal genetic control is the tetracycline (Tet)-inducible system (Fig. 5.2).

There are two major forms of this system: one in which Tet (or its derivative doxycycline, Dox) represses expression of a transgene ("TetOff"), and one in which Tet induces expression of a transgene ("TetOn"). There are five variants of these major forms, each of which will be discussed in detail below. These systems can be used to cycle gene expression by adding or removing Dox from the cell culture media. Expression levels can also be tuned based on Dox concentration.

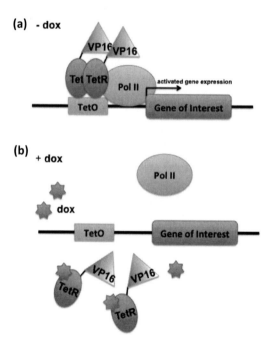

Figure 5.2 Tetracycline-OFF gene expression system. The Tet-controlled transcriptional activator (tTA) consists of the DNA binding domain of TetR fused to the transcriptional activation domain VP16. (a) tTA binds the Tet Operon (TetO) in the absence of Dox. This recruits RNA Polymerase II (PolII) to the target transgene and activates transcription. (b) Dox binds to TetR and prevents it from binding TetO, abolishing recruitment of PolII and inhibiting transcription of the transgene.

Tet-inducible systems are based on the *E. coli* Tn10 Tet resistance operon, which contains a Tet operator (TetO) DNA sequence and the Tet repressor protein (TetR), which binds the TetO DNA sequence, also known as the TRE, or Tet-responsive element [44]. In the different Tet-controllable systems, TetR has been modified via fusion to the transcriptional activation domain VP16 from the Herpes simplex virus, fusion to the transinhibitor protein Krüppel-associated box (KRAB), and/or genetically mutated to change its transcriptional effect. The Tet-inducible system is usually expressed within cells using two separate expression cassettes: one that expresses the Tet regulatory protein, typically constitutively, and one that contains multiple copies of the TRE upstream of a minimal hCMV promoter and the transgene of interest.

The simplest TetOff system involves a fusion protein containing TetR's DNA-binding domain fused to VP16, which is constitutively expressed from one DNA cassette. This fusion protein is referred to as the Tet-controlled transcriptional activator (tTA). Another DNA cassette contains seven copies of the TRE upstream of the minimal hCMV promoter and the transgene of interest. If no Dox is present, tTA remains bound to the TREs, which activates transcription of the downstream transgene. If Dox is present, it will bind to the TetR binding domain of tTR, changing TetR's conformation and causing it to dissociate from the TREs. This removes VP16 from the vicinity of the transgene and prevents it from activating transcription. Although the TetOff system functions in vitro [45] and in vivo [46], it is not extensively used for in vivo experiments because Dox must be present the entire time gene expression is desired to be "off." Consequently, repeated administrations of Dox are required, raising cost as well as concerns of off-target effects due to extended exposure to antibiotics. Furthermore, because Dox must be removed for the gene of interest to turn "on," induction kinetics are limited by the diffusion of Dox out of tissues and cells.

To address these limitations, Gossen and colleagues discovered four mutations in TetR that cause it to bind the TRE only in the presence of Dox [47]. Fusion of this reverse TetR mutant (rTetR) to VP16 creates a system in which the addition of Dox enables the reverse tTA (rtTA) fusion protein to bind to TRE and activate transcription. Although this initial rtTA protein required high concentrations of Dox for transgene activation and exhibited relatively high background transgene expression in the absence of inducer molecule, more rtTA mutants have been synthesized that improve the system's sensitivity and decrease background expression [48,49]. These enhancements, including amino acid changes, deletion of cryptic splice sites, and codon optimization, have led to extensive use of this TetOn system in vivo [44,49,50].

Another version of the TetOn system utilizes the TetR protein fused to the KRAB repressor domain; as with the other systems, this TetR-KRAB protein is constitutively expressed from one DNA cassette. On another cassette, the transgene of interest is cloned downstream of multiple copies of the TRE as well as a full CMV promoter. In the absence of Dox, TetR-KRAB binds the TRE and inhibits expression of the transgene. This occurs via recruitment and binding of KAP-1 by KRAB, which results in heterochromatin formation and gene silencing via recruitment of other factors [51,52]. When Dox is present, it binds to TetR and releases TetR-KRAB from the TRE. Since the CMV promoter drives constitutive activation of a downstream gene in the absence of repressors, the presence of Dox indirectly activates transcription. A major driving force behind the development of this system stemmed from concerns of toxicity of the VP16 domain; because VP16 is native to the Herpes simplex virus, there is potential for a triggered immune response to rtTA in vivo. However, despite replacement of VP16 with KRAB, there is still potential for an immune response to TetR [53].

Despite alterations to the TetOn systems that increase sensitivity to the inducer molecule and reduce leaky expression of the transgene, some basal transgene expression in the absence of Dox is still observed. While this is not necessarily problematic for many systems, low basal activity is of concern when the transgene product is toxic to the cell [54]. Freundlieb and colleagues circumvented this problem by engineering a Tet-responsive system containing both a Tet-repressor and a Tet-activator: a TetR-KRAB fusion protein and rtTA [54]. The transgene of interest is cloned downstream of TREs and the full CMV promoter. In the absence of Dox, the TetR-KRAB protein binds to the TREs and prevents transcription of the transgene. Under this condition, rtTA cannot bind the TREs and thus does not affect gene expression. Upon addition of Dox, the TetR-KRAB protein dissociates from the TREs and is replaced by rtTA, activating transcription via the VP16 activation domain. This system was shown to greatly reduce the basal activity of the Tet-responsive system, increasing the fold-induction of the transgene in the presence of Dox.

Lastly, the Tet-responsive system can be expressed via an autoregulatory loop [55]. The transgene and either rtTA or tTA are cloned downstream of multiple copies of the TRE and the minimal hCMV promoter. The two genes are joined by an internal ribosomal entry site (IRES), which causes the two genes to be transcribed as one transcript but translated as two separate proteins. In the autoregulatory TetOn system, the addition of Dox allows low, basally expressed levels of rtTA to bind the TREs, inducing expression of new rtTA, which continues to bind the TREs and activate transcription through a positive-feedback mechanism. Removal of Dox relieves expression. One benefit of this system is that high levels of rtTA are only present at the time of induction, thus decreasing potential of toxicity of the VP16 activation domain [44]. The autoregulatory TetOff system works in a similar way, except that the presence of Dox represses transgene expression. Depending on the system's application, another potential benefit is that the positive feedback mechanism converts the Tet-responsive system into a more distinct "on/off" switch instead of a dose-responsive, graded activation system. Cell populations that express the autoregulatory Tet system are often characterized by two populations: one in which the transgene is switched "on," and one in which the transgene is switched "off" [56]. This is in contrast to a cell population that has varying levels of transgene expression determined by Dox concentration.

Tetracycline-inducible systems have been successful in vivo in many types of tissues and organs, including muscle [57], retina [58], brain [59], liver [60], and cartilage [44]. When the system is delivered virally and integrated into the genome of live animals, sustained transgene expression can be achieved. For example, the macaque erythropoietin gene was cloned into an rtTA TetOn system [58]. Expression of rtTA was driven by either the CAG promoter, which is a constitutively active hybrid promoter consisting of the CMV early enhancer element and the chicken beta-actin promoter, or the RPE65 promoter, which is a tissue-specific promoter that only allows downstream gene expression in retinal pigmented epithelium (RPE) of the retina. These cassettes were packaged in rAAV2/4 or rAAV2/5 vectors, which exclusively transduce cells of the RPE or of the RPE and photoreceptors of the eye, respectively [61,62]. Repeated induction of the EPO transgene was possible following repeated Dox administration over 2.5 years. This gene therapy not only holds promise for the treatment of various degenerative retinal disorders, but also has a potential application for sustained, controllable gene expression in tissue engineering, both in vitro and in vivo.

In some cases gene expression may only be required for weeks or months, which requires a system that can be turned off when it is no longer needed. For example, much research has been dedicated to ex vivo gene therapy for the repair of critical bone defects, in which non-osteoblast cells are directly differentiated into osteoblasts via constitutive overexpression of osteogenic factors like BMPs and Runx2. However, this approach can lead to tumorigenesis and the over-production of bone at the defect site [63,64]. These deleterious effects were avoided in one study via transduction of primary skeletal myoblasts with retroviruses containing a tTA cassette and a "TetOff"-responsive *Runx2* transgene [64]. Modified cells were seeded onto a collagen scaffold and transplanted into the hind limb muscles of immunocompetent syngenic mice. Mice were fed drinking water that did or did not contain anhydrotetracycline (aTc), which is a derivative of Tet that has higher affinity for TetR but less antibiotic activity. As demonstrated by micro-computed tomography (micro-CT) and von Kossa staining, mice that received aTc did not have any bone mineralization above background levels at the implant site, whereas mice that did not receive aTc demonstrated mineralization throughout the constructs. Histochemical staining also revealed the presence of collagen only within constructs implanted in mice that did not receive aTc, which suggests that the *Runx2*-expressing implanted cells underwent matrix remodeling and deposition.

Tetracycline-controlled systems have also been used to generate transgenic animals for the development of tissue engineering and repair techniques. One group generated a mouse liver injury model to study hepatocyte engraftment and proliferation [60]. This technique is an attractive alternative to total liver transplants because it is cheaper, less invasive, and will reduce the current strain on the liver transplant waitlist. One commonly used liver injury mouse model is the albumin-urokinase-type plasminogen activator (Alb-uPA) mouse, which is genetically modified to express a hepatotoxic transgene in hepatocytes [65]. However, this phenotype causes half of hemizygous and almost all of homozygous mice to die shortly after birth. To overcome this disadvantage, immunodeficient transgenic mice were bred that contain an rtTA transgene driven by the liver-specific mouse albumin promoter (rtTA/SCID mice). The uPA gene was then delivered to the mice via adenoviral vector. Expression of rtTA only in the liver enabled Tet-dependent liver injury that could be delayed until any age of the mouse.

In addition to the Tet systems, a more recent antibiotic-induced system for genetic control is based on the pristinamycin-induced protein (Pip) [66]. Like TetR, Pip binds P_{PTR}, a known DNA sequence motif. Addition of the clinically approved antibiotic pristinamycin I (PI) causes Pip to dissociate from its target DNA sequence. This mechanism was used to engineer the PipON and PipOFF systems, in which Pip is fused to VP16 or KRAB, respectively, and the transgene of interest is cloned downstream of one or more copies of P_{PTR} alone or P_{PTR} with a constitutive promoter.

5.3.1.2 Small molecule–induced dimerizers

The modularity of eukaryotic gene regulators allows the separation of some transcription factors into separate DNA binding and activation domains that are expressed as distinct proteins. When these domains are separated within cells, they cannot induce transcriptional activation; however, co-localization of the two domains—either covalently or noncovalently—restores the native activity of the full protein (Fig. 5.3). One of the earliest examples of an effector protein that can be manipulated this way is the yeast transcriptional activator GAL4. Fields and Song developed a system to study protein–protein interactions based on the transcriptional activity of the full GAL4 protein [67]. They split the DNA-binding N-terminal domain, which binds the upstream activation sequence (UAS) of the *LacZ* gene, from the C-terminal transcriptional activation domain and fused each domain to SNF1 or SNF4, which are two yeast proteins known to interact. *LacZ* activation only occurred when both GAL4 fusion proteins were co-expressed within cells. This system can be used to regulate transgenes by inserting multiple copies of the UAS upstream of the gene of interest, and then fusing an activation domain, such as VP16, to the GAL4 DNA binding domain. This results in constitutive expression of the transgene. This system has been shown to be functional in eukaryotic cells and animals, such as zebra fish [68].

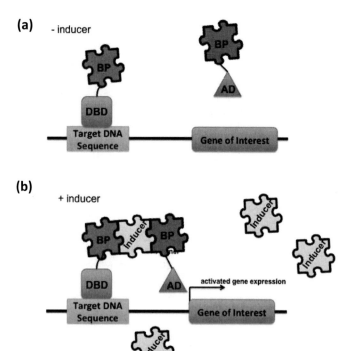

Figure 5.3 Chemically or hormonally induced dimerizers for temporal genetic control. Dimerizing systems are engineered that consist of a DNA-binding domain (DBD)/binding partner (BP) fusion protein and a transcriptional activator domain (AD)/binding partner (BP) fusion protein. The BPs can be homodimers or heterodimers. (a) In the absence of chemical or hormonal inducer, DBD-BP localizes to its target DNA sequence on a transgene or at an endogenous chromosomal site. (b) The inducer binds to both BPs, which translocates AD-BP to the target DNA sequence and activates transcription.

Building upon the idea of modular transcriptional effectors, Rivera and colleagues engineered the rapamycin-inducible system [69]. The human FKBP12 and FRAP proteins both bind the immunosuppressant drug rapamycin. Fusion of FKBP12 to the ZFHD1 DNA-binding domain and fusion of an 89-amino acid fragment of FRAP to the human transcriptional activator NF-κB p65 yields two chimeric proteins that heterodimerize only in the presence of rapamycin. When the ZFHD1 DNA recognition sequence is cloned upstream of a transgene, FRAP-ZFHD1 localizes to the transgene and dimerization between FKBP12 and FRAP translocates p65 to the transgene, leading to transcriptional activation. This system has been shown to function in mice and nonhuman primates [70]. Sequences encoding the two fusion proteins were cloned into a single AAV vector as a single transcriptional unit containing an IRES between the two transgenes. A second AAV vector contained the murine or rhesus monkey erythropoietin gene under control of a ZFHD1-activated promoter. Co-injection of these AAV vectors into skeletal muscle followed by rapamycin administration resulted in a 200-fold induction of plasma erythropoietin in mice for 6 months. An approximate 50-fold induction of plasma erythropoietin was observed in rhesus monkeys following intramuscular injection of the AAV vectors. Furthermore, there was no detectable basal expression of the transgene for 29 days following AAV delivery before rapamycin administration in the monkeys. However, one disadvantage of this system is that de-induction was slow: Erythropoietin levels did not decline to pre-rapamycin levels for 14 days following rapamycin withdrawal.

Systems similar to the rapamycin dimerization system have also been engineered. FK506, an immunosuppressant drug that also binds FKBP12, was chemically synthesized as a dimer (FK1012) [71]. Protein co-localization could then be achieved via homodimerization of FKBP12 fusion proteins. Fusion of FKBP12 to the intracellular Erythropoietin Receptor (EpoR) signaling domain allowed FK1012-dependent control over cell proliferation [72]. Normally, the native EpoR forms a dimer upon binding erythropoietin, which activates a cell proliferation pathway. Replacement of the erythropoietin domain with FKBP12 enabled FK1012 to act as the dimerizing inducer of erythropoietin signaling.

This system was adapted to enhance skeletal myoblast proliferation in vitro. Skeletal myoblasts can be used as grafts to replace scar tissue and repair the myocardium after an infarct, improving myocardial function [73]. However, achieving engraftment of enough cells to restore adequate function remains difficult. An alternative approach is to implant fewer cells and induce proliferation in vivo to achieve the necessary number cells. This has been done through administration of basic fibroblast growth factor (bFGF), which inhibits differentiation and induces cell proliferation. However, in vivo bFGF administration can also cause nontargeted host cells to proliferate, increasing the risk of fibrosis. As a means to circumvent this off-target effect, F36V, which binds FK506, was expressed as a fusion protein to the fibroblast growth factor receptor-1 cytoplasmic domain within skeletal myoblasts [74]. Addition of a dimeric mimic of FK506, AP20187, to cells in vitro induced receptor dimerization and resulted in delayed differentiation and increased proliferation compared to untreated cells. Such cellular modification prior to implantation may address problems of poor in vivo proliferation of skeletal myoblasts and off-target effects of administered bFGF and other growth factors.

Two other systems used by various groups involve cyclophilin or gyrase. The first system utilizes a cyclosporine A-derived dimer that binds cyclophilin, which is used as the dimerizing domain of fusion proteins [75]. The second chemical, coumermycin, is an antibiotic derived from *Streptomyces*; it is a natural dimerizer of the B subunit of bacterial DNA gyrase [76]. These systems follow a similar mechanism to the dimerizing systems mentioned above but have not been as widely used.

5.3.2 Hormone-Induced Systems

Natural hormone receptors are responsible for detecting the presence of a hormone and transducing the hormone's signal to the cell to activate a cellular pathway. Transmembrane receptors detect extracellular hormones via their extracellular domain. This signal is transmitted through the receptor's transmembrane domain to its intracellular domain, which interacts with intracellular proteins and initiates a signaling pathway. Alternatively, ligand-induced internalization of the receptor is required for downstream pathway activation, or as with the estrogen receptor, a receptor can reside completely in the cytoplasm of cells and detect lipid-soluble hormones.

Hormone receptor proteins typically act as dimers that are brought together by co-binding a signaling hormone (Fig. 5.3). As with the previously discussed dimerizing systems induced by chemicals, this dimerization mechanism can be manipulated to engineer fusion proteins that activate transcription of a target gene in response to an added ligand. Such fusion proteins have been made using the estrogen [77], ecdysone [77], glucocorticoid [78], and mineralocorticoid [79] receptors, among others [80,81].

Hollenberg, Cheng, and Weintraub engineered a conditional MyoD transcription factor to study the cellular effects of MyoD in muscle differentiation [81]. They fused MyoD to the glucocorticoid, thyroid, or estrogen hormone receptor. Stable expression of the MyoD fusion proteins in 3T3 and 10T½ cells resulted in hormone-responsive myotube formation and upregulation of myogenic markers. The presence of differentiated muscle cells was observed after 12 h of hormone treatment, and the cells remained differentiated after hormone was removed from the system. In addition to being used to characterize tissue differentiation and development, this system can potentially be used for engineering tissues when transcriptional activators are only needed at initial stages of differentiation. Thus, one can mimic the natural gene expression that occurs during tissue development to create more native-like tissues for implantation.

Another powerful application of hormone-induced systems involves the fusion of a synthetic zinc finger protein to hormone receptors to achieve hormone-induced activation or repression of endogenous genes [82–85]. Zinc finger proteins are DNA-binding proteins that are made up of two or more zinc finger domains. Each zinc finger domain recognizes a specific three base-pair DNA sequence; thus, assembly of multiple zinc finger domains in tandem enables specific targeting of longer, contiguous DNA base-pair sequences. It is possible to engineer a zinc finger protein to target almost any desired DNA sequence using synthetic zinc finger domains that target each DNA base pair triplet [86]; for example, a zinc finger protein that contains six zinc finger domains in tandem binds a contiguous 18 base-pair sequence with high specificity. Fusion of a gene-targeted zinc finger protein to a transcriptional activator or repressor enables constitutive activation or repression, respectively, of the targeted gene within cells [82].

Magnenat, Schwimmer, and Barbas III used estrogen receptor homodimerizaion or retinoid X receptor-α/ecdysone receptor heterodimerization to create hormone-responsive zinc finger transcription factors that regulated expression of intercellular adhesion molecule-1 (ICAM-1) or ErbB-2/HER-2 [84]. Six-finger zinc finger proteins that targeted the *ICAM-1* or *ErbB-2/HER2* gene promoters were fused to two estrogen receptor ligand-binding domains (LBDs) linked in tandem or to a retinoid X receptor-α LBD linked to an ecdysone receptor LBD. These constructs were then fused to either the VP16 or KRAB effector domain (ED), which created a four-part fusion protein: zinc finger-LBD-LBD-ED. Retroviral delivery of each construct to HeLa or A431 cells enabled regulation of the target genes in a ligand dose-dependent manner. This regulation was also reversible, was sustainable for up to 11 days, and demonstrated negligible basal activity in the absence of ligand.

Chemical- and hormone-controlled gene regulation systems have been extensively used to study gene function, protein interactions, and differentiation in vitro and in vivo. However, the potential of these systems goes beyond their use as tools for scientific discovery and characterization. Biomaterial scaffolds continue to be developed not only to improve cellular engraftment and behavior for engineering cardiac [87], neural [88], bone [89], cartilage [90], muscle [91], and other types of tissues, but also for controlled and sustained release of drugs [92], growth factors [93–95], and DNA vectors [96]. Recently, some research has focused on scaffold-mediated release of chemicals or hormones to control transgene expression in genetically modified, engrafted cells. In one study, B16 murine cells were genetically modified to express two fusion proteins: the ligand-binding domain of the ecdysone receptor fused to the GAL4 binding domain and the retinoid X receptor fused to VP16 [97]. Cells were transfected with a green fluorescent protein (GFP) reporter gene containing five upstream copies of the GAL4 binding site. In the presence of inducer drug, the ecdysone/retinoid X receptor fusion proteins formed a heterodimer and activated transcription of the reporter gene.

In the same study, poly(ester urethane) urea (PEUU) films were optimized for sustained release of the inducer drug; about 1–3% of loaded drug was released per week up to 10 months, and cells cultured on drug-loaded PEUU films expressed GFP for up to 3 weeks in vitro. Dose-dependent GFP expression was also observed based on the initial loading concentration (0–5 μM) of the drug into the PEUU film. This study is one example of the potential dual application of biomaterials as scaffolds for cellular proliferation and differentiation and depots of small molecules that can elicit a prescribed cellular response. As more is learned about the genetic requirements for proper cell differentiation and engraftment in implanted tissue constructs, it is likely that biomaterials will serve a crucial part in genetically controlling cell growth and tissue repair.

5.4 Spatiotemporal Gene Regulation Systems

Mimicking natural cell environments and tissues requires the control of cellular behavior in both space and time. This is particularly challenging when engineering tissues that naturally contain complex, organized structures of multiple cell types, such as three-dimensional heart, liver, and kidney tissues. These tissues contain vasculature that provides nutrients and oxygen that provides nutrients and oxygen and removes cellular waste products cellular waste products [98]. Tissue patterning during development and regeneration is driven by growth factor gradients and spatially patterned gene expression that direct cell differen-tiation and recruit specific cell types.

Systems have been developed that enable spatiotemporal control of gene expression. To date, these systems have been used to study protein–protein and cell–cell interactions as well as to spatially and temporally pattern gene expression in vitro and in vivo. Such control is typically not achieved through free addition of a small molecule because the molecule quickly diffuses throughout the cell media or animal tissue once it is administered, making it impossible to maintain spatial patterns of induction. Instead, spatiotemporal gene regulation systems employ other stimuli; the most common of these stimuli are heat, ultraviolet radiation, and light. It is also possible to achieve spatiotemporal control using a diffusible molecule by combining temporal gene regulation technology, such as the tetracycline-inducible system, with controlled-release scaffolds that have been loaded with the inducer molecule, such as Dox, in a defined pattern. Alternatively, chemical cell–cell communication systems can be engineered to create patterns of gene expression [99].

5.4.1 Heat-Inducible Gene Regulation

Heat-shock proteins (HSPs) comprise a large family of proteins that are up-regulated in response to elevated temperatures, exposure to metals or toxins, hypoxia, infection, and other stimuli [100,101]. There are many different HSPs, most of which are highly conserved across prokaryotes and eukaryotes. Insertion of HSP promoters upstream of a transgene of interest results in heat-induced transgene activation by endogenous proteins in response to elevated temperatures. In 1986, the *Drosophila Hsp70* promoter was cloned upstream of human growth hormone (hGH), chicken lysozyme (cL) or a human influenza haemagglutinin (HA) and was shown to upregulate expression of those genes over 1000-fold in mammalian cells [102]. Since then, HSP promoters have been used in a broad range of studies including the study of embryonic development and the determination of cell lineage commitment [103] and cancer therapy [104].

A major benefit of this system is that heat activation is non-invasive and can be directed to precise tissue locations using laser-equipped microscopes, temperature-controlled iron, or heating pads [103]. If extremely precise spatial activation is desired, implanted micro-scale fiber optics connected to an external laser can be used for heat delivery [105]. One study used MRI-guided focused ultrasound (MRI-FUS) to non-invasively deliver local heat and activate GFP in vivo [106]. A C6 glioma cell line was engineered that contained an integrated copy of the *GFP* gene downstream of the minimal human HSP70 promoter. These cells were implanted subcutaneously in immunodeficient mice and in Wistar rats, and upon tumor formation local hyperthermia was performed using FUS heating guided by MRI temperature maps. Tumors were removed 24 h after hyperthermia treatment and analyzed for endogenous HSP70 and exogenous GFP expression by Western blots and immunohistochemistry. Results showed elevations in GFP expression when tumors were heated over the range of 44–50°C for 180 s with no apparent toxicity to the cells. However, gene expression was heterogeneous throughout the tumor, and levels decreased with increasing distance to the focal point of heat delivery. Further refinement of this technology through optimization of HSP promoter sensitivity to hyperthermia, or of heat delivery methods, holds promise for non-invasively obtaining spatially and temporally controlled gene activation.

5.4.2 Ultraviolet Radiation-Induced Gene Expression

Photocaged biological molecules, such as small molecular inducers or ligands, oligonucleotides, or transcription factors, allow the control of cellular behavior with ultraviolet (UV) irradiation (Fig. 5.4). These biological molecules can be chemically modified such that they are covalently linked to a protecting group at an active site, thereby blocking their activity. The protecting, or "caging," group is often a 2-nitrobenzyl group; irradiation of the "caged" biological molecule with UV light breaks the covalent bond that links it to the effector, freeing the effector. As a result, the effector regains its activity [107]. When a photocaged effector is expressed within cells, irradiation in spatial patterns at varying intensities results in tunable, spatiotemporally controlled gene activation or repression depending on the type of biological molecule used.

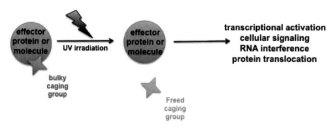

Figure 5.4   Spatiotemporal cellular control via caged molecules and effector proteins. A rationally placed caging group is incorporated into a protein or an RNA or inducer molecule, inhibiting the function of that protein or molecule. UV irradiation breaks the covalent bond between the caging group and the effector, releasing and activating it. This technology can be used to activate transcription, control cellular signaling, induce RNA interference, or control protein translocation within living cells.

Photocaging has been used with many different gene expression systems and technologies, including the tetracycline-controlled gene expression system, RNA interference (RNAi), and protein expression. Cambridge and others used the TetOn system along with photolabile Dox derivatives to achieve UV irradiation-dependent uncaging of Dox, which activated *Luciferase* or *GFP* transgene transcription in murine hippocampal slices and whole-embryos in vitro as well as *Xenopus* tadpoles in vivo [108]. Cells that were treated with 2 μM caged Dox and irradiated showed luciferase activity that was 73% of luciferase activity when cells were treated with 2 μM uncaged Dox. Although higher doses of caged Dox were required to achieve comparable gene expression levels as when uncaged Dox was used, the caged Dox showed no background activation of expression in the absence of irradiation. Furthermore, *GFP* activation was possible on a single-cell level in the hippocampal cultures, providing the opportunity to monitor cell migration and division over time. Similarly, another group patterned fluorescent markers and the expression of the cell surface ligand ephrin A5 using caged Dox and a Tet-responsive gene expression system [109]. Features as small as 300 µm were readily achievable.

Another way to achieve control of genetic repression in a spatiotemporal manner is by transfecting cells with photocaged small interfering RNA (siRNA). Chemical modification of the sugar-phosphate backbone of RNAi effectors allows attachment of caging groups like 1-(4,5-dimethoxy-2-nitrophenyl)-diazoethane (DMNPE) that block RNAi activity. One group tested the ability to knockdown GFP expression in BHK-21 cells using photocaged dsRNA [110]. When both the sense and antisense dsRNA strands were caged with DMNPE, about 10% of cells exhibited an RNAi response before UV irradiation; after irradiation, about 50% of cells showed an RNAi response. Similarly, zebra fish embryos co-injected with GFP plasmid and caged siRNAs targeted to GFP showed some GFP knockdown before irradiation as compared to embryos injected with GFP plasmid and no caged siRNA. However, GFP expression was significantly less in irradiated embryos co-injected with GFP plasmid and caged siRNA as compared to co-injected, non-irradiated embryos and GFP-only embryos. More work must be done to reduce RNAi activity when the molecules are caged (pre-UV irradiation) as well as to increase the efficiency of uncaging upon UV irradiation.

Another group synthesized caged dsRNA by incorporating four terminal phosphates on each duplex molecule and then covalently linking a molecule of cyclo-dodecyl dimethoxy nitro phenyl ethyl (CD-DMNPE) to each phosphate [111]. When inserted into human cells, UV-irradiation of the caged dsRNA molecules freed the dsRNA from CD-DMNPE and initiated RNA interference of a target gene. Spatial knock-down of GFP was achieved using a photomask by using caged GFP-targeted dsRNA.

A third application of photocaging is to control the activity of proteins within cells. Caged proteins can be made by chemical modification of isolated proteins [112] or by incorporation of caged amino acids using aminoacylated (caging) tRNAs in vitro [113]. Alternatively, cells can be genetically modified to incorporate a caged amino acid using an engineered suppressor tRNA/aminoacyl-tRNA synthetase pair that incorporates an exogenously supplied caged amino acid at amber (UAG) stop codons. Thus, delivery of a transgene that has been mutated to contain an amber stop codon at a key residue of an active site of the encoded protein results in cellular incorporation of the caged amino acid at that site. The bulkiness of the incorporated caging group blocks protein activity until it is covalently detached by UV irradiation of the cells. These photocaging methods have been used to control protein phosphorylation and nuclear export [114], activation of protein activity [115], and other protein functions.

Although photocaging methods provide the opportunity to control effector molecules on a single-cell level with high spatial and temporal precision, there are notable disadvantages to this technology that limit its use. First, photocaging is irreversible; once caging groups are removed from effectors by UV irradiation, effector activity cannot be reversed until the effector is degraded by the cell or exhausted. In addition, caged amino acids that are incorporated at amber stop codons of a transgene will likely also be incorporated at amber stop codons in endogenous transcripts. This may result in translational read-through of transcripts that are normally not expressed, raising concern of toxicity. Lastly, when a caged small molecule is used, the uncaged inducer can diffuse among cells and tissues, blurring the effects of spatial gene activation. Despite these disadvantages, however, photocaging remains a valuable tool for studying effector interactions within cells, and it may prove useful for tissue engineering when spatiotemporal activation of an "on-only" genetic switch is desired.

5.4.3 Light-Induced Gene Regulation Systems

Methods that control genes and proteins using visible light address the shortcomings of photocaging. Multiple gene switches ("photoswitches") have been engineered that allow one to turn a gene on or off at will or control protein–protein interactions using illumination at different wavelengths within the visible spectrum (Fig. 5.5, Table 5.1). Unlike photocaging, these systems are reversible, and the use of light as a stimulus reduces the risk of cell toxicity that may be associated with irradiation of cells with UV light. Furthermore, light-induced systems may prove superior to heat-induced systems, as heat is a less specific stimulus with respect to spatial control and has many other effects on cell signaling pathways.

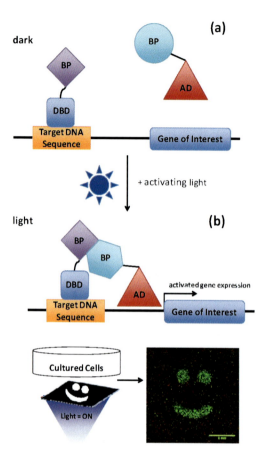

Figure 5.5 Light-inducible spatiotemporal gene expression. Gene regulatory systems are engineered that consist of a DNA-binding domain (DBD)/binding partner (BP) fusion protein and a transcriptional activator domain (AD)/binding partner (BP) fusion protein. The BPs can be homodimers or heterodimers. (a) In the dark, DBD-BP localizes to the target DNA sequence placed upstream of a transgene of interest. In the presence of activating light, one BP undergoes a conformational change that enables the two BPs to bind, translocating the AD to the transgene of interest and activating transcription. (b) Placement of a photomask (black) between the activating light (blue cone) and cells that express a light-inducible gene expression system results in a corresponding pattern of transgene activation. Here, expression of green fluorescent protein (GFP) was induced by illumination of cells with blue light in a happy face pattern (scale bar = 2 mm).

Table 5.1 Genetic systems for light-inducible control of living cells

Stimulus	Induced effector(s)	Output	Reference(s)
UV irradiation	Caged Dox	Dox-mediated activation of Tet-inducible transgene expression	108, 109
UV irradiation	Caged siRNA	RNA interference of target gene	110, 111
UV irradiation	Caged antibody	Antibody-antigen or antibody-receptor binding	112
UV irradiation	Caged amino acid	Activation of phosphorylation or gene transcription	113–115
Red light	PhyB and PIF3 heterodimers	Transgene expression	116
Blue light	LOV and GIGANTEA heterodimers	Transgene expression or protein translocation	117
Blue light	Cryptochrome 2 and CIB1 heterodimers	Transgene expression or protein translocation	118
Blue light	Vivid (VVD) homodimers	Transgene expression	119
Blue light	LOV-Rac1	Cell motility	121
Blue light	Melanopsin	Transgene expression	122

Numerous light-inducible gene regulation systems utilize plant protein homodimers or heterodimers that associate in response to red [116] or blue [117–119] light. These systems use modular fusion proteins, where one light-inducible binding partner is fused to a DNA-binding domain, such as the GAL4 DNA binding domain, and the other binding partner is fused to a transcriptional activation domain, such as VP16. Expression of these chimeric proteins in cells along with a transgene containing upstream copies of the DNA-binding domain's target sequence results in light-dependent transcriptional activation. In red-light responsive systems, one binding partner is usually a type of plant phytochrome, which is a protein covalently linked to a tetrapyrrole chromophore. Illumination with red light induces a conformational change in the phytochrome that converts it from its inactive Pr form to an active Pfr form. The Pfr form is able to dimerize with a binding partner; for instance, phytochromes phyA and phyB form dimers with the basic helix-loop-helix protein PIF3. Furthermore, red light–induced dimerization can be reversed by illumination with far-red light [116].

These interactions were explored by fusing the N-terminal domain of PhyB to the GAL4 DNA binding domain and PIF3 to the GAL4 activation domain [116]. Expression of these proteins in yeast, along with a GAL4 UAS-driven *LacZ* transgene, resulted in rapid *LacZ* induction after short pulses of red light: exposure of cells to red light for 1 min followed by incubation in the dark resulted in 2-fold, 4-fold, and 50-fold transgene induction after 5, 10, and 30 min, respectively. Furthermore, LacZ accumulation in photoactivated cells decreased within 10 min of a pulse of far-red light.

One drawback to systems that involve phytochromes is that the chromophore is only naturally found in plants. Thus, use of a phytochrome system in organisms other than plants requires purification and exogenous delivery of the chromophore, or the organism must be genetically engineered to make the chromophore. Current blue light–inducible systems use plant proteins that require cofactors that are naturally present in mammalian cells. For example, the proteins GIGANTEA and FKF1 from *Arabidopsis thaliana* form a heterodimer in the presence of blue light via the N-terminal light-oxygen-voltage (LOV) sensing domain of FKF1 [120]. A riboflavin that occurs naturally in plant and animal cells binds noncovalently within a pocket of LOV; the flavin molecule absorbs blue light energy, which initiates formation of a covalent bond between the flavin and a cysteine in FKF1. This causes a conformational change that allows the LOV domain to bind GIGANTEA. Yazawa and colleagues engineered two fusion proteins, GIGANTEA fused to the GAL4 binding domain and LOV fused to VP16, and achieved up to a fivefold increase in transgene expression after 30 min of blue light illumination (1.8 Joules) [117]. Furthermore, transgene activation was tunable based on the duration of illumination.

This group also showed that the GIGANTEA/FKF1 interaction could be used to control protein translocation and a cell signaling cascade. They fused FKF1 to Rac1, which is a GTPase that is activated and recruited to the plasma membrane upon binding GTP, resulting in lamellipodia formation and cellular movement. Rac1 was mutated such that it constitutively bound GTP but lacked the plasma membrane-localizing domain CAAX. Expression of this FKF1-Rac1 protein along with a GIGANTEA/CAAX fusion protein enabled light-induced recruitment of the active Rac1 mutant to the membrane, allowing control over where lamellipodia formed within cells. An earlier study similarly induced lamellipodia formation in metazoan cells, enabling control over the direction of cell movement [121]. However, this system did not involve dimerizing proteins; instead, the LOV domain from phototropin was fused via a helical linker peptide to Rac1. In the absence of blue light, the LOV domain sterically blocked Rac1 interactions with other cellular proteins and inhibited Rac1 activity. Illumination with blue light unwound the helical linker between LOV and Rac1, releasing steric hindrance and locally activating Rac1.

Another group used the blue light–inducible homodimer Vivid (VVD), which is the smallest known protein that contains a LOV domain, to achieve spatiotemporal transgene activation in vitro and in vivo [119]. The GAL4 DNA binding domain contains a DNA recognition motif and a dimerization domain; removal of the dimerization domain (Gal4 residues 1–65) abolishes GAL4's ability to dimerize and bind the UAS. Wang, Chen, and Yang fused VVD to the GAL4 DNA binding domain lacking the dimerization domain and the p65 or VP16 transcriptional activation domain to create GAL4-VVD-p65 and GAL4-VVD-VP16 fusion proteins. Expression of either of these chimeric proteins in human cells resulted in blue light-inducible activation of a transgene containing five upstream copies of the UAS by stimulating homodimerization of VVD, which also dimerized the two GAL4 DNA binding domains and enabled their binding to the UAS. As a result, the attached activation domain was translocated to the transgene for activation. Patterned illumination of cells containing a plasmid encoding GAL4-VVD-p65 and a reporter encoding the fluorescent protein mCherry downstream of five copies of the UAS resulted in a corresponding pattern of mCherry expression. Spatial activation was also possible in vivo; the GAL4-VVD-p65 expression vector and mCherry reporter vector were transferred into the livers of mice, and mice were illuminated with blue light from below their cage. This resulted in mCherry expression on the anterior side of the liver. Localized activation of mCherry within the liver was also possible by using optical fibers for targeted illumination.

Last, light-regulated systems have also been based upon light-sensitive membrane channels, such as melanopsin [122]. Melanopsin is a photopigment G protein-coupled receptor found in photosensitive retinal ganglion cells. Upon activation with blue light, melanopsin activates a cellular signaling cascade that ultimately results in a calcium influx through transient receptor potential cation channels (TRPCs). An intracellular increase in calcium concentration activates the NFAT transcription factor through the calmodulin pathway, which allows NFAT to enter the nucleus and bind NFAT-specific promoters (P_{NFAT}). Modification of HEK293 cells to constitutively express melanopsin and to contain a P_{NFAT}-driven *luciferase, human placental secreted alkaline phosphatase (SEAP),* or *glucagon-like peptide-1 variant* (shGLP-1) gene resulted in blue-light mediated induction of gene expression by over two orders of magnitude. Notably, melanopsin-expressing cells containing the P_{NFAT}-shGLP-1 transgene were microencapsulated and implanted subcutaneously into wild-type and diabetic db/db mice. Illumination of the animals for 48 h significantly increased insulin levels in both wild-type and diabetic db/db mice. A glucose-tolerance test showed significantly improved glucose homeostasis, suggesting that this technology could be used to remediate or treat type II diabetes.

Light-inducible systems enable tight spatial and temporal control over protein–protein interactions and gene expression. Further development of this relatively new technology will bring great advancements to all areas of science from experimental biology to biomedical and tissue engineering. The ability to reversibly control cells on a single-cell level may aid the development of patterned multicellular tissues through spatial activation of transcription factors that drive cellular differentiation.

5.4.4 Spatiotemporal Genetic Control Using Scaffolds

Spatiotemporal genetic control can be achieved through immobilization or encapsulation of inducer molecules, growth factors, and viral or nonviral DNA vectors on cellular scaffolds. As described above, spatially controlled activation of GFP was observed in cells that expressed the TetOn system and a TRE-driven GFP transgene. The cells were seeded onto porous PEUU scaffolds that were loaded with Dox only in the central region, resulting in GFP activation only in that region [97]. Replacement of the GFP transgene with a differentiation-driving transgene may facilitate the engineering of cell systems that mimic native tissues.

Another way to achieve spatiotemporal control of cellular activity is to immobilize nonviral or viral vectors on an implantable scaffold, resulting in in vivo genetic modification of cells. One major advantage of this method is that cells do not have to be genetically modified ex vivo, which greatly reduces the cost and time required to culture a patient's cells before implantation. Consequently, gene-loaded scaffolds provide the opportunity to manufacture "off-the-shelf" constructs that can be seeded with a patent's cells in an operating room and implanted immediately.

Despite low transfection efficiency when DNA plasmids are delivered without a vehicle like liposomes or viruses, immobilization of plasmids on scaffolds has resulted in observable upregulation of a transgene in implanted and host cells. Salvay, Zelivyanskaya, and Shea fabricated porous scaffolds using poly(D,L-lactide-co-glycolide) (PLG) and immobilized plasmids containing a constitutively expressed *luciferase*, *GFP*, or *Factor IX* gene [123]. Mice implanted with a subcutaneous scaffold containing the luciferase plasmid showed localized luciferase activity for up to 28 weeks in host cells. Luciferase activity was highest on day 1 post-implantation and then leveled out to 50% of this activity by 28 weeks. Thus, sustained and steady gene expression can be achieved using immobilized naked DNA.

To assess the spatial aspect of gene activation, PLG constructs containing Factor IX plasmids were implanted into mice, and systemic levels of Factor IX in the blood and tissue were measured using an enzyme-linked immunosorbent assay. Levels of Factor IX slightly above the assay's detection limit were observed in the blood at day 3 post-implantation, but by day 7 levels were not detectable. After 28 days tissue that was removed from the implant site was positive for Factor IX expression. Thus, plasmid immobilization to the PLG scaffold resulted in gene delivery that was locally restrained to the scaffold site after less than a week. Similar results have been similarly obtained by immobilizing viral particles to scaffolds [124]. The success of these methods in achieving localized gene delivery within scaffolds suggests that it may be possible to obtain patterned gene expression within the scaffold by spatially patterning DNA vectors within the construct. This idea was explored in one study that attempted to recapitulate the bone-soft tissue interface [125]. Phillips and colleagues attached retrovirus encoding Runx2/Cbfa1 in a gradient across a scaffold and then seeded fibroblasts onto the scaffold. This gave rise to a spatial pattern of Runx2/Cbfa1 expression, osteoblastic differentiation, and mineralized matrix deposition that corresponded to the gradient of attached retrovirus. The patterned phenotype of this construct persisted after being implanted in vivo.

5.5 Conclusion

Many different gene regulation systems have been engineered, each providing a unique level of cellular control and mode of induction. Depending on the application, a gene of interest can be constitutively expressed or repressed from a transgene or at an endogenous site within cells. Or, gene expression and protein interactions can be controlled in a temporal fashion using small molecular inducers like natural or synthetic antibiotics, drugs, or hormones. If a high level of regulation is required in both space and time, systems that are induced by heat, UV irradiation, light, or controlled-release scaffolds can be used. This extensive toolbox of regulatory systems has been used to discover the mechanisms behind cell differentiation, proliferation, and communication, and can serve as a key component to the engineering of tissues for clinical use.

Acknowledgments

This work was supported by an NSF CAREER Award (CBET-1151035), NIH Director's New Innovator Award (DP2-OD008586), NIH/NIAMS (R03-AR061042), an American Heart Association Scientist Development Grant (10SDG3060033), a Ralph E. Powe Junior Faculty Enhancement Award from Oak Ridge Associated Universities, and the Duke Biomedical Engineering McChesney Fellowship.

References

1. Hendriks, J., J. Riesle, and C. A. van Blitterswijk, Co-culture in cartilage tissue engineering. *J Tissue Eng Regen Med*, 2007. **1**(3): 170–178.
2. Khademhosseini, A., et al., Microscale technologies for tissue engineering and biology. *Proc Natl Acad Sci USA*, 2006. **103**(8): 2480–2487.
3. Shimizu, T., et al., Cell sheet engineering for myocardial tissue reconstruction. *Biomaterials*, 2003. **24**(13): 2309–2316.
4. Kaji, H., et al., Engineering systems for the generation of patterned co-cultures for controlling cell, Äìcell interactions. *Biochim Biophys Acta (BBA)—Gen Subj*, 2011. **1810**(3): 239–250.
5. Rivron, N. C., et al., Engineering vascularised tissues in vitro. *Eur Cells Mater*, 2008. **15**: 27–40.
6. Kielpinski, G., et al., Roadmap to approval: use of an automated sterility test method as a lot release test for Carticel, autologous cultured chondrocytes. *Cytotherapy*, 2005. **7**(6): 531–541.
7. Hidaka, C., et al., Acceleration of cartilage repair by genetically modified chondrocytes over expressing bone morphogenetic protein-7. *J Orthop Res*, 2003. **21**(4): 573–583.
8. Hidaka, C., et al., Enhanced matrix synthesis and in vitro formation of cartilage-like tissue by genetically modified chondrocytes expressing BMP-7. *J Orthop Res*, 2001. **19**(5): 751–758.
9. Nifuji, A., et al., Extracellular mdulators regulate bone morphogenic proteins in skeletal tissue. *J Oral Biosci*, 2010. **52**(4): 311–321.
10. Chen, F. H., K. T. Rousche, and R. S. Tuan, Technology insight: adult stem cells in cartilage regeneration and tissue engineering. *Nat Clin Pract Rheum*, 2006. **2**(7): 373–382.
11. Gimble, J., and F. Guilak, Adipose-derived adult stem cells: isolation, characterization, and differentiation potential. *Cytotherapy*, 2003. **5**(5): 362–369.
12. Longo, U. G., Petrillo, S., Franceschetti, E., Berton, A., Maffulli, N., and Denaro, V., Stem cells and gene therapy for cartilage repair, *Stem Cells Int*, 2012. **2012**, article ID 168385, 9 pages. doi:10.1155/2012/168385
13. Evans, C. H., et al., Gene transfer to human joints: progress toward a gene therapy of arthritis. *Proc Natl Acad Sci USA*, 2005. **102**(24): 8698–8703.

14. Evans, C. H., et al., Gene therapy with the interleukin-1 receptor antagonist for the treatment of arthritis. *Future Rheumatol*, 2006. **1**(2): 173–178.
15. Kuroda, R., et al., Cartilage repair using bone morphogenetic protein 4 and muscle-derived stem cells. *Arthritis Rheum*, 2006. **54**(2): 433–442.
16. Cirodde, A., et al., A retrospective study of the use of cultured epidermal autografts (CEA) in severe burn patients. *Burns*, 2009. **35, Suppl 1**(0): S19.
17. Tausche, A.-K., et al., An autologous epidermal equivalent tissue-engineered from follicular outer root sheath keratinocytes is as effective as split-thickness skin autograft in recalcitrant vascular leg ulcers. *Wound Repair Regen*, 2003. **11**(4): 248–252.
18. Verplancke, P., et al., Treatment of dystrophic epidermolysis bullosa with autologous meshed split-thickness skin grafts and allogeneic cultured keratinocytes. *Dermatology*, 1997. **194**(4): 380–382.
19. Andreadis, S., Gene-modified tissue-engineered skin, in *The Next Generation of Skin SubstitutesTissue Engineering II*, (K. Lee and D. Kaplan, eds.) 2007, Springer Berlin/Heidelberg. pp. 241–274.
20. Jang, J. H., D. V. Schaffer, and L. D. Shea, Engineering biomaterial systems to enhance viral vector gene delivery. *Mol Ther*, 2011. **19**(8): 1407–1415.
21. Gersbach, C. A., J. E. Phillips, and A. J. Garcia, Genetic engineering for skeletal regenerative medicine. *Annu Rev Biomed Eng*, 2007. **9**: 87–119.
22. Wang, C.-H. K., and S. H. Pun, Substrate-mediated nucleic acid delivery from self-assembled monolayers. *Trends Biotechnol*, 2011. **29**(3): 119–126.
23. Tyrone, J. W., et al., Collagen-embedded platelet-derived growth factor DNA plasmid promotes wound healing in a dermal ulcer model. *J Surg Res*, 2000. **93**(2): 230–236.
24. Beer, H.-D., M. T. Longaker, and S. Werner, Reduced expression of PDGF and PDGF receptors during impaired wound healing. *J Invest Dermatol*, 1997. **109**(2): 132–138.
25. Phillips, J. E., C. A. Gersbach, and A. J. Garcia, Virus-based gene therapy strategies for bone regeneration. *Biomaterials*, 2007. **28**(2): 211–229.
26. Payne, K. A., et al., Single intra-articular injection of adeno-associated virus results in stable and controllable in vivo transgene expression in normal rat knees. *Osteoarthritis Cartilage*, 2011. **19**(8): 1058–1065.

27. Watchko, J., et al., Adeno-associated virus vector-mediated mini-dystrophin gene therapy improves dystrophic muscle contractile function in mdx mice. *Hum Gene Ther*, 2002. **13**(12): 1451–1460.

28. Nathwani, A. C., et al., Long-term safety and efficacy following systemic administration of a self-complementary AAV vector encoding human FIX pseudotyped with serotype 5 and 8 capsid proteins. *Mol Ther*, 2011. **19**(5): 876–885.

29. Tian, J., et al., Regulated insulin delivery from human epidermal cells reverses hyperglycemia. *Mol Ther*, 2008. **16**(6): 1146–1153.

30. Berthod, F., and O. Damour, In vitro reconstructed skin models for wound coverage in deep burns. *Br J Dermatol*, 1997. **136**(6): 809–816.

31. Smiley, A. K., et al., Expression of human beta defensin 4 in genetically modified keratinocytes enhances antimicrobial activity. *J Burn Care Res*, 2007. **28**(1): 127–132.

32. Li, C. X., et al., Delivery of RNA interference. *Cell Cycle*, 2006. **5**(18): 2103–2109.

33. Lytton-Jean, A. K. R., R. Langer, and D. G. Anderson, Five years of siRNA delivery: spotlight on gold nanoparticles. *Small*, 2011. **7**(14): 1932–1937.

34. Rosi, N. L., et al., Oligonucleotide-modified gold nanoparticles for intracellular gene regulation. *Science*, 2006. **312**(5776): 1027–1030.

35. Lodish, H., et al., *The Molecular Cell Biology of Development*, in *Molecular Cell Biology* (K. Ahr, ed.), W. H. Freeman and Company: New York., 2007: pp. 949–1000.

36. Silva, J., and A. Smith, Capturing pluripotency. *Cell*, 2008. **132**(4): 532–536.

37. Takahashi, K., et al., Induction of pluripotent stem cells from adult human fibroblasts by defined factors. *Cell*, 2007. **131**(5): 861–872.

38. Brambrink, T., et al., Sequential expression of pluripotency markers during direct reprogramming of mouse somatic cells. *Cell Stem Cell*, 2008. **2**(2): 151–159.

39. Davis, R. L., H. Weintraub, and A. B. Lassar, Expression of a single transfected cDNA converts fibroblasts to myoblasts. *Cell*, 1987. **51**(6): 987–1000.

40. Berkes, C. A., and S. J. Tapscott, MyoD and the transcriptional control of myogenesis. *Semin Cell Dev Biol*, 2005. **16**(4–5): 585–595.

41. Eming, S. A., T. Krieg, and J. M. Davidson, Gene therapy and wound healing. *Clin Dermatol*, 2007. **25**(1): 79–92.

42. Margolis, D. J., et al., Phase I study of H5.020CMV.PDGF-beta to treat venous leg ulcer disease. *Mol Ther*, 2009. **17**(10): 1822–1829.
43. Katayama, K., et al., A novel PPAR γ gene therapy to control inflammation associated with inflammatory bowel disease in a murine model. *Gastroenterology*, 2003. **124**(5): 1315–1324.
44. Stieger, K., et al., In vivo gene regulation using tetracycline-regulatable systems. *Adv Drug Deliv Rev*, 2009. **61**: 527–541.
45. Gossen, M., and H. Bujard, Tight control of gene expression in mammalian cells by tetracycline-responsive promoters. *Proc Natl Acad Sci USA*, 1992. **89**(12): 5547–5551.
46. Vigna, E., et al., Robust and efficient regulation of transgene expression in vivo by improved tetracycline-dependent lentiviral vectors. *Mol Ther*, 2002. **5**(3): 252–261.
47. Gossen, M., et al., Transcriptional activation by tetracyclines in mammalian cells. *Science*, 1995. **268**(5218): 1766–1769.
48. Urlinger, S., et al., Exploring the sequence space for tetracycline-dependent transcriptional activators: novel mutations yield expanded range and sensitivity. *Proc. Natl. Acad. Sci.*, 2000. **97**: 7963–7968.
49. Stebbins, M. J., et al., Tetracycline-inducible systems for Drosophila. *Proc Natl Acad Sci*, 2001. **98**(19): 10775–10780.
50. Xiong, W., et al., Immunization against the transgene but not the TetON switch reduces expression from gutless adenoviral vectors in the brain. *Mol Ther*, 2008. **16**(2): 343–351.
51. Margolin, J. F., et al., Kruppel-associated boxes are potent transcriptional repression domains. *Proc Natl Acad Sci USA*, 1994. **91**(10): 4509–4513.
52. Schultz, D. C., et al., SETDB1: a novel KAP-1-associated histone H3, lysine 9-specific methyltransferase that contributes to HP1-mediated silencing of euchromatic genes by KRAB zinc-finger proteins. *Genes Dev*, 2002. **16**(8): 919–932.
53. Le Guiner, C., et al., Immune responses to gene product of inducible promoters. *Curr Gene Ther*, 2007. **7**(5): 334–346.
54. Freundlieb, S., C. Schirra-Müller, and H. Bujard, A tetracycline controlled activation/repression system with increased potential for gene transfer into mammalian cells. *J Gene Med*, 1999. **1**(1): 4–12.
55. Markusic, D., et al., Comparison of single regulated lentiviral vectors with rtTA expression driven by an autoregulatory loop or a constitutive promoter. *Nucleic Acids Res*, 2005. **33**(6): e63.

56. Becskei, A., B. Seraphin, and L. Serrano, Positive feedback in eukaryotic gene networks: cell differentiation by graded to binary response conversion. *EMBO J*, 2001. **20**(10): 2528–2535.
57. Grill, M. A., et al., Tetracycline-inducible system for regulation of skeletal muscle-specific gene expression in transgenic mice. *Transgenic Res*, 2003. **12**(1): 33–43.
58. Stieger, K., et al., Long-term doxycycline-regulated transgene expression in the retina of nonhuman primates following subretinal injection of recombinant AAV vectors. *Mol Ther*, 2006. **13**(5): 967–975.
59. Hong, H.-K., et al., Inducible and reversible *Clock* Gene expression in brain using the tTA system for the study of circadian behavior. *PLoS Genet*, 2007. **3**(2): e33.
60. Song, X., et al., A mouse model of inducible liver injury caused by tet-on regulated urokinase for studies of hepatocyte transplantation. *Am J Pathol*, 2009. **175**(5): 1975–1983.
61. Auricchio, A., et al., Exchange of surface proteins impacts on viral vector cellular specificity and transduction characteristics: the retina as a model. *Human Mol Genet*, 2001. **10**(26): 3075–3081.
62. Weber, W., and M. Fussenegger, Synthetic gene networks in mammalian cells. *Curr Opin Biotechnol*, 2010. **21**(5): 690–696.
63. Pratap, J., et al., Regulatory roles of Runx2 in metastatic tumor and cancer cell interactions with bone. *Cancer Metastasis Rev*, 2006. **25**(4): 589–600.
64. Gersbach, C. A., et al., Inducible regulation of Runx2-stimulated osteogenesis. *Gene Ther*, 2006. **13**(11): 873–882.
65. Rhim, J. A., et al., Replacement of diseased mouse liver by hepatic cell transplantation. *Science*, 1994. **263**(5150): 1149–1152.
66. Fussenegger, M., et al., Streptogramin-based gene regulation systems for mammalian cells. *Nat Biotechnol*, 2000. **18**(11): 1203–1208.
67. Fields, S., and O.-K. Song, A novel genetic system to detect protein-protein interactions. *Nature*, 1989. **340**(6230): 245–246.
68. Asakawa, K., and K. Kawakami, Targeted gene expression by the Gal4-UAS system in zebrafish. *Dev, Growth Differ*, 2008. **50**(6): 391–399.
69. Rivera, V. M., et al., A humanized system for pharmacologic control of gene expression. *Nat Med*, 1996. **2**(9): 1028–1032.
70. Ye, X., et al., Regulated delivery of therapeutic proteins after in vivo somatic cell gene transfer. *Science*, 1999. **283**(5398): 88–91.

71. Spencer, D. M., et al., Controlling signal transduction with synthetic ligands. *Science*, 1993. **262**(5136): 1019-1019.
72. Blau, C. A., et al., A proliferation switch for genetically, Ââmodified, Ââcells. *Proc Natl Acad Sci*, 1997. **94**(7): 3076-3081.
73. Taylor, D. A., et al., Regenerating functional myocardium: improved performance after skeletal myoblast transplantation. *Nat Med*, 1998. **4**(8): 929-933.
74. Whitney, M. L., et al., Control of myoblast proliferation with a synthetic ligand. *J Biol Chem*, 2001. **276**(44): 41191-41196.
75. Belshaw, P. J., et al., Controlling programmed cell death with a cyclophilin-cyclosporin-based chemical inducer of dimerization. *Chem Biol*, 1996. **3**(9): 731-738.
76. Farrar, M. A., J. Alberola-Ila, and R. M. Perlmutter, Activation of the Raf-1 kinase cascade by coumermycin-induced dimerization. *Nature*, 1996. **383**(6596): 178-181.
77. Eilers, M., et al., Chimaeras of myc oncoprotein and steroid receptors cause hormone-dependent transformation of cells. *Nature*, 1989. **340**(6228): 66-68.
78. Becker, D. M., S. M. Hollenberg, and R. P. Ricciardi, Fusion of adenovirus E1A to the glucocorticoid receptor by high-resolution deletion cloning creates a hormonally inducible viral transactivator. *Mol Cell Biol*, 1989. **9**(9): 3878-3887.
79. Fankhauser, C. P., P. A. Briand, and D. Picard, The hormone binding domain of the mineralocorticoid receptor can regulate heterologous activities in cis. *Biochem Biophys Res Commun*, 1994. **200**(1): 195-201.
80. Takebayashi, H., et al., Hormone-induced apoptosis by Fas-nuclear receptor fusion proteins: novel biological tools for controlling apoptosis in vivo. *Cancer Res*, 1996. **56**(18): 4164-4170.
81. Hollenberg, S. M., P. F. Cheng, and H. Weintraub, Use of a conditional MyoD transcription factor in studies of MyoD trans-activation and muscle determination. *Proc Natl Acad Sci USA*, 1993. **90**(17): 8028-8032.
82. Beerli, R. R., B. Dreier, and C. F. Barbas, Positive and negative regulation of endogenous genes by designed transcription factors. *Proc Natl Acad Sci*, 2000. **97**(4): 1495-1500.
83. Dent, C. L., et al., Regulation of endogenous gene expression using small molecule-controlled engineered zinc-finger protein transcription factors. *Gene Ther*, 2007. **14**(18): 1362-1369.

84. Magnenat, L., L. J. Schwimmer, and C. F. Barbas, III, Drug-inducible and simultaneous regulation of endogenous genes by single-chain nuclear receptor-based zinc-finger transcription factor gene switches. *Gene Ther*, 2008. **15**(17): 1223–1232.
85. Schwimmer, L. J., B. Gonzalez, and C. F. Barbas, III, Benzoate X receptor zinc-finger gene switches for drug-inducible regulation of transcription. *Gene Ther*, 2012. **19**(4): 458–462.
86. Beerli, R. R., and C. F. Barbas, III, Engineering polydactyl zinc-finger transcription factors. *Nat Biotechnol*, 2002. **20**(2): 135–141.
87. Segers, V. F. M., and R. T. Lee, Biomaterials to enhance stem cell function in the heart. *Circ Res*, 2011. **109**(8): 910–922.
88. Little, L., K. E. Healy, and D. Schaffer, Engineering biomaterials for synthetic neural stem cell microenvironments. *Chem Rev*, 2008. **108**(5): 1787–1796.
89. Holzwarth, J. M., and P. X. Ma, Biomimetic nanofibrous scaffolds for bone tissue engineering. *Biomaterials*, 2011. **32**(36): 9622–9629.
90. Awad, H. A., et al., Chondrogenic differentiation of adipose-derived adult stem cells in agarose, alginate, and gelatin scaffolds. *Biomaterials*, 2004. **25**(16): 3211–3222.
91. McCullen, S. D., A. G. Y. Chow, and M. M. Stevens, In vivo tissue engineering of musculoskeletal tissues. *Curr Opin Biotechnol*, 2011. **22**(5): 715–720.
92. Cartmell, S., Controlled release scaffolds for bone tissue engineering. *J Pharm Sci*, 2009. **98**(2): 430–441.
93. Whitaker, M. J., et al., Growth factor release from tissue engineering scaffolds. *J Pharm Pharmacol*, 2001. **53**(11): 1427–1437.
94. Chen, R. R., and D. J. Mooney, Polymeric growth factor delivery strategies for tissue engineering. *Pharm Res*, 2003. **20**(8): 1103–1112.
95. Elisseeff, J., et al., Controlled-release of IGF-I and TGF-β1 in a photopolymerizing hydrogel for cartilage tissue engineering. *J Orthop Res*, 2001. **19**(6): 1098–1104.
96. Salvay, D. M., and L. D. Shea, Inductive tissue engineering with protein and DNA-releasing scaffolds. *Mol BioSyst*, 2006. **2**(1): 36–48.
97. Baraniak, P. R., et al., Spatial control of gene expression within a scaffold by localized inducer release. *Biomaterials*, 2011. **32**(11): 3062–3071.
98. Kaully, T., et al., Vascularization—the conduit to viable engineered tissues. *Tissue Eng Part B Rev*, 2009. **15**(2): 159–169.
99. Basu, S., et al., A synthetic multicellular system for programmed pattern formation. *Nature*, 2005. **434**(7037): 1130–1134.

100. Ciocca, D. R., et al., Biological and clinical implications of heat shock protein 27,000 (Hsp27): a review. *J Natl Cancer Inst*, 1993. **85**(19): 1558–1570.

101. Walther, W., and U. Stein, Heat-responsive gene expression for gene therapy. *Adv Drug Deliv Rev*, 2009. **61**(7, Äì8): 641–649.

102. Dreano, M., et al., High-level, heat-regulated synthesis of proteins in eukaryotic cells. *Gene*, 1986. **49**(1): 1–8.

103. Shoji, W., and M. Sato-Maeda, Application of heat shock promoter in transgenic zebrafish. *Dev Growth Differ*, 2008. **50**(6): 401–406.

104. Braiden, V., et al., Eradication of breast cancer xenografts by hyperthermic suicide gene therapy under the control of the heat shock protein promoter. *Hum Gene Ther*, 2000. **11**(18): 2453–2463.

105. Placinta, M., et al., A laser pointer driven microheater for precise local heating and conditional gene regulation in vivo. Microheater driven gene regulation in zebrafish. *BMC Dev Biol*, 2009. **9**: 73.

106. Guilhon, E., et al., Spatial and temporal control of transgene expression in vivo using a heat-sensitive promoter and MRI-guided focused ultrasound. *J Gene Med*, 2003. **5**(4): 333–342.

107. Deiters, A., Light activation as a method of regulating and studying gene expression. *Curr Opin Chem Biol*, 2009. **13**(5, Äì6): 678–686.

108. Cambridge, S. B., et al., Doxycycline-dependent photoactivated gene expression in eukaryotic systems. *Nat Meth*, 2009. **6**(7): 527–531.

109. Sauers, D. J., et al., Light-activated gene expression directs segregation of co-cultured cells in vitro. *ACS Chem Biol*, 2010. **5**(3): 313–320.

110. Blidner, R. A., et al., Photoinduced RNA interference using DMNPE-caged 2[prime or minute]-deoxy-2[prime or minute]-fluoro substituted nucleic acids in vitro and in vivo. *Mol BioSyst*, 2008. **4**(5): 431–440.

111. Jain, P. K., S. Shah, and S. H. Friedman, Patterning of gene expression using new photolabile groups applied to light activated RNAi. *J Am Chem Soc*, 2010. **133**(3): 440–446.

112. Self, C. H., and S. Thompson, Light activatable antibodies: models for remotely activatable proteins. *Nat Med*, 1996. **2**(7): 817–820.

113. Ye, S., et al., Chemical aminoacylation of tRNAs with fluorinated amino acids for in vitro protein mutagenesis. *Beilstein J Organ Chem*, 2010. **6**: 40.

114. Lemke, E. A., et al., Control of protein phosphorylation with a genetically encoded photocaged amino acid. *Nat Chem Biol*, 2007. **3**(12): 769–772.

115. Deiters, A., et al., A genetically encoded photocaged tyrosine. *Angew Chem Int Ed*, 2006. **45**(17): 2728–2731.
116. Shimizu-Sato, S., et al., A light-switchable gene promoter system. *Nat Biotech*, 2002. **20**(10): 1041–1044.
117. Yazawa, M., et al., Induction of protein–protein interactions in live cells using light. *Nat Biotech*, 2009. **27**(10): 941–945.
118. Kennedy, M. J., et al., Rapid blue-light-mediated induction of protein interactions in living cells. *Nat Methods*, 2010. **7**(12): 973–975.
119. Wang, X., X. Chen, and Y. Yang, Spatiotemporal control of gene expression by a light-switchable transgene system. *Nat Meth*, 2012. **9**(3): 266–269.
120. Crosson, S., and K. Moffat, Structure of a flavin-binding plant photoreceptor domain: insights into light-mediated signal transduction. *Proc Natl Acad Sci*, 2001. **98**(6): 2995–3000.
121. Wu, Y. I., et al., A genetically encoded photoactivatable Rac controls the motility of living cells. *Nature*, 2009. **461**(7260): 104–108.
122. Ye, H., et al., A synthetic optogenetic transcription device enhances blood-glucose homeostasis in mice. *Science*, 2011. **332**(6037): 1565–1568.
123. Salvay, D. M., M. Zelivyanskaya, and L. D. Shea, Gene delivery by surface immobilization of plasmid to tissue-engineering scaffolds. *Gene Ther*, 2010. **17**(9): 1134–1141.
124. Shin, S., D. M. Salvay, and L. D. Shea, Lentivirus delivery by adsorption to tissue engineering scaffolds. *J Biomed Mater Res A*, 2010. **93**(4): 1252–1259.
125. Phillips, J. E., et al., Engineering graded tissue interfaces. *Proc Natl Acad Sci USA*, 2008. **105**(34): 12170–12175.

Chapter 6

Biomimetic Design of Extracellular Matrix-Like Substrate for Tissue Regeneration

Chao Jia,[a] Seyed Babak Mahjour,[b] Lawrence Chan,[b] Da-wei Hou,[b] and Hongjun Wang[b]

[a]*Department of Chemical Engineering and Materials Science, Stevens Institute of Technology, 507 River Street, McLean Building 100, Hoboken, NJ 07030, USA*
[b]*Department of Chemistry, Chemical Biology and Biomedical Engineering, Stevens Institute of Technology, 507 River Street, McLean Hall 416, Hoboken, NJ 07030, USA*

Hongjun.Wang@stevens.edu

Electrospinning, a high-voltage–driven spinning technique, has the ability to fabricate nanofibers with the dimension and morphology similar to native tissue extracellular matrix (ECM) fibers from various materials. Owing to relatively high production rate, low setup cost, and easy operation, electrospinning receives great attention in materials and life sciences, especially in the tissue engineering research. It is predominantly applied to polymeric materials, including synthetic and natural polymers. The possibility of temporospatially incorporating and releasing various bioactive molecules from electrospun nanofibers and yielding anisotropic fiber orientation enables the recapitulation of the major features of ECM in the scaffold design for tissue regeneration. In addition, three-dimensional cell–fiber constructs can be fabricated using either the layer-by-layer assembly approach or co-electrospraying to emulate the *in vivo* circumstances. Taken together, this review will highlight the particular application of electrospinning technique in creation of ECM-like environment favorable for functional tissue formation.

6.1 Introduction

Tissue engineering has been proved to be a promising alternative therapy in clinical practice (Langer and Vacanti, 1993) and can provide a well-defined *in vitro* model for drug screening or tissue-related studies (Griffith and Swartz, 2006). In tissue engineering, a scaffold is normally used. Apart from its primary function as a temporary substrate for cells to attach and grow, more and more efforts in scaffold design are also made to provide the cells with instructive external cues to guide the tissue formation (Lutolf and Hubbell, 2005). In the search for an ideal scaffold to enhance tissue formation, it remains a big challenge to satisfy the mechanical need along with the delivery of appropriate chemical cues to cells. Many approaches, e.g., rapid prototyping, melt extrusion, salt leaching, emulsion templating, or phase separation, have been taken to create 3D porous structures from biocompatible and biodegradable materials such as poly(lactic-*co*-glycolic acid) (PLGA) in order to accommodate both requirements (Chen et al., 2002). However, they are still far beyond ideal in terms of guiding the desirable cell function.

In normal tissues, cells are either embedded within or reside on top of the extracellular matrix (ECM) depending on cell types (Abrams et al., 2000), e.g., epithelial cells sit on the basement membrane consisting of tightly cross-linked ECM fibers with pores to form a continuous lining layer, while connective tissue cells like fibroblasts reside in a three-dimensional (3D) porous fiber network to control the ECM turnover (Lopez et al., 2008). Clearly, ECM is the major component to determine the shape and mechanical performance of tissues, and meanwhile provide physical supports for cells to attach and grow. More specifically, both ECM composition and tempo-spatial arrangement of anchored bioactive molecules greatly regulate the cell function, including cell migration, proliferation, and differentiation, as well as the synthesis of new ECM proteins via the cell/matrix interaction (Lane and Sage, 1994). Thus, ECM can be considered as a natural scaffold for residing cells. To appropriately maintain the cell phenotype during tissue engineering, it is desirable for the scaffold to maximally recapitulate the major features of native ECM on a multiscale, from the composition, morphology, topography, to spatial organization. To this end, we believe that nanofibrous scaffolds will be ideal as its similarity to ECM fibers in both dimension and morphology. Indeed, the advantages of nanofibrous scaffolds in promoting cell growth and maintaining proper cell phenotype have been demonstrated in a number of studies (Min et al., 2004; Chua et al., 2005; Ji et al., 2006; Li et al., 2007), which is a synergistic result of both nanotopography and chemical signaling (Wang et al., 2003; Patel et al., 2007; Zhang et al., 2009). Several approaches are available to fabricate nanofibers, including self-assembly (Zhang, Gelain et al., 2005), phase separation (Barnes et al., 2007; Li et al., 2007), and electrospinning (Michel, L'Heureux et al., 1999; Matthews et al., 2002; Telemeco et al., 2005; Pham et al., 2006). Among these approaches, electrospinning, a high voltage driven spinning technique, has received a great attention mainly due to its low setup cost, easy operation, and high production rate. As a result, extensive efforts have been made to explore the potential utilization of electrospun nanofibers for tissue regeneration. The electrospinning setup, various materials used for electrospinning and the potential applications of electrospun fibers for various tissue regenerations have been well documented (Ashammakhi et al., 2006). Thus, in this review, we are attempting to summarize the recent achievements in electrospinning, in particular with the focus on creation of artificial ECM-like scaffolds enabled by electrospinning.

6.2 Electrospinning and Electrospun Fibers

Electrospinning has received a tremendous attention recently due to its ease in setup and operation and most importantly its ability to produce nanofibers with similar dimensions as collagen fibers in the natural tissue matrix (Pham et al., 2006). Basically, the electrospinning apparatus mainly contains a spinneret, a syringe pump, a high-voltage supply, and a grounded conductive surface for fiber collection (Fig. 6.1a). With a typical electrospinning condition—at a flow rate (v) between 5 and 15 µL/min with electric field from 0.8 to 2.0 kV/cm and the electrospinning distance between 7 and 10 cm, the melt or solution from a variety of polymers such as PLGA, poly-L-lactide acid (PLLA), PCL, poly(ethylene oxide terephthalate)-poly(butylene terephthalate) (PEOT-PBT), collagen, chitosan, and composite materials (Matthews et al., 2002; Yoshimoto et al., 2003; Chua et al., 2005; Geng et al., 2005; Li et al., 2005; Moroni et al., 2006) has been successfully electrospun into micro- or nano-size fibers with the diameter ranging from 50 to 1000 nm. Further modifications of the electrospinning setup to satisfy different needs have been made (Agarwal et al., 2008). For example, in order to increase the mixing uniformity especially in the case of composite fibers or the incorporation of bioactive molecules, we have integrated a twin-extruder with the electrospinning setup, in which various components can be fed into the mixing chamber for a thorough mixing prior to electrospinning (Erisken et al., 2008). Multispinnerets are also often used to increase the electrospinning efficiency and uniform fiber distributions for large surface area (Madhugiri et al., 2003). We have also investigated the direct collection nanofibers onto grounded liquid surface (Yang et al., 2009), which has been similarly tested by other group (Smit et al., 2005).

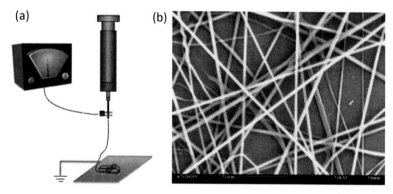

Figure 6.1   Illustration of the electrospinning setup (a) and scanning electron microscopy (SEM) image of electrospun 3:1 (w/w) polycaprolactone (PCL)/collagen nanofibers (b) (Yang et al., 2008).

Most of the electrospun fibers have smooth surface with a solid cross section. However, in order to achieve novel properties and specific functionalities, such as the incorporation of drug molecules for controlled release (Huang et al., 2006) and promotion of cell anchorage (Yashiki et al., 2001) to the surface, efforts have been made to create secondary unique structures in the electrospun fibers, e.g., core/shell composite fibers (He et al., 2005; Zhang, Lim et al., 2005), tubular fibers (Dosunmu et al., 2006), multichannel tubular structure (Zhao et al., 2007), and porous fibers (McCann et al., 2006). Many potential applications can be identified with these structures. To fabricate either tubular or core/shell composite fibers, coaxial electrospinning has been developed, in which a spinneret consisting of two coaxial capillaries with different diameters is used to accommodate two solutions for co-electrospinning. Inspired by this setup, a spinneret with multiple capillaries embedded in a plastic syringe at three vertexes of an equilateral triangle was fabricated for multifluidic compound jet electrospinning (Zhao et al., 2007). As an example, by using two immiscible viscous liquids (i.e., an ethanol solution of $Ti(OiPr)_4$ and poly(vinyl pyrrolidone)) and innocuous paraffin oil, multichannel tubular structure can be created as shown in Fig. 6.2. Porous fibers of a variety of polymers can be prepared through electrospinning using a bath of liquid nitrogen, which induces a phase separation between the polymer and the solvent (Nayani et al., 2011). In a particular humidity environment, electrospinning can also generate porous fibers, and the pore size could be adjusted by altering the humidity values (Casper et al., 2003). It has been reported that porous fibers can also be obtained when a highly volatile solvent is utilized in the electrospinning process (Celebioglu and Uyar, 2011). Following a similar approach above, attempt was also made to form porous fibers by electrospinning of mixtures composed of two immiscible polymers and a common solvent and selectively removing one polymer to yield the pores (Ma et al., 2009; Lyoo et al., 2005). In this process, a phase-separated structure needs to be formed within the electrospun fibers after the evaporation of the solvent. Different from the electrospinning of immiscible polymers, it is also possible to use nonsolvent/solvent combination to create porous fibers. For example, following the nonsolvent/solvent approach, in which alcohol was used as nonsolvent and dichloromethane as solvent, porous PLLA fibers could be obtained by varying the applied voltage and the ratio of nonsolvent/solvent (Lubasova and Martinova, 2011). Very often, only thick fibers can accommodate the additional nanostructures and it is not practical for nanofibers.

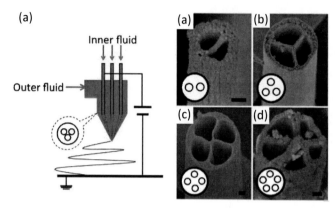

Figure 6.2 Left: Schematic illustration of the three-channel tube fabrication system. Right: SEM images of multichannel tubes with variable diameter and channel number (Zhao et al., 2007).

Depending on the materials used and electrospinning conditions, nonwoven fiber meshes with microscale variation, for instance, in pore size and fiber diameter (Pham et al., 2006), can be produced. It has been found that viscosity of the solution plays a determinant role in forming fibers or beads (Soares et al., 2011). In general, the thinner the electrospun fibers are, the smaller the pore size is (Park and Park, 2005). However, it is not possible to obtain the nanofibers with a uniform diameter; instead, they always appear as a range of distribution (Fig. 6.1b). Necessary to mention, the inter-fiber pore size is also to certain degree controlled by the size of collection surface when fiber diameters are comparable. Many reviews have comprehensively discussed the involvement of various parameters in controlling fiber diameters and inter-fiber distance (i.e., pore size) (Thompson et al., 2007; Milleret et al., 2011).

The control of inter-fiber pore size is an essential issue especially in the case of cell infiltration and tissue ingrowth. For most electrospun nanofiber meshes, the pore size is less than 5 μm (Fig. 6.1b), smaller than the cell size, which constrains the cells from penetrating into the meshes (Karageorgiou and Kaplan, 2005). The opportunity to increase the pore size by manipulating nanofiber diameter is very limited. In this regard, attempts have been made to improve the cell infiltration by using enzyme-degradable natural polymers (Puppi et al., 2010), or co-electrospinning with sacrificing nanofibers, which will be removed afterwards to generate large pores (Phipps et al., 2012). Recent methods used in enlarging pore size of electrospun nanofibers include salt leaching (Mikos et al., 1994; Lee et al., 2005; Nam, Huang et al., 2007), solid crystals on collection device (Simonet et al., 2007; Leong et al., 2009), wet electrospinning on bath collector (Ki et al., 2007; Yokoyama et al., 2009), nanofibers and microfibers combination (Kwon et al., 2005; Pham et al., 2006; Shim et al., 2009), laser/UV irradiation (Yixiang et al., 2008; Sundararaghavan et al., 2010), and electric field for controlling deposition of nanofibers (Zhang and Chang, 2008; Zhang et al., 2009; Vaquette and Cooper-White, 2011).

6.3 Incorporation of Various Biomolecules (Like ECM Molecules, Growth Factors) into Nanofibers

The advantage of electrospun nanofibers in promoting cell adhesion and maintaining cell phenotype, as a result of its dimensional similarities to ECM fibrils, has been reported (Min et al., 2004; Chua et al., 2005; Ji et al., 2006). As a temporary substrate to support cell growth and retain the tissue shape during new tissue formation, the nanofibrous scaffold should have both bioactivity and desired mechanical properties. Just like any other engineered construct, the choice of materials for ECM significantly depends on the specific properties required for the tissue. A number of synthetic and natural polymers such as PLGA, PLLA, PCL, semicrystalline poly(L-lactide-co-ε-caprolactone) (P(LLA-CL)), gelatin, chitosan, collagen, and silk protein can be used for scaffold fabrication. While it is possible to electrospin natural polymers especially in consideration of their good biocompatibility and biological activity; however, the fast degradation and weak mechanical properties often require a cross-linking step to maintain the structural integrity, which inevitably compromises the biological activity. On the other hand, many synthetic polymers have superior mechanical properties and tunable biodegradation rate. In this regard, a composite material composed of both natural and synthetic polymers will be ideal for both mechanical properties and biological properties. Actually, the advantages of incorporation of natural polymers into synthetic polymer fibers have been continuously highlighted (Orr et al., 2006). For example, the blend of collagen type I, a major ECM fiber protein of skin, into PCL can yield the PCL/collagen composite nanofibers. Its biological superiority has been evidenced by fibroblasts with a high cell adhesion (88.2%) and rapid cell spreading in spindle-like morphology on its surface (Yang et al., 2009). In comparison to PCL only, PCL/collagen nanofibers represent a better mimicking of the native ECM in both topology and composition. The advantages of PCL/collagen hybrid fibers have also been reported in other studies on the support of glial cells and fibroblasts (Venugopal et al., 2006; Schnell et al., 2007). The incorporation of other insoluble ECM molecules like elastin into nanofibers has also been investigated for vascular grafts (Ishii et al., 2005). The possible inclusion of various ECM components into nanofibers has been briefly summarized in Table 6.1. Furthermore, as frequently observed for synthetic polymers, PCL alone is unable to provide the osteoinductive and osteoconductive cues necessaries to guide cellular processes that underpin the genesis of new bone tissue. The integration of calcium phosphates particles, such as hydroxyapatite (HA), within PCL matrix has been one of the most investigated strategies to overcome such a limitation associated with "biological recognition" of PCL implants (Verderio et al., 2001). In fact, calcium phosphates are characterized by physical and chemical properties similar to the mineral phase of native bone tissue, and therefore may act as solid signals for cells, finally improving new-bone formation guided by PCL scaffolds. As a concomitant beneficial effect, these composites are often characterized by mechanical strength and stiffness similar to those of native bone.

The incorporation or immobilization of soluble biomolecules like growth factors into the polymeric nanofibers can better mimic the ECM function. Indeed, synergistic regulation of cell behavior by growth factors is critical for functional tissue formation (Frenz et al., 1994; Wei et al., 2007). Supplement of soluble bioactive molecules in the culture medium can deliver the stimulation to the cells; however, it is difficult to achieve a sustainable, separate, and temporal stimulation to multiple cell types in the same culture. Inclusion of bioactive molecules directly into scaffolds is considered as a practical solution to the aforementioned matter (Corden et al., 2000). Therefore, we hypothesize that specifically designed microenvironment can be formulated for different cells by combining the hierarchical spatial arrangement of nanofibers and incorporation of various bioactive molecules in the fibers.

Table 6.1 Fabrication of nanofibers containing various ECM components

Synthetic	Natural	Coat/ blend	Solvent	Method	Application	Reference
Poly(ε-caprolactone)	Collagen (type I)	Blend	DCM/DMF (75:25)	Electrospinning	For hMSCs support	(Srouji et al., 2007)
Poly(ethylene oxide)(PEO) Segmented polyurethane Styrenated gelatin	Collagen (type I)	Coat	Collagen and ST-gelatin: HFIP SPU (15.0 wt%): THF, PEO (1 to 4.5 wt%): chloroform	Mixing electrospinning Multi-layering electrospinning	Artificial and tissue-engineering devices	(Kidoaki et al., 2005)
Poly(ε-caprolactone)	Collagen (type I)	Blend	HFIP	Bottom-up, on-site layer-by-layer cell assembly	Form functional tissues composed of multiple types of cells,	(Yang et al., 2009)
Poly(ε-caprolactone)	Porcine skin type A Bovine type B gelatin	Blend	HFIP, TFE	Electrospinning	Design of unique properties of triple-helical collage	(Zeugolis et al., 2008)
Chitosan	Gelatin	Blend	TFA or mixture of TFA & DCM	Electrospinning	Potential application in skin regeneration.	(Dhandayuthapani et al., 2010)
Hydroxyapatite/ Chitosan	Collagen (type I)	Blend	HAC and DMSO	Electrospinning	Osteoregeneration-related applications	(Zhang et al., 2008)

(Continued)

Table 6.1 (Continued)

Synthetic	Natural	Coat/blend	Solvent	Method	Application	Reference
Poly(lactic-co-glycolic acid) (PLGA)	Collagen (type I)	Blend	HFIP	Electro-spinning	Bone tissue engineering applications	(Ngiam et al., 2009)
PHBV	Collagen (type I)	Blend	HFIP	Electro-spinning	Better cells adherence	(Meng et al., 2007)

Abbreviations: HFIP, 1,1,1,3,3,3-hexafluoro-2-propanol; DCM, dichloromethane; DMF, dimethylformamide; THF, tetrahydrofuran; TFE, 2,2,2-trifluoroethanol; TFA, trifluoroacetic acid; HAC, acetic acid; DMSO, dimethyl sulfoxide; hMSCs, human bone marrow-derived mesenchymal stem cells; PHBV, poly(3-hydroxybutyrate-co-3-hydroxyvalerate).

The most critical challenge to incorporate growth factors into nanofibers is how to preserve their bioactivity as they can easily denature during the chemical or physical processing. Second, how to maintain a sustainable or desirable release profile is another challenge. Although the lifetime for growth factors *in vivo* is short due to the presence of numerous proteolysis enzymes (Werle and Bernkop-Schnürch, 2006), continuous synthesis and secretion of new ones can provide non-stop guidance to the cells. However, this is not the case for the *in vitro* setting. Thus, it is essential for the scaffolds to maintain a desired temporospatial concentration of growth factors to guide tissue regeneration. Several possible pathways to incorporate growth factors have been established, including the physical absorption, coaxial electrospinning, blended electrospinning, covalent immobilization, and noncovalent binding. Table 6.2 summarizes all the possible ways to incorporate various growth factors into nanofibers. Although the physical absorption, i.e., soaking electrospun nanofibers in a growth factor solution can maximally preserve the bioactivity of growth factors, however, the uncontrollable adsorption efficiency and release rate suggest its limited application. The blended electrospinning allows a uniform distribution of growth factors across the fiber matrix and the procedure is simple. By controlling the mixing step, nanofibers with a gradient distribution of growth factors can be obtained along with electrospinning (Kim et al., 2004). Typically, a "burst" release would occur rapidly from the growth factor-containing nanofibers and then a slow release follows for rest of the time (Jha et al., 2009). The release kinetics greatly depends on the fiber diameter and initial loading. For instance, we have found the release of bovine serum albumin (BSA), a model protein, from fibers with the average diameter of 636.1 ± 211.8 nm is slower than that from the fibers of 322.6 ± 87.0 nm in diameter (Yang et al., 2008). However, the direct exposure to both solvent and high electric field may lead to the conformation change of growth factors, and therefore, lose their bioactivity (Ji et al., 2011). Coaxial electrospinning of two immiscible solutions, e.g., an organic polymer solution and an aqueous growth factor solution, on the other hand, is expected to form core–shell fibers with the growth factor in the core for a slow release. Similar to blended electrospun fibers, a "burst" release of growth factors also occurs to the core–shell fibers with a delayed release as a result of the controlled diffusion from the barrier shell. Surprisingly, the opportunity to preserve the bioactivity of growth factors through this approach is limited (Nair et al., 2010). Growth factors can be covalently immobilized onto electrospun fiber surface despite a possible alteration of the surface property. To controllably release the growth factor, enzyme-cleavable linkers can be used to trigger the release. For instance, Choi and Yoo (2007) reported the use of matrix metalloproteinases (MMPs)-cleavable linker for demanded release of target molecules from fiber surface. However, the complex reaction step involved and possible alteration of growth factor conformation constrains its wide application. Considering that many growth factors like vascular endothelial growth factor (VEGF), basic fibroblast growth factor (b-FGF) and epithelial growth factor (EGF) adhere to ECM *in vivo* via binding to specific domains in heparin a biomimetic design to mimic this process has been taken. That is, heparin is covalently immobilized onto the electrospun fibers and then allowing the binding of growth factors (Casper et al., 2005). In this approach, the bioactivity of growth factor is maximally preserved and the release of growth factor follows a fashion similar to physiological situation for better guidance of cellular functions. For example, the binding of FGF and EGF onto PLLA nanofibers via this approach can greatly guide the axon growth of ESC-derived neural cells (Xie et al., 2010). This strategy is clearly superior to others; however, it is only applicable to heparin-binding growth factors. More efforts in exploring other biomimetic mechanism to bind growth factors onto ECM-like fibers would be of great benefits in guiding cell function and consequently functional tissue regeneration.

Table 6.2 Incorporation of various growth factors into nanofibers

Materials	Growth factor	Methods	Application	Reference
Poly(ε-caprolactone) Poly(ethylene glycol)	NGF	NGF conjugated	Application in neural tissue engineering	(Cho et al., 2010)
Silk	BMP-2	Silk coated with BMP-2	Bone tissue engineering	(Li et al., 2006)
PLGA	IGF-1	Encapsulating IGF-1 into PLGA	Enhanced mesenchymal stem cell survival/ growth and orientation	(Wang et al., 2009)
Chitosan polyelectrolyte multilayers	FGF-2	FGF-2 was adsorbed on the PEM coated nanofibers	Stabilization of therapeutic growth factors for delivery *in vitro* and *in vivo*.	(Almodóvar and Kipper, 2011)
Dextran (DEX) as the core component PLGA as the shell polymer	VEGF	VEGF-loaded with dextran	Vascular tissue engineering	(Jia et al., 2011)
PLCL	NGF	Coaxial electrospinning	Nerve regeneration	(Liu et al., 2011)
PCL catalyzed by Sn(Oct)(2)/BDO	FGF2	FGF2 loaded in aqueous solution	Improve amount and morphology of cells	(Ye et al., 2011)
PCL/gelatin	EGF	EGF was chemically conjugated to the surface of nanofibers	Skin tissue-engineering applications	(Tigli et al., 2011)
Dextran (DEX) PLCL	PDGF-bb	Coaxial electrospinning	Membrane with fine core/shell	(Li et al., 2010)

			structure of fibers	
Collagen (type I) Gelatin	FGF-2	Coated with perlecan domain I (PlnDI) to improve binding of basic FGF-2	creating a successful tissue engineering scaffold	(Casper et al., 2007)

Abbreviations: PLCL, poly(L-lactide-co-ε-caprolactone); NGF, nerve growth factor; FGF-2, fibroblast growth factor 2; BMP-2, bone morphogenetic protein 2; VEGF, vascular endothelial growth factor; IGF-1, insulin-like growth factor; EGF, epidermal growth factor; PDGF-bb, platelet-derived growth factor-bb.

6.4 Control of Fiber Spatial Arrangement

In native tissue like bone, vessel, muscle, ligament, and tendon, alignment of ECM fiber is often observed, leading to the anisotropic mechanical performance. Thus, an important aspect in fabrication of ECM-like scaffolds is to control the spatial arrangement of fibers. During electrospinning process, the fibers can be collected onto a grounded stationary flat surface, on which the fibers are randomly oriented. On the other hand, fibers with aligned anisotropy can be achieved by using various collectors, such as a rotating drum, parallel electrodes, rotating discs, and square wire loop (Huang et al., 2003). As the fiber deposition onto a grounded surface is greatly controlled by the electric field, a gradient deposition of nanofibers on the collecting surface could be obtained by manipulating the intensity distribution of electric field. This control can also extend to further induce alignment by changing the ejection path from that of a spiral to that of a sinusoid or into a straight jet. Most of the time, more than one type of fibers, e.g., elastin fibers interpenetrate the collagen fibers, forms the ECM structure. In this regards, increasing efforts have been made to simultaneously deposit nanofibers of different compositions from multiple spinnerets, respectively (Fig 6.3). With manipulation of the feeding rate for each solution, a gradient distribution of each component with spatial control can be generated in the lateral direction.

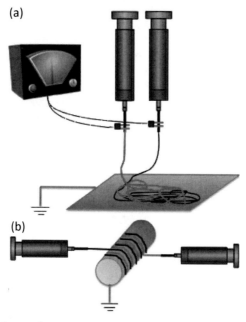

Figure 6.3 Setup for co-electrospinning for simultaneously collecting two types of nanofibers (red and black). Co-electrospinning for random nanofiber collection (a) or for aligned nanofiber collection (b).

We have investigated the formation of nanofibers with various 2D spatial arrangements based on a PCL/collagen blend. Figure 6.4 shows the PCL/collagen/BSA-FITC nanofibers collected on glass coverslips with different electric field modification. Without modifying the electric field, PCL/collagen nanofibers randomly deposited on the collecting surface. By manipulating the intensity distribution of electric field on the collecting surface, a gradient deposition of PCL/collagen nanofibers on the glass coverslips could be obtained. The alignment of PCL/collagen nanofibers was achieved by applying grounded parallel metal wires on the collecting surface described previously (Ball et al., 2004). The aligned fibers were deposited across the wires, and by changing the angle of parallel wires, the orientation of aligned fibers could be controlled. The cross-aligned fibers with two different compositions (PCL/Collagen/FITC-BSA, and PCL/Collagen/TRITC-BSA) were obtained by using parallel wires for the first TRITC fiber and then turning the wire pair 90° for the second FITC-fiber layer. The aligned fiber arrangement has been tested for their mechanical properties and found to be higher than the randomly aligned fibers (Li et al., 2007). A more elegant comparison was recently made by Garrigues' group (Garrigues et al., 2010), in which a multilayered electrospun nanofibrous scaffold, with each layer having its own fiber direction, was successfully created without the need of lamination. In this approach, they used rectangular and square insulating masks to control the geometry of the electric field, which controls the alignment of the fibers and generates mechanical anisotropy in the resulting scaffold. Testing mechanical properties in two orthogonal directions of resulting scaffolds revealed that aligned scaffolds, produced using a rectangular mask, were significantly stiffer in tension in the axial direction than the transverse direction at 0 strain (22.9 ± 1.3 MPa in axial, 16.1 ± 0.9 MPa in transverse), and at 0.1 strain (4.8 ± 0.3 MPa in axial, 3.5 ± 0.2 MPa in transverse). On the other hand, the use of a square mask resulted in nonaligned scaffolds with similar stiffness in the axial and transverse directions at 0 strain (19.7 ± 1.4 MPa axial, 20.8 ± 1.3 MPa transverse) and 0.1 strain (4.4 ± 0.2 MPa axial, 4.6 ± 0.3 MPa, transverse). The fiber orientation enables regional control of mechanical stress of scaffolds, allowing controllable deposition of new ECM molecules (Manwaring et al., 2004). The anisotropic mechanical properties of aligned fiber can be used to form the cross fibers with optimal strength (Budiansky and Cui, 1995), which is an important parameter for ECM emulation, especially for the tissues undergoing loading applications. The spatial orientation of nanofibers has significant effect on the cell attachment, morphology, migration, and new ECM deposition. For example, aligned PCL/collagen scaffolds induced the alignment of adipose stem cells near the expected axis on aligned scaffolds, while on the nonaligned scaffolds; their orientation showed more variation and was not along the expected axis (Fu and Wang, 2012). Other studies had mimicked the native tissue ECM and created aligned fibers that regulate cell behaviors by inducing cell orientation, examples include enhanced proliferation of nerve cells (Kijenska et al., 2012), better differentiation as well as proliferation of cardiac and skeletal muscle cells (Ricotti et al., 2011), and promoted fibroblast-to-myofibroblast differentiation (Huang et al., 2012). The effect of different fiber arrangements on cellular function is still under an extensive investigation with a clear indication of the involvement of integrins (Huang et al., 2012).

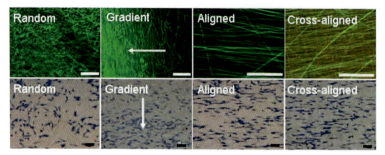

Figure 6.4 Cell growth on PCL/Collagen fibrous meshes with distinctive topographical patterns. Fluorescent images of nanofibers collected on glass coverslips (Top). Green fibers labeled with FITC-BSA and red fibers labeled with TRITC-BSA. Cells cultured overnight were stained with methylene blue (blue) (Bottom). Arrow indicates the gradient direction. Scale bar: 100 μm (Yang et al., 2008).

6.5 Formation of Multifunctional Hierarchical Structures Enabled by Nanofibers

6.5.1 Formation of Acellular Sandwiched Structures

Many *in vivo* tissues and organs exhibit hierarchical layered structures with distinct ECM composition and arrangement in each layer. These anisotropic ECM properties not only offer the cells with distinct signaling information, but also provide the tissues with a unique mechanical performance to coordinate with the physiological requirement. For example, three distinctive layers (ventricularis, spongiosa, and fibrosa) are clearly recognized in heart valve (Schoen and Levy, 1999). Densely packed collagen fibers are found in fibrosa layer to provide the predominant strength and stiffness, and prevent excessive stretching of valve. Spongiosa, composed of loosely arranged collagen and abundant hydrophilic glycosaminoglycans (GAG), lubricates the relative movement between ventricularis and fibrosa layers. Ventricularis is rich with elastin and shows radially aligned elastic fibers to enable the recoil and stretch of valve in response to diastole and systole of heart. Thus, it is highly desirable for the scaffolds to accommodate this hierarchical feature on a multiscale to achieve the subtle elaboration using electrospun nanofibers.

Electrospinning is a process that can not only generate fiber mesh scaffolds with high porosities, high surface area-to-volume ratios, and variable fiber diameters, but also allow the formation of tissue constructs sandwiched with multilayered cells. Electrospinning usually produces nonwoven sheet with a two-dimensional (2D) profile. If the electrospinning time is long enough, 3D fibrous meshes can be obtained from homopolymers or by using different polymers for different layers, or simultaneously ejecting different polymer solutions from different orifices (Fig. 6.3). Wan-Ju et al., evaluated the formation of thick 3D PCL nanofibrous scaffolds by extending the spinning time (Li et al., 2003). As a result, homogeneous PCL nanofibrous meshes with a thickness of 1 mm was formed on an aluminum foil surface with 14 mL of polymer solution at the rate of 0.4 mL/h. In order to test the cellular response, fetal bovine chondrocytes (FBCs) were seeded onto the electrospun PCL nanofibrous meshes. Gene expression analysis indicated that the biological activities of FBCs were crucially correlated with the architecture of extracellular scaffolds as well as the composition of culture medium. Moreover, the authors believed that PCL nanofibrous meshes acted as a biologically preferred substrate for chondrocytes in terms of cell proliferation and maintenance of chondrogenic phenotype, suggesting their suitability for cartilage tissue engineering.

How to assemble nanofibers into a 3D scaffold with a maximum match to the native environment is still under investigation. During electrospinning, either a planar structure or a vascular-like tubular structure of randomly oriented fibers can be obtained depending on the collecting setup. For instance, the collection of nanofibers onto a flat surface yields a flat tissue-like structure; on the other hand, fibers collected on a rotating mandrel turn to be a tubular structure. In either case, multilayered structures can be generated. It is possible to generate fibers with a wide range of diameters (e.g., 5 nm to 10 µm) by electrospinning. With this regard, Pham et al. attempted to create PCL multilayered scaffolds consisting of alternating layers of micro- and nanofibers following the sequential multilayering process (Pham et al., 2006). It was noted that as the fiber diameter increased, the average pore size of formed scaffolds increased (ranging from 20 to 45 µm) while remaining a constant porosity. By electrospinning the nanofiber layers for various times, the thickness of nanofiber layers could be modulated. The culture of rat marrow stromal cells on the multilayered scaffolds showed that cell attachment after 24 h did not change with the increase of nanofiber density, but the presence of nanofibers supported cell spreading as evidenced by F-actin staining with rhodamine phalloidin. Clearly, the alternated microfibers and nanofibers in the scaffolds favor cell infiltration while providing a physical mimicry of ECM by the nanofibers. In general, melt spinning and electrospinning are utilized separately. However, very recently these two techniques have been successfully combined to fabricate bioresorbable double-layered tubular structures (5 mm in diameter) from elastomeric 50:50 poly(L-lactide-co-ε-caprolactone) copolymers (Chung et al., 2010). This vascular-like structure contains both melt-spun macrofibers (<200 μm in diameter) and electrospun submicron fibers (>400 nm in diameter). Overall, the mechanical properties of prototype tubes exceeded the transverse tensile strength of natural arteries of similar caliber. In consideration of the anisotropic arrangement of ECM fibers from layer to layer in native tissues, Garrigues and coworkers (2010) recently created a multilayered electrospun scaffolds with specific fiber orientation for each layer. As described earlier, a rectangular insulating mask was used to regulate the geometry of electric field and therefore control the fiber alignment. This method provides a novel means of creating multilayered electrospun scaffolds with controlled anisotropy for each layer, potentially providing a way to mimic the complex mechanical properties of various native tissues.

Instead of only varying the fiber size and fiber orientation, adoption of various materials for the fiber layers would introduce more functionality to the scaffolds. The incorporation of fibers with various compositions can be realized through multilayering electrospinning or mixing electrospinning (Kidoaki et al., 2005). For example, Kidoaki et al. has recently generated a trilayered electrospun mesh, containing type I collagen, styrenated gelatin (ST-gelatin), segmented polyurethane (SPU) via sequentially layer-by-layer electrospinning the respective material solutions (Kidoaki et al., 2005). By simultaneously electrospinning onto a stainless steel mandrel with a high-speed rotation and traverse movement, a mixed electrospun-fiber mesh composed of intermingled SPU and PEO fibers was also prepared. As part of the demonstration, a bilayered tubular structure with a thick SPU microfiber mesh as the outer layer and a thin type I collagen nanofiber mesh as the inner layer was fabricated. We have also successfully demonstrated the capability of manipulating sequential deposition of different layers of fibers into a spatially graded nanofibrous scaffold by using PCL only and PCL/Collagen containing FITC-BSA (Yang et al., 2008). Similarly, the possibility of incorporating various small molecules like growth factors into various fiber layers would endorse the scaffolds with more cues for regulating cellular function. In addition, a gradient change for some components across the thickness without a clear borderline could be realized with the setup of twin-extruder electrospinning while continuous electrospinning (Erisken et al., 2008). A demonstration was made by incorporating β-TCP into PCL electrospun fibers, in which a gradient of TCP (0% to 15%) formed from the bottom to the top of the fiber mat. More and more efforts have been made to include multiple fibers into the scaffold design to achieve either mechanical or chemical superiority or both (Lutolf and Hubbell, 2005). It is expected that the mesoscopic spatial depositions and structural complexity can be of great benefits for new tissue formation particularly in formulating specific environments for various types of cells.

6.5.2 Formation of Cell/Fiber Multilayered Structure

Most tissues and organs of our body are composed of multiple types of cells and varying ECM, in which the cells are embedded in between 3D ECM fibers with various elaborate and hierarchical orders to achieve multiscale functions, and to mutually regulate the cellular activity by soluble bioactive molecules, cell–cell direct contact or cell–ECM interaction (Schwartz et al., 1998; Fukuhara et al., 2003; Kleinman et al., 2003; Stahl et al., 2004). The elaborate structure also provides individual cells with a defined microenvironment where the cells experience specific imparted cues and show corresponding responses.

Clearly, multifunctional electrospun nanofibers have many superior advantages in regulating cell functions. However, challenges are also recognized in using nanofibrous scaffolds, e.g., the difficulty of infiltrating cells into nanofibrous meshes despite various attempts to improve cell penetration (Zhang et al., 2007). In response to this particular challenge together with the spatial manipulation of cell arrangement and fiber arrangement, more innovative approaches are needed to incorporate the cells into fiber meshes. Srouji et al.

have examined the possibility of forming 3D constructs using nanofiber meshes seeded with cells, in which human bone marrow-derived mesenchymal stem cells (hMSCs) were cultured on nonwoven 1:1 PCL/collagen fiber meshes (100–200 µm in thickness) for 24 h and then stacked into a 3D construct and cultured under perfusion (Srouji et al., 2007). Although the cell penetration is not a big issue in this study as a result of large pores (>50 µm), it suggests a possible approach to incorporate cells into fiber meshes. However, in the case of stacking thin fiber meshes into 3D constructs it can be of a tremendous challenge for the operator. In this regard, Yang et al. in our group has developed a novel approach toward 3D multilayered tissue formation by using a bottom-up layer-by-layer cell assembly while electrospinning (Yang et al., 2009). Briefly, a thin layer (5–10 µm) of 3:1 PCL/collagen nanofibers was collected on the surface of medium, onto the fiber surface normal human fibroblasts (used as model cells) were evenly seeded and then a thin layer of nanofibers was electrospun onto the cell surface again. By repeating this process, 3D multilayer fibroblast/nanofiber constructs was created right along electrospinning, similar to *in vivo* tissues where cells were embedded in ECM fibers. During this layer-by-layer tissue rebuilding, it is flexible to vary cell seeding density and cell type for each cell layer and the composition for each nanofiber layer. With the opportunity to precisely control fiber layer thickness, fiber diameter and orientation, as well as to include bioactive molecules into the fibers for each fiber layer it is possible to create a specific 3D microenvironment for each cell type within the same construct. This approach has marked potentials to form functional tissues composed of multiple types of cells, heterogeneous scaffold composition, and customized specific microenvironment for cells. Instead of manual seeding cells, it is possible to electrospray cells through one of the spinnerets concurrently with electrospun nanofibers, which has been successfully demonstrated by stankus et al. in the microintegration of smooth muscle cells into a biodegradable, elastomeric poly(ester urethane) urea (PEUU) fiber matrix (Stankus et al., 2006). Cell electrospraying shows promises in bringing cells inside the fiber meshes, yet with some drawbacks, including less control of cell distribution as well as the potential cell damage from high voltage during cell electrospraying.

6.5.3 Three-Dimensional Tissue Formation from the Assembled Cell/Fiber Structure

The successful formation of cell/fiber structure offers a great opportunity to form 3D tissue. Indeed, further culture of the 10-layer fibroblast-PCL/collagen fiber constructs assembled as shown above for 3 and 7 days could result in the formation of dermal-like tissues. The exploration of forming epidermal/dermal bi-layer skin grafts was similarly made by layer-by-layer assembling fibroblasts and keratinocytes together with PCL/collagen nanofibers into a multilayer cell/fiber structure (18 layers of fibroblast/fiber in the lower part and 2 layers of keratinocyte/fiber on the top) and then culturing for additional days. The seeded keratinocytes remained on the surface and formed a continuous epidermal layer, and fibroblasts retained in the lower part with a uniform distribution. A tight binding formed between epidermal layer and dermal layer. Similarly, we recently assembled mouse osteoblasts together with PCL/chitosan nanofibers layer-by-layer into 3D cell/fiber structures. The culture of such structures for 14 days resulted in the formation of bone-like tissues, in which mineralization occurs across the full-thickness of the construct (Yang et al., 2009). Although it was labour consuming, Ishii et al. overlaid layers of PCL fiber meshes (10 µm thick and 15 mm in diameter) cultured with neonatal rat cardiomyocytes for 5–7 days into 3D structures and then cultured for 14 days (Ishii et al., 2005). Thick cardiac-like grafts with a uniform cell distribution and synchronized beating were obtained, indicating the proper retention of cardiomyocyte phenotype. Following the established electrospraying/electrospinning approach, Stankus et al. continued their effort to electrospray smooth muscle cells concurrently with electrospun PEUU fibers into a small diameter conduit (4.7 mm in diameter). Upon dynamic culture in spinner flask (15 rpm) for 3 days, the obtained conduits were strong and flexible with mechanical performance similar to those of native arteries, including static compliance of $1.6 \pm 0.5 \times 10^{-3}$ mmHg^{-1}, dynamic compliance of $8.7 \pm 1.8 \times 10^{-4}$ mmHg^{-1}, burst strengths of 1750 ± 220 mmHg, and suture retention (Stankus et al., 2008). It is necessary to mention that many of these approaches are only applicable to those layered tissues with simple geometry and shape.

6.6 Future Perspectives

The simple and easy setup of electrospinning has initiated a wide effort in fabricating fibers from various materials with the diameter in nanometers/micrometers, or with a secondary structure like nanopores or nanochannels within the fibers. Multilayering electrospinning or coelectrospinning offers a further dimension to functionalize the scaffold with more composition diversity and spatial arrangement. With all the capabilities, it is possible for us to design and fabricate an ECM-like scaffold to match the target tissue for optimal tissue regeneration. However, in reality different tissues have a great variation in ECM composition and structure, for instance, bone tissue contains mainly type I collagen and hydroxyapatite while cartilage is mainly composed of type II collagen and glycosaminoglycans (GAG). Furthermore, even in the same tissue subtle variation of ECM can be also recognized, e.g., various zones in articular cartilage (Tchetina, 2011), which determines the tissue function. Additionally, the dynamic ECM turnover while tissue development adds more complexity to our attempt to establish a standardized formulation recipe for 3D ECM-like scaffolds. Along with the extensive characterization of subtle composition and elaborate structure of various tissues and insightful understanding of the critical role of each ECM component in regulating cellular function, especially at the molecular level, it is possible for us to capture the major physiological features of each tissue matrix in scaffold design. However, extensive efforts will be needed to confirm that such scaffolds are sufficient to maintain the desired cell phenotype.

Compared to the formation of nanofibers via self-assembly of peptides, electrospinning offers a rapid and massive production of nanofibers. However, it remains a challenge to fabricate fibers with uniform and well-controlled diameters. Considering the composition complexity of ECM fibers in tissues, it would be of a great benefit to develop a fully automated and programmable electrospinning platform, in which it is free to control flow rate and switch the electrospinning solutions. In this way, the composition of nanofibers can be customized for different ECM while electrospinning.

6.7 Conclusion

Electrospinning offers a great opportunity to produce a variety of fibers with various diameters from a spectrum of materials, which can result in the formation of an ECM-like scaffold with diverse functionality and tunable spatial distribution of bioactive molecules. Together with the capability of incorporating cells directly into multilayered fiber structures, it is possible to formulate customized microenvironment specific for each type of cells. The development of nanofiber-assisted cell layering in a layer-by-layer manner or by co-electrospraying means enables 3D tissue formation. Electrospun nanofibers would provide a useful avenue to fabricate tissues with complex hierarchical architecture and an *in vitro* physiological platform to study cell–cell or cell–matrix interaction.

Acknowledgment

The authors are grateful for the financial support from NIAMS (Grant Number: 1R21 AR056416) and from National Science Foundation (Grant Number: CBET1033742).

References

Abrams, G. A., S. L. Goodman, et al. (2000). Nanoscale topography of the basement membrane underlying the corneal epithelium of the rhesus macaque. *Cell Tissue Res* **299**(1): 39–46.

Agarwal, S., J. H. Wendorff, et al. (2008). Use of electrospinning technique for biomedical applications. *Polymer* **49**(26): 5603–5621.

Almodóvar, J., and M. J. Kipper (2011). Coating electrospun chitosan nanofibers with polyelectrolyte multilayers using the polysaccharides heparin and N,N,N-trimethyl chitosan. *Macromol Biosci* **11**(1): 72–76.

Ashammakhi, N., A. Ndreu, et al. (2006). Biodegradable nanomats produced by electrospinning: expanding multifunctionality and potential for tissue engineering. *J Nanosci Nanotechnol* **6**(9–10): 2693–2711.

Ball, S. G., A. C. Shuttleworth, et al. (2004). Direct cell contact influences bone marrow mesenchymal stem cell fate. *Int J Biochem Cell Biol* **36**(4): 714–727.

Barnes, C. P., S. A. Sell, et al. (2007). Nanofiber technology: designing the next generation of tissue engineering scaffolds. *Adv Drug Deliv Rev* **59**(14): 1413–1433.

Budiansky, B., and Y. L. Cui (1995). Toughening of ceramics by short aligned fibers. *Mechan Mater* **21**(2): 139–146.

Casper, C. L., J. S. Stephens, et al. (2003). Controlling surface morphology of electrospun polystyrene fibers: Effect of humidity and molecular weight in the electrospinning process. *Macromolecules* **37**(2): 573–578.

Casper, C. L., N. Yamaguchi, et al. (2005). Functionalizing electrospun fibers with biologically relevant macromolecules. *Biomacromolecules* **6**(4): 1998–2007.

Casper, C. L., W. Yang, et al. (2007). Coating electrospun collagen and gelatin fibers with perlecan domain I for increased growth factor binding. *Biomacromolecules* **8**(4): 1116–1123.

Celebioglu, A., and T. Uyar (2011). Electrospun porous cellulose acetate fibers from volatile solvent mixture. *Mater Lett* **65**(14): 2291–2294.

Chen, G., Ushida, T., and T. Tateishi (2002). Scaffold design for tissue engineering. *Macromol. Biosci.* **2**: 67–77.

Cho, Y. I., J. S. Choi, et al. (2010). Nerve growth factor (NGF)-conjugated electrospun nanostructures with topographical cues for neuronal differentiation of mesenchymal stem cells. *Acta Biomater* **6**(12): 4725–4733.

Chua, K., W. Lim, et al. (2005). Stable immobilization of rat hepatocyte spheroids on galactosylated nanofiber scaffold. *Biomaterials* **26**(15): 2537–2547.

Chung, S., N. P. Ingle, et al. (2010). Bioresorbable elastomeric vascular tissue engineering scaffolds via melt spinning and electrospinning. *Acta Biomater* **6**(6): 1958–1967.

Chung, S., A. K. Moghe, et al. (2009). Nanofibrous scaffolds electrospun from elastomeric biodegradable poly(L-lactide-co-ε-caprolactone) copolymer. *Biomed Mater* **4**(1): 015019.

Corden, T. J., I. A. Jones, et al. (2000). Physical and biocompatibility properties of poly-epsilon-caprolactone produced using in situ polymerisation: a novel manufacturing technique for long-fibre composite materials. *Biomaterials* **21**(7): 713–724.

Dhandayuthapani, B., U. M. Krishnan, et al. (2010). Fabrication and characterization of chitosan-gelatin blend nanofibers for skin tissue engineering. *J Biomed Mater Res Part B: Appl Biomater* **94**(1):264–272.

Dosunmu, O. O., G. G. Chase, et al. (2006). Electrospinning of polymer nanofibres from multiple jets on a porous tubular surface. *Nanotechnology* **17**(4): 1123–1127.

Erisken, C., D. M. Kalyon, et al. (2008). Functionally graded electrospun polycaprolactone and β-tricalcium phosphate nanocomposites for tissue engineering applications. *Biomaterials* **29**(30): 4065–4073.

Frenz, D. A., W. Liu, et al. (1994). Induction of chondrogenesis: requirement for synergistic interaction of basic fibroblast growth factor and transforming growth factor-beta. *Development* **120**(2): 415–424.

Fu, X., and H. Wang (2012). Spatial arrangement of polycaprolactone/collagen nanofiber scaffolds regulates the wound healing related behaviors of human adipose stromal cells. *Tissue Eng Part A* **18**(5–6):631–642.

Fukuhara, S., S. Tomita, et al. (2003). Direct cell–cell interaction of cardiomyocytes is key for bone marrow stromal cells to go into cardiac lineage *in vitro*. *J Thorac Cardiovasc Surg* **125**(6): 1470–1480.

Garrigues, N. W., D. Little, et al. (2010). Use of an insulating mask for controlling anisotropy in multilayer electrospun scaffolds for tissue engineering. *J Mater Chem* **20**(40): 8962.

Geng, X., O. Kwon, et al. (2005). Electrospinning of chitosan dissolved in concentrated acetic acid solution. *Biomaterials* **26**(27): 5427–5432.

Griffith, L. G., and M. A. Swartz (2006). Capturing complex 3D tissue physiology *in vitro*. *Nat Rev Mol Cell Biol* **7**(3): 211–224.

He, W., Z. Ma, et al. (2005). Fabrication of collagen-coated biodegradable polymer nanofiber mesh and its potential for endothelial cells growth. *Biomaterials* **26**(36): 7606–7615.

Huang, C., X. Fu, et al. (2012). The involvement of integrin β1 signaling in the migration and myofibroblastic differentiation of skin fibroblasts on anisotropic collagen-containing nanofibers. *Biomaterials* **33**(6): 1791–1800.

Huang, Z. M., C. L. He, et al. (2006). Encapsulating drugs in biodegradable ultrafine fibers through co-axial electrospinning. *J Biomed Mater Res A* **77**(1): 169–179.

Huang, Z.-M., Y.-Z. Zhang, et al. (2003). A review on polymer nanofibers by electrospinning and their applications in nanocomposites. *Composites Sci Technol* **63**(15): 2223–2253.

Ishii, O., M. Shin, et al. (2005). *In vitro* tissue engineering of a cardiac graft using a degradable scaffold with an extracellular matrix-like topography. *J Thorac Cardiovasc Surg* **130**(5): 1358–1363.

Jha, A. K., W. Yang, et al. (2009). Perlecan domain I-conjugated, hyaluronic acid-based hydrogel particles for enhanced chondrogenic differentiation via BMP-2 release. *Biomaterials* **30**(36): 6964–6975.

Ji, W., Y. Sun, et al. (2011). Bioactive electrospun scaffolds delivering growth factors and genes for tissue engineering applications. *Pharm Res* **28**(6): 1259–1272.

Ji, Y., K. Ghosh, et al. (2006). Electrospun three-dimensional hyaluronic acid nanofibrous scaffolds. *Biomaterials* **27**(20): 3782–3792.

Jia, X., C. Zhao, et al. (2011). Sustained release of VEGF by coaxial electrospun dextran/PLGA fibrous membranes in vascular tissue engineering. *J Biomater Sci Polym Ed* **22**(13): 1811–1827.

Karageorgiou, V., and D. Kaplan (2005). Porosity of 3D biomaterial scaffolds and osteogenesis. *Biomaterials* **26**(27): 5474–5491.

Ki, C. S., J. W. Kim, et al. (2007). Electrospun three-dimensional silk fibroin nanofibrous scaffold. *J Appl Polym Sci* **106**(6): 3922–3928.

Kidoaki, S., I. Kwon, et al. (2005). Mesoscopic spatial designs of nano- and microfiber meshes for tissue-engineering matrix and scaffold based on newly devised multilayering and mixing electrospinning techniques. *Biomaterials* **26**(1): 37–46.

Kijenska, E., M. P. Prabhakaran, et al. (2012). Electrospun bio-composite P(LLA-CL)/collagen I/collagen III scaffolds for nerve tissue engineering. *J Biomed Mater Res B Appl Biomater* **100**(4): 1093–1102.

Kim, K., Y. K. Luu, et al. (2004). Incorporation and controlled release of a hydrophilic antibiotic using poly(lactide-*co*-glycolide)-based electrospun nanofibrous scaffolds. *J Control Release* **98**(1): 47–56.

Kleinman, H. K., D. Philp, et al. (2003). Role of the extracellular matrix in morphogenesis. *Curr Opin Biotechnol* **14**(5): 526–532.

Kwon, I. K., S. Kidoaki, et al. (2005). Electrospun nano- to microfiber fabrics made of biodegradable copolyesters: structural characteristics, mechanical properties and cell adhesion potential. *Biomaterials* **26**(18): 3929–3939.

Lane, T., and E. Sage (1994). The biology of SPARC, a protein that modulates cell–matrix interactions. *FASEB J* **8**(2): 163–173.

Langer, R., and J. P. Vacanti (1993). Tissue engineering. *Science* **260**(5110): 920–926.

Lee, Y. H., J. H. Lee, et al. (2005). Electrospun dual-porosity structure and biodegradation morphology of Montmorillonite reinforced PLLA nanocomposite scaffolds. *Biomaterials* **26**(16): 3165–3172.

Leong, M. F., M. Z. Rasheed, et al. (2009). In vitro cell infiltration and in vivo cell infiltration and vascularization in a fibrous, highly porous poly(D,L-lactide) scaffold fabricated by cryogenic electrospinning technique. *J Biomed Mater Res Part A* **91A**(1): 231–240.

Li, C., C. Vepari, et al. (2006). Electrospun silk-BMP-2 scaffolds for bone tissue engineering. *Biomaterials* **27**(16): 3115–3124.

Li, D., G. Ouyang, et al. (2005). Collecting electrospun nanofibers with patterned electrodes. *Nano Lett* **5**(5): 913–916.

Li, H., C. Zhao, et al. (2010). Controlled release of PDGF-bb by coaxial electrospun dextran/poly(L-lactide-co-ε-caprolactone) fibers with an ultrafine core/shell structure. *J Biomater Sci Polym Ed* **21**(6–7): 803–819.

Li, W., R. Mauck, et al. (2007). Engineering controllable anisotropy in electrospun biodegradable nanofibrous scaffolds for musculoskeletal tissue engineering. *J Biomechan* **40**(8): 1686–1693.

Li, W. J., K. G. Danielson, et al. (2003). Biological response of chondrocytes cultured in three-dimensional nanofibrous poly(epsilon-caprolactone) scaffolds. *J Biomed Mater Res A* **67**(4): 1105–1114.

Liu, J. J., C. Y. Wang, et al. (2011). Peripheral nerve regeneration using composite poly(lactic acid-caprolactone)/nerve growth factor conduits prepared by coaxial electrospinning. *J Biomed Mater Res A* **96**(1): 13–20.

Lopez, J. I., J. K. Mouw, et al. (2008). Biomechanical regulation of cell orientation and fate. *Oncogene* **27**(55): 6981–6993.

Lubasova, D., and L. Martinova (2011). Controlled morphology of porous polyvinyl butyral nanofibers. *J Nanomater* **2011**:292516.

Lutolf, M. P., and J. A. Hubbell (2005). Synthetic biomaterials as instructive extracellular microenvironments for morphogenesis in tissue engineering. *Nat Biotech* **23**(1): 47–55.

Lyoo, W. S., J. H. Youk, et al. (2005). Preparation of porous ultra-fine poly(vinyl cinnamate) fibers. *Mater Lett* **59** (28): 3558–3562.

Ma, G., D. Yang, et al. (2009). Preparation of porous ultrafine polyacrylonitrile (PAN) fibers by electrospinning. *Polym Adv Technol* **20**(2): 147–150.

Madhugiri, S., A. Dalton, et al. (2003). Electrospun MEH-PPV/SBA-15 composite nanofibers using a dual syringe method. *J Am Chem Soc* **125**(47): 14531–14538.

Manwaring, M. E., J. F. Walsh, et al. (2004). Contact guidance induced organization of extracellular matrix. *Biomaterials* **25**(17): 3631–3638.

Matthews, J. A., G. E. Wnek, et al. (2002). Electrospinning of collagen nanofibers. *Biomacromolecules* **3**(2): 232–238.

McCann, J. T., M. Marquez, et al. (2006). Highly porous fibers by electrospinning into a cryogenic liquid. *J Am Chem Soc* **128**(5): 1436–1437.

Meng, W., S.-Y. Kim, et al. (2007). Electrospun PHBV/collagen composite nanofibrous scaffolds for tissue engineering. *J Biomater Sci Polym Ed* **18**(1): 81–94.

Michel, M., N. L'Heureux, et al. (1999). Characterization of a new tissue-engineered human skin equivalent with hair. *In vitro Cell Dev Biol Anim* **35**(6): 318–326.

Mikos, A. G., A. J. Thorsen, et al. (1994). Preparation and characterization of poly(l-lactic acid) foams. *Polymer* **35**(5): 1068–1077.

Milleret, V., B. Simona, et al. (2011). Tuning electrospinning parameters for production of 3D-fiber-fleeces with increased porosity for soft tissue engineering applications. *Eur Cell Mater* **21**: 286–303.

Min, B., M. G. Lee, et al. (2004). Electrospinning of silk fibroin nanofibers and its effect on the adhesion and spreading of normal human keratinocytes and fibroblasts *in vitro*. *Biomaterials* **25**(7–8): 1289–1297.

Moroni, L., R. Licht, et al. (2006). Fiber diameter and texture of electrospun PEOT/PBT scaffolds influence human mesenchymal stem cell proliferation and morphology, and the release of incorporated compounds. *Biomaterials* **27**(28): 4911–4922.

Nair, A., P. Thevenot, et al. (2010). Novel polymeric scaffolds using protein microbubbles as porogen and growth factor carriers. *Tissue Eng Part C Methods* **16**(1): 23–32.

Nam, J., Y. Huang, et al. (2007). Improved cellular infiltration in electrospun fiber via engineered porosity. *Tissue Eng* **13**(9): 2249–2257.

Nayani, K., H. Katepalli, et al. (2011). Electrospinning combined with nonsolvent-induced pohase separation to fabricate highly porous and hollow submicrometer polymer fibers. *Ind Eng Chem Res* **51**(4): 1761–1766.

Ngiam, M., S. Liao, et al. (2009). The fabrication of nano-hydroxyapatite on PLGA and PLGA/collagen nanofibrous composite scaffolds and their effects in osteoblastic behavior for bone tissue engineering. *Bone* **45**(1): 4–16.

Orr, A. W., M. H. Ginsberg, et al. (2006). Matrix-specific suppression of integrin activation in shear stress signaling. *Mol Biol Cell* **17**(11): 4686–4697.

Park, H.-S., and Y. Park (2005). Filtration properties of electrospun ultrafine fiber webs. *Korean J Chem Eng* **22**(1): 165–172.

Patel, S., K. Kurpinski, et al. (2007). Bioactive nanofibers: synergistic effects of nanotopography and chemical signaling on cell guidance. *Nano Lett* **7**(7): 2122–2128.

Pham, Q. P., U. Sharma, et al. (2006a). Electrospinning of polymeric nanofibers for tissue engineering applications: a review. *Tissue Eng* **12**(5): 1197–1211.

Pham, Q. P., U. Sharma, et al. (2006b). Electrospun poly(ε-caprolactone) microfiber and multilayer nanofiber/microfiber scaffolds: characterization of scaffolds and measurement of cellular infiltration. *Biomacromolecules* **7**(10): 2796–2805.

Phipps, M. C., W. C. Clem, et al. (2012). Increasing the pore sizes of bone-mimetic electrospun scaffolds comprised of polycaprolactone, collagen I and hydroxyapatite to enhance cell infiltration. *Biomaterials* **33**(2): 524–534.

Puppi, D., F. Chiellini, et al. (2010). Polymeric materials for bone and cartilage repair. *Prog Polym Sci* **35**(4): 403–440.

Ricotti, L., A. Polini, et al. (2011). Nanostructured, highly aligned poly(hydroxy butyrate) electrospun fibers for differentiation of skeletal and cardiac muscle cells. *Conf Proc IEEE Eng Med Biol Soc* **2011**: 3597–3600.

Schnell, E., K. Klinkhammer, et al. (2007). Guidance of glial cell migration and axonal growth on electrospun nanofibers of poly-epsilon-caprolactone and a collagen/poly-epsilon-caprolactone blend. *Biomaterials* **28**(19): 3012–3025.

Schoen, F. J., and R. J. Levy (1999). Tissue heart valves: Current challenges and future research perspectives. *J Biomed Mater Res* **47**(4): 439–465.

Schwartz, J. D., S. Monea, et al. (1998). Soluble factor(s) released from neutrophils activates endothelial cell matrix metalloproteinase-2. *J Surg Res* **76**(1): 79–85.

Shim, I. K., W. H. Suh, et al. (2009). Chitosan nano-/microfibrous double-layered membrane with rolled-up three-dimensional structures for chondrocyte cultivation. *J Biomed Mater Res A* **90**(2): 595–602.

Simonet, M., O. D. Schneider, et al. (2007). Ultraporous 3D polymer meshes by low-temperature electrospinning: Use of ice crystals as a removable void template. *Polymer Eng Sci* **47**(12): 2020–2026.

Smit, E., U. Buttner, et al. (2005). Continuous yarns from electrospun fibers. *Polymer* **46**(8): 2419–2423.

Soares, R. M. D., V. L. Patzer, et al. (2011). A novel globular protein electrospun fiber mat with the addition of polysilsesquioxane. *Int J Biol Macromol* **49**(4): 480–486.

Srouji, S., T. Kizhner, et al. (2007). 3D Nanofibrous electrospun multilayered construct is an alternative ECM mimicking scaffold. *J Mater Sci Mater Med* **19**(3): 1249–1255.

Stahl, A., A. Wenger, et al. (2004). Bi-directional cell contact-dependent regulation of gene expression between endothelial cells and osteoblasts in a three-dimensional spheroidal coculture model. *Biochem Biophys Res Commun* **322**(2): 684–692.

Stankus, J. J., D. O. Freytes, et al. (2008). Hybrid nanofibrous scaffolds from electrospinning of a synthetic biodegradable elastomer and urinary bladder matrix. *J Biomater Sci Polym Ed* **19**(5): 635–652.

Stankus, J. J., J. Guan, et al. (2006). Microintegrating smooth muscle cells into a biodegradable, elastomeric fiber matrix. *Biomaterials* **27**(5): 735–744.

Suk Choi, J., and H. Sang Yoo (2007). Electrospun nanofibers surface-modified with fluorescent proteins. *J Bioactive Compatible Polymers* **22**(5): 508–524.

Sundararaghavan, H. G., R. B. Metter, et al. (2010). Electrospun fibrous scaffolds with multiscale and photopatterned porosity. *Macromol Biosci* **10**(3): 265–270.

Tchetina, E. V. (2011). Developmental mechanisms in articular cartilage degradation in osteoarthritis. *Arthritis* **2011**: 683970.

Telemeco, T. A., C. Ayres, et al. (2005). Regulation of cellular infiltration into tissue engineering scaffolds composed of submicron diameter fibrils produced by electrospinning. *Acta Biomater* **1**(4): 377–385.

Tigli, R. S., N. M. Kazaroglu, et al. (2011). Cellular behavior on epidermal growth factor (EGF)-immobilized PCL/gelatin nanofibrous scaffolds. *J Biomater Sci Polym Ed* **22**(1–3): 207–223.

Thompson, C. J., G. G. Chase, et al. (2007). Effects of parameters on nanofiber diameter determined from electrospinning model. *Polymer* **48**: 6913–6922.

Vaquette, C., and J. J. Cooper-White (2011). Increasing electrospun scaffold pore size with tailored collectors for improved cell penetration. *Acta Biomater* **7**(6): 2544–2557.

Venugopal, J. R., Y. Zhang, et al. (2006). In vitro culture of human dermal fibroblasts on electrospun polycaprolactone collagen nanofibrous membrane. *Artif Organs* **30**(6): 440–446.

Verderio, E., A. Coombes, et al. (2001). Role of the cross-linking enzyme tissue transglutaminase in the biological recognition of synthetic biodegradable polymers. *J Biomed Mater Res* **54**(2): 294–304.

Wang, F., Z. Li, et al. (2009). Fabrication and characterization of prosurvival growth factor releasing, anisotropic scaffolds for enhanced mesenchymal stem cell survival/growth and orientation. *Biomacromolecules* **10**(9): 2609–2618.

Wang, H., E. Shimizu, et al. (2003). Inducible protein knockout reveals temporal requirement of CaMKII reactivation for memory consolidation in the brain. *Proc Natl Acad Sci USA* **100**(7): 4287–4292.

Wei, D., Z. Jin, et al. (2007). Survival, synaptogenesis, and regeneration of adult mouse spiral ganglion neurons *in vitro*. *Dev Neurobiol* **67**(1): 108–122.

Werle, M., and A. Bernkop-Schnürch (2006). Strategies to improve plasma half life time of peptide and protein drugs. *Amino Acids* **30**(4): 351–367.

Xie, J., M. R. MacEwan, et al. (2010). Electrospun nanofibers for neural tissue engineering. *Nanoscale* **2**(1): 35–44.

Yang, X., X. Chen, et al. (2009). Acceleration of osteogenic differentiation of preosteoblastic cells by chitosan containing nanofibrous scaffolds. *Biomacromolecules* **10**(10): 2772–2778.

Yang, X., K. R. Ogbolu, et al. (2008). Multifunctional nanofibrous scaffold for tissue engineering. *J Exp Nanosci* **3**(4): 329–345.

Yang, X., J. D. Shah, et al. (2009). Nanofiber enabled layer-by-layer approach toward three-dimensional tissue formation. *Tissue Eng Part A* **15**(4): 945–956.

Yashiki, S., R. Umegaki, et al. (2001). Evaluation of attachment and growth of anchorage-dependent cells on culture surfaces with type I collagen coating. *J Biosci Bioeng* **92**(4): 385–388.

Ye, L., X. Wu, et al. (2011). Heparin-conjugated PCL scaffolds fabricated by electrospinning and loaded with fibroblast growth factor 2. *J Biomater Sci Polym Ed* **22**(1–3): 389–406.

Yixiang, D., T. Yong, et al. (2008). Degradation of electrospun nanofiber scaffold by short wave length ultraviolet radiation treatment and its potential applications in tissue engineering. *Tissue Eng Part A* **14**(8): 1321–1329.

Yokoyama, Y., S. Hattori, et al. (2009). Novel wet electrospinning system for fabrication of spongiform nanofiber 3-dimensional fabric. *Mater Lett* **63**(9–10): 754–756.

Yoshimoto, H., Y. M. Shin, et al. (2003). A biodegradable nanofiber scaffold by electrospinning and its potential for bone tissue engineering. *Biomaterials* **24**(12): 2077-2082.

Zeugolis, D. I., S. T. Khew, et al. (2008). Electro-spinning of pure collagen nano-fibres—Just an expensive way to make gelatin? *Biomaterials* **29**(15): 2293-2305.

Zhang, D., and J. Chang (2008). Electrospinning of three-dimensional nanofibrous tubes with controllable architectures. *Nano Lett* **8**(10): 3283-3287.

Zhang, K., X. Wang, et al. (2009). Bionic electrospun ultrafine fibrous poly(L-lactic acid) scaffolds with a sscale structure. *Biomed Mater* **4**(3): 035004.

Zhang, S., F. Gelain, et al. (2005). Designer self-assembling peptide nanofiber scaffolds for 3D tissue cell cultures. *Semin Cancer Biol* **15**(5): 413-420.

Zhang, Y., C. T. Lim, et al. (2005). Recent development of polymer nanofibers for biomedical and biotechnological applications. *J Mater Sci Mater Med* **16**(10): 933-946.

Zhang, Y., J. R. Venugopal, et al. (2008). Electrospun biomimetic nanocomposite nanofibers of hydroxyapatite/chitosan for bone tissue engineering. *Biomaterials* **29**(32): 4314-4322.

Zhang, Y. Z., B. Su, et al. (2007). Biomimetic and bioactive nanofibrous scaffolds from electrospun composite nanofibers. *Int J Nanomed* **2**(4): 623-638.

Zhao, Y., X. Cao, et al. (2007). Bio-mimic multichannel microtubes by a facile method. *J Am Chem Soc* **129**(4): 764-765.

Chapter 7

Degradable Elastomers for Tissue Regeneration

G. Rajesh Krishnan, Michael J. Hill, and Debanjan Sarkar

Department of Biomedical Engineering, University at Buffalo,
State University of New York at Buffalo,
316 Bonner Hall, Buffalo, NY 14260, USA

debanjan@buffalo.edu

7.1 Introduction

Biomaterial-based tissue engineering strategies to repair, restore, and improve tissue functions represent a viable strategy for treating defective tissues and organs. These approaches involve biomaterial-based artificial matrices, which are designed to provide structural and functional support to cells for organizing into effective tissues. Polymeric biomaterials, particularly synthetic polymers, have been developed for tissue engineering applications. Synthetic polymers can alleviate the complexities of processing, purification, immunogenicity, and pathogen transmissions that are usually associated with natural polymers [1,2]. Recent advancements in material science and engineering have triggered the development of synthetic polymers with defined functionalities to present appropriate physicochemical and physicomechanical

---

Tissue and Organ Regeneration: Advances in Micro- and Nanotechnology
Edited by Lijie Grace Zhang, Ali Khademhosseini, and Thomas J. Webster
Copyright © 2014 Pan Stanford Publishing Pte. Ltd.
ISBN 978-981-4411-67-7 (Hardcover), 978-981-4411-68-4 (eBook)
www.panstanford.com

microenvironments [3]. The niches developed from synthetic polymers can spatially and temporally coordinate cell–matrix interactions to induce proper signaling events [1,4]. Essential characteristics of a synthetic material are biocompatibility (i.e., to induce appropriate cellular and tissue response without any toxic effect) and biodegradability (i.e., to degrade within a clinically relevant timescale into nontoxic materials). These features usually pertain to physical and chemical characteristics, but recent studies have shown that mechanical characteristics of synthetic polymers influence tissue regeneration at cellular and tissue level [5–7]. It is, therefore, important to design synthetic polymers that are mechanically compatible for tissue regeneration. Particularly regeneration of soft tissues under dynamic mechanical environment requires synthetic polymers that are designed to match the tissue modulus and to recover from mechanical strains. This has led to the development of elastomeric polymers as synthetic degradable biomaterials for regenerative applications.

This chapter describes the development and application of degradable elastomers as biomaterials for tissue regeneration. Typically, elastomers undergo large reversible elongation when an external force is applied, i.e., these materials are stretchable, like a rubber band. The force required for elongation is small and some elastomers can undergo 1000% elongation by a small force [8,9]. Thus, in generic term, elastomeric features of a material are characterized by stretchability and elongation at break (maximum deformation at rupture). Inter- and intramolecular interactions between the polymer segments and chains contribute to the elastomeric character and, therefore, the elastomeric behavior is regulated by physical and chemical characteristics of the polymer. And from biological and clinical perspective, elastomeric polymers should be biocompatible and biodegradable to induce appropriate interactions in a biological milieu.

7.2 Characteristics of Elastomers

Elastomeric properties of synthetic polymers are significant in designing biomimetic artificial matrix. Thus, understanding the structure-property relationship is an important tool in designing degradable elastomers for engineering tissue regeneration.

The physiocomechanical characteristics of elastomers are best explained in terms of "rubber elasticity" and "viscoelasticity." These theories are based on time-independent and time-dependent recovery of polymer chain orientation and structure, respectively. Stretchability of elastomers is often described by the elastomeric force, which is developed on stretching. Elastomers are highly extensible and the entropic component of the elastomeric force explains the retractile behavior [10,11]. Large free volume and lower degree of cross-linking in the material allows them to respond to external forces with rapid rearrangement of polymer chains. Different theoretical and experimental models have been developed to explain the elastomeric behavior. Deviations from "rubber-like" elastic behavior have been observed when the polymer chains undergo significantly high extensions. These deviations are described by phenomenological treatments to explain the macroscopic behavior of the polymer. Thus, from structural perspective, polymer structure and composition entailing large free volume and less cross-links (both physical and chemical) will contribute to more elastomeric properties [9].

However, time-dependent properties of elastomers can be described by "viscoelasticity," which considers the fluid-like characteristics of polymer chains in a mechanically active condition [11]. As mechanical stress (or strain) leads to time-dependent strain (or stress) and the polymer chains move, the behavior is termed viscoelastic. Increased flow-properties of polymer chains and segments contribute to time-dependent alignment of polymer chains. Viscoelasticity of elastomers is important when an elastomer is designed for use at temperatures close to the glass-transition temperature of the polymer (a temperature that characterizes the transition of polymers from glassy solid to leathery rubber with increased chain mobility). Therefore, development of synthetic degradable polymers with elastomeric properties is related to the polymer design and condition of use. Important design parameters for developing elastomers are: composition monomer/co-monomer, molecular weight, cross-linking density, and extent of swelling [9]. Furthermore, additional design criterion should include the tunable structure (and functionality), degradability, and compatibility of these materials for tissue engineering applications.

7.3 Design of Biodegradable Elastomers

A biodegradable elastomer should exhibit high extensibility, biodegradability, and biocompatibility under a given physiological or pathophysiological condition. Synthetic polymers are designed as elastomers with different structure and composition for regenerative applications. Biodegradability of the elastomers is achieved through the presence of linkages, which degrade due to breakdown of the covalent bonds in polymers by bioactive molecules, reactive chemical species and enzymes present in biological microenvironments. Additionally, general design principles should consider the use of non-toxic monomers, which can be metabolized or excreted by the host. Elastomers can be categorized on the basis of chemical architectures, cross-linking design and source [12–14]. Chemically elastomers are classified according to the functional group present in the polymer, e.g., ester, urethane, amide. In addition to the chemical characteristics, cross-links of polymer chains elastomers are characterized as either physical entanglements or chemical cross-links. Finally, depending on the source, elastomers can be natural, synthetic, or semi-synthetic in origin. Elastomers based on the chemical structure are described in the following sections and will be appropriately classified in other categories.

7.3.1 Polyesters

Polymers with ester functionality constitute a major section of biodegradable elastomers for tissue regeneration. Polyesters are formed by polycondensation reaction between dicarboxylic acids and diols. They can also be synthesized by ring-opening polymerization of lactones. A general scheme of synthesis of polyesters is shown in Fig. 7.1.

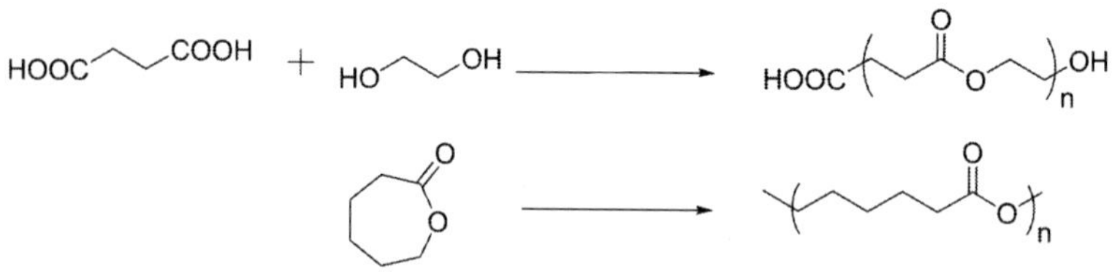

Figure 7.1 General scheme of synthesis of polyesters.

Detailed instructions for the preparation of the book using MS Word, including notes on preparing text, which comprises parts, chapters, section headings; lists; floats that include tables and figures; mathematics; miscellaneous; and references are described elaborately in this chapter.

Polymers with ester functionality constitute a major section of biodegradable elastomers for tissue regeneration. Polyesters are formed by polycondensation reaction between dicarboxylic acids and diols. They can also be synthesized by ring-opening polymerization of lactones. A general scheme of synthesis of polyesters is shown in Fig. 7.1.

Recent development of polyesters as degradable elastomers has expanded repertoire of synthetic elastomeric biomaterials. Linear polyester chains participate in physical cross-links through ionic interactions of ester group and can form hydrogen bond if functional groups such as hydroxyl, carboxylic acid are present. Chemical cross-linking (curing) of linear polyester chains into network structure can occur through thermal- or photopolymerization.

Polyesters based on sebacic acid and polyols with multiple hydroxyl groups are developed through esterification of acid and alcohol group in polycondenstaion reaction. Poly(glycerol-sebacate) (PGS) is an elastomer formed by condensation of glycerol and sebacic acid and contains pendant hydroxyl group attached to the backbone (Fig. 7.2) [15]. Elastomeric property of PGS is contributed by flexible hydrocarbon unit and the physical cross-links formed by hydrogen bonds through the hydroxyl group. Degradation characteristics of PGS are investigated in-vitro [16]. This polymer primarily degrades by surface erosion, which gives a linear degradation profile of mass, preservation of geometry and intact surface, and retention of mechanical strength. To enhance mechanical characteristics, PGS is thermally cured into

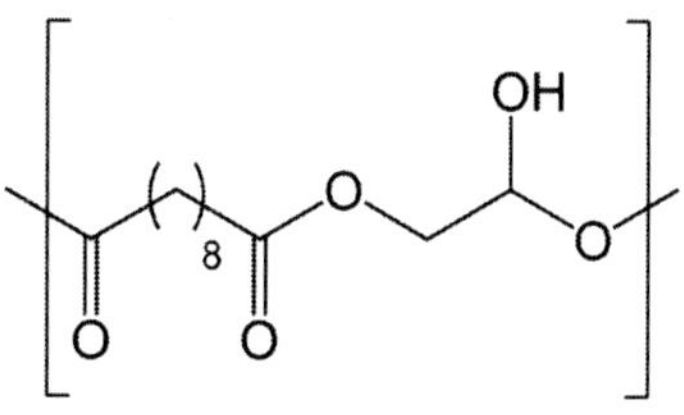

Figure 7.2 Chemical structure of poly-glycerol-sebacate (PGS).

thermosetting elastomer with tensile Young's modulus between 0.3 and 1.4 MPa, ultimate tensile strength (UTS) and a maximum elongation of 0.4 to 0.7 MPa and 125% to 160%, respectively.

However, the limitation of thermally cross-linked PGS to encapsulate cell and temperature sensitive molecules during curing has led to development photo-cross-linkable version of PGS with pendant acrylate group [17]. Acrylated- PGS (Acr-PGS) macromers are capable of cross-linking through free radical initiation mechanisms to form a polyester network. Alterations in the molecular weight and degree of acrylation of the Acr-PGS led to changes in network mechanical properties. In general, Young's modulus increased with degree of acrylation and the elongation at break increased with molecular weight when the degree of acrylation was held constant. These materials were investigated for in vitro and in vivo degradation and biocompatibility. The scaffold was associated with a moderate inflammatory response. Moreover, fibrous scaffolds of Acr-PGS and a carrier polymer, poly(ethylene oxide), were prepared via an electrospinning and photopolymerization technique and the fiber morphology was dependent on the ratio of these components [18]. This system provided biodegradable elastomeric polymers with tunable properties and enhanced processing capabilities toward the advancement of approaches in engineering soft tissues. The family sebacic acid–based biodegradable elastomer is further extended based on polycondensation reactions of xylitol with sebacic acid, referred to as poly(xylitol sebacate) (PXS) elastomers [19]. In vivo behavior of PXS elastomers were compared with poly(L-lactic-co-glycolic acid) (PLGA). PXS elastomers displayed a high level of structural integrity and form stability during degradation. The in vivo half-life ranged from approximately 3 to 52 weeks. PXS elastomers exhibited increased biocompatibility compared with PLGA implants.

In addition to PGS, copolymers of PGS have been developed as elastomeric degradable materials. Poly(1,3-diamino-2-hydroxypropane-co-polyol sebacate) is a copolymer of sebacic acid, polyol and amino alcohol 1,3-diamino-2-hydroxypropane, a new class of synthetic, biodegradable elastomeric poly(ester amide)s shown in Fig. 7.3 [20]. Presence of ester and amide linkages within the polymer provides tuning of degradability through defined mechanism. These cross-linked networks feature tensile Young's modulus on the order of 1 MPa and reversible elongations up to 92%. These polymers exhibited in vitro and in vivo biocompatibility and showed degradation half-lives up to 20 months in vivo. Mechanical properties and degradation kinetics of this elastomer can be influenced by adjusting polymer composition [21]. The tunable mechanical properties, biodegradability over a wide range and biocompatibility shows the potential of this material as degradable elastomer. Another derivative of PGS has been developed by incorporating lactic acid as co-monomer, which resulted in a degradable elastomer with defined degradation kinetics, biocompatibility, and mechanical characteristics [22].

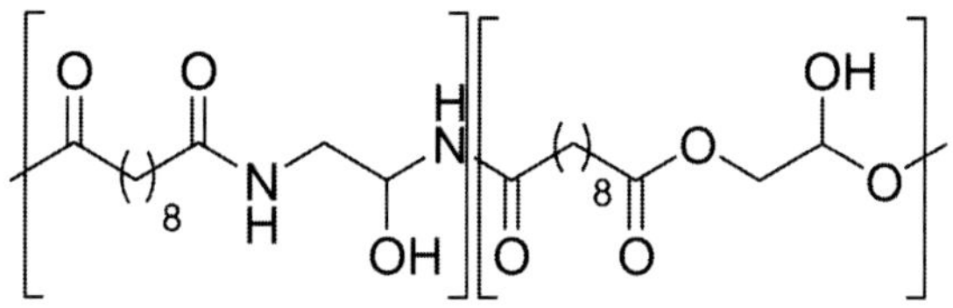

Figure 7.3 Chemical structure of PGS-based copolymer poly(1,3-diamino-2-hydroxypropane-co-polyol sebacate).

A new family of polyester-based degradable elastomers has been developed from the formulation based on citric acid and diols. Polycondensation reaction between citric acid and different diols resulted in the formation poly(diol-citrate) [23,24]. Similar to the synthesis of PGS, citric acid is reacted with aliphatic diols: hexanediol, octanediol, or decanediol to form a prepolymer that can be chemically cross-linked through thermal curing. Chemical characteristics of these polymers and the cross-linking induce the elastomeric properties. The mechanical properties, degradation, and surface characteristics of poly(diol citrates) can be controlled by diol characteristics and cross-link density of the polyester network. Various types of poly(diol citrate) scaffolds were fabricated to demonstrate their processing potential. These scaffolds were soft and could recover from deformation. In vitro and in vivo evaluation of the material, using cell culture and subcutaneous implantation respectively, confirmed cell and tissue compatibility. Among the different poly(diol-citrates), poly(1,8-octanediol-co-citrate) has been examined as degradable elastomers due to the mechanical properties: Young's modulus ranging from 0.92 to 16.4 MPa, ultimate tensile strength of 6.1 MPa and elongation at break of 117–265%. Additionally, degradation of poly(1,8-octanediol-co-citrate) results in the formation of octanediol, which is water soluble with no reported toxic effect. This poly(diol-citrate) has been used to design a nanoporous structure for controlling the mechanical and degradation properties of the elastomer. This nanoporous elastomer is biocompatible and a promising platform technology for engineering soft tissues [25]. The potential of this elastomer as tissue engineering scaffold was shown by engineering of small-diameter blood vessels [24]. Poly(1,8-octanediol-co-citrate) was also used to modify the surface of polytetrafluoroethylene (ePTFE) grafts in vitro, which reduced macrophage infiltration on the ePTFE grafts [26]. To improve the degradability and degradation time of poly(diol-citrate), poly (PEG-co-CA) was synthesized by condensation of poly(ethylene glycol) (PEG) as diol and citric acid (CA) under atmospheric pressure without any catalyst [27]. Like other poly(diol-citrate), the first step involved the synthesis of a pre-polymer by controlled condensation reaction between PEG and citric acid. This prepolymer was then post-polymerized and simultaneously cross-linked at 120°C in a mold. A series of polymers were prepared at different post-polymerization time and with different monomer ratios. Measurements on the mechanical properties of these polymers showed that the polymers are elastomeric with low hardness and high elongation. Hydrolytic degradation of the polymer films in a buffer of pH 7.4 at 37°C showed the hydrolytic degradability of these polymers. The different post-polymerization time and monomer ratio significantly influenced the degradation rates and mechanical performances. The material was showed to be useful for controlled drug delivery and other biomedical applications.

Photo-cross-linkable version of citric acid–based polyester, poly(octamethylene maleate citrate) (POMC), was developed through copolymerization of citric acid, octanediol, and maleic acid, which preserves pendant hydroxyl and carboxylic functionalities after cross-linking for the potential conjugation of biologically active molecules (Fig. 7.4) [28]. The prepolymers can be cross-linked by photopolymerization to yield a network structure that is soft and elastic with an initial modulus of 0.07 to 1.3 MPa and an elongation-at-break between 38% and 382%. POMC films demonstrated a wide range of physicomechanical properties, which show the potential of this material as degradable elastomer.

Another photo-cross-linkable citric acid-based polyester was developed by condensation of citric acid, 1,8-octanediol, and unsaturated monomers such as glycerol 1,3-diglycerolate diacrylate and bis(hydroxypropylfumarate) [29]. The polyesters were further cross-linked thermally in presence of a radical initiator. The cross-linked elastomeric network exhibited mechanical properties like Young's modulus, tensile strength, and elongation at break over a wide range. The mechanical properties of fumarate-containing elastomers were dependent on the content of 1-vinyl-2-pyrrolidinone used for cross-linking. Addition of a secondary cross-link network is a viable method to increase the range of mechanical properties of citric acid-based biodegradable elastomers.

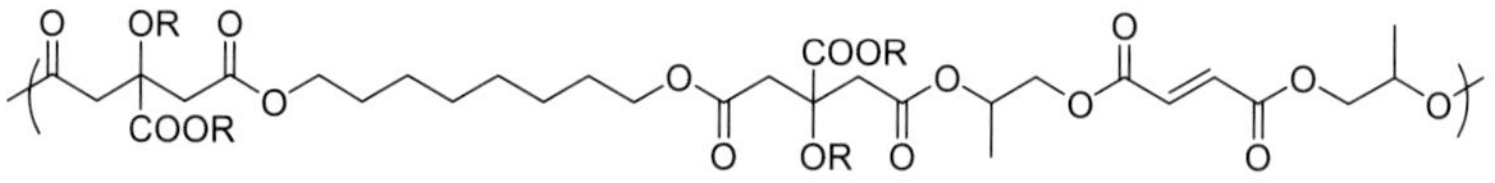

Figure 7.4 Citric acid–based biodegradable polyester with cross-linkable group.

Polyhydroxy alkanoates (PHA) are a family of thermoplastic polymers with wide ranging properties from rigid plastic to elastomers [30]. Polyhydroxy alkanoates can be homopolymers or copolymers in which the two or more hydroxyalkanoates are randomly arranged or occur in blocks and have been developed as degradable elastomers. The tensile strength of PHAs ranges between 20 and 50 MPa with elongations at break from 5–850%. PHAs degrade by surface erosion with a rate that can be tuned and the materials have demonstrated biocompatible characteristics. Among different PHAs, poly(3-hydroxybutyrate) (P3HB), co-polymers of 3 hydroxybutyrate and 3-hydroxyvalerate (PHBV), poly (4-hydroxybutyrate) (P4HB), copolymers of 3-hydroxybutyrate and 3-hydroxyhexanoate (PHBHHx), and poly 3-hydroxyoctanoate (PHO) have been studied in regenerative medicine applications [31–33].

Caprolactone-based polymers represent a versatile group of polyester-based degradable elastomers. A biodegradable star copolymer was prepared by ring-opening polymerization of D,L-lactide and ε-caprolactone initiated with glycerol and catalyzed by stannous 2-ethylhexanoate [34]. The star copolymers were synthesized of varying molecular weight and monomer composition and cross-linked by compression molding using bis(e-caprolactone-

4-yl)propane dissolved in ε-caprolactone monomer. The change in their physical properties during in vivo degradation in rats after subcutaneous implantation over a 12 week period was studied. Elastomers with high cross-link density exhibited degradation behavior consistent with a surface erosion mechanism, and degraded at the same rate in vivo as observed in vitro. Young's modulus and the stress at break of these elastomers decreased linearly with the degradation time, while the strain at break decreased slowly. Elastomers with low cross-link density exhibited degradation mechanism consistent with bulk erosion. Young's modulus and the stress at break of these elastomers decreased slowly initially, followed by a marked loss in mechanical strength after 4 weeks. The elastomers were well tolerated by rats over a 12 week period in vivo [35]. Similarly, a multiblock elastomer has been developed by copolymerizing L-lactide and ε-caprolactone as monomers. A series of polymers with various structures was synthesized. The basic structure is that of a diblock, with each block being modified by the addition of co-monomer. The synthesized polymers exhibited a range of mechanical properties from a typical thermoplastic polymer to that approaching a elastomer [36].

The potential disadvantages of thermally cured polyester have been addressed by the development of photo-cross-linkable version of caprolactone-based polymer. One formulation includes the polycondensation of ε-caprolactone with 4,4'-(adipoyldioxy)dicinnamic acid, which is used as a chain extender [37]. The mechanical and degradation properties can be altered through varying the degree of cross-links formed through photo-polymerization. However, to avoid the use potentially toxic photoinitiator, poly(caprolactone) has been functionalized with photosensitive coumarin, which undergoes photo-reversible dimerization to yield shape-memory biodegradable polymers with elastomeric properties [38].

7.3.2 Polyamides/Peptides

Polyamides are formed by a condensation reaction between acids and amines. In addition, they can be synthesized by ring-opening reactions of lactones (Fig. 7.5). Polyamides are an important class of polymers and include biological molecules like proteins and synthetic polymers like nylon 6 and nylon 6,6. Polyamides like nylon are used as surgical sutures but these polymers are less exploited in tissue engineering applications compared to polyesters and polyurethanes due to reduced degradability.

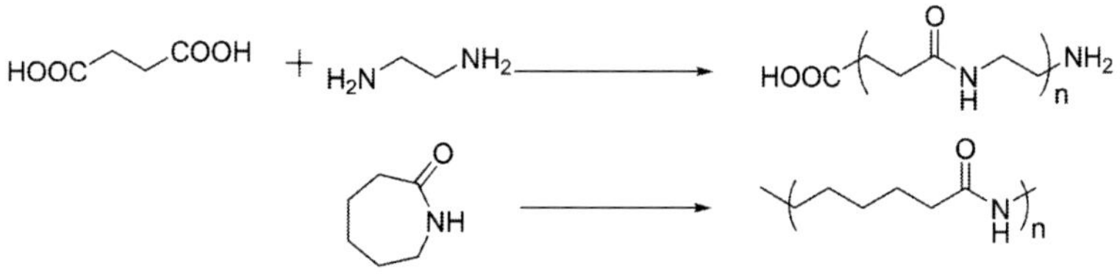

Figure 7.5 General scheme of synthesis of polyamides.

Porous nanohydroxyapatite/polyamide 66 (n-HA/PA66) scaffold material implanted into muscle and tibiae of rabbits to showed biocompatibility, osteogenesis, and osteoinductivity in vivo [39]. It is shown that nylon-3 modified surfaces enhance fibroblast attachment [40]. Three-dimensional scaffolds made from woven fabric of nylon-6,6 shown to enhance human osteoblast proliferation [41]. The behavior of human embryonic stem cell derived neural progenitors was evaluated on a synthetic, randomly oriented, three-dimensional nanofibrillar matrix composed of electrospun polyamide nanofibers. Homogenous, expandable, and self-renewable neural progenitors can be easily generated from human embryonic stem cells; and they can undergo differentiation to neurons and glials [42]. Similarly, electrospun polyamide nanofibres were shown to enhance retinal pigment epithelium proliferation [43].

Proteins are natural polymers of amino acids linked through amide bonds. Although synthetic polymers have advantageous properties compared to natural polymers, several proteins have emerged as elastomeric biomaterial for regenerative application. These elastomeric proteins have demonstrated potential to engineer tissue regeneration. Elastomeric proteins contain distinct domains, which comprise elastic repeated sequences and cross-links formed between sites in the nonelastic domains [44]. Elastin is one of the elastomeric proteins that has been extensively studied and characterized as the biomaterial for the regeneration of soft and elastic tissues [45]. Similarly, genetically engineered proteins similar to elastin have also been developed [46]. Several other proteins have been used as elastomeric materials, e.g., elastic spider silk, which has been recently used in nerve tissue engineering applications [47,48].

7.3.3 Polyurethanes

Polyurethanes represent a versatile family of biodegradable elastomers that have been extensively investigated and used in regenerative application due to their ease of synthesis and wide range of tunable properties. Polyurethanes are formed by the reaction between diisocyanates and diols (typically long-chain diols) in the presence of a catalyst. Polyurethanes are characterized by the presence of carbamate (urethane) bonds that connect monomers together as shown in Fig. 7.6.

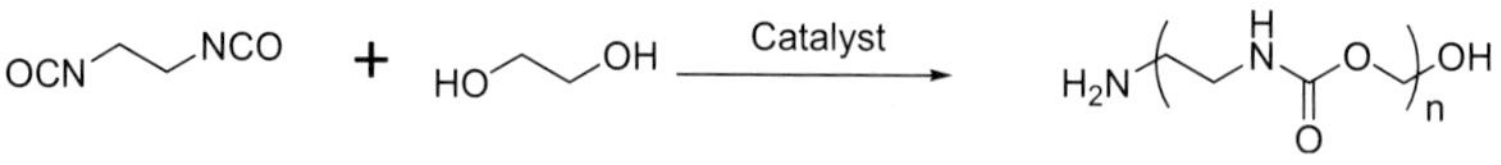

Figure 7.6 General scheme of synthesis of polyurethanes.

However, polyurethanes are further extended with a third component, known as chain extender to yield a biphasic polymer. The resultant polyurethanes polymers are composed of alternating "soft" amorphous segments of long-chain diols, and "hard" segments of diisocyanate and chain extender sections. The hard segments function as physical cross-links between the soft segments to prevent the chains from flowing apart when they are stretched under applied stress. The stretched polymer segments can then reshape elastically when stress is released [49,50]. Hence, polyurethanes are elastomeric in character. Mechanical properties of polyurethanes can be varied over a wide range: Young's modulus and ultimate tensile strength (UTS) of several tens of MPa, and large elongation at break in the range of 100–1000%. Moreover, by selecting appropriate segments, biodegradable and biocompatible polyurethanes can be designed for regenerative applications [51].

A library of biodegradable elastomeric polyurethanes was developed from polyether and polyester diols with aliphatic diisocyanate and amino acid–based chain extender from phenylalanine [52]. Detailed structure–function relationship was studied for this group of polyurethanes as elastomeric material and it was shown that polyurethane segments control the mechanical and degradation properties [53]. This study underlined the importance of segmental polyurethanes as degradable elastomeric material and demonstrated that by tuning the polyurethane structure, physicomechanical properties of the material can be modulated. This group further investigated the properties and application of degradable polyurethanes for various tissue engineering applications with scaffolds and fibers. For example, polyurethanes were synthesized from poly(hexamethylene carbonate)diol hexamethylene diisocyanate and chain extended using 1,4-butanediol. This polymer was fabricated into fibrous scaffolds by electrospinning. The surface of these scaffolds was modified with recombinant elastin-like polypeptide-4 (ELP4). These surface-modified scaffolds were used as substrates for smooth muscle cell culture. ELP4 surface-modified materials demonstrated enhanced smooth muscle cell (SMC) adhesion and maintenance of cell numbers over a 1 week period relative to controls [54]. Similar electrospun fibrous scaffold was made from a polyurethane synthesized from polycaprolcatone diol, lysine-based diisocyanate and a phenylalanine-based chain extender. These scaffold were used to differentiate phenotype of murine ESC-derived cardiomyocytes (mESCDCs). It was observed that both fiber alignment and pre-treatment of scaffolds with fibroblasts improve the differentiation of mESCDCs and were important parameters for developing engineered myocardial tissue constructs using ESC-derived cardiac cells [55]. Another example of amino acid–based polyurethane was developed from L-tyrosine-based chain extender with poly(ethylene glycol) and poly(caprolactone) and aliphatic diisocyantes [56]. A peptidomimetic structure was derived from L-tyrosine-based chain extender used in these polyurethanes as shown in Fig. 7.7. Being a peptide, the chain extender undergoes biodegradation easily and these polymers contribute to the class of biodegradable polyurethanes [57]. Furthermore, mechanical characteristics of the polyurethane were tuned over a wide range and studies have shown to be compatible in presence of cells [58]. Several other biodegradable polyurethanes have been designed from L-tyrosine-based chain extenders [59].

Guelcher and co-workers showed the importance of polyurethanes as biodegradable elastomers by a number studies. They showed that injectable lysine-derived polyurethane (PUR)/allograft biocomposites promoted bone healing in critical-size rabbit calvarial defects. Once injected, the material cured within 10–12 min to form a tough, elastomeric solid that maintained mechanical integrity during the healing process. When injected into a critical-size calvarial defect in rabbits, the biocomposites supported ingrowth of new bone [60]. The same research group used injectable polyurethane scaffolds as depot for delivering siRNA, drugs, and growth factors [61,62].

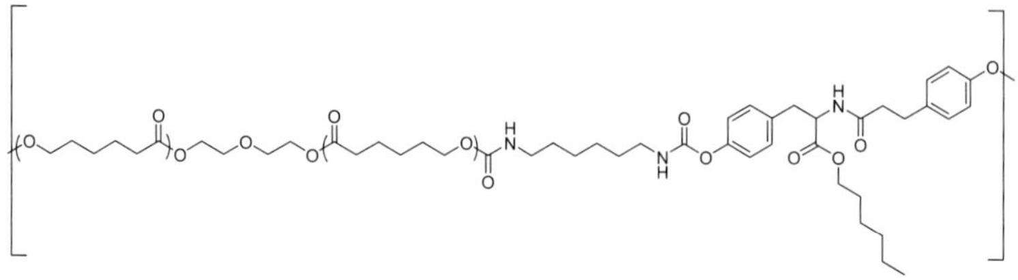

Figure 7.7 Polyurethane having biodegradable peptidomimetic links.

The family degradable polyurethanes was further extended by the inclusion of polyurethanes containing urea linkages and enzyme sensitive linkage for degradation (Fig. 7.8) [63,64]. These polyurethanes have been processed as three-dimensional scaffolds in the form of porous structure, fibers, and sheets and have been used for engineering tissue regeneration [65,66]. Biodegradable, elastomeric poly(ester urethane)urea (PEUU) scaffolds were explored as depots for the delivery of bioactive insulin-like growth factor-1 (IGF-1) and hepatocyte growth factor (HGF). Long-term in vitro IGF-1 release kinetics was investigated in both saline and saline with 100 units/mL lipase to simulate in vivo degradation. Cellular assays were used to confirm the bioactivity of released IGF-1 and HGF. Lipase-accelerated scaffold degradation led to delivery of >90% protein over 9 weeks. The bioactivity of IGF-1 and HGF was confirmed [67].

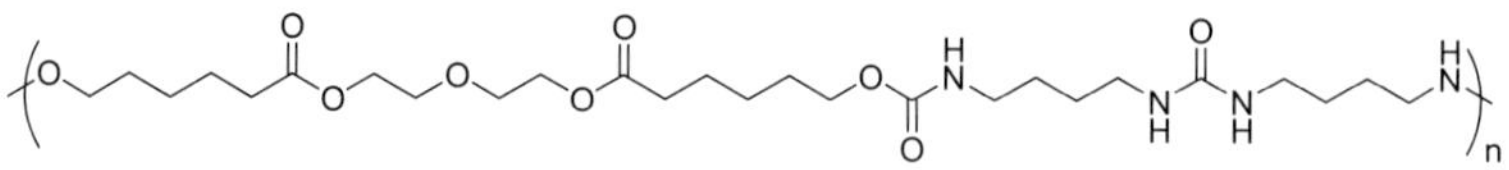

Figure 7.8 Poly(ester urethane urea) used for bioactive molecule delivery.

Versatility of polyurethanes has led to development hybrid polymeric system where non-urethane polymers are modified with urethane linkages through post-polymerization modifications or copolymerization techniques. Polyester prepared from octane diol and citric acid was further converted into polyurethane on reacting with hexamethylene diisocyantes in presence of octylstanane as the catalyst. Post-polymerization modification of this polymer, which includes thermally induced formation of cross-linking, produced biodegradable cross-linked urethane-doped polyesters (CUPEs). Mechanical properties and degradation rates of CUPE can be controlled by varying diol, polymerization conditions, as well as the concentration of urethane bonds in the polymer. The polymers demonstrated in vitro and in vivo biocompatibilities. Preliminary hemocompatibility evaluation indicated that CUPE adhered and activated lesser number of platelets compared to poly(L-lactic acid) (PLLA). Good mechanical properties and easy processability are the advantages that made these materials a good choice for soft tissue engineering applications [68]. In another study, injectable reverse thermal gels were developed with an amine-functionalized ABA type block copolymer, poly(ethylene glycol)-poly(serinol hexamethylene urethane) [69]. This reverse thermal gel consists of a hydrophobic block poly(serinol hexamethylene urethane) and a hydrophilic block poly(ethylene glycol). This gel demonstrated good biocompatibility and shows the potential to be an elastomeric gel for engineering tissue regeneration.

7.3.4 Hydrogels

Hydrogels are water-swellable but water-insoluble cross-linked networks that exhibit high water content and tissue-like elastic properties. These three-dimensional hydrophilic polymeric networks can absorb a large amount of water or biological fluids and maintain their semisolid morphology. Hydrogels are attractive materials for various biomedical applications like drug delivery and tissue engineering. A wide range of natural and synthetic polymers has been developed as hydrogels where the polymer chains are either chemically cross-linked or physically entangled to form a network structure with high water content [70,71]. Hydrogels have emerged as elastomeric biomaterials due to their ability to undergo reversible deformations under external stress [9]. Additionally, hydrogels can mechanically behave as a tough or a soft material depending on the chemical structure, cross-links, and water content. Hydrogels can be designed as degradable material under a given condition if degradable linkages are present and physicochemical features of the gels provides accessibility to the degradation agents. Thus, hydrogels have emerged as degradable elastomeric materials and have been investigated for many tissue regeneration applications.

Polyethylene glycol (PEG)-based hydrogels are most explored for tissue engineering and biomedical applications due to the biocompatibility of PEG. Photopolymerizable hydrogels derived from PEG and its derivatives have been developed from acrylate and methacrylate chemistries and rendered degradable through specific linkages [72–74]. Typically, chemical cross-linking of a PEG derivative with photo-cross-linkable group is used develop variety of PEG gels (Fig. 7.9). These gels have found widespread application in engineering cartilage, cardiac tissues, muscle tissues, and neural tissues, which typically require a mechanically compliant material to induce appropriate cell–matrix interactions [75]. Hybrid hydrogel systems with PEG have also been developed by combining urethane polymers with PEG-diacrylates [76].

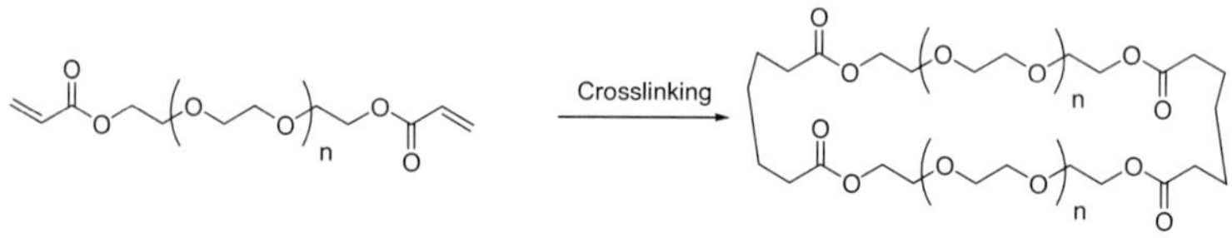

Figure 7.9 PEG diacrylate for cross-linked hydrogel.

Non-PEG–based synthetic gels have also been developed for tissue engineering applications. Hydrogels derived by the copolymerization of acrylamide and acryloyl amino acids have shown control over stem cell adhesion, migration, and differentiation. The cell–matrix interaction on these hydrophobic hydrogels was controlled by the matrix characteristics showing that hydrophobicity of these gels induces significant effect on the function mesenchymal stem cells [77]. In a different study, it was shown that thermosensitive hydrogels, based on N-isopropylacrylamide, N-acryloxysuccinimide, acrylic acid, and hydroxyethyl methacrylate-poly(trimethylene carbonate), are capable of differentiating mesenchymal stem cells into cardiomyocyte-like cells. The hydrogel was highly flexible at body temperature. When mesenchymal stem cells (MSCs) were encapsulated in the hydrogel and cultured under normal culture conditions, the cells differentiated into cardiomyocyte-like cells. On the other hand, the differentiation was retarded, and even diminished, under low-nutrient and low-oxygen conditions, which are typical of the infarcted heart. Once the hydrogels were loaded with a pro-survival growth factor (bFGF), MSC survival and differentiation in the hydrogel under the low-nutrient and low-oxygen conditions was enhanced considerably. This example shows the importance of combination of hydrogels and growth factors for the effective differentiation of cells [78].

Similarly, hydrogels made from natural polymer has gained significant importance. Alginate-based hydrogels has been developed and extensively characterized for tissue regeneration [79,80]. Tunable mechanical and degradation characteristics of alginates depend on molecular weight, cross-linking, and other physicochemical characteristics of the polymer. Alginate gels have been used for delivery of cells, biomolecules, and controlling of cell–matrix interactions [81,82]. The potential of alginates as degradable elastomeric biomaterial signifies its relevance in tissue regeneration. Guan and co-workers developed a saccharide-peptide hydrogel for encapsulating and culturing chondrocytes in three dimensions (Fig. 7.10). The polymers were synthesized from a galactaric acid-lysine co-polymer as the starting material. Four polymers were synthesized by valine, cysteine, tyrosine, and vinyl sulphone as side chains. Hydrogels were prepared from a solution containing one of the peptide polymers and vinyl sulphone polymers. In vitro studies using encapsulated chondrocytes showed that hydrophilicity of the side chain improved the biocompatibility and the hydrophilic tyrosine containing hydrogels assisted in cell proliferation and differentiation compared to hydrophobic valine polymer [83]. Hydrogels derived from hyaluronic acid were shown to enhance cell proliferation and differentiation. It is shown that the stiffening of the hydrogel is able to regulate the differentiation of human mesenchymal stem cells [84].

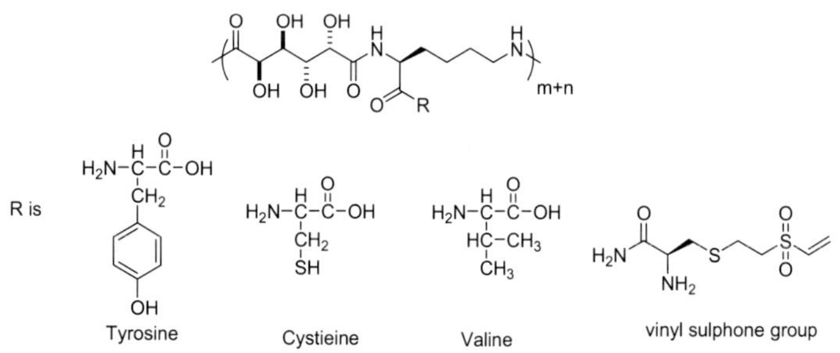

Figure 7.10 Saccharide-peptide hydrogel for cell encapsulation.

7.4 Applications of Biodegradable Elastomers in Tissue Regeneration

Development biodegradable elastomers have paved the way to engineer tissues with a mechanically compliant polymer. Particularly, soft tissues and tissues under dynamic environment require an artificial polymer that can mechanically match the native tissue. Engineering of these tissues has witnessed the use of degradable elastomers for effective and synchronized regeneration. Some of these examples are briefly described in this section.

7.4.1 Blood Vessels

Cardiovascular disease is one of the leading causes of mortality in developed countries, and especially, coronary artery disease increases with aging population and increasing obesity. Replacing arteries with autologous vessels, allografts, and synthetic grafts is the most common method for treatment. However, these grafts have limited applications when an inner diameter of arteries is less than 6 mm due to low availability, thrombotic complications, compliance mismatch, and late intimal hyperplasia. To overcome these limitations, tissue engineering has been successfully applied as a promising alternative to develop small-diameter arterial constructs that mimic natural healthy artery. Elastomers are particularly useful for the tissue engineering of blood vessels because of the elastic properties of these polymers, which resemble that of blood vessels to a great extent. Particularly, the elastomeric materials are able to withstand large radial strains during vascular perfusions. These materials can demonstrate biodegradability and cytobiocompatibility necessary for engineering vascular structures. Moreover, due to the advancements in micro/nano-fabrication techniques, it is possible to fabricate polymers into finely tubular scaffolds, which are particularly useful in the tissue engineering of fine blood vessel capillaries. Synthetic and tissue-engineered grafts are yet to show clinical effectiveness in arteries smaller than 5 mm in diameter, but they offer a promising future for elastomers in tissue engineering of blood vessels. Some of the recent advances in the tissue engineering of blood vessels using elastomers are described as follows.

Wang et al. designed cell-free biodegradable elastomeric grafts by covering a porous tube made of poly(glycerol sebacate) with electrospun sheet of poly(caprolactone). This scaffold degraded rapidly to yield neoarteries nearly free of foreign materials 3 months after interposition grafting in rat abdominal aorta. Three months after implantation, the neoarteries showed regular, strong, and synchronous pulsation, a confluent endothelium, contractile smooth muscle layers, expression of elastin, collagen, and glycosaminoglycan and tough and compliant mechanical properties, which are comparable to native arteries. This method is really promising because of the direct, cell free implantation of the polymeric material [85]. The adhesion, proliferation, and phenotypic and morphologic properties of primary baboon endothelial progenitor cells and baboon smooth muscle cells cultured on poly(glycerol sebacate) films and scaffolds were examined by the same research group. Phase contrast microscopy indicated that both types of cells showed normal morphology on the polymer films. Immunofluorescent staining revealed that von Willebrand factor and alpha-smooth muscle actin were expressed by endothelial cells and smooth muscle cells, respectively. Both types of cells proliferated well on PGS surfaces. When cultured in three-dimensional scaffolds, the muscle cells were distributed throughout the scaffolds and synthesized extracellular matrix. Immuno-fluorescent staining of co-cultured constructs indicated that the smooth muscle cells seeded constructs provided suitable surfaces for endothelial cells adhesion, and both types of cells maintained their specific phenotypes [86]. Poly(glycerol sebacate) was also used for fabricating porous tubular scaffolds using salt fusion method. Adult primary baboon smooth muscle cells were seeded on the lumen of scaffolds, which cultured for 3 weeks to get a tissue-engineered blood capillary analogue that had consistent thickness and randomly distributed macro- and micro-pores [87]. Degradable polar hydrophobic ionic polyurethane porous scaffolds were synthesized using a lysine-based divinyl oligomer. The scaffold properties were manipulated through the introduction of a lysine-based cross-linker. Preliminary study with vascular smooth muscle cells showed that these scaffolds demonstrated the ability to support cell adhesion and growth during 2 weeks of culture. It is possible to tailor the cell-material interaction and ultimately functional tissue regeneration and so these materials is a promising contribution in vascular tissue engineering [88]. Poly(ester urethane urea)-based small diameter, bilayered, biodegradable, elastomeric scaffold was prepared by thermally induced phase separation process. The scaffold incorporates a highly porous inner layer, allowing cell integration and growth, and an external, fibrous reinforcing layer of the same polymer deposited by electrospinning. These scaffolds were then seeded with adult stem cells using a rotational vacuum seeding device to obtain a tissue-engineered vascular graft, cultured under dynamic conditions for 7 days and evaluated for cellularity. The scaffold showed firm integration of the two polymeric layers with no delamination. This scaffold showed consistent mechanical properties under physiological conditions and maintained a high level of cellular density throughout dynamic culture [89]. Recent developments in microfluidic vascularized network structures with elastomeric polymers, e.g., poly-glycerol-sebacate and its derivatives have shown the potential of these materials [90]. Although the ultimate success of any vascular engineering strategy is dependent on its effective and functional integration, but these studies indicate that degradable elastomers have potential as a synthetic material for effective vessel regeneration.

7.4.2 Bladder

Degradable elastomers are leading candidate materials for efficient reconstruction of bladder tissues. It is critical to mimic the mechanical characteristics, particularly elastic property of bladder tissues and the dynamic flow environment in bladder for effective regeneration. Thus, elastomeric biomaterials represent a better alternative to traditional thermoplastic materials for bladder reconstruction.

Elastomeric degradable polyester poly-diol-citrate films have been used to with mesenchymal stem cell and urothelial cells for regeneration of bladder muscle. The mechanical characteristic of this construct demonstrated high uniaxial elastic potential, which indicates the significance of elastomeric polyester material [91]. Three-dimensional, porous, nanostructured poly(ether urethane) matrices too were found to be useful in bladder tissue-engineering. Cytocompatibility experiments using human bladder smooth muscle cells provided evidence that compared to conventionally used, micro-dimensional polyurethane scaffolds, these novel, nanodimensional scaffolds showed increased cell adhesion, growth, and extra cellular matrix protein production [92]. A hybrid electrospun scaffold composed of a biodegradable poly(ester-urethane)urea (PEUU) and a porcine extracellular matrix (ECM) scaffold (urinary bladder matrix) was fabricated and characterized for its bioactive and physical properties both in vitro and in vivo. Increasing amounts of PEUU led to linear increases in both tensile strength and breaking strain while ECM incorporation led to improved in vitro smooth muscle cell adhesion and proliferation and in vitro mass loss. Subcutaneous implantation of the hybrid scaffolds resulted in increased scaffold degradation and a large cellular infiltrate when compared with electrospun PEUU alone. This new scaffold possesses both bioactivity and mechanical features of its individual components [93]. Although these studies are at the preliminary level and additional studies are required for complete analysis, but the potential of elastomeric materials for bladder reconstruction seems promising.

7.4.3 Cardiac Tissue Engineering

Tissue engineering strategies for cardiac tissue require biomaterials that have structural, mechanical, and electrical features of native tissue. Scaffolds designed from biomaterial should match the physiologic mechanical properties, provide low mechanical resistance to accommodate large contractile deformations cardiac tissue, and provide signals to organize cells into a higher tissue superstructure. Biodegradable elastomers are suitable for this purpose and can provide appropriate physicomechanical signals to regenerate effective cardiac tissues.

Polyester-based elastomer developed from PGS has been investigated in different cardiac tissue engineering application due to elastomeric and degradable characteristics of the material. Three scaffolds were fabricated from the photo-cross-linkable PGS, with changes in fiber alignment (non-aligned (NA) versus aligned (AL)) and the introduction of a poly (ethylene oxide) (PEO) sacrificial polymer population to the AL scaffold (composite (CO)). PEO removal led to an increase in scaffold porosity and maintenance of scaffold anisotropy, CO scaffolds were completely degraded as early as 16 days, whereas NA and AL scaffolds had ~90% mass loss after

21 days when monitored in vitro. Neonatal cardiomyocytes, used as a representative cell type, that were seeded onto the scaffolds maintained their viability and aligned along the surface of the AL and CO fibers. When implanted subcutaneously in rats, CO scaffolds were completely integrated at 2 weeks, whereas ~13% and ~16% of the NA and AL scaffolds, respectively, remained acellular. AL scaffolds were completely populated with cells at 4 weeks post-implantations [94]. In vivo studies were performed with elastomeric nanofiber scaffold processed from acrylated poly(glycerol sebacate) (Acr-PGS) macromers processed using electrospinning, with gelatin as a carrier polymer that facilitated adhesion of mesenchymal stem cells. The resulting scaffolds were also diverse with respect to their mechanics (tensile modulus ranging from approximately 60 kPa to 1 MPa) and degradation (approximately 45–70% mass loss by 12 weeks). The scaffolds showed similar diversity when implanted on the surface of hearts in a rat model of acute myocardial infarction and demonstrated a dependence on the scaffold thickness and chemistry in the host response [95].

A hybrid heart patch engineered from poly(glycerol sebacate) supplemented with cardiomyocytes differentiated from human embryonic stem cells (hESCs). The PGS patch material without gelatin coating was found to satisfactorily support cardiomyocyte viability and attachment, with active cell beating for periods longer than 3 months until interrupted. Dynamic culture studies revealed that cells detached more efficiently from the uncoated surface of PGS than from gelatin-coated PGS. No significant differences were detected between the beating rates of human embryonic stem cell-derived cardiomyocytes on tissue culture plate and the pre-conditioned and gelatin-uncoated PGS. PGS patches sutured over the left ventricle of rats in vivo remained intact over a 2 week period without any deleterious effects on ventricular function [96]. In addition, three-dimensional structures from degradable elastomers are used for cardiac applications. Porous PGS scaffolds were prepared by salt leaching method. The scaffold contains an array of channels providing conduits for medium perfusion and sized to provide efficient transport of oxygen to the cells by a combination of convective flow and molecular diffusion over short distances between the channels. The channel constructs were seeded with myocytes and endothelial cells. It was determined that a linear perfusion velocity of 1.0 mm/s resulted in seeding efficiency of 87% ± 26% within 2 h. When applied to seeding of channeled scaffolds with neonatal rat cardiac myocytes, these conditions also resulted in high efficiency (77.2% ± 23.7%) of cell seeding. Uniform spatial cell distributions were obtained when scaffolds were stacked on top of one another in perfusion cartridges, effectively closing off the channels during perfusion seeding. Perfusion seeding of single scaffolds resulted in preferential cell attachment at the channel surfaces, and was employed for seeding scaffolds with rat aortic endothelial cells [97]. Similarly, micromolded scaffolds made from poly(glycerol sebacate) were found to assist the proliferation of cardiac muscle cells [92].

Skeletal myoblasts isolated and expanded from newborn Lewis rats were seeded on polyurethane (PU) scaffolds and transfected with DNA of VEGF-A, HGF, SDF-1, or Akt1. The seeded scaffolds were transplanted onto damaged myocardium of Lewis rats 2 weeks after myocardial infarction. After 6 weeks, primary rat skeletal myoblasts seeded on PU scaffolds were efficiently transfected, achieving transfection rates of 20%. A significant increase in expression of VEGF-A, HGF, SDF-1, and Akt1 after transfection was observed in vitro. In vivo studies showed that transplantation of growth factor-producing myoblast-seeded scaffolds resulted in enhanced angiogenesis (VEGF-A, HGF, and Akt1) or a reduced infarction zone (SDF-1 and Akt1) in the ischemically damaged myocardium [98]. Polyurethane-based cardiac patches have been developed with elastomeric and biodegradable, polyester urethane urea (PEUU). This patch was implanted on the heart in sub-acute infarction stage (2 weeks after infarction) and it was subsequently confirmed that this PEUU implantation could interrupt the adverse remodeling and improve cardiac function [99]. Collectively, these results indicate elastomeric biomaterial can effective comply with mechanical and biological microenvironment of cardiac tissue to restore and regenerate tissue function.

7.4.4 Tracheal, Neural, and Retinal

Development of biodegradable elastomers has provided significant advancement in the tissue regeneration strategy of trachea, neuron, and retina. The mechanical characteristics of these tissues indicate the importance of elastomeric biomaterial for effectively engineering the regeneration process.

Porous poly(ethylene oxide terephthalate)-poly(butylene terephthalate) scaffold and biodegradable polyester-urethane foam were used in preparation of tissue-engineered trachea. These polymers were found to enhance epithelial cell proliferation and tissue formation [100,101]. Use of degradable elastomers in neural tissue engineering is significant because extremely soft and delicate tissues in nerve. Sebacic acid elastomeric polyester, PGS, has been used for guided regeneration of the peripheral nerve through conduit structures [102]. Several other elastomeric polymers—poly-caprolactone-based elastomers based on copolymers of caprolactone and lactic acid, poly(hydroxyl alkanoates)—have shown promise to augment the nerve regeneration [13]. Degradable elastomers are also finding use in retinal applications. Regeneration of retina using polyester-based degradable elastomer poly-glycerol-sebacate (PGS) and retinal cells has the feasibility of such approaches [103]. Films of biodegradable polyurethanes containing poly(caprolactone) and/or poly(ethylene glycol) as soft segments, and isophorone diisocyanate and hydrazine as hard segments were used to study the interaction of retinal pigment epithelium cells with polymers. In addition, in vivo ocular biocompatibility of these polyurethane films was evaluated. The cells adhered to and proliferated onto the polyurethane supports, thus establishing cell–polymer surface interactions. Upon confluence, the cells formed an organized monolayer, exhibited a polygonal appearance, and displayed actin filaments, which ran along the upper cytoplasm. At 15 days of seeding, the occluding expression was confirmed between adjacent cells, representing the barrier functionality of epithelial cells on polymeric surfaces and the establishment of cell-cell interactions. Results from the in vivo study indicated that polyurethanes exhibited a high degree of short-term intraocular biocompatibility [104].

In addition to these specific applications, biodegradable elastomers have been developed as adhesives and for drug delivery applications [105,106]. Particularly micro- and nanostructured materials, devices, and particles have been designed from these materials for application in regenerative medicine [107–110]. Clearly, the usefulness of these materials is expanding in different fields of regenerative medicine. Degradable elastomers are potential biomaterials that can provide a biologically and mechanically compliant polymer for various tissue engineering applications.

7.5 Conclusion

Biodegradable elastomers continue to emerge as a versatile class of synthetic biomaterials with many applications in tissue engineering and regenerative medicine. Due to the continuous advances in the chemistry and materials science of polymers, a number of methods are available for the synthesis and processing of elastomers with defined range of properties, which can be tuned easily. These polymers can be processed into defined three-dimensional structures. Recent understanding in molecular and cellular characteristics has enabled to elucidate the interaction of these materials in a biological environment. Furthermore, advances in stem cell research provided an impetus in tissue engineering, which can be effective integrated with functional materials for effective and synchronized tissue regeneration. Combination of stem cells and elastomers will create an impressive future for tissue engineering and regenerative therapy.

References

1. Lutolf, M. P., and Hubbell, J. A. (2005). Synthetic biomaterials as instructive extracellular microenvironments for morphogenesis in tissue engineering, *Nat. Biotech.* **23**, 47–55.
2. Langer, R., and Tirrell, D. A. (2004). Designing materials for biology and medicine, *Nature* **428**, 487–492.
3. Okada, M. (2002). Chemical syntheses of biodegradable polymers, *Pro. Polym. Sci.* **27**, 87–133.
4. Place, E. S., Evans, N. D., and Stevens, M. M. (2009). Complexity in biomaterials for tissue engineering, *Nat. Mater.* **8**, 457–470.
5. Ingber, D. (2002). Mechanical signaling. *Ann. New York Acad. Sci.* **961**, 162–163.
6. Ingber, D. E., Dike, L., Hansen, L., Karp, S., Liley, H., and Maniotis, A. (1994). Cellular tensegrity: exploring how mechanical changes in the cytoskeleton regulate cell growth, migration, and tissue pattern during morphogenesis, *Int. Rev. Cytol.* **150,** 173–224.

7. Engler, A. J., Sen, S., Sweeney, H. L., and Discher, D. E. (2006). Matrix elasticity directsstem cell lineage specification, *Cell* **126**, 677–689.
8. Odian, G. (2004). *Principles of Polymerization*, 4th ed. (Wiley Interscience, New Jersey).
9. Anseth, K. S., Bowman, C. N., and Brannon-Peppas, L. (1996). Mechanical properties of hydrogels and their experimental determination, *Biomaterials* **17**, 1647–1657.
10. Mark, J. E., and Erman, B. (2007). *Rubber Like Elasticity: A Molecular Primer* (Cambridge University Press, Cambridge).
11. Treloar, L. R. G. (1958). *The Physics of Rubber Elasticity* (Oxford University Press, New York).
12. Amsden, B. (2007). Curable, biodegradable elastomers: emerging biomaterials for drug delivery and tissue engineering, *Soft Mat.* **3**, 1335–1348.
13. Serrano, M. C., Chung, E. J., and Ameer, G. A. (2010). Advances and applications of biodegradable elastomers in regenerative medicine, *Adv. Funct. Mater.* **20**, 192–208.
14. Bettinger, C. J. (2011). Biodegradable elastomers for tissue engineering and cell–biomaterial interactions, *Macromol. Biosci.* **11**, 467–482.
15. Wang, Y., Ameer, G. A., Sheppard, B. J., and Langer, R. A. (2002). Tough biodegradable elastomer, *Nat. Biotech.* **20**, 602–606.
16. Wang, Y., Kim, Y. M., and Langer, R. (2003). In vivo degradation characteristics of poly(glycerol sebacate), *J. Biomed. Mater. Res. A.* **66A**, 192–197.
17. Nijst, C. L. E., Bruggeman, J. P., Karp, J. M., Ferreira, L., Zumbuehl, A., Bettinger, C. J., and Langer, R. (2007). Synthesis and characterization of photocurable elastomers from poly(glycerol-co-sebacate), *Biomacromolecules.* **8**, 3067–3073.
18. Ifkovits, J. L., Padera, R. F., and Burdick, J. A. (2008). Biodegradable and radically polymerized elastomers with enhanced processing capabilities, *Biomed Mater.* **3**, 034104.
19. Bruggeman, J. P., Bettinger, C. J., and Langer, R. (2010). Biodegradable xylitol-based elastomers: in vivo behavior and biocompatibility, *J. Biomed. Mater. Res. A.* **95A**, 92–104.
20. Bettinger, C. J., Bruggeman, J. P., Borenstein, J. T., and Langer, R. (2008). Amino alcohol-based degradable poly(ester amide) elastomers, *Biomaterials* **29**, 2315–2325.
21. Bettinger, C. J., Bruggeman, J. P., Borenstein, J. T., and Langer, R. (2009). In vitro and in vivo degradation of poly(1,3-diamino-2-hydroxypropane-

co-polyol sebacate) elastomers, *J. Biomed. Mater. Res. A.*, **91A**, 1077–1088.

22. Chen, Q., Liang, S., and Thouas, G. A. (2011). Synthesis and characterisation of poly(glycerol sebacate)-co-lactic acid as surgical sealants, *Soft. Matter.*, **7**, 6484–6492.

23. Yang, J., Webb, A. R., Pickerill, S. J., Hageman, G., and Ameer, G. A. (2006). Synthesis and evaluation of poly(diol citrate) biodegradable elastomers *Biomaterials* **27**, 1889–1898.

24. Yang, J., Webb, A. R., and Ameer, G. A. (2004). Novel citric acid-based biodegradable elastomers for tissue engineering, *Adv. Mater.* **16**, 511–516.

25. Hoshi, R. A., Behl, S., and Ameer, G. A. (2009). Nanoporous biodegradable elastomers, *Adv. Mater.* **21**, 188–192.

26. Yang, J., Motlagh, D., Allen, J. B., Webb, A. R., Kibbe, M. R., Aalami, O., Kapadia, O., Carroll, T. J., and Ameer, A. G. (2006). Modulating expanded polytetrafluoroethylene vascular graft host response via citric acid-based biodegradable elastomers, *Adv. Mater.* **18**, 1493–1498.

27. Ding, T., Liu, Q., Shi, R., Tian, M., Yang, J., and Zhang, L. (2005). Synthesis, characterization and in vitro degradation study of a novel and rapidly degradable elastomer. *Polym. Degrad. Stab.* **91**, 733–739.

28. Gyawali, D., Tran, R. T., Guleserian, K. J., Tang, L., and Yang, J. (2010). Citric-acid-derived photo-cross-linked biodegradable elastomers, *J. Biomater. Sci. Polym. Ed.* **21**, 1761–1782.

29. Zhao, H., and Ameer, G. A. (2009). Modulating the mechanical properties of poly(diol citrates) via the incorporation of a second type of crosslink network, *J. Appl. Polym. Sci.* **114**, 1464–1470.

30. Lee, S. Y. (1996). Bacterial polyhydroxyalkanoates, *Biotech. Bioeng.* **49**, 1–14.

31. Sevastianov, V. I., Perova, N. V., Shishatskaya, E. I., Kalacheva, G. S., and Volova, T. G. (2003). Production of purified polyhydroxyalkanoates (PHAs) for applications in contact with blood, *J. Biomater. Sci. Polym. Ed.* **14**, 1029–1042.

32. Zhao, K., Deng, Y., Chen J. C., and Chen, G. Q. (2003). Polyhydroxyalkanoate (PHA) scaffolds with good mechanical properties and biocompatibility, *Biomaterials* **24**, 1041–1045.

33. Borkenhagen, M., Stoll, R. C., Neuenschwander, P., Suter, U. W., and Aebischer, P. (1998). In vivo performance of a new biodegradable polyester urethane system used as a nerve guidance channel, *Biomaterials* **19**, 2155–2165.

34. Amsden, B., Wang, S., and Wyss, U. (2004). Synthesis and characterization of thermoset biodegradable elastomers based on star-poly (ε-caprolactone-co-D,L-lactide), *Biomacromolecules* **5**, 1399–1404.

35. Amsden, B. G., Tse, M. Y., Turner, N. D., Knight, D. K., and Pang, S. C. (2005). In vivo degradation behavior of photo-cross-linked star-poly(ε-caprolactone-co-D,L-lactide) elastomers, *Biomacromolecules* **7**, 365–372.

36. Lipik, V. T., Kong, J. F., Chattopadhyay, S., Widjaja, L. K., Liow, S. S., Venkatraman, S. S., and Abadie, M. J. (2010). Thermoplastic biodegradable elastomers based on ε-caprolactone and L-lactide block co-polymers: a new synthetic approach, *Acta Biomater.* **6**, 4261–4270.

37. Nagata, M., and Sato, Y. (2004). Biodegradable elastic photocured polyesters based on adipic acid, 4-hydroxycinnamic acid and poly(epsilon-caprolactone) diols, *Polymer* **45**, 87–93.

38. Nagata, M., and Yamamoto, Y. (2009). Synthesis and characterization of photocrosslinked poly(ε-caprolactone)s showing shape-memory properties, *J. Polym. Sci. A: Polym. Chem.* **7**, 2422–2433.

39. Xu, Q., Lu, H., Zhang, J., Lu, G., Deng, Z., and Mo, A. (2010). Tissue engineering scaffold material of porous nanohydroxyapatite/polyamide 66, *Int. J. Nanomed.* **13**, 331–335.

40. Liu, R., Masters, K. S., and Gellman, S. H. Polymer chain length effects on fibroblast attachment on nylon-3-modified surfaces, *Biomacromolecules* **13**, 1100–1105.

41. Moczulska, M., Bitar, M., Święszkowski, W., Bruinink, A. (2012). Biological characterization of woven fabric using two- and three-dimensional cell cultures, *J. Biomed. Mater. Res. A.* **100A**, 882–893.

42. Shahbazi, E., Kiani, S., Gourabi, H., and Baharvand, H. (2011). Electrospun nanofibrillar surfaces promote neuronal differentiation and function from human embryonic stem cells, *Tissue Eng. A.* **17**, 3021–3031.

43. Thieltges, F., Stanzel, B. V., Liu, Z., and Holz, F. G. (2011). A nanofibrillar surface promotes superior growth characteristics in cultured human retinal pigment epithelium, *Ophthalmic Res.* **46**, 133–140.

44. Tatham, A. S., and Shewry, P. R. (2000). Elastomeric proteins: biological roles, structures and mechanisms, *Trends Biochem. Sci.* **25**, 567–571.

45. Daamen, W. F., Veerkamp, J. H., van Hest, J. C. M., and van Kuppevelt, T. H. (2007). Elastin as a biomaterial for tissue engineering, *Biomaterials*, **28**, 4378–4398.

46. Betre, H., Setton, L. A., Meyer, D. E., and Chilkoti, A. (2002). Characterization of a genetically engineered elastin-like polypeptide for cartilaginous tissue repair, *Biomacromolecules* **3**, 910–916.
47. Gosline, J. M., Denny, M. W., and DeMont, M. E. (1984). Spider silk as rubber, *Nature* **309**, 551–552.
48. Radtke, C., Allmeling, C., Waldmann, K. H., Reimers, K., Thies, K., Schenk, H. C., Hillmer, A., Guggenheim, M., Brandes, G., and Vogt, P. M. (2011). Spider silk constructs enhance axonal regeneration and remyelination in long nerve defects in sheep, *PLoS ONE*. **6**, e16990.
49. Guelcher, S. A. (2008). Biodegradable polyurethanes: synthesis and applications in regenerative medicine, *Tissue Eng. B Rev.* **14**, 3–17.
50. Petrović, Z. S., and Ferguson, J. (1991). Polyurethane elastomers, *Progr. Polym. Sci.* **116**, 695–836.
51. Santerre, J. P., Woodhouse, K., Laroche, G., and Labow, R. S. (2005). Understanding the biodegradation of polyurethanes: from classical implants to tissue engineering materials, *Biomaterials* **26**, 7457–7470.
52. Skarja, G. A., and Woodhouse, K. A. (1998). Synthesis and characterization of degradable polyurethane elastomers containing an amino acid-based chain extender, *J. Biomater. Sci. Polym. Ed.* **9**, 271–295.
53. Skarja, G. A., and Woodhouse, K. A. (2000). Structure-property relationships of degradable polyurethane elastomers containing an amino acid-based chain extender, *J. Appl. Polym. Sci.* **75**, 1522–1534.
54. Blit, P. H., Battiston, K. G., Yang, M., Paul Santerre, J., and Woodhouse, K. A. (2012). Electrospun elastin-like polypeptide enriched polyurethanes and their interactions with vascular smooth muscle cells, *Acta Biomater.* **8**, 2493–2503.
55. Parrag, I. C., Zandstra, P. W., and Woodhouse, K. A. (2012). Fiber alignment and coculture with fibroblasts improves the differentiated phenotype of murine embryonic stem cell-derived cardiomyocytes for cardiac tissue engineering, *Biotech. Bioeng.* **109**, 813–822.
56. Sarkar, D., Yang, J. C., and Lopina, S. T. (2008). Structure-property relationship of L-tyrosine-based polyurethanes for biomaterial applications, *J. Appl. Polym. Sci.* **108**, 2345–2355.
57. Sarkar, D., and Lopina, S. T. (2007). Oxidative and enzymatic degradations of L-tyrosine based polyurethanes, *Polym. Degrad. Stab.* **92**, 1994–2004.
58. Shah, P. N., and Yun Y. H. (2011). Cellular interactions with biodegradable polyurethanes formulated from L-tyrosine, *J. Biomater. Appl.* **27**, 1017–1031.

59. Guelcher, S. A., Gallagher, K. M., Didier, J. E., Klinedinst, D. B., Doctor, J. S., Goldstein, A. S. Wilkes, G. L., Beckman, E. J., and Hollinger, J. O. (2005). Synthesis of biocompatible segmented polyurethanes from aliphatic diisocyanates and diurea diol chain extenders, *Acta Biomater.* **1**, 471–484.

60. Dumas, J. E., Brownbaer, P. B., Prieto, E. M., Guda, T., Hale, R. G., Wenke, J. C., and Guelcher, S. A. (2012). Injectable reactive biocomposites for bone healing in critical-size rabbit calvarial defects, *Biomed Mater.* **7**, 024112.

61. Nelson, C. E., Gupta, M. K., Adolph, E. J., Shannon, J. M., Guelcher, S. A, Duvall, C. L. (2012). Sustained local delivery of siRNA from an injectable scaffold, *Biomaterials* **33**, 1154–1161.

62. Wenke, J. C., and Guelcher, S. A. (2011). Dual delivery of an antibiotic and a growth factor addresses both the microbiological and biological challenges of contaminated bone fractures, *Expert Opin. Drug Del.* **8**, 1555–1569.

63. Guan, J., Sacks, M. S., Beckman, E. J., and Wagner, W. R. (2002). Synthesis, characterization, and cytocompatibility of elastomeric, biodegradable poly(ester-urethane)ureas based on poly(caprolactone) and putrescine, *J. Biomed. Mater. Res.* **61**, 493–503.

64. Guan, J., and Wagner, W. R. (2005). Synthesis, characterization and cytocompatibility of polyurethaneurea elastomers with designed elastase sensitivity, *Biomacromolecules* **6**, 2833–2842.

65. Guan, J., Fujimoto, K. L., Sacks, M. S., and Wagner, W. R. (2005). Preparation and characterization of highly porous, biodegradable polyurethane scaffolds for soft tissue applications, *Biomaterials* **26**, 3961–3971.

66. Hong, Y., Fujimoto, K., Hashizume, R., Guan, J., Stankus, J. J., Tobita K., and Wagner, W. R. (2008). Generating elastic, biodegradable polyurethane/poly(lactide-*co*-glycolide) fibrous sheets with controlled antibiotic release via two-stream electrospinning, *Biomacromolecules* **9**, 1200–1207.

67. Nelson, D., Baraniak, P., Ma, Z., Guan, J., Mason, N., and Wagner, W. (2011). Controlled release of IGF-1 and HGF from a biodegradable polyurethane scaffold, *Pharm. Res.* **28**, 1282–1293.

68. Dey, J., Xu, H., Shen, J., Thevenot, P., Gondi, S. R., Nguyen, K. T., Sumerlin, B. S., Tang, L., and Yang, L. (2008). Development of biodegradable crosslinked urethane-doped polyester elastomers, *Biomaterials* **29**, 4637–4649.

69. Park, D., Wu, W., and Wang, Y. (2011). A functionalizable reverse thermal gel based on a polyurethane/PEG block copolymer, *Biomaterials* **32**, 777–786.
70. Hoffman, A. S. (2002). Hydrogels for biomedical applications, *Adv. Drug Del. Rev.* **54**, 3–12.
71. DeForest, C. A., and Anseth, K. S. (2012). Advances in bioactive hydrogels to probe and direct cell fate, *Ann. Rev. Chem. Biomol. Eng.* **3**, 421–444.
72. Nguyen, K. T., and West, J. L. (2002). Photopolymerizable hydrogels for tissue engineering applications, *Biomaterials* **23**, 4307–4314.
73. Lin-Gibson, S., Jones, R. L., Washburn, N. R., and Horkay, F. (2005). Structure–property relationships of photopolymerizable poly(ethylene glycol) dimethacrylate hydrogels, *Macromolecules* **38**, 2897–2902.
74. Halstenberg, S., Panitch, A., Rizzi, S., Hall, H., and Hubbell, J. A. (2002). Biologically engineered protein-graft-poly(ethylene glycol) hydrogels: a cell adhesive and plasmin-degradable biosynthetic material for tissue repair, *Biomacromolecules* **3**, 710–723.
75. Drury, J. L., and Mooney, D. J. (2003). Hydrogels for tissue engineering: scaffold design variables and applications, *Biomaterials* **24**, 4337–4351.
76. Lin-Gibson, S., Bencherif, S., Cooper, J. A., Wetzel, S. J., Antonucci, J. M., Vogel, B. M., Horkay, F., and Washburn, N. R. (2004). Synthesis and characterization of PEG dimethacrylates and their hydrogels., *Biomacromolecules* **5**, 1280–1287.
77. Ayala, R., Zhang, C., Yang, D., Hwang, Y., Aung, A., Shroff, S. S., Arce, F. T., Lal, R., Arya, G., and Varghese, S. (2011). Engineering the cell–material interface for controlling stem cell adhesion, migration, and differentiation, *Biomaterials* **32**, 3700–3711.
78. Li, Z., Guo, X., and Guan, J. A. (2012). Thermosensitive hydrogel capable of releasing bFGF for enhanced differentiation of mesenchymal stem cell into cardiomyocyte-like cells under ischemic conditions, *Biomacromolecules* **13**, 1956–1964.
79. Augst, A. D., Kong, H. J., and Mooney, D. J. (2006). Alginate hydrogels as biomaterials, *Macromol. Biosci.* **6**, 623–633.
80. Rowley, J. A., Madlambayan, G., and Mooney, D. J. (1999). Alginate hydrogels as synthetic extracellular matrix materials, *Biomaterials.* **20**, 45–53.
81. Hao, X., Silva, E. A., Månsson-Broberg, A., Grinnemo, K. H., Siddiqui, A. J., Dellgren, G., Wardell, E., Brodin, L. A., Mooney, D. J., and Sylven, C. (2007). Angiogenic effects of sequential release of VEGF-A165 and PDGF-BB

with alginate hydrogels after myocardial infarction, *Cardiovas. Res.* **75**, 178–185.

82. Huebsch, N., Arany, P. R., Mao, A. S., Shvartsman, D., Ali, O. A., Bencherif, S. A., Rivera-Feliciano, J., and Mooney, D. J. (2010). Harnessing traction-mediated manipulation of the cell/matrix interface to control stem-cell fate, *Nat. Mater.* **9**, 518–526.

83. Chawla, K., Yu, T. B., Stutts, L., Yen, M., and Guan, Z. (2012). Modulation of chondrocyte behavior through tailoring functional synthetic saccharide–peptide hydrogels, *Biomaterials* **33**, 6052–6060.

84. Guvendiren, M., and Burdick, J. A. (2012). Stiffening hydrogels to probe short- and long-term cellular responses to dynamic mechanics, *Nat. Commun.* **3**, 792.

85. Wu, W., Allen, R. A., and Wang, Y. (2012). Fast-degrading elastomer enables rapid remodeling of a cell-free synthetic graft into a neoartery, *Nat. Med.* advance online publication.

86. Gao, J., Ensley, A. E., Nerem, R. M., and Wang, Y. (2007). Poly(glycerol sebacate) supports the proliferation and phenotypic protein expression of primary baboon vascular cells, *J. Biomed. Mater. Res. A.* **83A**, 1070–1075.

87. Lin, S., Sandig, M., and Mequanint, K. (2011). Three-dimensional topography of synthetic scaffolds induces elastin synthesis by human coronary artery smooth muscle cells, *Tissue Eng. A.* **17**, 1561–1571.

88. Sharifpoor, S., Labow, R. S., and Santerre, J. P. (2009). Synthesis and characterization of degradable polar hydrophobic ionic polyurethane scaffolds for vascular tissue engineering applications, *Biomacromolecules* **10**, 2729–2739.

89. Soletti, L., Hong, Y., Guan, J., Stankus, J. J., El-Kurdi, M. S., Wagner, W. R., and Vorp, D. A. (2010). A bilayered elastomeric scaffold for tissue engineering of small diameter vascular grafts, *Acta Biomater.* **6**, 110–122.

90. Bettinger, C. J., Weinberg, E. J., Kulig, K. M., Vacanti, J. P., Wang, Y., Borenstein, J. T., and Langer, R. (2005). Three-dimensional microfluidic tissue-engineering scaffolds using a flexible biodegradable polymer, *Adv. Mater.* **18**, 165–169.

91. Sharma, A. K., Hota, P. V., Matoka, D. J., Fuller, N. J., Jandali, D., Thaker, H., Ameer, G. A., and Cheng, E. Y. (2010). Urinary bladder smooth muscle regeneration utilizing bone marrow derived mesenchymal stem cell seeded elastomeric poly(1,8-octanediol-co-citrate) based thin films, *Biomaterials* **31**, 6207–6217.

92. Pattison, M. A., Webster, T. J., and Haberstroh, K. M. (2006). Select bladder smooth muscle cell functions were enhanced on three-dimensional, nano-structured poly(ether urethane) scaffolds, *J. Biomater. Sci. Poly. Ed.* **17**, 1317–1332.
93. Stankus, J. J., Freytes, D. O., Badylak, S. F., and Wagner W. R. (2008). Hybrid nanofibrous scaffolds from electrospinning of a synthetic biodegradable elastomer and urinary bladder matrix, *J. Biomater. Sci. Poly. Ed.* **19**, 635–652.
94. Ifkovits, J. L., Wu, K., Mauck, R. L., and Burdick, J. A. (2010). The influence of fibrous elastomer structure and porosity on matrix organization, *PLoS ONE* **5**, e15717.
95. Ifkovits, J. L., Devlin, J. J., Eng, G., Martens, T. P., Vunjak-Novakovic, G., and Burdick, J. A. (2009). Biodegradable fibrous scaffolds with tunable properties formed from photo-cross-linkable poly(glycerol sebacate), *ACS Appl. Mater. Interfaces* **1**, 1878–1886.
96. Chen, Q. Z., Ishii, H., Thouas, G. A., Lyon, A. R., Wright, J. S., Blaker, J. J. Chrzanowski, W., Boccaccini, A. R., Ali, N. N., Knowles, J. C., and Harding, S. E. (2010). An elastomeric patch derived from poly (glycerol sebacate) for delivery of embryonic stem cells to the heart, *Biomaterials*, **31**, 3885–3893.
97. Maidhof, R., Marsano, A., Lee, E. J., and Vunjak-Novakovic, G. (2010). Perfusion seeding of channeled elastomeric scaffolds with myocytes and endothelial cells for cardiac tissue engineering, *Biotech. Progr.* **26**, 565–572.
98. Blumenthal, B., Golsong, P., Poppe, A., Heilmann, C., Schlensak, C., Beyersdorf, F., and Siepe, M. (2010). Polyurethane scaffolds seeded with genetically engineered skeletal myoblasts: A promising tool to regenerate myocardial function, *Artific. Org.* **34**, E46–E54.
99. Fujimoto, K. L., Tobita, K., Merryman, W. D., Guan, J., Momoi, N., Stolz, D. B., Sacks, M. S., Keller, B. B., and Wagner, W. R. (2007). An elastic, biodegradable cardiac patch induces contractile smooth muscle and improves cardiac remodeling and function in subacute myocardial infarction, *J. Am. Coll. Cardiol.* **49**, 2292–2300.
100. Tan, Q., El-Badry, A. M., Contaldo, C., Steiner, R., Hillinger, S., Welti, M., Hilbe, M., Spahn, D. R., Jaussi, R., Hiquera, G., van Blitterswijk, C. A., Luo, Q., and Weder, W. (2009). The effect of perfluorocarbon-based artificial oxygen carriers on tissue-engineered trachea, *Tissue Eng. A.* **15**, 2471–2480.
101. Yang, L., Korom, S., Welti, M., Hoerstrup, S. P., Zünd, G., Jung, F. J., Neuenschwander, P., and Weder, P. (2003). Tissue engineered cartilage

generated from human trachea using DegraPol® scaffold, *Eur. J. Cardiothorac. Surg.* **24**, 201–207.

102. Sundback, C. A., Shyu, J. Y., Wang, Y., Faquin, W. C., Langer, R. S., Vacanti, J. P., and Hadlock, T. A. (2005). Biocompatibility analysis of poly(glycerol sebacate) as a nerve guide material, *Biomaterials* **26**, 5454–5464.

103. Neeley, W. L., Redenti, S., Klassen, H., Tao, S., Desai, T., Young, M. J., and Langer, R. (2008). A microfabricated scaffold for retinal progenitor cell grafting, *Biomaterials* **29**, 418–426.

104. da Silva, G. R., Junior Ada, S., Saliba, J. B., Berdugo, M., Goldenberg, B. T., Naud, M. C., Ayres, E., Orefice, R. L., and Cohen, F. B. (2011). Polyurethanes as supports for human retinal pigment epithelium cell growth, *Int. J. Art. Organs.* **34**, 198–209.

105. Mahdavi, A., Ferreira, L., Sundback, C., Nichol, J. W., Chan, E. P., Carter, D. J., Bettinger, C. J., Patanvanich, S., Chignozha, L., Ben-Jospeh, E., Galakatos, A., Pryor, H., Pomerantseva, I., Masiakos, P. T., Faquin, W., Zumbuehl, A., Hong, S., Hong, S., Borenstein, J., Vacanti, J., Langer, R., and Karp, J. M. (2008). A biodegradable and biocompatible gecko-inspired tissue adhesive, *Proc. Natl. Acad. Sci.* **105**, 2307–2312.

106. Amsden, B. G. (2008). Biodegradable elastomers in drug delivery, *Exp. Opin. Drug Deliv.* **5**, 175–187.

107. Wang, J., Bettinger, C. J., Langer, R. S., and Borenstein, J. T. (2010). Biodegradable microfluidic scaffolds for tissue engineering from amino alcohol-based poly(ester amide) elastomers, *Organogenesis* **6**, 212–216.

108. Engelmayr, G. C., Cheng, M., Bettinger, C. J., Borenstein, J. T., Langer, R., and Freed, L. E. (2008). Accordion-like honeycombs for tissue engineering of cardiac anisotropy, *Nat. Mater.* **7**, 1003–1010.

109. Olson, D. A., Gratton, S. E. A., DeSimone, J. M., and Sheares, V. V. (2006). Amorphous linear aliphatic polyesters for the facile preparation of tunable rapidly degrading elastomeric devices and delivery vectors, *J. Am. Chem. Soc.* **128**, 13625–13633.

110. Lynn, D. M., and Langer, R. (2000). Degradable poly(β-amino esters): Synthesis, characterization and self-assembly with plasmid DNA, *J. Am. Chem. Soc.* **122**, 10761–1078.

Chapter 8

Protein Engineering Strategies for Modular, Responsive, and Spatially Organized Biomaterials

Ian Wheeldon

Chemical and Environmental Engineering, University of California, Riverside, 900 University Avenue, Riverside, CA 92521, USA

wheeldon@ucr.edu

When applied to biomaterials design, protein engineering provides a powerful set of tools to create systems with modularity, environmental responsiveness, and nanoscale control over the presentation of bioactive molecules. These functionalities stem from the ability of protein and peptide domains to self-assemble via non-covalent interactions, an ability that is governed by the structure–function relationships of the protein or peptide. When readily available molecular biology techniques are used to create new and engineer existing proteins and peptides an approach emerges where one can control the macroscopic properties of a biomaterial through molecular-level design. In this chapter we review a number of examples of protein- and peptide-based biomaterials that exemplify this approach, and in doing so attempt to provide a general overview of the field and its potential for advancing tissue and organ engineering.

Tissue and Organ Regeneration: Advances in Micro- and Nanotechnology
Edited by Lijie Grace Zhang, Ali Khademhosseini, and Thomas J. Webster
Copyright © 2014 Pan Stanford Publishing Pte. Ltd.
ISBN 978-981-4411-67-7 (Hardcover), 978-981-4411-68-4 (eBook)
www.panstanford.com

8.1 Introduction

There is an extensive set of engineering tools that have been used to control the interface between cells and their environment. These tools, among others, include nano- and micro-scale engineering [1,2], polymeric hydrogels [3,4], and synthetic polymer cell scaffolds [5]. Common to the application of these tools is the connection that cells make to the engineered environment, a connection that is made through thousands of protein cell-surface receptors: Extracellular proteins, peptides, (bio)polymers, and small molecules bind to protein receptors on the cell surface and initiate (or suppress) biochemical signals that dictate cellular activity and behavior. These interactions between bioactive ligands and cell surface receptors are dynamic and are driven by non-covalent interactions. As the extracellular environment changes, existing protein–ligand interactions on the cell surface may also change and new binding events occur as cells respond to newly presented ligands and external cues. This dynamic, molecular-level exchange between cells and their environment highlights three important aspects of biomaterials design that are enabled through protein engineering: (1) cell–materials interactions are mediated through protein–ligand interactions, (2) protein–ligand interactions are non-covalent, and (3) these interactions can be dynamic. These three aspects are the driving forces behind the design of new protein- and peptide-based biomaterials that leverage protein functions to create useful systems that respond to the surrounding environment, self-assemble in a predictable and organized manner, and display biologically active epitopes and ligands that can initiate, mediate, and suppress cellular activity.

At the core of the protein engineering approach to biomaterials design is the use of proteins and peptides as building blocks to create complex, functional biomaterials that are tunable at the molecular level. When we consider polypeptides as polymer systems, control at the macroscopic level is attained by control over the DNA sequence encoding the desired polypeptides, as DNA is transcribed to RNA and RNA is translated to the encoded protein. The protein primary sequence (the amino acid sequence) dictates the secondary, tertiary, and quaternary structure, which in turn controls protein function, including enzymatic activity, biological signaling, self-assembly, and ligand binding. Protein and peptide production by recombinant expression in a microbial host such as *Escherichia coli* allows for tight control over the polymer length, is reliable and repeatable for a given system, and production in large quantities can occur with accompanying purification to high level of homogeneity. The steps involved in the protein engineering approach to functional biomaterials are schematically shown in Fig. 8.1.

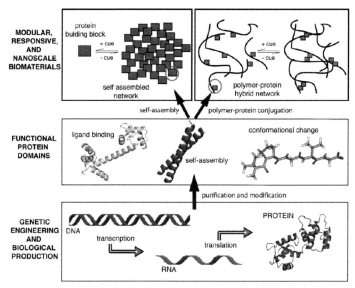

Figure 8.1 The protein engineering methodology of biomaterials design. Molecular design of the biomaterials begins with genetic engineering of the DNA sequence that encodes the desired functional protein. The functional proteins and peptides are then used to create modular hydrogels, hydrogels with stimuli and environmental responsiveness, and biomaterials that can control the nanoscale presentation of bioactive cues. Reproduced and modified with permission from Banta, Wheeldon, and Blenner, *Ann Rev Biomed Eng* 2010, **12**, 167–186.

There are many good reviews that cover the vast field of biomaterials, including synthetic polymer hydrogels for biomaterials [3,4,6,7] and biomaterials design [8]. Protein, peptide, and hybrid protein–polymer hydrogel systems have also been the focus of a number of general reviews. We do not intend to provide an extensive overview of the field as is covered elsewhere and direct the reader to comprehensive publications for such treatments as is found in references [9–11]. There has also been a significant focus on protein engineering of biopolymers for the development of tissue engineering scaffolds, including engineering recombinant extracellular matrix proteins with tunable properties. These efforts have been reviewed elsewhere (see reference [12]) and are not the focus of this review.

In this chapter we focus on novel protein engineering efforts to design and create functional biomaterials, including (i) the modular design of multi-functional hydrogels, (ii) stimuli and environmental responsiveness, and (iii) nanoscale spatial organization of bioactive signals. In each case we review a number of examples that best demonstrate the capabilities of the given functionality and the application of protein engineering to develop the system. In discussing and reviewing these example we attempt to provide a general overview of the potential range of solutions that protein-based materials can provide to current problems in tissue and organ regeneration, including cell-compatible hydrogels, systems for studying cellular behaviors with controlled experimental conditions, and systems with potential for responsive growth factor delivery, and stimuli-responsive gelation. Each of these applications an important focus for tissue and organ engineering.

8.2 Modular Design of Multi-Functional and Bioactive Hydrogels

Engineering modularity into a biomaterials system, i.e., engineering a system that can seamlessly include functionally distinct units within the same biomaterials system, is advantageous as it allows for (1) the design of systems with multiple functions and (2) control over the number and identity of the biologically active signals within a given system. These two engineering features allow for the fabrication of biomaterials systems that can be used to isolate individual parameters in controlled studies of cell–materials interactions. For example, when studying the proliferation or differentiation of cells on natural ECM components such as collagen, fibronectin, or the ECM extract Matrigel, it is difficult (if not impossible) to accurately control the number and identity of cell binding ligands presented in the cell substrate or hydrogel. An engineered modular system would allow for the independent tuning of each of the bioactive signals present in the hydrogel thus allowing for the isolation of the biological effects due to each signal.

In synthetic polymeric hydrogels a network of polymer chains is made by covalently linking between chains. For example, a common cross-linking scheme is to initiate free radical polymerization of methacrylated poly(ethylene glycol) (PEG) chains with UV light. The result is a PEG network with multiple covalent bonds between chains. In a protein-based system cross-linking is non-covalent and physical in nature driven by hydrophobic interactions, hydrogen bonding, and van der Waals interactions. The general scheme for creating modular protein-based materials is to create protein building block with different functionalities but with compatible cross-linking domains. An excellent example of this scheme is cross-linking with the hydrophobically driven coiled coil protein domain. The coiled coil is a basic folding motif where two or more peptides with α-helical secondary structure come together to form a superhelix, or coiled coil. Such a strategy was used to create multi-functional protein hydrogels with self-assembly, catalytic, and bioactive functionalities from protein building blocks with compatible α-helical coiled coil cross-linking domains [13–15].

There is rich history in studying and engineering the structure and function of α-helical coiled coils [10,16–18] culminating, with respect to biomaterials engineering, in an extensive set of designed helices with known and predictable aggregation number, binding partner specificity, orientation (i.e., parallel and anti-parallel), and stability [19,20]. The first works to demonstrate hydrogel cross-linking with coiled coils were published in 1998 and 1999 (see references [21,22]), and have since been replicated and the concept extended to a number of applications, including enzymatic hydrogels [23,24], protein hydrogels with integrated cell binding ligands [13,25,26], stimuli-responsive hydrogels [27–29], and protein hydrogels with tunable erosion rate [30], among others. In a similar strategy, hybrid protein-PEG hydrogels were self-assembled using a coiled coil motif identified from fibrin. Trimeric cross-linking junctions were formed by modifying the ends of PEG chains with α-helical domains that naturally form trimeric coiled coil bundles in fibrin fibers [31]. Engineering of α-helical peptides and proteins has also extended into the design and fabrication of protein fibers. In this scheme, helices are engineered to self-assemble not into coiled coil bundles but into coiled coils with overlapping ends that assemble into long, microscale fibers. This strategy has been reviewed in publications dedicated to the discussion of protein fibers (see references [32] and [33]) and will be discussed in Section 8.4 of this chapter with respect to the nanoscale engineering of bioactive ligand presentation.

Here, we describe one example in detail that uses α-helical coiled coil cross-links to create hydrogels comprising polypeptide chains that themselves are series of globular protein domains. We describe this example as it effectively demonstrates the capabilities of a protein engineering approach for biomaterials design: building protein-based hydrogels from the genetic level up through the expression of protein building blocks and the assembly of functional biomaterials. This example also represents an important advancement in the capabilities of protein-based hydrogels as it demonstrates the ability to create self-assembling hydrogels that are modular at the polypeptide chain level and also within the internal structure of each polypeptide chain. To this end, Cao and Li demonstrate a tandem, modular hydrogel of a self-assembled network of triblock polypeptide with terminal α-helices separated by a series of eight GB1 IgG antibody binding domain [34]. Aqueous solutions of 7 wt% triblock polypeptide self-assemble into a self-supporting hydrogel network at near neutral pH. The network is created through physical cross-links of tetrameric coiled coil bundles that are stable to approximately 60°C. Schematic representations of the polypeptide chain and the self-assembled network are shown in Fig. 8.2.

In a subsequent work the same research group extended their work to a two-component system with two different but compatible polypeptide chains with terminal α-helices that form heterodimeric coiled coils [35]. The fact that the hydrogels are made water soluble from a series of globular proteins is an important demonstration and represents significant potential toward engineering self-assembling polypeptide chains with repeat units of biologically active globular domains. For example, the authors express their goal of creating protein hydrogels that mimic the ECM, and one can envision that a series of biologically active proteins (e.g., growth factors or ECM domains) can be strung together with α-helical cross-linking domains at each end. Genetic engineering of the polypeptides will allow for the control of the amino acid sequence, and consequently the structure and function of each of the globular units that make up the polypeptide. Cross-linking will be controlled by the terminal α-helices and the cross-linking density controlled by the aggregation number of the coiled coil bundles.

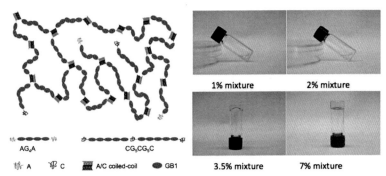

Figure 8.2   Tandem, modular protein-based hydrogels. (Left) Schematic representation of the two protein components and the assembly of a hydrogel network. (Right) Photographs of mixtures of AG4A and CG5CG5C components of varying concentrations. The photographs show that 1 and 2% mixtures do not form hydrogels but at 3.5% and 7% hydrogels are formed. Adapted with permission from Lv, Cao, and Li, *Langmuir* 2012, **28**, 2269–2274. Copyright (2012) American Chemical Society.

Modular construction of bioactive hydrogels has also been demonstrated using a two-component polypeptide system that cross-links into a stable hydrogel via peptide–peptide associations [36]. In this system a series of WW domains (a 31–40 amino acid domain named for its conserved tryptophan residues; the single letter representation of tryptophan is W) are genetically linked within a long polypeptide chain. A hydrogel is formed when the WW containing polypeptide is mixed with a second polypeptide containing proline-rich repeats (with a PPxY motif) that bind to the WW domains of the first component. This system is aptly referred to as mixing-induced, two-component hydrogels or MITCH. The components and the assembly of the system are schematically shown in Fig. 8.3.

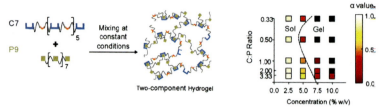

Figure 8.3 Protein engineering of mixing-induced, two component hydrogels (MITCH). (Left) C7 and P9 two components of the MITCH system. C7 indicates seven repeats of the CC43 WW domain and P9 indicates nine repeats of the proline-rich ligand. Mixtures of the two components assemble into a hydrogel network. (Right) A sol-gel phase diagram indicating the conditions where a two-component hydrogel is formed. Reprinted with permission from Mulyasasmita, Lee, and Heilshorn, *Biomacromolecules* 2011, **12**, 3406–3411. Copyright (2011) American Chemical Society.

As each component in the MITCH system is genetically engineered, the polypeptide chains are tunable at the molecular level thus allowing for control over the number of each functional protein domain and ligand. Tuning of the binding strength of the interaction between WW domains and proline-rich ligands is also possible as structure–function studies have indentified the important residues in binding and engineering of the binding affinity between ~1 and ~10 mM is possible [37]. Tuning of these molecular-level design parameters (i.e., the binding affinity of WW domains and the number of binding domain within a single polypeptide chain) results in control over the macroscopic viscoelelastic properties (micro-rheological experiments demonstrate tuning of the storage modulus from ~9 to ~50 Pa). Further investigation into the relationship between the number of cross-linking domains and the sol-gel transition has lead to the ability to predict gel mechanic and sol-gel behavior based on the molecular-level design [38]. Protein engineering of the MITCH system also allows for the inclusion of bioactive ligands in each component. Similar to the strategy used in designing cell-compatible α-helical triblock polypeptides [13], the two component WW/proline-rich ligand system incorporates the cell binding ligand ariginine-glycine-aspartic acid (RGD) into each polypeptide component. When the RGD ligand is included, the MITCH system has be shown to support three-dimensional (3D) culture and proliferation of human umbilical vein endothelial cells

(HUVECs) and murine adult neural stem cells (NSCs). Additionally, culture and proliferation of neuronal-like PC-12 cells was demonstrated for a period of six days [36].

8.3 Protein Engineering of Stimuli-Responsive Hydrogels

There are a wide variety of polymer-based strategies for engineering stimuli- and environmental responsiveness; these strategies have been reviewed extensively [6,39,40]. In this chapter we focus on protein-based systems and discuss the protein domains that are responsible for the stimulus-responsive action. Most often the responsiveness is mediated by ligand binding or protein-protein interactions and these non-covalent interactions are modulated to alter the cross-linking within the material. Such systems find utility in tissue and organ engineering as shear thinning and injectable hydrogels and as hydrogels that undergo phase transition or swelling in response to changing environmental conditions or the presence of specific biomarkers.

A beneficial effect of the non-covalent interactions that form cross-links in MITCH [36,38] and other protein- and peptide-based hydrogels [41,42] is that they are often shear thinning and undergo a sol-gel transition with the application of sufficient shear stress. Under applied shear stress the weak non-covalent interactions that support the network can be broken. The physical cross-links reform when the shear stress is reduced. This breaking and reforming of the physical cross-links allows the hydrogels to be extruded through a small-bore needle only to be reformed once injected. Another example of shear thinning due to protein-based cross-linking is a two-component system that uses the docking functionality of cAMP-dependent protein kinase A and the dimerization functionality of A-kinase anchoring proteins to create physically cross-linked cell-compatible hydrogels [42]. This system was shown to undergo repeated sol-gel transitions, where after each 4 min period of high shear stress the hydrogel quickly recovered from a liquid-like state to a self-supporting hydrogel. Additionally, the inclusion of RGD ligands into the system produces a cell compatible hydrogel supporting high viability of human mesenchymal stem cells after injection into a collagen gel after 3 days. Shear thinning in protein-based and tissue engineering hydrogels has recently been reviewed in detail (see reference [43] and references therein for more examples) and is discussed here as it is a property that originates in the molecular-level design of these systems.

With respect to hydrogels responsive to chemical changes in the environment, the calmodulin protein has been used to create peptide and calcium responsive hydrogels that undergo reversible swelling [44,45]. The reversible action is due to the three distinct conformations that calmodulin takes on in response to a binding event. In the presence of Ca^{2+} ions the extended structure (Fig. 8.4, left) binds Ca^{2+} and folds into an extended barbell conformation (Fig. 8.4, middle). In this state the protein is available to bind specific peptide ligands. Upon binding, the protein collapses around the peptide taking on a globular structure (Fig. 8.4, right). This change in conformation causes a change in end-to-end distance of approximately 3.5 nm [46,47]. In two different hybrid polymer–protein systems, the change in the physical dimensions of calmodulin and the binding specificity are exploited to produce large changes in hydrogel volume [44,45,48–50]. Calmodulin conjugated to the backbone of a polymer hydrogel modulates the total internal cross-linking of the material as the protein binds to peptide ligands that are also conjugated to the polymer hydrogel. In the presence of freely diffusing peptide ligands the cross-links are broken and the hydrogel swells. Swelling is reversed in the absence of freely diffusing ligands. Responsive action can also be modulated by Ca^{2+} ions as calmodulin is unable to bind the peptide ligand in the absence of Ca^{2+}. In one example, the release rate of the vascular endothelialgrowth factor (VEGF) entrapped within the hydrogel is modulated by the presence and absence of a specific peptide

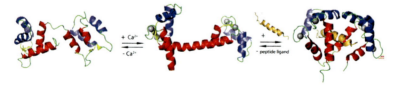

Figure 8.4 Conformational change of the calmodulin protein in response to calcium and peptide ligand binding. Crystal structures of non-ligand binding (1DMO), extended "dumbbell" conformation with bound Ca^{2+} (3CLN), and globular structure with bound ligand (2BBM).

biomarker [49]. In the presence of the biomarker VEGF-laden hydrogels are collapsed and the VEGF payload is released over 10 h. In the absence of the biomarker hydrogels are swollen and the VEGF is released over a longer time period reaching full release after >20 h.

A peptide-based cross-linking scheme similar to that used in the calmodulin-based hydrogels is used to self-assemble a modular protein-hydrogel systems created from tetratricopeptide repeats (TPR) [51]. This system is an excellent example of the capabilities of genetic control of the protein building block structure and function to produce novel macroscopic properties and functions. The basic unit of TPRs is a 34 amino acids sequence that takes on a helix-turn-helix structure. In long polypeptide chains with many TPR units, the tandem helices stack to form rigid superhelical structures with eight repeats per superhelical turn [52]. In nature, TPR domains promote the assembly of macromolecular complexes as TPR modules bind a variety of different peptide ligands. This functionality has been used to engineer dynamic cross-links in TPR-polymer hydrogel systems. This system is powerful in that (i) it is modular, and (ii) the functionality and properties of each module can be manipulated. For example, the stability of the superhelical structure can be predicted from the amino acid sequences of the TPR modules that make up the structure [51], ligand binding affinity and specificity can be engineered [53,54], the TPR units are themselves modular and can include modules that bind different peptides or that do not bind peptides and act as spacer modules, and the number and order of the TPR units can be arbitrarily designed and the architecture of an array of units can be altered [55]. In this systems ligands that bind to the TPR units are conjugated to a polymer backbone and cross-linking occurs when the TPR units are mixed with the ligand-modified polymers (Fig. 8.5). The interaction between peptide ligand and TPR unit is primarily electrostatic and is therefore sensitive to changes in ionic strength. This fact was exploited to create a salt responsive controlled release system where the rate hydrogel erosion can vary from >>600 h to <24 [51]. In a demonstrate of this system TPR-based hydrogels responsive to ionic-strength that release anti-cancer drug payloads in a tunable manner were created [55]. The gels themselves were shown to be non-toxic, but the anti-cancer drug (1,6-dimethyl-3-propylpyrimido[5,4-e][1,2,4]triazine-5,7-dione) released from the hydrogel killed HER2-positive BT-474 breast cancer cells over a

24 h period. One can envision the novel application of this modular and stimuli-responsive hydrogel system, including, controlled growth factor release or controlled stiffness of a cell-encapsulation matrix.

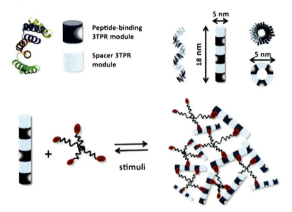

Figure 8.5 Design and assembly of TPR-based hydrogels. (Top, left) Crystal structure of TPR unit and schematic of peptide-binding and spacer 3TPR modules. (Top, right) Assembly of multiple 3TPR modules. (Bottom) Assembly of hydrogel networks with PEG-peptide and TPR-based components. Adapted with permission from Grove et al., *JACS* 2010, **132**, 14024–14026. Copyright (2010) American Chemical Society.

Another example of controlling macroscopic properties by engineering at the molecular level is a Ca^{2+} sensitive protein hydrogel with engineered protein-protein cross-links [56]. This system uses polypeptide chains with bifunctional terminal protein domains. At one end of a highly soluble, randomly coiled polypeptide is an α-helical domain, while at the other end is a Ca^{2+} sensitive β-roll domain. In the presence of Ca^{2+} the β-roll folds from an unstructured chain into a β-helix consisting of two short β-sheet faces separated by turns. Populating one face of the β-roll amino acid residues with hydrophobic side chain (in this case leucine residues) creates a hydrophobic patch that can create stable protein-protein interactions with other similarly modified β-rolls. In the presence of Ca^{2+} the β-roll ends of the polypeptides form cross-links with other β-rolls and the α-helical ends form coiled coils, thus creating a network of polypeptide chains. Similarly, a triblock polypeptide with calmodulin and α-helical terminal domains on a highly soluble polypeptide has been shown to create Ca^{2+}-sensitive hydrogels [57].

The bifunctional α-helix/β-roll and α-helix/calmodulin polypeptides as well as the coiled coil cross-links in protein and hybrid hydrogels are also pH and temperature sensitive due to the nature of the cross-linking interactions. There has been a number of works describing this type of behavior, i.e., pH and temperature sensitive protein hydrogels [21,22,58]. In many of these cases, the responsive action occurs when the α-helical domains lose tertiary and secondary structure when denatured at high pH or elevated temperatures. Varying α-helical domain length and amino acid sequence can alter the transition pH and temperature, thus making the sol-gel response tunable. The reader is directed to comprehensive reviews on engineered α-helical domains for more detailed discussion of these systems [10,59].

The examples discussed here do not represent all of the demonstrated protein-based and protein–polymer hybrid responsive hydrogels, but are a representative cross-section of the field and are discussed in detail as they are some of the best examples of the capabilities of the protein engineering approach to functional materials design. In the case of the calmodulin mediated Ca^{2+} and peptide responsiveness the detailed studies identifying the mutation necessary for altering Ca^{2+} binding affinity [60,61] and ligand specificity have been identified [62]. As described in the previous section on modular protein hydrogels, extensive work has been done in engineering coiled coils and α-helical bundles [10,20]. The engineered β-roll domains demonstrate that site selective mutagenesis can be used to create hydrophobic interactions to drive cross-linking within a hydrogel system. Lastly, engineered TPRs are strong examples of the modular nature of a protein system and the ability to control ligand binding specificity and domain stability. Other interesting examples include temperature-responsive elastin-like peptides which have been proposed for a wide range of biomedical application, including drug delivery and injectable hydrogels (see reference [10] and references therein), and antibody-antigen pairs for reversible swelling hydrogels [63,64]. In the following section we discuss peptide- and protein-based systems that have capabilities to present bioactive signals (e.g., peptide sequences, epitopes, and peptide mimics of growth factors) with spatial control at the nanometer scale. Many of these systems, such as peptide-based fibers and hydrogels, are also responsive to environmental conditions. Some of these systems are also modular in that different protein or peptide building blocks with compatible self-assembly or cross-linking modes can be seamlessly included or exchanged within a single hydrogel. Similar to the examples discussed in Section 8.2 and in this section, the examples discussed below have application as cell-encapsulation matrices and injectable therapies, among others.

8.4 Nanoscale Spatial Organization of Bioactive Signals in Protein Hydrogels

The ECM is a complex, highly heterogeneous composite material comprising protein fibers, polysaccharides, glycosaminoglycans (GAGs), and bioactive protein and peptide signals. One of the main goals of biomaterials design for tissue engineering and regenerative medicine is to re-create this complex natural medium in a controlled manner. Cells respond to and interact with the nanoscale architecture of the ECM and the bioactive signals contained within the ECM are information that cells receive and respond to. In this section we discuss and review protein and peptide engineering toward the development of hydrogels and protein systems that can replicate some of the nanoscale features and bioactive cues in the ECM. We focus on those technologies that have the ability to control the nanoscale spatial organization of bioactive signals, including peptide fibers made from peptide amphiphiles (PA), β-sheet peptide fibers, self-assembling α-helical fibers, and a protein engineering effort to control the spatial organization of carbohydrates on an self-assembled protein substrate.

One of the most successful examples of mimicking the nanoscale structure of the ECM is the PA hydrogels developed by Stupp and co-workers [65–68]. Bioactive hydrogels are made from 3D networks of nanoscale fibers comprising peptides modified with an alkyl tail. Fibers are assembled as the hydrophobic alkyl tails of the PA align to create the core of the fiber and the hydrophilic peptides align along the outer shell of the fiber (Fig. 8.6). The long nanoscale fibers branch and entangle to create a 3D, self-supporting hydrogel with the peptides creating one or more polyvalent bioactive signals on the surface of the fibers. Two of the first demonstrations of this system showed the ability to create bioactive hydrogels that have instructive cues for mineralization of hydroxyapatite and for selective differentiation of neural progenitor cells [65,68]. These two works exemplify the ability of this system to create hydrogels with structural fibers with nanoscale diameter and microscale length and the ability to control the amino acid sequence of a polyvalent bioactive peptide signal on the surface of the fibers. In the first example, a phosphoserine residue is included in the peptide sequence thus creating a highly phosphorylated fiber surface to promote hydroxyapatite mineralization [65]. In the second example, the bioactive laminin epitope IKVAV (letters indicate the single letter amino acid code) was included at the end of the PA to create a 3D hydrogel displaying a neurite-promoting signal [68].

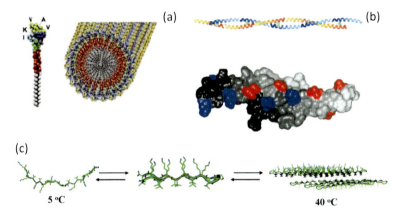

Figure 8.6 Self-assembling peptide fiber hydrogels with capabilities for nanoscale presentation of bioactive ligands. (a) Peptide amphiphile (PA) and a PA nanofiber with cell binding ligand IKVAV from Silva et al., *Science* 2004, **303**, 1352–1355. Reprinted with permission from AAAS. (b) Sticky-end self-assembling peptide fiber with corresponding molecular model of a single α-helix. Reprinted with permission from Pandya et al., *Biochemistry* 2000, **39**, 8728–8734. Copyright (2000) American Chemical Society. (c) Self-assembly of a thermally responsive β-sheet peptide fiber. Reprinted with permission from Pochan et al., *JACS* 2003, **125**(39), 11802–11803. Copyright (2003) American Chemical Society.

The PA hydrogel system has since been extended to a number of different applications [69,70] and has recently been used to create a novel injectable hydrogel therapy for promoting ischemic tissue repair [71]. The peptide sequence KLTWQELYQLKYKGI-NH2 is known to mimic VEGF through the activation of its cell surface receptors [72]. This VEGF epitope was included as a bioactive signal in the peptide portion of the PA system to create hydrogels with high-density VEGF-mimetic peptide fibers. Three days after injection of the hydrogel into a chicken embryo model, blood vessel density was shown in increase by >225% in the area surrounding the hydrogel. Additionally, in a mouse hind-limb ischemia model significant improvement in the motor function and tissue salvage scores as well as the perfusion ratio were demonstrated 28 days after injection of the hydrogel [71]. This work along with the other examples of PA hydrogels show that this system is capable of mimicking some the nanoscale structural features of the natural ECM and has the powerful ability to tune the bioactive nature of the fiber surface through the inclusion of polyvalent peptide signals.

A different approach to creating bioactive nanoscale fibers is the self-assembling of β-sheet motifs. In this case, fibers are assembled from peptides that self-associate through β-sheet interactions where short peptides align side-by-side creating long microscale-length fibers with width and thickness governed by the length and height of the peptides. For example, the Pochan and Scheider groups have created peptides that fold into a β-turn motif and self-assemble into peptide fibers and 3D hydrogels [41,73]. The Zhang group has also developed an extensive set of peptides that self-assemble into peptide fibers and entangled hydrogels that are cell compatible [74,75]. Additionally, Collier and co-workers have produced a number of works describing and investigating bioactive hydrogels made from a self-assembling peptide named Q11 [76]. The peptide, QQKFQFQFEQQ, can be modified to include bioactive peptide sequences that assemble into β-sheet fibers decorated with signals such as the RGD cell adhesion peptide, IKVAV, or other bioactive sequences [77–79]. We focus on the engineering of this system as it exemplifies the abilities of self-assembling peptide fibers to control the nanoscale presentation of bioactive signals and mimic structural features of natural ECM. Additionally, this system demonstrates the ability to produce modular and multi-functional hydrogels as the most basic component of the systems (i.e., the self-assembling peptide with bioactive signal) can be assembled with other similarly structured peptides with different bioactivity. Inclusion of the bioactive signal does not prohibit hydrogel formation or significantly alter the macroscale hydrogel properties [77,78]. This modular ability also allows for the tuning of the concentration of bioactive ligands through mixtures of self-assembling peptides with and without the modified peptide epitopes.

In one example, the Q11 β-sheet fibers were used to create hydrogels with cell adhesion peptides, including IKVAV and RGD to encapsulate and support the proliferation and spreading of HUVECs [76]. Exploiting the modular nature of this system, this work was extended to create a multi-factorial optimization of endothelial cell growth using four different cell adhesion peptides that mimic natural epitopes in the ECM [78]. This combinatorial approach revealed significant binary and tertiary interaction between the ECM mimics on the growth of HUVECs seeded on self-assembled hydrogels. This work also identified an optimized hydrogel composition for HUVEC growth with 8 mM RGDS-Q11 and 3 mM IKVAV-Q11 peptides. An important extension to this work was the development of a hydrogel preparation method that allows of the control of fiber composition when multiple bioactive peptides are used [77]. This method allows for the controlled fabrication of heterogeneous hydrogels with each fiber containing only one bioactive signal or with each fiber containing a mixture of two or more bioactive signals.

In addition to the PA and β-sheet fibrillizing hydrogels, there has also been significant work put toward the development of self-assembling hydrogels made from α-helical coiled coil fibers. This hydrogel system pioneered by Woolfson and co-workers has nanoscale structural features that mimic the composition of the ECM but also has the ability to decorate fibers with peptide ligands. Alpha-helical coiled coil peptides, similar to those discussed above in Section 8.2, come together to form microscale long fibers with diameters in the tens of nanometers. The fibers assemble lengthwise as two α-helical peptides form a coiled coil with "sticky-ends" that overlap with other coiled coils [80]. Aggregates of the thin fibers form thicker bundles to produce microscale length fibers with diameters between 40 and 70 nm [81]. Woolfson and co-workers have developed a peptide tagging method of immobilizing peptide epitopes along the length of the fibers at the edge of

4 nm striations across the fiber [82]. The tagging method takes advantage of the local charge at the junction between overlapping coiled coils to non-covalently attach an external peptide tag. This self-assembling fiber system is extensively reviewed elsewhere and has great potential for future use as biocompatible hydrogels with nanoscale spatial organization of bioactive ligands [32,83].

One exciting protein engineering approach to the controlled nanoscale presentation of bioactive ligands is the engineering of crystalline cell surface proteins, or S-layer proteins. In many different prokaryotic organisms S-layer proteins self-assemble on the outer layer of the organisms to form a monomolecular crystalline envelop [84]. These proteins are being used to engineer new bioactive materials, including micro- and nanoparticle coatings for immunotherapies, vaccines, and diagnostic sensors, as well as immobilization platforms for biocatalysis [85]. With respect to biomaterials development for tissue and organ engineering, this platform offers valuable capabilities that are not replicated in the protein and peptide engineering technologies previously discussed: S-layer proteins have the capability to display nanoscale arrays of carbohydrate chains. As mentioned at the outset of this section, the ECM is a complex, highly heterogeneous environment containing protein and peptide fibers, growth factors and signaling molecules, but also containing carbohydrates and GAGs. With the "bottom-up" design of S-layer biomaterials it is possible to genetically engineer the base S-layer protein unit at distinct positions without interfering with self-assembly of the resulting crystalline sheet to create spatially organized biomolecular arrays. To this end, SgsE S-layer proteins from *Geobacillus stearothermophilus*, which are naturally O-glycosylated, have been engineered to self-assemble into periodic nanoarrays of neoglycoproteins [86]. Such a system allows for the controlled study of the nanoscale presentation of glycoproteins and carbohydrates. The main focus of many existing protein and peptide-based biomaterials is the controlled presentation of ECM proteins and growth factors. This system of engineered S-layer proteins presents new possibilities to expand controlled studies of the effects of ECM components on cellular behavior to include interesting and relevant glycoproteins and carbohydrates.

8.5 Future Direction of Protein and Peptide Biomaterials

In this chapter we have reviewed and discussed a number of protein- and peptide-based biomaterials that have potential for use in tissue and organ engineering. The hydrogels and biomaterials are classified into three areas: (i) modular and multi-functional hydrogels, (ii) stimuli- and environmentally-responsive systems, and (iii) protein and peptide biomaterials for the nanoscale spatial organization of bioactive signals. In each section we reviewed in detail one or more examples that best exemplifies the category. For example, the MITCH system represents an excellent example of molecular-level engineering of a modular, multi-functional hydrogel with tunable bioactivity and physical properties. The TPR-based hydrogels are also excellent examples of modularity, but this system was discussed in the context of stimuli responsiveness because one of the main applications of this system was the controlled release of encapsulated anti-cancer drugs. This overlap in classification is important to note as it is common to many of the examples discussed here. The inherent properties of protein- and peptide-based biomaterials, i.e., non-covalent but specific interactions between building blocks, are responsible for the functionality in each of the classifications, including modularity, responsiveness, and nanoscale spatial organization, and often in designing one functionality another arises.

We foresee the future of protein- and peptide-based biomaterials to be focused on the development of expanded sets of modular building blocks that mimic the many functions and components of the ECM, including fibrous ECM protein (collagens I–IV, vitronectin, and others), growth factors (TGFβ, BMP, PDGF, and others), and GAGs. We also foresee the development of protein-based systems that are responsive to multiple biological signals and that can release bioactive payloads or alter their physical properties at multiple time points that match the time scales of different cellular behaviors. For example, it would be useful to have hydrogel systems that release a set of growth factors during the initial stages of cell seeding and release a second set of growth factors at longer time scales as tissue functions begin to develop. Many of the examples reviewed here have been demonstrated in vitro and as the field of tissue and organ engineering matures and the tools and experimental investigations of that use these tools must also mature. In this respect, we anticipate that the future of protein and peptide biomaterials will include many more investigations in vivo using animal models and eventually in human trails. A number of the systems discussed in this chapter have already begun such advanced studies and are showing great promise in the development of new angiogenetic therapies and in biomaterials systems for tissue and organ engineering.

Acknowledgments

This work was supported by the Bourns College of Engineering at the University of California, Riverside. I thank Dr. Shilpa Sant for her valuable comments and edits to the manuscript.

References

1. Khademhosseini, A., R. Langer, J. Borenstein, and J. P. Vacanti, Microscale technologies for tissue engineering and biology. *Proc. Natl. Acad. Sci. U.S.A.*, 2006. **103**(8): 2480–2487.
2. Wheeldon, I., A. Farhadi, A. G. Bick, E. Jabbari, and A. Khademhosseini, nanoscale tissue engineering: spatial control over cell–materials interactions. *Nanotechnology*, 2011. **22**(21): 212001.
3. Lee, K. Y., and D. J. Mooney, Hydrogels for tissue engineering. *Chem. Rev.*, 2001. **101**(7): 1869–1879.
4. Van Vlierberghe, S., P. Dubruel, and E. Schacht, Biopolymer-based hydrogels as scaffolds for tissue engineering applications: a review. *Biomacromolecules*, 2011. **12**(5): 1387–1408.
5. Yang, S. F., K. F. Leong, Z. H. Du, and C. K. Chua, The design of scaffolds for use in tissue engineering. Part 1. Traditional factors. *Tissue Eng.*, 2001. **7**(6): 679–689.
6. Gupta, P., K. Vermani, and S. Garg, Hydrogels: from controlled release to pH-responsive drug delivery. *Drug Discov. Today*, 2002. **7**(10): 569–579.
7. Ratner, B. D., and S. J. Bryant, Biomaterials: where we have been and where we are going. *Ann. Rev. Biomed. Eng.*, 2004. **6**: 41–75.
8. Lutolf, M. P., and J. A. Hubbell, Synthetic biomaterials as instructive extracellular microenvironments for morphogenesis in tissue engineering. *Nat. Biotechnol.*, 2005. **23**(1): 47–55.

9. Jonker, A. M., D. W. P. M. Lowik, and J. C. M. van Hest, Peptide- and protein-based hydrogels. *Chem. Mater.*, 2012. **24**(5): 759–773.
10. Banta, S., I. R. Wheeldon, and M. Blenner, Protein engineering in the development of functional hydrogels. *Ann. Rev. Biomed. Eng.*, 2010. **12**: 167–186.
11. Ulijn, R. V., N. Bibi, V. Jayawarna, P. D. Thornton, S. J. Todd, R. J. Mart, A. M. Smith, and J. E. Gough, Bioresponsive hydrogels. *Mater. Today*, 2007. **10**(4): 40–48.
12. Gomes, S., I. B. Leonor, J. F. Mano, R. L. Reis, and D. L. Kaplan, Natural and genetically engineered proteins for tissue engineering. *Prog. Polym. Sci.*, 2012. **37**(1): 1–17.
13. Mi, L. X., S. Fischer, B. Chung, S. Sundelacruz, and J. L. Harden, Self-assembling protein hydrogels with modular integrin binding domains. *Biomacromolecules*, 2006. **7**(1): 38–47.
14. Wheeldon, I. R., S. C. Barton, and S. Banta, Bioactive proteinaceous hydrogels from designed bifunctional building blocks. *Biomacromolecules*, 2007. **8**(10): 2990–2994.
15. Wheeldon, I. R., J. W. Gallaway, S. C. Barton, and S. Banta, Bioelectrocatalytic hydrogels from electron-conducting metallopolypeptides coassembled with bifunctional enzymatic building blocks. *Proc. Natl. Acad. Sci. U.S.A.*, 2008. **105**(40): 15275–15280.
16. Marsden, H. R., and A. Kros, Self-assembly of coiled coils in synthetic biology: inspiration and progress. *Angew. Chem. Int. Edit.*, 2010. **49**(17): 2988–3005.
17. Meier, M., J. Stetefeld, and P. Burkhard, The many types of interhelical ionic interactions in coiled coils: an overview. *J. Struct. Biol.*, 2010. **170**(2): 192–201.
18. Oshea, E. K., K. J. Lumb, and P. S. Kim, Peptide velcro: design of a heterodimeric coiled-coil. *Curr. Biol.*, 1993. **3**(10): 658–667.
19. Bromley, E. H. C., K. Channon, E. Moutevelis, and D. N. Woolfson, Peptide and protein building blocks for synthetic biology: from programming biomolecules to self-organized biomolecular systems. *ACS Chem. Biol.*, 2008. **3**(1): 38–50.
20. Fletcher, J. M., A. L. Boyle, M. Bruning, G. J. Bartlett, T. L. Vincent, N. R. Zaccai, C. T. Armstrong, E. H. C. Bromley, P. J. Booth, R. L. Brady, A. R. Thomson, and D. N. Woolfson, A basis set of de novo coiled-coil peptide oligomers for rational protein design and synthetic biology. *ACS Synth. Biol.*, 2012. **1**(6): 240–250.

21. Petka, W. A., J. L. Harden, K. P. McGrath, D. Wirtz, and D. A. Tirrell, Reversible hydrogels from self-assembling artificial proteins. *Science*, 1998. **281**(5375): 389–392.
22. Wang, C., R. J. Stewart, and J. Kopecek, Hybrid hydrogels assembled from synthetic polymers and coiled-coil protein domains. *Nature*, 1999. **397**(6718): 417–420.
23. Lu, H. D., I. R. Wheeldon, and S. Banta, Catalytic biomaterials: engineering organophosphate hydrolase to form self-assembling enzymatic hydrogels. *Protein Eng. Des. Sel.*, 2010. **23**(7): 559–566.
24. Wheeldon, I. R., E. Campbell, and S. Banta, A chimeric fusion protein engineered with disparate functionalities-enzymatic activity and self-assembly. *J. Mol. Biol.*, 2009. **392**(1): 129–142.
25. Fischer, S. E., X. Y. Liu, H. Q. Mao, and J. L. Harden, Controlling cell adhesion to surfaces via associating bioactive triblock proteins. *Biomaterials*, 2007. **28**(22): 3325–3337.
26. Fischer, S. E., L. X. Mi, H. Q. Mao, and J. L. Harden, Biofunctional coatings via targeted covalent cross-linking of associating triblock proteins. *Biomacromolecules*, 2009. **10**(9): 2408–2417.
27. Xu, C. Y., V. Breedveld, and J. Kopecek, Reversible hydrogels from self-assembling genetically engineered protein block copolymers. *Biomacromolecules*, 2005. **6**(3): 1739–1749.
28. Xu, C. Y., L. Joss, C. Wang, M. Pechar, and J. Kopecek, The influence of fusion sequences on the thermal stabilities of coiled-coil proteins. *Macromol. Biosci.*, 2002. **2**(8): 395–401.
29. Xu, C. Y., and J. Kopecek, Genetically engineered block copolymers: influence of the length and structure of the coiled-coil blocks on hydrogel self-assembly. *Pharm. Res.*, 2008. **25**(3): 674–682.
30. Shen, W., K. C. Zhang, J. A. Kornfield, and D. A. Tirrell, Tuning the erosion rate of artificial protein hydrogels through control of network topology. *Nat. Mater.*, 2006. **5**(2): 153–158.
31. Jing, P., J. S. Rudra, A. B. Herr, and J. H. Collier, Self-assembling peptide-polymer hydrogels designed from the coiled coil region of fibrin. *Biomacromolecules*, 2008. **9**(9): 2438–2446.
32. Gunasekar, S. K., J. S. Haghpanah, and J. K. Montclare, Assembly of bioinspired helical protein fibers. *Polym. Adv. Technol.*, 2008. **19**(6): 454–468.
33. Morris, K., and L. Serpell, From natural to designer self-assembling biopolymers, the structural characterisation of fibrous proteins & peptides using fibre diffraction. *Chem. Soc. Rev.*, 2010. **39**(9): 3445–3453.

34. Cao, Y., and H. B. Li, Engineering tandem modular protein based reversible hydrogels. *Chem. Commun.*, 2008(35): 4144–4146.
35. Lv, S. S., Y. Cao, and H. B. Li, Tandem modular protein-based hydrogels constructed using a novel two-component approach. *Langmuir*, 2012. **28**(4): 2269–2274.
36. Wong Po Foo, C. T., J. S. Lee, W. Mulyasasmita, A. Parisi-Amon, and S. C. Heilshorn, Two-component protein-engineered physical hydrogels for cell encapsulation. *Proc. Natl. Acad. Sci. U.S.A.*, 2009. **106**(52): 22067–22072.
37. Russ, W. P., D. M. Lowery, P. Mishra, M. B. Yaffe, and R. Ranganathan, Natural-like function in artificial WW domains. *Nature*, 2005. **437**(7058): 579–583.
38. Mulyasasmita, W., J. S. Lee, and S. C. Heilshorn, Molecular-level engineering of protein physical hydrogels for predictive sol-gel phase behavior. *Biomacromolecules*, 2011. **12**(10): 3406–3411.
39. Alarcon, C. D. H., S. Pennadam, and C. Alexander, Stimuli responsive polymers for biomedical applications. *Chem. Soc. Rev.*, 2005. **34**(3): 276–285.
40. Stuart, M. A. C., W. T. S. Huck, J. Genzer, M. Muller, C. Ober, M. Stamm, G. B. Sukhorukov, I. Szleifer, V. V. Tsukruk, M. Urban, F. Winnik, S. Zauscher, I. Luzinov, and S. Minko, Emerging applications of stimuli-responsive polymer materials. *Nat. Mater.*, 2010. **9**(2): 101–113.
41. Haines-Butterick, L., K. Rajagopal, M. Branco, D. Salick, R. Rughani, M. Pilarz, M. S. Lamm, D. J. Pochan, and J. P. Schneider, Controlling hydrogelation kinetics by peptide design for three-dimensional encapsulation and injectable delivery of cells. *Proc. Natl. Acad. Sci. U.S.A.*, 2007. **104**(19): 7791–7796.
42. Lu, H. D., M. B. Charati, I. L. Kim, and J. A. Burdick, Injectable shear-thinning hydrogels engineered with a self-assembling Dock-and-Lock mechanism. *Biomaterials*, 2012. **33**(7): 2145–2153.
43. Guvendiren, M., H. D. Lu, and J. A. Burdick, Shear-thinning hydrogels for biomedical applications. *Soft Mat.*, 2012. **8**(2): 260–272.
44. Ehrick, J. D., S. K. Deo, T. W. Browning, L. G. Bachas, M. J. Madou, and S. Daunert, Genetically engineered protein in hydrogels tailors stimuli-responsive characteristics. *Nat. Mater.*, 2005. **4**(4): 298–302.
45. Mohammed, J. S., and W. L. Murphy, Bioinspired design of dynamic materials. *Adv. Mater.*, 2009. **21**(23): 2361–2374.
46. Tan, R. Y., Y. Mabuchi, and Z. Grabarek, Blocking the Ca^{2+}-induced conformational transitions in calmodulin with disulfide bonds. *J. Biol. Chem.*, 1996. **271**(13): 7479–7483.

47. Zhang, M. J., and T. Yuan, Molecular mechanisms of calmodulin's functional versatility. *Biochem. Cell Biol.*, 1998. **76**(2-3): 313-323.
48. Ehrick, J. D., S. Stokes, S. Bachas-Daunert, E. A. Moschou, S. K. Deo, L. G. Bachas, and S. Daunert, Chemically tunable lensing of stimuli-responsive hydrogel microdomes. *Adv. Mater.*, 2007. **19**(22): 4024-4027.
49. King, W. J., J. S. Mohammed, and W. L. Murphy, Modulating growth factor release from hydrogels via a protein conformational change. *Soft Mat.*, 2009. **5**(12): 2399-2406.
50. Murphy, W. L., W. S. Dillmore, J. Modica, and M. Mrksich, Dynamic hydrogels: translating a protein conformational change into macroscopic motion. *Angew. Chem.-Int. Edit.*, 2007. **46**(17): 3066-3069.
51. Grove, T. Z., C. O. Osuji, J. D. Forster, E. R. Dufresne, and L. Regan, Stimuli-responsive smart gels realized via modular protein design. *J. Am. Chem. Soc.*, 2010. **132**(40): 14024-14026.
52. Cortajarena, A. L., J. M. Wang, and L. Regan, Crystal structure of a designed tetratricopeptide repeat module in complex with its peptide ligand. *FEBS J.*, 2010. **277**(4): 1058-1066.
53. Cortajarena, A. L., T. Y. Liu, M. Hochstrasser, and L. Regan, Designed proteins to modulate cellular networks. *ACS Chem. Biol.*, 2010. **5**(6): 545-552.
54. Jackrei, M. E., R. Valverde, and L. Regan, Redesign of a protein-peptide interaction: characterization and applications. *Prot. Sci.*, 2009. **18**(4): 762-774.
55. Grove, T. Z., J. Forster, G. Pimienta, E. Dufresne, and L. Regan, A modular approach to the design of protein-based smart gels. *Biopolymers*, 2012. **97**(7): 508-517.
56. Dooley, K., Y. H. Kim, H. D. Lu, R. Tu, and S. Banta, Engineering of an environmentally responsive beta roll peptide for use as a calcium-dependent cross-linking domain for peptide hydrogel formation. *Biomacromolecules*, 2012. **13**(6): 1758-1764.
57. Topp, S., V. Prasad, G. C. Cianci, E. R. Weeks, and J. P. Gallivan, A genetic toolbox for creating reversible Ca^{2+}-sensitive materials. *J. Am. Chem. Soc.*, 2006. **128**(43): 13994-13995.
58. Yang, J. Y., C. Y. Xu, C. Wang, and J. Kopecek, Refolding hydrogels self-assembled from N-(2-hydroxypropyl) methacrylamide graft copolymers by antiparallel coiled-coil formation. *Biomacromolecules*, 2006. **7**(4): 1187-1195.

59. Kopecek, J., Hydrogel biomaterials: A smart future? *Biomaterials*, 2007. **28**(34): 5185–5192.
60. Ikura, M., Calcium binding and conformational response in EF-hand proteins. *Trends Biochem. Sci.*, 1996. **21**(1): 14–17.
61. McPhalen, C. A., N. C. J. Strynadka, and M. N. G. James, Calcium-binding sites in proteins: A structrual perspective. *Adv. Protein Chem.*, 1991. **42**: 77.
62. Ikura, M., and J. B. Ames, Genetic polymorphism and protein conformational plasticity in the calmodulin superfamily: Two ways to promote multifunctionality. *Proc. Natl. Acad. Sci. U.S.A.*, 2006. **103**(5): 1159–1164.
63. Miyata, T., N. Asami, and T. Uragami, A reversibly antigen-responsive hydrogel. *Nature*, 1999. **399**(6738): 766–769.
64. Miyata, T., T. Uragami, and K. Nakamae, Biomolecule-sensitive hydrogels. *Adv. Drug Deliv. Rev.*, 2002. **54**(1): 79–98.
65. Hartgerink, J. D., E. Beniash, and S. I. Stupp, Self-assembly and mineralization of peptide-amphiphile nanofibers. *Science*, 2001. **294**(5547): 1684–1688.
66. Hartgerink, J. D., E. Beniash, and S. I. Stupp, Peptide-amphiphile nanofibers: A versatile scaffold for the preparation of self-assembling materials. *Proc. Natl. Acad. Sci. U.S.A.*, 2002. **99**(8): 5133–5138.
67. Niece, K. L., J. D. Hartgerink, J. J. J. M. Donners, and S. I. Stupp, Self-assembly combining two bioactive peptide-amphiphile molecules into nanofibers by electrostatic attraction. *J. Am. Chem. Soc.*, 2003. **125**(24): 7146–7147.
68. Silva, G. A., C. Czeisler, K. L. Niece, E. Beniash, D. A. Harrington, J. A. Kessler, and S. I. Stupp, Selective differentiation of neural progenitor cells by high-epitope density nanofibers. *Science*, 2004. **303**(5662): 1352–1355.
69. Aida, T., E. W. Meijer, and S. I. Stupp, Functional supramolecular polymers. *Science*, 2012. **335**(6070): 813–817.
70. Zhang, S. M., M. A. Greenfield, A. Mata, L. C. Palmer, R. Bitton, J. R. Mantei, C. Aparicio, M. O. de la Cruz, and S. I. Stupp, A self-assembly pathway to aligned monodomain gels. *Nat. Mater.*, 2010. **9**(7): 594–601.
71. Webber, M. J., J. Tongers, C. J. Newcomb, K. T. Marquardt, J. Bauersachs, D. W. Losordo, and S. I. Stupp, Supramolecular nanostructures that mimic VEGF as a strategy for ischemic tissue repair. *Proc. Natl. Acad. Sci. U.S.A.*, 2011. **108**(33): 13438–13443.

72. D'andrea, L. D., G. Iaccarino, R. Fattorusso, D. Sorriento, C. Carannante, D. Capasso, B. Trimarco, and C. Pedone, Targeting angiogenesis: structural characterization and biological properties of a de novo engineered VEGF mimicking peptide. *Proc. Natl. Acad. Sci. U.S.A.*, 2005. **102**(40): 14215–14220.

73. Schneider, J. P., D. J. Pochan, B. Ozbas, K. Rajagopal, L. Pakstis, and J. Kretsinger, Responsive hydrogels from the intramolecular folding and self-assembly of a designed peptide. *J. Am. Chem. Soc.*, 2002. **124**(50): 15030–15037.

74. Zhang, S. G., Fabrication of novel biomaterials through molecular self-assembly. *Nat. Biotechnol.*, 2003. **21**(10): 1171–1178.

75. Zhang, S. G., D. M. Marini, W. Hwang, and S. Santoso, Design of nanostructured biological materials through self-assembly of peptides and proteins. *Curr. Opin. Chem. Biol.*, 2002. **6**(6): 865–871.

76. Jung, J. P., A. K. Nagaraj, E. K. Fox, J. S. Rudra, J. M. Devgun, and J. H. Collier, Co-assembling peptides as defined matrices for endothelial cells. *Biomaterials*, 2009. **30**(12): 2400–2410.

77. Gasiorowski, J. Z., and J. H. Collier, Directed intermixing in multicomponent self-assembling biomaterials. *Biomacromolecules*, 2011. **12**(10): 3549–3558.

78. Jung, J. P., J. V. Moyano, and J. H. Collier, Multifactorial optimization of endothelial cell growth using modular synthetic extracellular matrices. *Integrat. Biol.*, 2011. **3**(3): 185–196.

79. Rudra, J. S., Y. F. Tian, J. P. Jung, and J. H. Collier, A self-assembling peptide acting as an immune adjuvant. *Proc. Natl. Acad. Sci. U.S.A.*, 2010. **107**(2): 622–627.

80. Ryadnov, M. G., and D. N. Woolfson, Engineering the morphology of a self-assembling protein fibre. *Nat. Mater.*, 2003. **2**(5): 329–332.

81. Papapostolou, D., A. M. Smith, E. D. T. Atkins, S. J. Oliver, M. G. Ryadnov, L. C. Serpell, and D. N. Woolfson, Engineering nanoscale order into a designed protein fiber. *Proc. Natl. Acad. Sci. U.S.A.*, 2007. **104**(26): 10853–10858.

82. Mahmoud, Z. N., D. J. Grundy, K. J. Channon, and D. N. Woolfson, The non-covalent decoration of self-assembling protein fibers. *Biomaterials*, 2010. **31**(29): 7468–7474.

83. Woolfson, D. N., and M. G. Ryadnov, Peptide-based fibrous biomaterials: some things old, new and borrowed. *Curr. Opin. Chem. Biol.*, 2006. **10**(6): 559–567.

84. Sara, M., and U. B. Sleytr, S-layer proteins. *J. Bacteriol.*, 2000. **182**(4): 859–868.
85. Ilk, N., E. M. Egelseer, and U. B. Sleytr, S-layer fusion proteins: construction principles and applications. *Curr. Opin. Biotechnol.*, 2011. **22**(6): 824–831.
86. Steiner, K., A. Hanreich, B. Kainz, P. G. Hitchen, A. Dell, P. Messner, and C. Schaffer, Recombinant glycans on an S-layer self-assembly protein: a new dimension for nanopatterned biomaterials. *Small*, 2008. **4**(10): 1728–1740.

Part 2

Tissue and Organ Regeneration

Chapter 9

Design and Fabrication of Biomimetic Microvascular Architecture

Thomas M. Cervantes and Joseph P. Vacanti

Center for Regenerative Medicine, Department of Surgery,
Massachusetts General Hospital, 185 Cambridge St, Boston, MA 02114, USA

jvacanti@partners.org

9.1 Introduction

9.1.1 Clinical Need for Whole Organ Fabrication

Organ transplantation is needed for patients suffering end-stage organ failure. In 2011 alone, over 50,000 patients were added to the waiting list to receive an organ for transplantation (Organ Procurement and Transplantation Network, accessed May 2012). Of these patients, close to 16,500 died, became too sick to transplant, or could not be matched to a donor. The demand for viable organs is far greater than the current supply. Currently, the only sources for transplant organs are from living donors and deceased donors. In 2011 living donors accounted for just over 6,000 transplanted organs, while deceased donor organs comprised the remaining 22,500; this sum accounts for far less than the 50,000 patients

---

Tissue and Organ Regeneration: Advances in Micro- and Nanotechnology
Edited by Lijie Grace Zhang, Ali Khademhosseini, and Thomas J. Webster
Copyright © 2014 Pan Stanford Publishing Pte. Ltd.
ISBN 978-981-4411-67-7 (Hardcover), 978-981-4411-68-4 (eBook)
www.panstanford.com

added to the wait list that year (Organ Procurement and Transplantation Network, accessed May 2012). The remaining demand must be supplied by deceased donor organs. Since 1988, the total number of deceased donors has increased thanks to improved protocols for deceased donor organ harvest and transplantation (Perera and Bramhall, 2011; Goldstein et al., 2012; Pavlakis and Hanto, 2012; Ojo et al., 2004). However, in order to satisfy the needs of all patients requiring a transplant, whole organ fabrication approaches are required.

The disparity between organ supply and demand led to emergence of the field of Tissue Engineering in the late 1980s (Vacanti et al., 1988). According to Langer and Vacanti, "tissue engineering is an interdisciplinary field that applies the principles of engineering and the life sciences toward the development of biological substitutes that restore, maintain, or improve tissue function" (Langer and Vacanti, 1993). Several engineered tissues have been designed in labs throughout the world and have been proven successful in clinical trials, including skin (Gómez et al., 2011), cartilage (Kreuz et al., 2009), and vascular grafts (McAllister et al., 2009). Significant growth in the tissue engineering and stem cell industry from 2007 reflects successful results from these academic research efforts (Jaklenec et al., 2012). Despite this progress, the goal of whole organ fabrication has yet to be realized. Certain fundamental limitations must be overcome in order to scale from engineered tissues up to whole organ replacement.

9.1.2 Mass Transport and Manufacturing Limitations

The first limitation to overcome arises from mass transport properties in engineered tissues. Aerobic respiration in these cells consumes oxygen and glucose and creates waste products such as carbon dioxide and urea. Mass transport of these molecules to and from the cell is accomplished through passive diffusion along concentration gradients. Oxygen has the highest metabolic rate and diffusional resistance of these molecules, and therefore can be considered as the limiting factor in mass transport (Malda et al., 2007). Consumption of oxygen during aerobic respiration occurs at an average rate of 4×10^{17} mol/cell-sec, depending on cell type (Chow et al., 2001a; Collins et al., 1998; Kunz-Schughart et al., 2000). Tissues without sufficient oxygen to support their metabolic needs are in a state of hypoxia, which can lead to necrosis (Smith and Mooney, 2007).

The cardiovascular system enables convective transport of oxygen and other molecules to each of the trillions of cells within the human body. Most cells are within 100–200 µm from a capillary lumen (Ishaug-Riley et al., 1998; Suzuki et al., 1998). The minimum distance between a cell and an oxygen source, the oxygen diffusion distance limit, is dependent upon (1) the rate of cellular oxygen consumption and (2) the diffusion rate of oxygen through tissue. Dimensional analysis of these quantities shows that the following relationship must be observed in order to avoid necrosis within a tissue (Muschler et al., 2004):

$$[\text{Cell}] < \frac{2D_{O2}C_0}{Q_{\text{Cell}}L^2}, \qquad (9.1)$$

where [Cell] is the cellular concentration in the scaffold, D_{O2} is the diffusion coefficient of oxygen, C_0 is the oxygen concentration at the surface of the tissue, Q_{cell} is oxygen consumption rate of each cell, and L is the diffusion distance to the center of the tissue. D_{O2} and C_0 are constants that have been measured experimentally (Chow et al., 2001b). An inverse square relationship is evident; $[\text{Cell}] \propto 1/L^2$.

The implications for engineered tissues are evident; according to the relationship defined in Eq. 9.1, if the characteristic dimension of a tissue-engineered construct is scaled by a factor of N, the theoretical limit of cellular density is decreased by a factor of N^2. An intrinsic vascular network is thus necessary in order to increase the size of engineered tissues while maintaining minimum oxygen diffusion distances. This concept has been recognized, and several attempts have been made to incorporate vascularization into scaffolds for cellular growth. As early as 2000, microfluidic devices were used as platforms for cell culture, manufactured using photolithography technology adapted from the semiconductor industry (Kaihara et al., 2000; Pimpin and Srituravanich, 2012). Typical designs contain two-dimensional microchannel arrays and can be theoretically adapted for whole organ scaffolds. However, organs are inherently three-dimensional, and their vascular organization must reflect this. The evolutionary development of capillary systems has favored specific vascular designs and fluidic properties for different organ functions. The emerging field of biomimetic vascular design utilizes these principles found in natural vascular architectures to create models for tissue-engineered scaffolds of whole organs. Fabrication of such intricate networks would be challenging when using traditional photolithography techniques. Several microfabrication technologies have been developed that are capable of achieving the geometric complexity of organ capillary networks.

9.2 Biomimetic Vascular Design Principles

The field of biomimetic design has developed as an engineering approach that attempts to recapitulate the form and function of biological systems. Living organism structures have developed through years of evolution in order to survive in specific ecosystems; their adaptations to the environment can yield unique design solutions for engineering problems. For example, the hooked spines found on plant burs, which allow them to cling to animal fur and be dispersed, led to the development of Velcro products (Hagland, 2012). The self-cleaning and water-repellent surface of the lotus leaf inspired the creation of water-repellent paint (Barthlott and Neinhuis, 1997). The unique properties of the Gecko's footpads, which allow the animal to traverse walls and ceilings, have spurred the creation of surgical bandages (Cho et al., 2012) and wall-climbing robots (Kim et al., 2008).

Recently, biomimetic design principles have been used in the creation of vascular networks for engineered tissues (Hoganson et al., 2010; Huh et al., 2012). Branching patterns and fluidic properties of native vasculature drove the development of a lung assist device with improved gas exchange properties and reduced risk of thrombus formation (Hoganson et al., 2011). Cyclic expansion of alveoli during respiration led to the development of a lung bioreactor that applies cyclic mechanical strain to an alveolar capillary structure (Huh et al., 2010). The radial organizational structure of liver tissue vasculature inspired the design of a microfluidic hepatocyte bioreactor (Hoganson et al., 2010). In each of these examples, fundamental design principles of native vasculature were identified and incorporated into engineered tissue constructs.

Several fundamental design principles have been identified for the development of biomimetic vascular architecture based on analytical modeling and experimental observations. This section explores each of these principles in depth, reviewing the theoretical and experimental methods that have been used in their derivation.

9.2.1 Functional Motif

Every tissue has a set of defining functional motifs that influences its form and functionality. These functional motifs encompass design parameters such as spatial organization, transport specifications, and chemical and physical microenvironments (Huh et al., 2012). Biomimetic microvascular designs begin by identifying one or more of these functional motifs to recapitulate using microfabrication techniques. For example, a well-known feature of microvasculature of the liver is the radial organization of the liver sinusoids. This specific geometry is known to influence the organization of hepatocytes into three distinct zones, each performing a unique metabolic function (Gebhardt, 1992). This radial architecture was used as a functional motif in the design of a biomimetic microdevice to improve the in vivo functionality of hepatocytes (Hoganson et al., 2010).

An example of a transport motif is the exchange of oxygen and carbon dioxide within the alveolar sacs of the lungs. Alveolar capillary structures have a high density of vessels in order to optimize blood gas flux for a given blood volume and the cardiac output necessary to drive pulmonary blood flow. Using this functional motif, a high-density microvascular network was developed as a biomimetic lung assist device (Hoganson et al., 2011). The physiologic blood flow within this vascular design has potential to reduce the propensity for clotting that is observed in current membrane oxygenator systems (Federspiel and Henchir, 2004).

The physical microenvironment of alveolar capillaries is another functional motif that has been incorporated into a microvascular device. During the breathing cycle, repeated expansion of the alveoli imparts a cyclic strain to the airway epithelium and vascular endothelium. This has implications for cellular morphology and transport of macromolecules. The cyclic strain environment was incorporated into a biomimetic lung-on-a-chip and was shown to influence the uptake of various chemicals (Huh et al., 2010).

The human intestine experiences a similar type of physical microenvironment; peristaltic contractions apply strain to intestinal epithelium that affects their morphology and unctionality.

This functional motif was incorporated into a gut-on-a-chip microdevice that was shown to promote spontaneous self-assembly of villi-like formations in a human intestinal epithelium cell line (Kim et al., 2012). In another study, the high-aspect-ratio geometry of villi structures was directly fabricated into a biomimetic gastrointestinal tract device (Sung et al., 2011).

Kidney nephrons have a unique microvascular structure and chemical microenvironment that affect the osmoregulatory function of the tissue. Mass transport throughout the renal corpuscle serves to main a homeostatic balance of water and solutes in the blood. These functional motifs were incorporated into a multi-layer microfluidic device for culture and analysis of renal tubular cells (Jang and Suh, 2010). Renal tubular cells were grown on a porous membrane separating an outer tubular compartment (blood stream) and inner tubular fluid (urine precursor) with flow at a specified shear stress. This biomimetic design demonstrated improved cellular morphology and molecular transport over static culture designs.

These examples illustrate the plurality of biomimetic functional motifs that can be incorporated into microfluidic vascular architecture. Similar design principles have also been applied to the creation of biomimetic devices for bone, breast, eye, and brain tissues (Huh et al., 2011). A functional motif is the foundation for biomimetic design around which all other principles are organized. Therefore, it is important to carefully consider the intended function and performance environment of the microvascular device.

9.2.2 Pressure and Flow Conditions

Pressure and flow rate are important biomimetic design parameters that can affect mass transport, cell viability, and overall functional capacity of a tissue-engineered microvascular device. Pressure boundary conditions can be defined based on the physiologic values of the target tissue. For example, a biomimetic lung device was designed with an inlet pressure of the pulmonary artery (19 mmHg) and an outlet pressure of the left atrium (3 mmHg) (Hoganson et al., 2011). A biomimetic liver device was designed based on the inlet pressure of the hepatic portal vein (10 mmHg) and outlet pressure of the inferior vena cava (3 mmHg) for the target population of patients with liver disease (Hoganson et al., 2010). Pressures above or below physiologic values can disrupt the desired mass transport properties and have deleterious effects on cell growth. For example, hepatocytes are known to be sensitive to parenchymal fluid pressure (PFP); in a rat liver, PFP was measured at 2.86 mmHg (Moran et al., 2012). Evaluation of a bioartificial liver device in an in vivo rat model reported adverse effects on hepatocyte health when the PFP exceeded 11 mmHg (Hsu et al., 2010). This sensitivity underscores the importance of pressure as a biomimetic design parameter to ensure function and viability of the target tissue.

Flow rate affects the functional capacity and energy costs of an engineered microvascular network. For example, diffusion of gases through a permeable membrane is known to increase at higher flow rates (Bassett et al., 2011). Similarly, the linear distribution of nutrients along a vessel length becomes more uniform as flow is increased (Inamdar et al., 2011). However, increased flow corresponds with increased wall shear stress (see Eq. 9.4b), which can lead to platelet activation. Furthermore, high flow rates cause an increase in pressure drop, as defined by Poiseuille's relationship (White, 2008):

$$\Delta P = \frac{128\mu L Q}{\pi D^4}, \tag{9.2}$$

where ΔP is pressure drop, μ is blood viscosity, L is vessel length, Q is the volumetric flow rate, and D is the vessel diameter.

Thus, high flow rates require greater pumping power to operate, an important consideration when available cardiac output is a limiting factor.

The flow profile within a vessel is also affected by the flow rate. A laminar flow profile is important to reduce risk of platelet activation and maintain optimal distribution of cells and macromolecules within vessel. The Reynolds number, a dimensionless ratio of inertial forces to viscous forces, is commonly used to quantify flow conditions (Incropera et al., 2007). For laminar flow, the Reynolds number must be below 2300. Using this limit, an upper boundary for flow rate can be estimated based on vessel diameter:

$$\mathrm{Re}_{max} = \frac{4Q}{\pi \nu D^4}, \tag{9.3}$$

where Re_{max} is the maximum Reynolds number for laminar flow (2300), Q is the volumetric flow rate, ν is the kinematic viscosity of blood (average value = 4×10^{-6} m^2/s), and D is the diameter of the vascular channel. The value of v was estimated by dividing the estimates of blood viscosity (4 cP) and density (1 g/cm^2) (Baskurt and Meiselman, 2003). Using this relationship, order-of-magnitude estimates can be made; a vessel with diameter 1 mm has a maximum flow of ~10 µL/min, while a vessel with a diameter of 10 µm has a maximum flow of ~10 µL/min. In the early stages of device design, this relationship can provide useful estimates of scale.

9.2.3 Shear Stress

Luminal shear stress has important implications for the development and maintenance of patent microvasculature. Vessel size and arrangement throughout all levels of the cardiovascular system are influenced by shear stress values (Zamir, 1976b). Endothelial cells within microfabricated vascular channels exhibit morphological and biochemical when subjected to shear stress. Several studies report shear-induced stretching and re-arrangement of the endothelial cytoskeleton along the axis of flow, as well as the formation of focal adhesions and adherens junctions (Ensley et al., 2012; Esch et al., 2011; Malek et al., 1999). Anticoagulant and platelet inhibitory factors produced by endothelial cells are upregulated in response to physiologic shear values (Nagel et al., 1999). This response mediates shear-induced platelet activation and adhesion. Exposure to regions of high shear stress, such as a narrowing due to atherosclerosis, can cause platelet activation (Kroll et al., 1996), whereas platelet adhesions are known to occur in regions of low shear values, such as the outer walls of a branched bifurcation (Caro et al., 1971). Commonly cited values for physiologic shear stresses are between 10 and 70 dynes/cm^2 for normal arteries (Malek et al., 1999).

Shear stress as a physical property, depicted in Fig. 9.2, is dependent on the dynamic viscosity of the fluid medium and the velocity gradient within a cross-sectional area of flow (White, 2008). The maximum value of shear stress is at the luminal surface of the vessel, where the fluid velocity is zero as defined by the no-slip boundary condition. Poiseuille's law can be used to calculate the luminal shear stress for Newtonian fluids in laminar flow (Wootton and Ku, 1999); the magnitude of shear stress at any point in the fluid can then be extrapolated. These relationships are described in Eqs. 9.4a–9.4c:

$$\tau_r = -\mu \frac{\partial u}{\partial r} \qquad (9.4a)$$

$$\tau_w = \frac{32\mu Q}{\pi D^3} \qquad (9.4b)$$

$$\tau_r = 2\tau_w \frac{r}{D} \qquad (9.4c)$$

where τ is shear stress, μ is dynamic viscosity, u is fluid velocity, r is radial distance from the center of the vessel, τ_w is luminal shear stress, Q is volumetric flow rate, and D is vessel diameter.

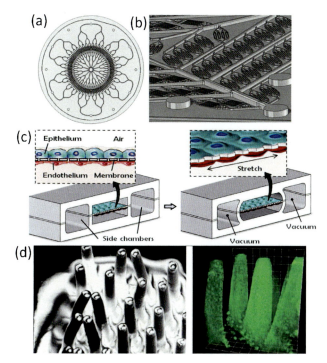

Figure 9.1 Examples of tissue-specific functional motif incorporated into biomimetic microfluidic networks. (a) Microfluidic liver scaffold with a radial pattern reflecting the architecture of the liver sinusoid. (b) High-density capillary networks increase area for gas exchange in a lung oxygenator device, mimicking the function of alveoli. (c) Cyclic strain imposed on a biomimetic lung-on-a-chip device recreates the physical microenvironment of the alveoli (Huh et al., 2010). (d) High-aspect-ratio microscale structures molded into a hydrogel to model the architecture of intestinal villi (Sung et al., 2011).

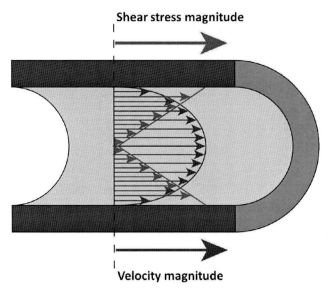

Figure 9.2 Shear stress within a circular lumen. The velocity magnitude at the wall is zero, as defined by the no-slip condition, and reaches a maximum in the center of the lumen (laminar flow). The shear stress magnitude is greatest at the wall, and decreases due to the radial change in velocity magnitude (as defined by Eq. 9.4a).

Blood is known to be a non-Newtonian fluid and exhibits shear thinning (Wells and Merrill, 1961; White 2008). As shear rate increases, the fluid viscosity decreases (similar to the behavior of tomato ketchup, another pseudoplastic fluid (Rani and Bains, 1986); this effect is exacerbated in micro-scale geometries. Non-linear variations in blood viscosity are commonly accounted for using the Herschel–Bulkley model (Herschel and Bulkley, 1926):

$$\mu = k\dot{\gamma}^{n-1} + \frac{\tau_0}{\dot{\gamma}}, \tag{9.5}$$

where k is the consistency coefficient, $\dot{\gamma}$ is the strain rate, n is the power-law index, and τ_0 is the yield stress. The determination of these parameter values for blood flow has been described by several authors (Kim, 2002; Valencia et al., 2008; Hoganson et al., 2011).

Shear stress is an important criterion for the design of microvascular networks in engineered tissues. Vascular occlusion due to thrombosis is a catastrophic failure mode for a tissue-engineered device. Acellular vascular configurations, such as extracorporeal membrane oxygenator devices (Hoganson et al., 2011; Federspiel and Svitek, 2004), are especially susceptible to occlusion due to the absence of anti-coagulant factors produced by endothelial cells. Microvascular geometries should be designed to maintain physiologic levels of shear stress throughout the vascular network.

9.2.4 Aspect Ratio

A defining feature of biomimetic networks is that all vessel cross-sectional geometries have a 1:1 aspect ratio, meaning that all cross sections must be circular or square. The motivation for this design principle is derived from an analysis of wall shear stress. Channel geometries with a 1:1 aspect ratio exhibit uniform shear stress distribution on all channel walls. Non-uniform shear variation can lead to platelet activation and thrombosis. Shear stress is dependent on the thickness of the fluid boundary layer, as is evident in Eq. 9.4a. Laminar, fully developed internal flows thus have minimum shear stress at the fluid center, and maximum shear stress at the fluid boundaries. For a circular cross section, all boundaries are equidistant from the fluid center by definition, and thus have uniformly distributed shear stress. Square cross-sectional geometries exhibit a small but evenly distributed shear variation at the corners. Native vasculature exhibits circular cross-sectional geometry, and this is the preferred configuration for biomimetic networks. Square cross sections, however, are a more feasible configuration for many fabrication techniques, and retain the same branching optimality relationships derived for circular cross sections (discussed in detail in a later section) (Emerson et al., 2006).

Rectangular geometries exhibit a higher degree of shear variation, but are commonly seen in microfluidic devices utilizing standard Photolithography fabrication techniques (Hoganson et al., 2011). This becomes problematic when large networks are created with a uniform channel depth. Consider the case where the largest vessel is 300 μm in height and width, but the smallest is 30 μm wide. The 10:1 aspect ratio causes significant shear variation, putting the network at risk of clot formation in the smallest channels. This situation can be avoided by designing microvascular networks with a uniform 1:1 aspect ratio, using advanced microfabrication technologies (see Section 9.3). Examples of wall shear stress for various blood vessel geometries are shown in Fig. 9.3.

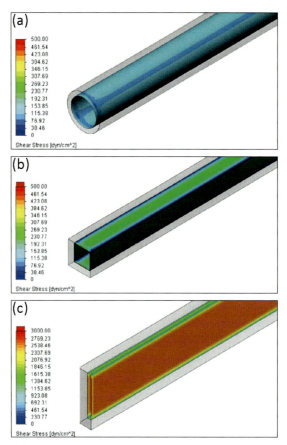

Figure 9.3 Wall shear stresses for (a) circular, (b) square, and (c) rectangular geometries. The rectangular geometry has a 10:1 aspect ratio. All cross sections have equal perimeter length, and all vessels have the same volumetric flow rate. SolidWorks Flow Simulation CFD software (SolidWorks Corp., Concord, MA) was used for flow analysis. The circular channel has a uniform shear stress distribution, an ideal physiological condition. The square cross section exhibits small shear variation at the corners, but the majority of the wall has uniform wall shear. The 10:1 aspect ratio rectangular geometry exhibits a high degree of shear variation (as well as larger magnitudes), and is unsuitable for a biomimetic vascular configuration.

9.2.5 Vessel Length

Vessel length of microscale capillary structures can influence mass transport and the flow profile. As a general rule, smaller diameter vessels tend to be shorter. Tables comparing vessel diameters and length have been published and can be used as a guideline for biomimetic designs (Milnor, 1989; Hoganson et al., 2011). An experimental study evaluating resin castings of a human coronary artery tree suggests an upper limit of $L = 35 * D$, (L = vessel length, D = vessel diameter) with a rough mean of $L = 10D$ as a suggested approximation (Zamir, 1999). A micro-CT analysis of a rat hepatic portal vein tree determined a weak correlation ($R^2 = 0.31$) of $L = 8.8 * D^0.76$ (Buijs et al., 2006). It is important to note, however, that these experimental findings display a wide degree of variation.

A deterministic approach to biomimetic vessel length can be driven by considering the fundamental relationships governing mass transport and flow profiles. At the microvascular scale, an important functional requirement is the exchange of blood gasses and macromolecules. Given the initial concentration of a solute at the vessel entrance, the concentration gradient along the vessel length can be modeled using differential equations that take into account cellular density and the metabolic rate of specific cell types (Inamdar et al., 2011). If a uniform distribution is desired, the vessel length can be adjusted appropriately. In scenarios where a gradient is desired, such as the liver sinusoids (Allen et al., 2005), the length can be set to achieve the desired distribution.

As mentioned previously, a laminar flow profile is an important functional requirement for biomimetic vascular designs. Disturbances to laminar flow can occur at branched connections; to ensure return of laminar flow, the entry length can be considered. Entry length is defined as the length of flow necessary to establish fully developed flow (that is, the flow profile does not change axially). The correlation for laminar flow entry length in a circular duct is defined as follows (Shah and London, 1978):

$$L_{entry} = D_h \left[\left(\frac{0.60}{0.035 Re + 1} \right) + 0.056 Re \right], \qquad (9.6)$$

where L_{entry} is the entry length, D is the vessel diameter, and Re is the Reynolds number (see Eq. 9.3).

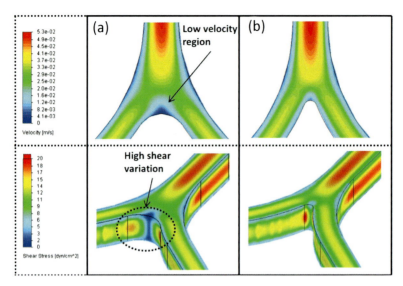

Figure 9.4 Iterative optimization of the boundary layer profile at a branched intersection using CFD software (SolidWorks Flow Simulation). Velocity and shear stress scales are identical for pre-optimized and optimized geometries. (a) A large low velocity region is observed in the region of the bifurcation, as well as significant shear stress variation, increasing the risk of platelet activation. (b) The fillet radius of the branching corner was decreased, eliminating the low velocity region and reducing the shear variation.

In practice, many biomimetic microvascular designs are space-limited by the capabilities of microfabrication techniques, such as for in vitro microfluidic tissue networks. For these scenarios, the best practice is often to define a biomimetic length for the smallest vessels, and then adjust the lengths of larger vessels to fit within the design. Often, maintaining the overarching functional motif supersedes strict adherence to the length correlations described above, which can explain the significant variation observed in experimental studies.

9.2.6 Diameter Relationships

The branching configuration of the cardiovascular system exhibits remarkable adherence to fractal scaling laws, suggesting a common underlying mechanism of development (West et al., 1997).

Theoretical physiologists have long sought to define general laws that govern the geometry of branched connections in vascular trees. In 1926, Murray proposed a model to describe the relationship between the diameters of parent and daughter vessels (Murray, 1926). Using the principle of minimum work, he optimized the energy required to overcome viscous drag forces and the metabolic energy required to maintain a given blood volume (Sherman, 1981). In this scenario, the luminal shear stress is uniform throughout all levels of the network. The resulting equation is applicable for both symmetric and asymmetric bifurcations:

$$D_0^3 = \sum_{i=1}^{n} D_i^3, \qquad (9.7)$$

where D_0 is the diameter of the parent vessel, n is the number of daughter vessels, and D_i is the diameter of the ith daughter vessel. This relationship was calculated for vessels with circular geometry; theoretical calculations by Emerson and colleagues have extrapolated results to arbitrary vessel geometries (Emerson et al., 2006).

The simplicity of the cubed power–law relationship and repeated experimental validation have led to Murray's law as a widely accepted tenet of biomimetic design principles (Buijs et al., 2006). However, it is noted that the value of the power index had differs for larger arteries where turbulent flows can dominate (e.g., the aorta), or the smallest capillaries where the shear thinning effects of blood are exacerbated (Sherman, 1981; Zamir et al., 1992). Various alternate models have been developed that aim to extrapolate scaling relationships that apply to arbitrary vessel sizes and vascular trees for specific tissues (Kassab, 2006; Zhou et al., 1999). In practice, these differences are small and can be ignored when the scale of an engineered network does not vary greatly. Murray's law is a valuable design tool and has been incorporated into several biomimetic microvascular devices (Lim et al., 2003; Vozzi et al., 2004; Hoganson et al., 2010, 2011).

9.2.7 Branching Angle

Branching angles within the cardiovascular system influence the overall vascular architecture of a tissue and can affect the shear stress profile at branched intersections. Theoretical and analytical approaches have been applied to understand the relationships that govern branching angles. Zamir and colleagues applied optimality principles to the parameters of luminal surface area, blood volume, pumping power, and viscous drag forces (Zamir, 1976a,b).

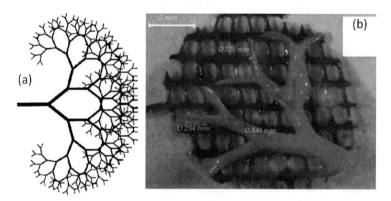

Figure 9.5 Computational techniques can be used to generate biomimetic architecture with a high degree of complexity. (a) A kidney vasculature model generated using a Lindenmayer system approach (Zamir, 2001). (b) Branched 3D microstructure designed with a Lindenmayer system and fabricated in a polyethylene glycol diacrylate (PEGDA)-based hydrogel (Yasar et al., 2009).

For each parameter, optimum branching geometry was calculated. From these results, it was determined that larger daughter vessels have a smaller branching angle from the direction of the parent artery than do smaller branches, which have an branching angle that approaches 90°.

Experimental measurements of branch angles in human and primate arterial trees have confirmed the predicted trend that the branch angle of the larger daughter vessel is considerably smaller than form smaller daughter vessels (Zamir and Brown, 1982; Zamir and Medeiros, 1982). Recently, micro-CT analysis has been used to perform high-resolution measurements of branching parameters within a rat hepatic portal vein tree (Buijs et al., 2006). Within this vascular tree, branching angles varied between values predicted by minimum pumping power and minimum viscous drag. The branching angle between daughter vessels had an average value of 88.3°, which in practice can be approximated as a right angle. Considerable variation of branching angles was observed, but the data suggest a simultaneous optimization of luminal surface area, blood volume, pumping power, and viscous forces.

Biomimetic vascular networks can be constructed using theoretical equations predicted by Zamir and colleagues (Zamir, 1976a; Zamir and Brown, 1982). In practice, adjustments form theoretical values may be necessary in order to adhere to the organizing functional motif of the structure. During final stages of network preparation, computational design tools can be used to identify branch intersections with significant flow disruptions and iteratively optimize the branching angle to correct them (see Sections 9.2.8 and 9.2.9).

9.2.8 Boundary Layer Profile at Intersections

Another important fluidic consideration for biomimetic vascular design is the profile of the boundary layer at branch intersections. The boundary layer of blood flow within a vascular conduit is the region in which the magnitude of velocity varies in the radial direction for a given cross section. This phenomenon is the result of viscous forces that dominate in Laminar flow, and the no-slip condition of the lumen wall. The speed of the fluid at the wall is defined to be zero, and at the center of the vessel the blood is flowing at a maximum velocity. The region in between these locations is the boundary layer, and is where variations in velocity occur.

A physiologic boundary layer profile is symmetric about the axis of flow. However, branched intersections are at high risk for disturbances to the boundary layer, which can lead to platelet activation (Dewey, 2002). Numerical studies have shown that large branching angles correlate with a high probability of boundary layer separation and flow reversal (Tadjfar, 2004), adverse situations that promote thrombosis formation and cause large fluctuations in shear stress. Several studies have identified a strong correlation between regions of large shear variation and regions at high risk for atherosclerosis (DePaola et al., 1992; Nagel et al., 1999).

In practice, branched intersections with a non-uniform boundary layer profile can corrected using an iterative approach (Hoganson et al., 2011). The primary parameters affecting boundary layer distribution are the fillets at the inner and outer intersection points. Using numerical methods, these fillet values can be adjusted until uniform flow profiles are achieved.

9.2.9 Computational Design Tools

The biomimetic design principles described here can be synthesized to create vascular architectures that recapitulate organ functions. For small-scale networks, these parameters can be easily incorporated into the design. However, for large-scale constructs, such as whole-organ vasculature, the many mass transport and fluid flow relationships can become quite complex. Computational Fluid Dynamics (CFD) is a powerful numerical analysis tool that can be used to drive the design of large, intricate networks. Numerical results can be used in an iterative approach to change vessel parameters incrementally until optimal biomimetic flow is achieved. CFD packages such as FloWorks (SolidWorks Corp., Concord, MA) and Fluent (Ansys Inc., Canonsburg, PA) interface with modeling software that allow full control of vessel dimensions. This iterative CFD approach has been widely used to design and analyze biomimetic microvascular devices (Lim et al., 2003; Hoganson et al., 2010, 2011).

An alternative approach to network design utilizes mathematical algorithms to generate vascular networks computationally based on a defined set of parameters. These algorithms, known as Lindenmayer systems (L-systems) were originally created in the 1960s to model the development of the branched topology in plants (Prusinkiewicz and Lindenmayer, 1996). Since then, L-systems have been applied to a variety of scenarios including linguistics, computer graphics, microfluidic heat sinks (Kobayashi, 2010). To generate a vascular network, the production rules of an L-system are defined based on the biomimetic design parameters and spatial limitations. Vascular geometry is then created based on a recursive algorithm that accounts for the production rules at each step. An adaptation of this approach has been shown to mimic the structure and variability of native vascular architecture (Zamir, 2001). A three-dimensional biomimetic vascular network was also designed and fabricated using an L-system approach (Yasar et al., 2009). The recursive approach has strong potential to generate complex, biomimetic designs, but further work is needed to fully understand and specify parameters that govern variability within the cardiovascular system (Zamir, 2001).

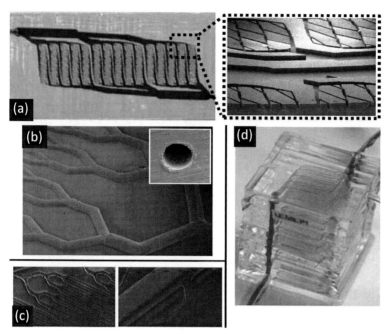

Figure 9.6 (a) Microfluidic network created using traditional photolithography (Carraro et al., 2008). All channels have the same depth regardless of width, resulting in high aspect ratios at the smallest channels. (b) A positive mold for hot embossing fabricated using patterned gap electroplating (Borenstein et al., 2010). Vessel height decreases with the width, resulting in a constant uniform aspect ratio. The embossed polystyrene sheets were sealed together, creating enclosed circular channels. (c) A biomimetic lung architecture created with micromilling technology (Hoganson et al., 2011). The five-axis mill control is capable of maintaining a uniform aspect ratio, as well as machining three-dimensional contours and fillets at bifurcation points. (d) Example of microfluidic networks assembled in a stacked configuration to increase functional capacity (Kniazeva et al., 2011).

9.3 Microfabrication Technologies

In 1959, the physicist Richard Feynman delivered a talk titled "There's Plenty of Room at the Bottom," in which he discussed the concept miniaturizing machines to perform tasks at the micro and nanoscale level (Feynman, 1960). Interestingly, he mused that "small machines might be permanently incorporated in the body to assist some inadequately functioning organ." In the following decades, micro and nanotechnologies were developed for a wide variety of applications, including miniaturized gas chromatography devices (Terry et al., 1979), high resolution microscopy (Giessibl, 2003), and integrated circuit components (van Lintel et al., 1988). Later, these technologies were adapted to create fluidic "lab on a chip" devices, eventually leading to the emergence of cell-based microfluidics (Manz et al., 1990). Microfabrication technologies have been successfully employed to study tumor cell migration (Polacheck et al., 2011), measure cellular density (Grover et al., 2011), and identify genetic disorders (Fan et al., 2009). Tissue-engineered scaffolds have also been fabricated using the same fabrication methods, reminiscent of Feynman's concept for miniaturized implantable machines. Although many different fabrication strategies have been employed, only certain approaches are capable of producing vascular structures that comply with the biomimetic principles discussed previously. These biomimetic fabrication technologies can be grouped into four broad categories: Micromolding, Direct Fabrication, Sacrificial Molding, and Bioprinting. This section reviews studies that have used microfabrication technologies to incorporate one or more biomimetic design principles.

9.3.1 Micromolding

Micromolding strategies have been utilized to create microfluidic devices since the 1970s (Aumiller et al., 1974), and have been increasingly adapted for biological research since the turn of the century (Berthier et al., 2012). The fabrication of a microfluidic device using this approach is accomplished in three stages. In the first stage, the desired microchannel geometry is fabricated as a positive feature pattern on a master substrate. In the second stage, the pattern of the master mold is transferred to a scaffold material. A variety of materials have been incorporated into this strategy, including PDMS (Duffy et al., 1998; Lee et al., 2003; Wu and Hjort, 2009), polystyrene, collagen (Liu et al., 2011), and a range of biodegradable polymers (Liu et al., 2012). The final stage of fabrication involves the assembly of the patterned secondary substrate into an enclosed microfluidic device. Devices can be combined in multiple layers to increase functional capacity (Marentis et al., 2009; Kniazeva et al., 2011). The resolution of vascular networks in micromolded devices is dependent upon the capabilities of the technology used to fabricate the master patterned substrate.

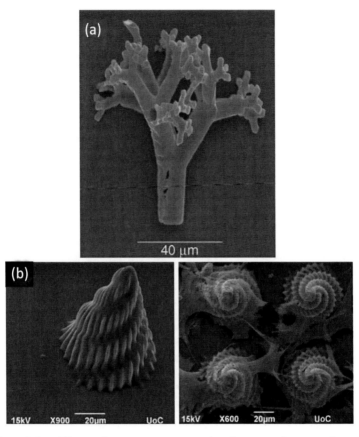

Figure 9.7 Microscale structures created using two-photon polymerization (2PP). (a) A vascular tree-like structure was printed with micron-level resolution (Osvianikov et al., (2007). (b) Sea-shell structures created by 2PP, highlighting the arbitrary three-dimensional control of the technology (Melissinaki et al., 2011). The biocompatible structures were used to support neuronal growth.

Photolithography is one of the most widely used techniques for fabricating micropatterned molds (Berthier et al., 2012). Originally developed for the semiconductor industry (Terry et al., 1979), this process is capable of resolutions on the order of 100 nm, much smaller than the minimum feature size for biomimetic vascular designs (Whitesides et al., 2001). As early as 2000, photoli-thography has been used to create molds for vascular networks with physiologic shear stresses (Kaihara et al., 2000). These early networks supported endothelial cell growth in scaffolds made from PDMS (Shin et al., 2004) and PGS, a biodegradable elastomer (Fidkowski et al., 2005), and were later adapted for in vitro and in vivo hepatocyte growth (Carraro et al., 2008; Hsu et al., 2010). Despite the high resolution of the photolithography process, certain limitations prevent adherence to biomimetic design principles. For example, in a biomimetic lung network, channel size may range from 100–3000 µm (Hoganson et al., 2011). However, standard photolithography methods are only capable of patterns with uniform height, resulting in channels without a uniform aspect ratio (see Section 9.2.4). Depth variation can be achieved with specialized techniques (Lai et al., 2013), but channel contours at intersections cannot be controlled, resulting in regions prone to boundary layer disturbances and flow separation (see Section 9.2.8). Due to these limitations, researchers have sought improved methods to fabricate micropatterned molds.

Micropatterned molds with three-dimensional features can be fabricated using specialized fabrication techniques. A generalized bifurcating vascular network (minimum diameter = 200 µm) was created using a patterned-gap electroplating process (Borenstein et al., 2010). The resulting copper molds were used to hot-emboss the microchannel features into polystyrene sheets, which were then bonded to create enclosed circular channels. The device supported endothelial cell growth into confluent monolayers. This fabrication method is capable of 1:1 channel aspect ratios and smoothed intersection contours, an improvement over standard photolithographic methods. However, the 3D geometry is dependent upon the growth rate and isotropic expansion of copper during the electroplating process, and cannot be directly controlled.

Electron discharge machining (EDM) was used to create a biomimetic network to model the liver sinusoid (Hoganson et al., 2010). Layered PDMS devices with the radial liver deign (minimum diameter = 267 µm) were constructed from the resulting stainless steel molds using soft lithography techniques. Flow behavior was verified by in vitro testing with whole blood and comparison to computational fluid dynamics analysis. Although the EDM fabricated mold had 1:1 channel aspect ratios and smoothed intersection contours, the positioning accuracy was 5–10 µm, which is substantially less than photolithography. Furthermore, the surface finish was very rough, which could have an adverse affect on blood flow.

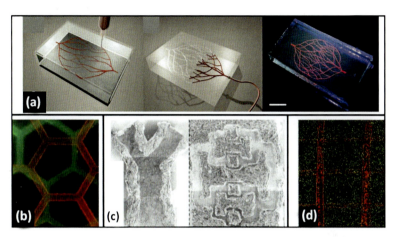

Figure 9.8 Biomimetic vascular scaffolds created using sacrificial molding strategies. (a) Omnidirectional printing of a fugitive ink within a gel reservoir (Wu et al., 2011). After the ink is deposited (left panel), the gel matrix is photochemically cross-linked. The ink is then removed via vacuum (center panel), resulting in an enclosed vascular network with three-dimensional geometry. (b) Multiplanar vascular structures within a collagen gel (Golden and Tien, 2007). The network design was fabricated in gelatin, encapsulated within the collagen gel, and subsequently flushed to leave an enclosed network. (c) Vascular structures within a collagen scaffold created using a sacrificial mold (Sachlos et al., 2003). First, the mold was fabricated using 3D printing technology. Collagen was cast in the mold cavity, and then the mold material was removed in an ethanol bath, leaving the collagen scaffold with internal channels. (d) Endothelial cells seeded within channels of a fibrin gel, created by dissolving patterned carbohydrate glass within the scaffold material (Miller et al., 2012).

High feature resolution and three-dimensional contour control of micropatterned features can be created using micromilling (Dornfeld et al., 2006). Positioning accuracies of 1 µm can be achieved, with tool diameters as small as 25 µm. This technology was used to create a biomimetic lung network (Hoganson et al., 2011). A three axis micromilling machine (Microlution Inc, Chicago, IL) was used to create the positive feature substrate (minimum diameter = 100 µm) with 1:1 channel aspect ratios and smooth intersection contours. The high accuracy and precision of the micromilling approach resulted in a high fidelity mold, with a relative difference of 0.6% from the original design. The three-dimensional control afforded by this technique is superior to photolithography, patterned-gap electroplating, and EDM. As this technology is developed and becomes more widely available, it will be an attractive option for micropatterning applications.

Micromolding techniques are capable of producing microfluidic devices with biomimetic vascular networks. Micromolding has been successfully utilized by several research groups to validate proof-of-concept designs for biomimetic networks.

9.3.2 Direct Fabrication

Arbitrary dimensional control of biomimetic vascular networks can be achieved through direct fabrication strategies. In this approach, the internal microchannel geometries are built within a scaffold structure without the need for secondary patterning and assembly steps, as is required for micromolding. However, formation of patent channels within a scaffold material requires a high degree of accuracy and precision.

Layer-by-layer rapid prototyping techniques have been applied to direct fabrication of scaffolds containing internal vascular structures. Selective laser sintering (SLS) uses a laser beam to selectively fuse small particles into a three-dimensional shape, and is capable of accuracy on the order of 100 µm. A bifurcating microchannel perfusion scaffold (minimum diameter = 1 mm) was created using SLS with poly(η-caprolactote) particles (Niino et al., 2011). The particles were combined with a NaCl porogen, resulting in a matrix with porosity of 89%. Hepatocytes cultured within the vascular scaffold demonstrated improved growth and function compared to those grown in avascular scaffolds (Huang et al., 2007). Other rapid prototyping processes have greater dimensional accuracy and smaller channel sizes. Stereolithography (SLA) uses a laser beam to selectively cure a vat of resin, and can achieve parts with three-dimensional accuracy up to 20 µm (Melchels et al.,

2010). Biodegradable SLA resins have been developed with a variety of mechanical properties, could be used to fabricate scaffolds with internal biomimetic vascular channels (Cooke et al., 2003; Elomaa et al., 2011; Sharifi et al., 2012). Projection SLA was used to create computationally derived biomimetic designs in a poly(ethylene glycol)-diacrylate (PEGDA) hydrogel with a feature size of 50 μm (Yasar et al., 2009).

Direct fabrication of scaffolds with feature sizes less than 100 nm can be achieved with two photon polymerization (2PP) methods (Ovsianikov and Chichkov, 2012). As the name implies, two femtosecond focused laser pulses are applied to a liquid solution containing monomers and photosensitizers. Polymerization occurs only in a narrow region of multiphoton absorption, allowing for full three-dimensional control of features (Raimondi et al., 2012). The volumetric resolution of this process is proportional to the cube of the laser wavelength (Cumpston et al., 1999), and the polymerization rate is proportional to the square of laser intensity (Lee et al., 2006). 2PP was used to create a biomimetic scaffold for neural tissue engineering that incorporated microchannels to direct axon growth (Melissinaki et al., 2011). Other applications have utilized biodegradable resins to create mesh scaffold structures, including enclosed microchannels with a width of 100 μm (Zhou et al., 2002; Claeyssens et al., 2009; Osvianikov et al., 2011; Koskela et al., 2012).

9.3.3 Sacrificial Molding

Sacrificial molding strategies are capable of producing arbitrarily complex microchannels within a matrix structure. A vascular structure is fabricated and then encapsulated within a scaffold material. The vascular structure is then sacrificed, leaving a hollow microfluidic architecture within the scaffold material that can be seeded with cells and support flow. Sacrificial methods exploit differences in the chemical and/or physical properties of the vascular structure and encapsulating materials. The conditions of the sacrificial technique are important to consider; the process of removing the sacrificial material must not impair the remaining scaffold structure. For example, Reed et al. embedded polycarbonate microstructures within various encapsulate materials including glass, a thermoplastic polymer, and a thermoset polymer (Reed et al., 2001). The polycarbonate was then decomposed by increasing the temperature up to 300°C. Although this approach yielded high-fidelity microchannels, the temperature conditions are not suitable for biocompatible polymers.

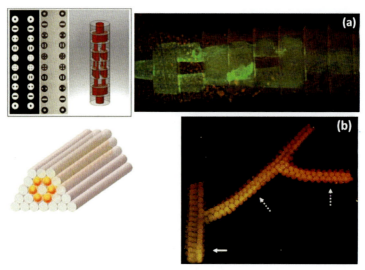

Figure 9.9   Scaffolds created using directed-assembly and bioprinting strategies. (a) Self-assembled hydrogel structure containing vascular channels (Du et al., 2011) (b) A bioprinting approach (left panel) based on the deposition of agarose rods and multicellular spheroids (Norotte et al., 2009). Using this method, a branched structure was produced (right panel) with diameters of 1.2 mm (solid arrow) and 0.9 mm (dashed arrows).

Chemical sacrificial conditions are more appropriate for many scaffold biomaterials. For example, phosphate-based glass fibers between 10 and 50 μm were fabricated and embedded in collagen construct. The fibers were then simply dissolved in deionized water to create patent internal channels (Nazhat et al., 2007). A similar approach was taken by Golden and colleagues. First, a simple branching microfluidic network was fabricated out of gelatin using traditional soft lithography techniques. This structure was then encapsulated within a hydrogel comprised of type I collagen, fibrinogen, and Matrigel. After polymerization of the hydrogel, the branched gelatin matrix was "sacrificed" by flushing with PBS. Endothelial cells were then seeded into the resulting microfluidic scaffold and assembled into a confluent monolayer along the channel walls (Golden and Tien, 2007). This approach yielded a patent internal microvascular structure, but was limited by the 2D constraints of the soft lithography technique used to create the branched gelatin structure.

Three-dimensional internal microchannels were created by Wu and colleagues using an omnidirectional printing method (Wu et al., 2011). A fugitive ink was deposited into a photocurable gel reservoir using a nozzle capable of translation in three dimensions. The gel holds the ink in place as arbitrary patterns are written by the syringe. When the gel is photochemically cross-linked, the ink remains liquid and is removed by vacuum, leaving an intrinsic microvascular structure. This approach is capable of three-dimensional and biomimetic architecture with a minimum vessel diameter of 18 μm. Ideally, these same techniques could be utilized with a biodegradable hydrogel material capable of supporting cell growth for whole-organ regeneration.

Other groups have applied sacrificial molding techniques using natural and synthetic extracellular matrix (ECM) materials. A bifurcating vascular network was 3D printed out organic compounds, with a minimum vessel diameter of 200 μm. The network was then encased in a collagen dispersion and frozen. The vascular structure was removed by immersion in an ethanol bath, followed by a critical point drying process, yielding a collagen matrix with patent microvascular channels (Sachlos et al., 2003). Using a similar approach, hydroxyapatite was incorporated into the collagen mesh to create a vascularized scaffold for bone growth (Sachlos et al., 2006). Although cell culture was not attempted in these devices, collagen is known to be an excellent material to promote cell growth (Lynn et al., 2004).

Perfused cell culture was demonstrated in a microfluidic ECM scaffold manufactured with sacrificial molding techniques. Rigid microscale networks were created using an optically clear, cytocompatible carbohydrate glass (Miller et al., 2012). These networks were then successfully encapsulated within five different ECM materials. After the ECM material was set, the carbohydrate glass was dissolved by immersion in an aqueous solution, resulting in a patent microchannel network. Endothelial cells seeded into the structure formed a confluent monolayer throughout the channels. Another structure fabricated in this manner was able to support high-density growth of primary rat hepatocytes. The carbohydrate glass sacrificial lattice was 3D printed using a nozzle extrusion technique and produced channel diameters ranging from 150 µm to 1 mm. However, a similar extrusion method was used to create a fractal branching network in a PLGA matrix with channel diameters as small as 16 µm (Vozzi et al., 2004), suggesting that the channel resolution of this approach can be increased.

9.3.4 Self-assembly and Bioprinting

Tissue engineering strategies typically incorporate a porous scaffold as a matrix to support cellular growth. Tissues with complex architecture and composition often require similarly complex scaffolds in order to recapitulate the target function. Recently, self-assembly and bioprinting methods have emerged as strategies for direct fabrication of tissues using cellular materials, precluding the need for a scaffold structure (Chung et al., 2012; Marga et al., 2012). Cells encapsulated in a hydrogel or ink medium are deposited in guided patterns, which then assemble into free-standing tissue structures. These approaches have been employed to create constructs that incorporate biomimetic vascular architecture.

Vascular microchannels were fabricated in cell-laden PEGDA (poly(ethylene glycol)-diacrylate) hydrogels by Du and colleagues using a modular directed-assembly approach (Du et al., 2011). Repeating annular units (300 µm thick) of the hydrogels were aligned and photochemically cross-linked. Internal channels remained patent, with diameters of 250 µm. Cellular viability was demonstrated with constructs containing concentric rings of endothelial cells and smooth muscle cells. Branching patterns can be achieved by changing the internal geometry of individual repeating units.

Another group patterned single cells into a capillary network using a laser guided direct writing (LGDW) approach (Nahmias et al., 2005). Cells were contained within a weakly focused laser beam and deposited with micrometer accuracy in arbitrary patterns within a Matrigel substrate. Human umbilical vein endothelial cells (HUVECs) were deposited in radial structures to mimic the liver sinusoid. The HUVECs assembled into tubular conformations and were combined with hepatocytes to create biomimetic co-cultures that tested positive for albumin production.

Small diameter vascular tubes were created by Norotte et al. using bioprinting technology (Norotte et al., 2009). Multicellular cylinders were extruded into a bioink material. The cylindrical bioink was then deposited in conjunction with agarose rods to form tubular structures. The agarose acts as a mold to support the vessel and maintain patency during cellular maturation and assembly. Using this approach, vessels with diameters ranging from 0.9 to 2.5 mm were fabricated. Simple branched structures with varying diameters were also created using this approach.

References

Allen, J., Khetani, S., and Bhatia, S. (2005). In vitro zonation and toxicity in a hepatocyte bioreactor, *Toxicol. Sci.* **84**, 1, 110–119.

Aumiller, G., Chandros, E., Tomlinson, W., and Weber, H. (1974). Submicrometer resolution replication of relief patterns for integrated optics, *J. Appl. Phys.* **45**, 10, 4557–4562.

Baskurt, O., and Meiselman, H. (2003). Blood rheology and hemodynamics, *Semin. Thromb. Hemost.* **29**, 5, 435–450.

Bassett, E. K., Hoganson, D. M., Lo, J. H., Penson, E. J., and Vacanti, J. P. (2011). Influence of vascular network design on gas transfer in lung assist device technology, *ASAIO J.* **57**, 6, 533–538.

Berthier, E., Young, E. W. K., and Beebe, D. (2012). Engineers are from pdms-land, biologists are from polystyrenia, *Lab Chip* **12**, 7, 1224–1137.

Borenstein, J. T., Tupper, M. M., Mack, P. J., Weinberg, E. J., Khalil, A. S., Hsiao, J., and García-Cardenã, G. (2010). Functional endothelialized microvascular networks with circular cross-sections in a tissue-culture substrate, *Biomed. Microdevices* **12**, 1, 71–79.

Buijs, J. O. D., Bajzer, Z., and Ritman, E. L. (2006). Branching morphology of the rat hepatic portal vein tree: a micro-CT study, *Ann. Biomed. Eng.* **34**, 9, 1420–1428.

Caro, C., Fitz-Gerald, J., and Schroter, R. (1971). Atheroma and arterial wall shear observation, correlation, and proposal of shear dependent mass transfer mechanism for atherogenesis, *Proc. R. Soc. Lond. B Biol. Sci.* **177**, 1046, 109–159.

Carraro, A., Hsu, W.-M., Kulig, K. M., Cheung, W. S., Miller, M. L., Weinberg, E. J., Swart, E. F., Kaazempur-Mofrad, M., Borenstein, J. T., Vacanti, J. P., and Neville, C. (2008). In vitro analysis of a hepatic device with intrinsic microvascular-based channels, *Biomed. Microdevices* **10**, 6, 795–805.

Chow, D., Wenning, L., Miller, W., and Papoutsakis, E. (2001a). Modeling pO_2 distributions in the bone marrow hematopoietic compartment. I. Krogh's model, *Biophys. J.* **81**, 675–684.

Chow, D., Wenning, L., Miller, W., and Papoutsakis, E. (2001b). Modeling pO_2 distributions in the bone marrow hematopoietic compartment. II. Modified Kroghian models, *Biophys. J.* **81**, 685–696.

Cho, W. K., Ankrum, J. A., Guo, D., Chester, S. A., Yang, S. Y., Kashyap, A., Campbell, G. A., Wood, R. J., Rijal, R. K., Karnik, R., Langer, R., and Karp, J. M. (2012). *Proc. Natl. Acad. Sci.* **109**, 52, 21289–21294.

Chung, B., Lee, K., Khademhosseini, A., and Lee, S. (2012). Microfluidic fabrication of microengineered hydrogels and their application in tissue engineering, *Lab Chip* **12**, 1, 45–59.

Claeyssens, F., Hasan, E. A., Gaidukeviciute, A., Achilleos, D. S., Ranella, A., Reinhardt, C., Ovsianikov, A., Shizhou, X., Fotakis, C., Vamvakaki, M., Chichkov, B. N., and Farsari, M. (2009). Three-dimensional biodegradable structures fabricated by two-photon polymerization, *Langmuir* **25**, 5, 3219–3223.

Collins, P., Nielsen, L., Patel, S., Papoutsakis, E., and Miller, W. (1998). Characterization of hematopoietic cell expansion, oxygen uptake, and glycolysis in a controlled, stirred-tank bioreactor system, *Biotechnol Prog.* **14**, 466–472.

Cooke, M. N., Fisher, J. P., Dean, D., Rimnac, C., and Mikos, A. G. (2003). Use of stereolithography to manufacture critical-sized 3D biodegradable scaffolds for bone ingrowth, *J. Biomed. Mater. Res. Part B: Appl. Biomater.* **64**, 2, 65–69.

Cumpston, B. H., Ananthavel, S. P., Barlow, S., Dyer, D. L., Ehrlich, J. E., Erskine, L. L., Heikal, A. A., Kuebler, S. M., Lee, I. Y. S., McCord-Maughon, D., Qin, J. Q., Röckel, H., Rumi, M., Wu X.-L., Marder, S. R. and Perry, J. W. (1999). Two-photon polymerization initiators for three-dimensional optical data storage and microfabrication, *Nature* **398**, 51–54.

DePaola, N., Gimbrone, Jr., M. A., Davies, P. F., and Dewey, Jr., C. F. (1992). Vascular endothelium responds to fluid shear stress gradients, *Arterioscler. Thromb.* **12**, 1254–1257.

Dewey, Jr., C. F. (2002). Haemodynamic flow: symmetry and synthesis, *Biorheology* **39**, 3–4, 541–549.

Dornfeld, D., Min, S., and Takeuchi, Y. (2006). Recent advances in mechanical micromachining, *CIRP Ann. Manuf. Technol.* **55**, 2, 745–768.

Du, Y., Ghodousi, M., Qi, H., Haas, N., Xiao, W., and Khademhosseini, A. (2011). Sequential assembly of cell-laden hydrogel constructs to engineer vascular-like microchannels, *Biotechnol. Bioeng.* **108**, 7, 1693–1703.

Duffy, D. C., McDonald, J. C., Schueller, O. J., and Whitesides, G. M. (1998). Rapid prototyping of microfluidic systems in poly(dimethylsiloxane), *Anal. Chem* **70**, 23, 4974–4984.

Elomaa, L., Teixeira, S., Hakala, R., Korhonen, H., Grijpma, D. W., and Seppälä, J. V. (2011). Preparation of poly(η-caprolactone)-based tissue engineering scaffolds by stereolithography, *Acta Biomater.* **7**, 11, 3850–3856.

Emerson, D. R., Ciéslicki, K., Gu, X., and Barber, R. W. (2006). Biomimetic design of microfluidic manifolds based on a generalized Murray's law, *Lab Chip* **6**, 447–454.

Ensley, A. E., Nerem, R. M., Anderson, D. E., Hanson, S. R., and Hinds, M. T. (2012). Fluid shear stress alters hemostatic properties of endothelial outgrowth cells, *Tissue Eng. Part A* **18**, 1–2, 127–136.

Esch, M. B., Post, D. J., Shuler, M. L., and Stokol, T. (2011). Characterization of in vitro endothelial linings grown within microfluidic channels, *Tissue Eng. Part A* **17**, 23–24, 2965–2971.

Fan, H., Blumfield, Y., El-Sayed, Y., Chueh, J., and Quake, S. (2009). Microfluidic digital pcr enables rapid prenatal diagnosis of fetal aneuploidy, *Am. J. Obstet. Gynecol.* **200**, 5, 543.e1–7.

Federspiel, W. J., and Henchir, K. A. (2004). *Lung, Artificial: Basic Principles and Current Applications* (Marcel Dekker, Inc.), pp. 910–921.

Federspiel, W. J., and Svitek, R. G. (2004). *Lung, Artificial: Current Research and Future Directions* (Marcel Dekker, Inc.), pp. 922–931.

Feynman, R. (1960). There's plenty of room at the bottom, *Eng. Sci.* **23**, 5, 22–36.

Fidkowski, C., Kaazempur-Mofrad, M. R., Borenstein, J., Vacanti, J. P., Langer, R., and Wang, Y. (2005). Endothelialized microvasculature baed on a biodegradable elastomer, *Tissue Eng.* **11**, 1–2, 302–309.

Gebhardt, R. (1992). Metabolic zonation of the liver: regulation and implications for liver function, *Pharmacol. Ther.* **53**, 275–354.

Giessibl, F. (2003). Advances in atomic force microscopy, *Rev. Mod. Phys.* **75**, 3, 949–983.

Golden, A. P., and Tien, J. (2007). Fabrication of microfluidic hydrogels using molded gelatin as a sacrificial element, *Lab Chip* **7**, 720–725.

Goldstein, M. J., Lubezky, N., Yushkov, Y., Bae, C., and Guarrera, J. V. (2012). Innovations in organ donation, *Mt. Sinai J. Med.* **79**, 3, 351–364.

Gómez, C., Galán, J., Torrero, V., Ferreiro, I., Pérez, D., Palao, R., Martínez, E., Llames, S., Meana, A., and Holguín, P. (2011). Use of an autologous bioengineered composite skin in extensive burns: clinical and functional outcomes. A multicentric study, *Burns* **37**, 580–589.

Grover, W., Bryan, A., Diez-Silva, M., Suresh, S., Higgins, J., and Manalis, S. (2011). Measuring single-cell density, *Proc. Natl. Acad. Sci.* **108**, 27, 10992–10996.

Hagland, M. (2012). Got velcro? Heading into 2013, the healthcare industry could use the ingenuity of inventors like George de Mestral, *Healthc. Inform.* **29**, 10, 6

Herschel, W. H., and Bulkley, R. (1926). Konsistenzmessungen von gummi-benzollosungen, *Kolloid Zeitschrift* **39**, 4, 291–300.

Hoganson, D. M., Pryor II, H. I., Bassett, E. K., Spool, I. D., and Vacanti, J. P. (2011). Lung assist device technology with physiologic blood flow developed on a tissue engineered scaffold platform, *Lab Chip* **11**, 700–707.

Hoganson, D. M., Pryor II, H. I., Spool, I. D., Burns, O. H., Gilmore, J. R., and Vacanti, J. P. (2010). Principles of biomimetic vascular network design applied to a tissue-engineered liver scaffold, *Tissue Eng. Part A* **16**, 5, 1469–1477.

Hsu, W.-M., Carraro, A., Kulig, K. M., Miller, M. L., Kaazempur-Mofrad, M., Weinberg, E., Entabi, F., Albadawi, H., Watkins, M. T., Borenstein, J. T., Vacanti, J. P., and Neville, C. (2010). Liver-assist device with a microfluidics-based vascular bed in an animal model, *Ann. Surg.* **252**, 351–357.

Huang, H., Oizumi, S., Kojima, N., Niino, T., and Sakai, Y. (2007). Avidin-biotin binding-based cell seeding and perfusion culture of liver-derived cells in a porous scaffold with a three-dimensional interconnected flow-channel network, *Biomaterials* **28**, 26, 3815–3823.

Huh, D., Hamilton, G. A., and Ingber, D. E. (2011). From 3D cell culture to organs-on-chips, *Trends Cell Biol.* **21**, 12, 745–754.

Huh, D., Matthews, B. D., Mammoto, A., Montoya-Zavala, M., Hsin, H. Y., and Ingber, D. E. (2010). Reconstituting organ-level functions on a chip, *Science* **328**, 1662–1668.

Huh, D., Suke Torisawa, Y., Hamilton, G. A., Kim, H. J., and Ingber, D. E. (2012). Microengineered physiological biomimicry: organs-on-chips, *Lab Chip* **12**, 2156–2164.

Inamdar, N. K., Griffith, L. G., and Borenstein, J. T. (2011). Transport and shear in a microfluidic membrane bilayer device for cell culture, *Biomicrofluidics* **5**, 022213.

Incropera, F. P., DeWitt, D. P., Bergman, T. L., and Lavine, A. S. (2007). *Fundamentals of Heat and Mass Transfer*, 6th edn. (John Wiley & Sons, Hoboken, NJ).

Ishaug-Riley, S., Crane-Kruger, G., Yaszemski, M., and Mikos, A. (1998). Three-dimensional culture of rat calavarial osteoblasts in porous biodegradable polymers, *Biomaterials* **19**, 1405–1412.

Jaklenec, A., Stamp, A., Deweerd, E., Sherwin, A., and Langer, R. (2012). Progress in the tissue engineering and stem cell industry. Are we there yet?, *Tissue Eng. Part B Rev.* **18**, 3, 155–166.

Jang, K.-J., and Suh, K.-Y. (2010). A multi-layer microfluidic device for efficient culture and analysis of renal tubular cells, *Lab Chip* **10**, 1, 36–42.

Kaihara, S., Borenstein, J., Koka, R., Lalan, S., Ochoa, E. R., Ravens, M., Pien, H., Cunningham, B., and Vacanti, J. P. (2000). Silicon micromachining to tissue engineer branched vascular channels for liver fabrication, *Tissue Eng.* **6**, 2, 105–117.

Kassab, G. S. (2006). Scaling laws of vascular trees: of form and function, *Am. J. Physiol. Heart Circ. Physiol.* **290**, H894–H903.

Kim, H. J., Huh, D., Hamilton, G., and Ingber, D. E. (2012). Human gut-on-a-chip inhabited by microbial flora that experiences intestinal peristalsis-like motions and flow, *Lab Chip* **12**, 2165–2174.

Kim, S. (2002). *A Study of Non-Newtonian Viscosity and Yield Stress of Blood in a Scanning Capillary-Tube Rheometer*, Ph.D. thesis, Drexel University, Philadelphia, PA, USA.

Kim, S., Spenko, M., Trujillo, S., Heyneman, B., Santos, D., and Cutkosky, M. R. (2008). Smooth vertical surface climbing with directional adhesion. *IEEE* **24**, 1, 65–74.

Kniazeva, T., Hsiao, J. C., Charest, J. L., and Borenstein, J. T. (2011). A microfluidic respiratory assist device with high gas permeance for artificial lung applications, *Biomed. Microdevices* **13**, 315–323.

Kobayashi, M. H. (2010). On a biologically inspired topology optimization method, *Commun. Nonlinear Sci. Numer. Simulat.* **15**, 3, 787–802.

Koskela, J. E., Turunen, S., Ylä-Outinen, L., Narkilahti, S., and Kellomäki, M. (2012). Two-photon microfabrication of poly(ethylene glycol) diacrylate and a novel biodegradable photopolymer–comparision of processability for biomedical applications, *Polym. Adv. Technol.* **23**, 6, 992–1001.

Kreuz, P. C., Muller, S. M., Ossendorf, C., Kaps, C., and Erggelet, C. (2009). Treatment of focal degenerative cartilage defects with polymer-based autologous chondrocyte grafts: four-year clinical results, *Arthritis Res. Ther.* **11**, 2, R33.

Kroll, M. H., Hellums, D. J., McIntire, L. V., Shafer, A. I., and Moake, J. L. (1996). Platelets and shear stress, *Blood* **88**, 5, 1525–1541.

Kunz-Schughart, L., Doetsch, J., Mueller-Klieser, W., and Groebe, K. (2000). Proliferative activity and tumorigenic conversion: impact on cellular metabolism in 3D culture, *Am. J. Physiol. Cell Physiol.* **278**, C765–C780.

Langer, R., and Vacanti, J. P. (1993). Tissue engineering, *Science* **260**, 920–926.

Lai, Y., Chen, J., Zhang, T., Gu, D., Zhang, C., Li, Z., Lin, S., Fu, X., and Schultze-Mosqau, S. (2013). Effect of 3D microgroove surface topography on plasma and cellular fibronectin of human gingival fibroblasts, *J. Dent.* **41**, 11, 1109–1121.

Lee, J. N., Park, C., and Whitesides, G. M. (2003). Solvent compatibility of poly(dimethylsiloxane)-based microfluidic devices, *Anal. Chem.* **75**, 23, 6544–6554.

Lee, K.-S., Yang, D.-Y., Park, S. H., and Kim, R. H. (2006). Recent developments in the use of two-photon polymerization in precise 2D and 3D microfabrications, *Polym. Adv. Technol.* **17**, 2, 72–82.

Lim, D., Kamotani, Y., Cho, B., Mazumder, J., and Takayama, S. (2003). Fabrication of microfluidic mixers and artificial vasculatures using a high-brightness diode-pumped Nd:YAG laser direct write method, *Lab Chip* **3**, 4, 318–323.

Liu, X., Holzwarth, J. M., and Ma, P. X. (2012). Functionalized synthetic biodegradable polymer scaffolds for tissue engineering, *Macromol. Biosci.* **12**, 7, 911–919.

Liu, Y., Markov, D. A., Wikswo, J. P., and McCawley, L. J. (2011). Microfabricated scaffold-guided endothelial morphogenesis in three-dimensional culture, *Biomed. Microdevices* **13**, 837–846.

Lynn, A., Yannas, I., and Bonfield, W. (2004). Antigenicity and immunogenicity of collagen, *J. Biomed. Mater. Res. B Appl. Biomater.* **71**, 343–354.

Malda, J., Klein, T. J., and Upton, Z. (2007). The roles of hypoxia in the in vitro engineering of tissues, *Tissue Eng.* **13**, 9, 2153–2162.

Malek, A. M., Alper, S. L., and Izumo, S. (1999). Hemodynamic shear stress and its role in atherosclerosis, *JAMA* **282**, 21, 2035–2042.

Manz, A., Graber, N., and Widmer, H. (1990). Miniaturized total chemical analysis systems: a novel concept for chemical sensing, *Sens. Actuators* **1**, 1–6, 244–248.

Marentis, T. C., Vacanti, J. P., Hsiao, J. C., and Borenstein, J. T. (2009). Elastic averaging for assembly of three-dimensional constructs from elastomeric micromolded layers, *J. Microelectromechanical. Syst.* **18**, 3, 531–538.

Marga, F., Jakab, K., Khatiwala, C., Shepherd, B., Dorfman, S., Hubbard, B., Colbert, S., and Gabor, F. (2012). Toward engineering functional organ modules by additive manufacturing, *Biofabrication* **4**, 2, 022001.

McAllister, T. N., Marusewski, M., Garrido, S. A., Wystrychowski, W., Dusserre, N., Marini, A., Zagalski, K., Fiorillo, A., Avila, H., Manglano, X., Antonelli, J., Kotcher, A., Zembala, M., Cierpka, L., de la Fuente, L. M., and L'Heureux, N. (2009). Effectiveness of haemodialysis access with an autologous tissue-engineered vascular graft: a multicentre study, *Lancet* **373**, 1440–1446.

Melchels, F. P., Feijen, J., and Grijpma, D. W. (2010). A review on stereolithography and its applications in biomedical engineering, *Biomaterials* **31**, 24, 6121–6130.

Melissinaki, V., Gill, A. A., Ortega, I., Vamvakaki, M., Ranella, A., Haycock, J., Fotakis, C., Farsari, M., and Claeyssens, F. (2011). Direct laser writing of 3D scaffolds for neural tissue engineering applications, *Biofabrication* **3**, 4, 045005.

Miller, J. S., Stevens, K. R., Yang, M. T., Baker, B. M., Nguyen, D. H. T., Cohen, D. M., Toro, E., Chen, A. A., Gaile, P. A., Yu, X., Chaturvedi, R., Bhatia, S. N., and Chen, C. S. (2012). Rapid casting of patterned vascular networks for perfusable engineered three-dimensional tissues, *Nat. Mater.* **11**, 9, 768–774.

Milnor, W. (1989). *Hemodynamics* (Williams & Wilkins, Baltimore).

Moran, E., Baptista, P., Evans, D., Soker, S., and Sparks, J. (2012). Evaluation of parenchymal fluid pressure in native and decellularized liver tissue, *Biomed. Sci. Instrum.* **48**, 303–309.

Murray, C. D. (1926). The physiological principle of minimum work. I. the vascular system and the cost of blood volume, *Proc. Natl. Acad. Sci.* **12**, 207–214.

Muschler, G. F., Nakamoto, C., and Griffith, L. G. (2004). Engineering principles of clinical cell-based tissue engineering, *J. Bone Joint Surg. Am.* **86-A**, 7, 1541–1558.

Nagel, T., Resnick, N., Dewey, Jr., C., and Gimbrone, Jr., M. (1999). Vascular endothelial cells respond to spatial gradients in fluid shear stress by enhanced activation of transcription factors, *Arterioscler. Thromb. Vasc. Biol.* **19**, 8, 1825–1834.

Nahmias, Y., Schwartz, R. E., Verfaillie, C. M., and Odde, D. J. (2005). Laser-guided direct writing for three-dimensional tissue engineering, *Biotechnol. Bioeng.* **92**, 2, 129–136.

Nazhat, S. N., Neel, E. A. A., Kidane, A., Ahmed, I., Hope, C., Kershaw, M., Lee, P. D., Stride, E., Saffari, N., Knowles, J. C., and Brown, R. A. (2007). Controlled microchannelling in dense collagen scaffolds by soluble phosphate glass fibers, *Biomacromolecules* **8**, 2, 543–551.

Neinhuis, C., and Barthlott, W. (1997). Characterization and distribution of water-repellent, self-cleaning plant surfaces, *Ann. Bot.* **79**, 6, 667–677.

Niino, T., Hamajima, D., Montagne, K., Oizumi, S., Naruke, H., Huang, H., Sakai, Y., Kinoshita, H., and Fujii, T. (2011). Laser sintering fabrication of three-dimensional tissue engineering scaffolds with a flow channel network, *Biofabrication* **3**, 3, 034104.

Norotte, C., Marga, F., Niklason, L., and Forgacs, G. (2009). Scaffold-free vascular tissue engineering using bioprinting, *Biomaterials* **30**, 30, 5910–5917.

Ojo, A. O., Heinrichs, D., Emond, J. C., McGowan, J. J., Guidinger, M. K., Delmonico, F. L., and Metzger, R. A. (2004). Organ donation and utilization in the USA, *Am. J. Transplant.* **4**, Suppl. 9, 27–37.

Organ Procurement and Transplantation Network (Accessed May 2012). National data reports, http://optn.transplant.hrsa.gov/data.

Osvianikov, A., Deiwick, A., Van Vlierberghe, S., Dubruel, P., Mölloer, L., Dräger, G., and Chichkov, B. (2011). Laser fabrication of three-dimensional CAD scaffolds from photosensitive gelatin for applications in tissue engineering, *Biomacromolecules* 12, 851–858.

Osvianikov, A., Schlie, S., Ngezahayo, A., Haverich, A., and Chichkov, B. (2007). Two-photon polymerization technique for microfabrication of CAD-designed 3D scaffolds from commercially available photosensitive materials, *J. Tissue Eng. Regen. Med.* **1**, 6, 443–449.

Ovsianikov, A., and Chichkov, B. N. (2012). Three-dimensional microfabrication by two-photon polymerization technique, *Methods Mol. Biol.* **868**, 311–325.

Pavlakis, M., and Hanto, D. W. (2012). Clinical pathways in transplantation: a review and examples from Beth Israel Deaconess Medical Center, *Clin. Transplant.* **26**, 382–386.

Perera, M. T. P., and Bramhall, S. R. (2011). Current status and recent advances of liver transplantation from donation after cardiac death, *World J. Gastrointest. Surg.* **3**, 11, 167–176.

Pimpin, A., and Srituravanich, W. (2012). Review on micro- and nano-lithography techniques and their applications, *Eng. J.* **16**, 1, 37–55.

Polacheck, W., Charest, J., and Kamm, R. (2011). Interstitial flow influences direction of tumor cell migration through competing mechanisms, *Proc. Natl. Acad. Sci.* **108**, 27, 11115–111120.

Prusinkiewicz, P., and Lindenmayer, A. (1996). *The Algorithmic Beauty of Plants* (Springer-Verlag, New York), http:// algorithmicbotany.org/papers/abop/abop.pdf.

Raimondi, M. T., Eaton, S. M., Nava, M. M., Laganá, M., Cerullo, G., and Osellame, R. (2012). Two-photon laser polymerization: from fundamentals to biomedical application in tissue engineering and regenerative medicine. *J. Appl. Biomater. Biomech.* **4**, 1, 55–65.

Rani, U., and Bains, G. (1986). Flow behaviour of tomato ketchups, *Texture Stud.* **18**, 2, 125–135.

Reed, H. A., White, C. E., Rao, V., Bidstrup Allen, S. A., Henderson, C. L., and Kohl, P. A. (2001). Fabrication of microchannels using polycarbonates as sacrificial materials, *J. Micromech. Microeng.* **11**, 6, 733–737.

Sachlos, E., Gotora, D., and Czernuszka, J. T. (2006). Collagen scaffolds reinforced with biomimetic composite nano-sized carbonate-substituted hydroxyapatite crystals and shaped by rapid proto-typing to contain internal microchannels, *Tissue Eng.* **12**, 9, 2479–2487.

Sachlos, E., Reis, N., Ainsley, C., Derby, B., and Czernuszka, J. (2003). Novel collagen scaffolds with predefined internal morphology made by solid free form fabrication, *Biomaterials* **24**, 8, 1487–2003.

Shah, R., and London, A. (1978). *Laminar Flow Forced Convection in Ducts: a Source Book for Compact Heat Exchanger Analytical Data* (Academic Press, New York).

Sharifi, S., Blanquer, S. B. G., van Kooten, T. G., and Grijpma, D. W. (2012). Biodegradable nanocomposite hydrogel structures with enhanced mechanical properties prepared by photo-crosslinking solutions of poly(trimethylene carbonate)-poly(ethylene glycol)-poly(trimethylene carbonate) macromonomers and nanoclay particles, *Acta Biomater.* **8**, 12, 4233–4243.

Sherman, T. F. (1981). On connecting large vessels to small. The meaning of Murray's Law, *J. Gen. Physiol.* **78**, 431–453.

Shin, M., Matsuda, K., Ishii, O., Terai, H., Kaazempur-Mofrad, M., Borenstein, J., Detmar, M., and Vacanti, J. P. (2004). Endothelialized networks with a vascular geometry in microfabricated poly(dimethyl siloxane), *Biomed. Microdevices* **6**, 4, 269–278.

Smith, M. K., and Mooney, D. J. (2007). Hypoxia leads to necrotic hepatocyte death, *J. Biomed. Mater. Res. A* **80A**, 520–529.

Sung, J. H., Yu, J., Luo, D., Shuler, M. L., and March, J. C. (2011). Microscale 3D hydrogel scaffold for biomimetic gastrointestinal GI tract model, *Lab Chip* **11**, 3, 389–392.

Suzuki, K., Bonner-Weir, S., Hollister-Lock, J., Colton, C., and Weir, G. (1998). Number and volume of islets transplanted in immunobarrier devices, *Cell Transplant.* **7**, 47–52.

Tadjfar, M. (2004). Branch angle and flow into a symmetric bifurcation, *J. Biomech. Eng.* **126**, 4, 516–518.

Terry, S., Jerman, J., and Angell, J. (1979). A gas chromatographic air analyzer fabricated on a silicon wafer, *IEEE Trans. Electron. Devices* **26**, 12, 1880–1886.

Vacanti, J. P., Morse, M. A., Saltzman, W. M., Domb, A. J., Perez-Atayde, A., and Langer, R. (1988). Selective cell transplantation using bioabsorbable artificial polymers as matrices, *J. Pediatr. Surg.* **23**, 1, 3–9.

Valencia, A., Morales, H., Rivera, R., Bravo, E., and Galvez, M. (2008). Blood flow dynamics in patient-specific cerebral aneurysm models: the relationship between wall shear stress and aneurysm area index, *Med. Eng. Phys.* **30**, 329–340.

van Lintel, H., van De Pol, F., and Bouwstra, S. (1988). A piezoelectric micropump based on micromachining of silicon, *Sens. Actuators* **15**, 2, 153–167.

Vozzi, G., Previti, A., Ciaravella, G., and Ahluwalia, A. (2004). Microfabricated fractal branching networks, *J. Biomed. Mater. Res. A* **71**, 2, 326–333.

Wells, R. E., and Merrill, E. W. (1961). Shear rate dependance of the viscosity of whole blood and plasma, *Science* **133**, 3455, 763–764.

West, G. B., Brown, J. H., and Enquist, B. J. (1997). A general model for teh origin of allometric scaling laws in biology, *Science* **276**, 122–126.

White, F. M. (2008). *Fluid Mechanics*, 6th ed. (McGraw-Hill, New York).

Whitesides, G. M., Ostuni, E., Takayama, S., Jiang, X., and Ingber, D. E. (2001). Soft lithography in biology and biochemistry, *Annu. Rev. Biomed. Eng.* **3**, 335–373.

Wootton, D. M., and Ku, D. N. (1999). Fluid mechanics of vascular systems, diseases, and thrombosis, *Annu. Rev. Biomed. Eng.* **01**, 299–329.

Wu, W., DeConinck, A., and Lewis, J. A. (2011). Omnidirectional printing of 3D microvascular networks, *Adv. Mater* **23**, 24, H178–H183.

Wu, Z., and Hjort, K. (2009). Surface modification of pdms by gradient-induced migration of embedded Pluronic, *Lab Chip* **9**, 1500–1503.

Yasar, O., Lan, S.-F., and Starly, B. (2009). A Lindenmayer system-based approach for the design of nutrient delivery networks in tissue constructs, *Biofabrication* **1**, 4, 045004.

Zamir, M. (1976a). Optimality principles in arterial branching, *J. Theor. Biol.* **62**, 1, 227–251.

Zamir, M. (1976b). The role of shear forces in arterial branching, *J. Gen. Physiol.* **67**, 213–222.

Zamir, M. (1999). On fractal properties of arterial trees, *J. Theor. Biol.* **197**, 517–526.

Zamir, M. (2001). Arterial branching within the confines of fractal L-system formalism, *J. Gen. Physiol.* **118**, 3, 267–276.

Zamir, M., and Brown, N. (1982). Arterial branching in various parts of the cardiovascular system, *Am. J. Anat.* **163**, 4, 295–307.

Zamir, M., and Medeiros, J. (1982). Arterial branching in man and monkey, *J. Gen. Physiol.* **79**, 3, 353–360.

Zamir, M., Sinclair, P., and Wonnacott, T. (1992). Relation between diameter and flow in major branches of the arch of the aorta, *J. Biomech.* **25**, 11, 1303–1310.

Zhou, W., Kuebler, S. M., Braun, K. L., Yu, T., Cammack, J. K., Ober, C. K., Perry, J. W., and Marder, S. R. (2002). An efficient two-photon-generated photoacid applied to positive-tone 3D microfabrication, *Science* **296**, 5570, 1106–1109.

Zhou, Y., Kassab, G. S., and Molloi, S. (1999). On the design of the coronary arterial tree: a generalization of Murray's law, *Phys. Med. Biol.* **44**, 2929–2945.

Chapter 10

Tissue Engineering of Human Bladder

Anthony Atala

Wake Forest Institute for Regenerative Medicine,
Wake Forest University School of Medicine,
5th Floor, Watlington Hall, Medical Center Boulevard,
Winston-Salem, NC 27157, USA

aatala@wfubmc.edu

There are a number of conditions of the bladder that can lead to loss of function. Many of these require reconstructive procedures. However, current techniques may lead to a number of complications. Replacement of bladder tissues with functionally equivalent ones created in the laboratory could improve the outcome of reconstructive surgery. A number of animal studies and several landmark clinical experiences show that it is possible to reconstruct the bladder using tissues and neo-organs produced in the laboratory. Current research suggests that the use of biomaterial-based, bladder-shaped scaffolds seeded with autologous urothelial and smooth muscle cells is currently the best option for bladder tissue engineering. However, materials that could be used to create functionally equivalent urologic tissues in the laboratory, especially embryonic stem cells, have many ethical and technical limitations. Further research to develop novel biomaterials and cell sources,

---

Tissue and Organ Regeneration: Advances in Micro- and Nanotechnology
Edited by Lijie Grace Zhang, Ali Khademhosseini, and Thomas J. Webster
Copyright © 2014 Pan Stanford Publishing Pte. Ltd.
ISBN 978-981-4411-67-7 (Hardcover), 978-981-4411-68-4 (eBook)
www.panstanford.com

as well as information gained from developmental biology, signal transduction studies, and studies of the wound healing response would be beneficial.

10.1 Introduction

Congenital disorders, cancer, trauma, infection, inflammation, iatrogenic injuries, or other conditions of the genitourinary system can lead to bladder damage. Most of these situations require eventual reconstructive procedures. These procedures can be performed with native non-urologic tissues (skin, gastrointestinal segments, or mucosa), heterologous tissues or substances (bovine collagen), or artificial materials (silicone, polyurethane, Teflon). Currently, gastrointestinal segments are most commonly used as tissues for bladder replacement or repair. However, gastrointestinal tissues are designed to absorb specific solutes, whereas bladder tissue is designed for the excretion of these same solutes. As a result, when gastrointestinal tissue is placed within the urinary tract, multiple complications may ensue. These include infection, metabolic disturbances, urolithiasis, perforation, increased mucus production, and malignancy [1-4]. Because of the problems encountered with the use of gastrointestinal segments, numerous investigators have attempted alternative reconstructive procedures for bladder replacement or repair. These include autoaugmentation [5,6] and ureterocystoplasty [7-9]. In addition, novel methods for bladder reconstruction based on regenerative medicine, such as cell transplantation and tissue engineering, are being explored. This review focuses specifically on these novel regenerative medicine strategies for bladder reconstruction.

10.2 Basics of Tissue Engineering

Tissue engineering employs aspects of cell biology and transplantation, materials science, and biomedical engineering to develop biological substitutes that can restore and maintain the normal function of damaged tissues and organs. These include injection of functional cells into a nonfunctional site to stimulate regeneration and the use of biocompatible materials to create new tissues and organs. These biomaterials can be natural or synthetic matrices, often termed scaffolds, which encourage the body's natural ability to repair itself and assist in determination of the orientation and direction of new tissue growth. Often, tissue engineering uses a combination of both of these techniques. For example, biomaterial matrices seeded with cells can be implanted into the body to encourage the growth or regeneration of functional tissue.

10.2.1 Biomaterials Used in Genitourinary Tissue Construction

Synthetic materials have been used widely for urologic reconstruction. Silicone prostheses have been used for the treatment of urinary incontinence with the artificial urinary sphincter and detachable balloon system, for treatment of vesicoureteral reflux with silicone microparticles, and for impotence with penile prostheses [10–13]. There has also been a major effort directed toward the construction of artificial bladders made with silicone. In some disease states, such as urinary incontinence or vesicoureteral reflux, artificial agents (Teflon paste, glass microparticles) have been used as injectable bulking substances; however, these substances are not entirely biocompatible [14].

For regenerative medicine purposes, there are clear advantages to using degradable, biocompatible materials that can function as cell delivery vehicles, and/or provide the structural parameters needed for tissue replacement. Biomaterials in genitourinary regenerative medicine function as an artificial extracellular matrix (ECM) and elicit biologic and mechanical functions of native ECM found in tissues in the body. Native ECM brings cells together into tissue, controls the tissue structure, and regulates the cell phenotype [15]. Biomaterials facilitate the localization and delivery of cells and/or bioactive factors (e.g., cell adhesion peptides, growth factors) to desired sites in the body, define a three-dimensional space for the formation of new tissues with appropriate structure, and guide the development of new tissues with appropriate function [16]. Direct injection of cell suspensions without biomaterial matrices has been used in some cases [17,18], but it is difficult to control the localization of transplanted cells. In addition, the majority of mammalian cell types are anchorage dependent and will die if not provided with an appropriate cell adhesion substrate.

10.2.2 Design and Selection of Biomaterials

The design and selection of a biomaterial for use in regenerative medicine is critical for the proper development of engineered genitourinary tissues. The selected biomaterial must be capable of controlling the structure and function of the engineered tissue in a predesigned manner by interacting with transplanted cells and/or host cells. In addition, it should be biocompatible, able to promote cellular interaction and tissue development, and it should possess the proper mechanical and physical properties required for tissue support and function in the body site of interest.

Appropriate biomaterials should be biodegradable and bioresorbable to support the reconstruction of a completely normal tissue without inflammation. Thus, the degradation rate and the concentration of degradation products in the tissues surrounding the implant must be maintained at a tolerable level [19]. Such behavior avoids the risk of inflammatory or foreign-body responses that is often associated with the permanent presence of a foreign material in the body.

In addition, the biomaterial should provide appropriate regulation of cell behavior (e.g., adhesion, proliferation, migration, differentiation) in order to promote the development of functional new tissue. Cell behavior in engineered tissues is regulated by multiple interactions with the microenvironment, including interactions with cell-adhesion ligands [20] and with soluble growth factors [21]. Cell adhesion–promoting factors (e.g., Arg-Gly-Asp [RGD]) can be presented by the biomaterial itself or incorporated into the biomaterial in order to control cell behavior through ligand-induced cell receptor signaling processes [22,23]. As an example, a scaffold used to create an engineered bladder must be able to support the adhesion and proliferation of a number of cell types, including urothelial cells on the luminal side and smooth muscle cells surrounding the urothelial barrier, and it must be able to direct proper tissue development in order to form a functional bladder. In order to accomplish this, composite scaffolds consisting of both collagen and synthetic materials have been produced for hollow organ engineering [24].

In vivo, the biomaterials must provide temporary mechanical support sufficient to withstand forces exerted by the surrounding tissue and maintain a potential space for tissue development. In the case of bladder replacement, the biomaterial used to form the engineered organ must be able to withstand forces resulting from urine storage and filling/emptying. In addition, the biomaterial must be able to withstand the forces exerted on it by the pelvic muscles as the patient goes about daily activities. The mechanical support of the biomaterials should be maintained until the engineered tissue has sufficient mechanical integrity to support itself [25]. This can be achieved by an appropriate choice of mechanical and degradative properties of the biomaterials [16].

Finally, the chosen biomaterial must have properties that allow it to be processed into specific configurations. For example, it must be molded into a tubular shape for urethral replacement, or it must be shaped into a hollow, spherical configuration for bladder replacement. A large ratio of surface area to volume is often desirable to allow the delivery of a high density of cells. A high-porosity, interconnected pore structure with specific pore sizes promotes tissue ingrowth from the surrounding host tissue. Several techniques, such as electrospinning, have been developed, and they allow precise control of porosity, pore size, and pore structure [26–31].

10.2.3 Types of Biomaterials

Generally, three classes of biomaterials have been used for engineering of genitourinary tissues: naturally derived materials, such as collagen and alginate; acellular tissue matrices, such as bladder submucosa (BSM) and small-intestinal submucosa (SIS); and synthetic polymers, such as polyglycolic acid (PGA), polylactic acid (PLA), and poly(lactic-co-glycolic acid) (PLGA). These classes of biomaterials have been tested to determine their biocompatibility with primary human urothelial and bladder muscle cells [32]. Naturally derived materials and acellular tissue matrices have the potential advantage of biologic recognition. However, synthetic polymers can be produced quickly and reproducibly on a large scale with controlled properties of strength, degradation rate, and microstructure.

Collagen is the most abundant and ubiquitous structural protein in the body, and it may be readily purified from both animal and human tissues with an enzyme treatment and salt/acid extraction [33]. Collagen has long been known to exhibit minimal inflammatory and antigenic responses [34], and it has been approved by the U.S. Food and Drug Administration (FDA) for many types of medical applications, including wound dressings and artificial skin [35]. Intermolecular cross-linking reduces the degradation rate by making the collagen molecules less susceptible to enzymatic attack. Intermolecular cross-linking can be accomplished by various physical (e.g., ultraviolet radiation, dehydrothermal treatment) or chemical (e.g., glutaraldehyde, formaldehyde, carbodiimides) techniques [33]. Collagen contains cell-adhesion domain sequences (e.g., RGD) that exhibit specific cellular interactions. This may help to retain the phenotype and activity of many types of cells, including fibroblasts [36] and chondrocytes [37]. This material can be processed into a wide variety of structures such as sponges, fibers, and films [38–40].

Alginate, a polysaccharide isolated from seaweed, has been used as an injectable cell delivery vehicle [41] and a cell immobilization matrix [159] owing to its gentle gelling properties in the presence of divalent ions such as calcium. Alginate is a family of copolymers of D-mannuronate and L-guluronate. The physical and mechanical properties of alginate gel are strongly correlated with the proportion and length of the polyguluronate block in the alginate chains [41]. Efforts have been made to synthesize biodegradable alginate hydrogels with mechanical properties that are controllable in a wide range by intermolecular covalent cross-linking and with cell-adhesion peptides coupled to their backbones [42].

Recently, natural materials such as alginate and collagen have been used as "bio-inks" in a newly developed bioprinting technique based on inkjet technology [43,44]. Using this technology, these scaffold materials can be "printed" into a desired scaffold shape using a modified inkjet printer. In addition, several groups have shown that living cells can also be printed using this technology [45,46]. This exciting technique can be modified so that a three-dimensional construct containing a precise arrangement of cells, growth factors, and extracellular matrix material can be printed [47–49]. Such constructs may eventually be implanted into a host to serve as the backbone for a new tissue or organ.

Acellular tissue matrices are collagen-rich matrices prepared by removing cellular components from tissues. The most common tissue that has been used for this purpose has been bladder tissue. The matrices are prepared by removing the cellular material from a segment of bladder tissue using mechanical and chemical processes [50–53]. The resulting matrix can be used alone or seeded with cells. The matrices slowly degrade after implantation and are replaced and remodeled by ECM proteins synthesized and secreted by transplanted or ingrowing cells. Acellular tissue matrices support cell ingrowth and regeneration of several genitourinary tissue types, including urethra and bladder, with no evidence of immunogenic rejection [53,54]. Because the structures of the proteins (e.g., collagen, elastin) in acellular matrices are well conserved and normally arranged, the mechanical properties of the acellular matrices are not significantly different from those of native bladder submucosa [50].

Polyesters of naturally occurring α-hydroxy acids, including PGA, PLA, and PLGA, are widely used in regenerative medicine. These polymers have gained FDA approval for human use in a variety of applications, including sutures [55]. The degradation products of PGA, PLA, and PLGA are nontoxic, natural metabolites that are eventually eliminated from the body in the form of carbon dioxide and water [55]. Because these polymers are thermoplastics, they can easily be formed into a three-dimensional scaffold with a desired microstructure, gross shape, and dimension by various techniques, including molding, extrusion [56], solvent casting [57], phase separation techniques, and gas foaming techniques [58]. More recently, techniques such as electrospinning have been used to quickly create highly porous scaffolds in various conformations [28–30,59].

Many applications in genitourinary regenerative medicine require a scaffold with high porosity and a high ratio of surface area to volume. This need has been addressed by processing biomaterials into configurations of fiber meshes and porous sponges using the techniques described previously. A drawback of the synthetic polymers is lack of biologic recognition. As an approach toward incorporating cell recognition domains into these materials, copolymers with amino acids have been synthesized [22,23,60]. Other biodegradable synthetic polymers, including poly(anhydrides) and poly(ortho-esters), can also be used to fabricate scaffolds for genitourinary regenerative medicine with controlled properties [61]. In addition, composite scaffolds consisting of both natural and synthetic materials have been developed and may be useful in genitourinary tissue engineering. In particular, these scaffolds may be useful for engineering organs that are composed of layers of cells, such as the bladder (urothelial layer surrounded by smooth muscle cells) [24].

Nanotechnology, which is the use of small molecules that have distinct properties on a small scale, has been used to create "smart biomaterials" for regenerative medicine [62,63]. Nanoscaffolds have been manufactured specifically for bladder applications [64]. The manufacturing of nanostructured biomaterials has also led to enhanced cell alignment and tissue formation [28].

10.2.4 Cells for Urogenital Tissue Engineering Applications

Often, when cells are used for tissue engineering, donor tissue is removed and dissociated into individual cells, which are implanted directly into the host or expanded in culture, attached to a support matrix, and then implanted. The implanted tissue can be heterologous, allogeneic, or autologous. Ideally, this approach allows lost tissue function to be restored or replaced in to with limited complications [65–70].

Autologous cells are the ideal choice, as their use circumvents many of the inflammatory and rejection issues associated with a non-self-donor. In the past, one of the limitations of applying cell-based regenerative medicine techniques to organ replacement was the inherent difficulty of growing certain human cell types in large quantities. However, the discovery of native targeted progenitor cells in virtually every organ of the body has led to improved culture techniques that have overcome this problem for a number of cell types. Native targeted progenitor cells are tissue-specific unipotent cells derived from most organs. By noting the location of the progenitor cells, as well as by exploring the conditions that promote differentiation and/or self-renewal, it has been possible to overcome some of the obstacles that limit cell expansion in vitro. For example, urothelial cell culture has been improved in this way. Urothelial cells could be grown in the laboratory setting in the past, but only with limited success. It was believed that urothelial cells had a natural senescence that was hard to overcome. Several protocols have been developed over the last two decades that have improved urothelial growth and expansion [71–74]. A system of urothelial cell harvesting was developed that does not use any enzymes or serum and has a large expansion potential. Using these methods of cell culture, it is possible to expand a urothelial strain from a single specimen that initially covers a surface area of 1 cm^2 to one covering a surface area of 4202 m^2 (the equivalent area of one football field) within 8 weeks [71].

An advantage of native targeted progenitor cells is that they are already programmed to become the cell type needed, and no in vitro differentiation steps are required for their use in the organ of origin. An additional advantage in using native cells is that they can be obtained from the specific organ to be regenerated, expanded, and used in the same patient without rejection, in an autologous manner. [52,65-68,71,75-86].

Bladder, ureter, and renal pelvis cells can all be harvested, cultured, and expanded in a similar fashion. Normal human bladder epithelial and muscle cells can be efficiently harvested from surgical material, extensively expanded in culture, and their differentiation characteristics, growth requirements, and other biologic properties can be studied [71,73,74,80,81,87-94]. Major advances in cell culture techniques have been made within the past decade, and these techniques make the use of autologous cells possible for clinical application.

Another major concern has been that in cases where cells must be expanded from a diseased organ, there may no longer be enough normal cells present in that organ to begin the process. Recent research suggests that this may not be the case, however. For example, one study has shown that cultured neuropathic bladder smooth muscle cells possess and maintain different characteristics than normal smooth muscle cells in vitro, as demonstrated by growth assays, contractility and adherence tests in vitro [95]. Despite these differences, when neuropathic smooth muscle cells were cultured in vitro, and then seeded onto matrices and implanted in vivo, the tissue engineered constructs showed the same properties as the constructs engineered with normal cells [96]. It is now known that genetically normal progenitor cells, which are the reservoirs for new cell formation, are present even in diseased tissue. These normal progenitors are programmed to give rise to normal tissue, regardless of whether they reside in a normal or diseased environment. Therefore, the stem cell niche and its role in normal tissue regeneration remains a fertile area of ongoing investigation.

10.2.5 Stem Cells and Other Pluripotent Cell Types

As discussed, most current strategies for tissue engineering depend upon a sample of autologous cells from the diseased organ of the host. In some instances, primary autologous human cells cannot be expanded from a particular organ, such as the pancreas, or there is not enough normal tissue remaining in the diseased organ to use for the procedures described above. In these situations, pluripotent human stem cells are envisioned to be an ideal source of cells, as they can differentiate into nearly any replacement tissue in the body.

Embryonic stem cells exhibit two remarkable properties: the ability to proliferate in an undifferentiated, but still pluripotent state (self-renewal), and the ability to differentiate into a large number of specialized cell types [97]. They can be isolated from the inner cell mass of the embryo during the blastocyst stage, which occurs 5 days post-fertilization. These cells have been maintained in the undifferentiated state for at least 80 passages when grown using current published protocols [98]. In addition, many protocols for differentiation into specific cell types in culture have been published. However, there are several problems associated with the use of ES cells in tissue engineering. Importantly, these cells tend to form teratomas when implanted in vivo due to their multipotent state, and this risk of tumor formation limits their clinical application. In addition, many uses of these cells are currently banned in a number of countries due to the ethical dilemmas that are associated with the manipulation of embryos in culture.

Adult stem cells, especially hematopoietic stem cells, are the best understood cell type in stem cell biology [99]. Despite this, adult stem cell research remains an area of intense study, as their potential for therapy may be applicable to a myriad of degenerative disorders. Within the past decade, adult stem cell populations have been found in many adult tissues other than the bone marrow and the gastrointestinal tract, including the brain [100,101], skin, [102] and muscle [103]. Many other types of adult stem cells have been identified in organs all over the body and are thought to serve as the primary repair entities for their corresponding organs [104]. The discovery of such tissue-specific progenitors has opened up new avenues for research.

A notable exception to the tissue-specificity of adult stem cells is the mesenchymal stem cell, also known as the multipotent adult progenitor cell. This cell type is derived from bone marrow stroma [105,106]. Such cells can differentiate in vitro into numerous tissue types [107,108] and can also differentiate developmentally if injected into a blastocyst. Multipotent adult progenitor cells can develop into a variety of tissues including neuronal [109], adipose [103], muscle [103,110], liver [111,112], lungs [113], spleen [114], and gut tissue [106], but notably not bone marrow or gonads.

Research into adult stem cells has, however, progressed slowly, mainly because investigators have had great difficulty in maintaining adult non-mesenchymal stem cells in culture. Some cells, such as those of the liver, pancreas, and nerve, have very low proliferative capacity in vitro, and the functionality of some cell types is reduced after the cells are cultivated. Isolation of cells has also been problematic, because stem cells are present in extremely low numbers in adult tissue [111,115]. While the clinical utility of adult stem cells is currently limited, great potential exists for future use of such cells in tissue-specific regenerative therapies. The advantage of adult stem cells is that they can be used in autologous therapies, thus avoiding any complications associated with immune rejection.

The isolation of multipotent human and mouse amniotic-fluid and placental-derived stem (AFPS) cells that are capable of extensive self-renewal and give rise to cells from all three germ layers was reported in 2007 [116]. AFPS cells represent approximately 1% of the cells found in the amniotic fluid and placenta. The undifferentiated stem cells expand extensively without a feeder cell layer and double every 36 h. Unlike human embryonic stem cells, the AFPS cells do not form tumors in vivo. Lines maintained for over 250 population doublings retained long telomeres and a normal complement of chromosomes. AFPS cell lines can be induced to differentiate into cells representing each embryonic germ layer, including cells of adipogenic, osteogenic, myogenic, endothelial, neural-like and hepatic lineages. In addition to the differentiated AFPS cells expressing lineage-specific markers, such cells can have specialized functions. Cells of the hepatic lineage secreted urea and α-fetoprotein, while osteogenic cells produced mineralized calcium. In this respect, they meet a commonly accepted criterion for multipotent stem cells, without implying that they can generate every adult tissue.

AFS cells represent a new class of stem cells with properties somewhere between those of embryonic and adult stem cell types, probably more agile than adult stem cells, but less so than embryonic stem cells. Unlike embryonic and induced pluripotent stem cells, however, AFPS cells do not form teratomas, and if preserved for self-use, avoid the problems of rejection. The cells could be obtained from either amniocentesis or chorionic villous sampling in the developing fetus, or from the placenta at the time of birth. They could be preserved for self-use, and used without rejection, or they could be banked. A bank of 100,000 specimens could potentially supply 99% of the US population with a perfect genetic match for transplantation. Such a bank may be easier to create than with other cell sources, since there are approximately 4.5 million births per year in the United States.

Since the discovery of the AFPS cells, other groups have published on the potential of the cells to differentiate to other lineages, such as cartilage [117], kidney [118], and lung [119]. Muscle differentiated AFPS cells were also noted to prevent compensatory bladder hypertrophy in a cryo-injured rodent bladder model [120].

Nuclear transfer, or cloning, can serve as another source of pluripotent, "stem" cells that could possibly be used for regenerative medicine therapies. Unlike reproductive cloning, nuclear transfer produces an embryo that is genetically identical to the donor nucleus, but these are used to generate blastocysts that are explanted and grown in culture, rather than in utero, to produce embryonic stem cell lines. These autologous stem cells have the potential to become almost any type of cell in the adult body, and thus would be useful in tissue and organ replacement applications [121]. Therefore, somatic cell nuclear transfer may provide an alternative source of transplantable cells that are identical to the patient's own cells.

Recently, exciting reports of the successful transformation of adult cells into pluripotent stem cells through a type of genetic "reprogramming" have been published. Reprogramming is a technique that involves de-differentiation of adult somatic cells to produce patient-specific pluripotent stem cells, without the use of embryos. Cells generated by reprogramming would be genetically identical to the somatic cells (and thus, the patient who donated these cells) and would not be rejected. Yamanaka was the first to discover that mouse embryonic fibroblasts (MEFs) and adult mouse fibroblasts could be reprogrammed into an "induced pluripotent state (iPS)" [122]. They examined 24 genes that were thought to be important for embryonic stem cells and identified 4 key genes that were required to bestow embryonic stem cell-like properties on fibroblasts—Oct3/4, Sox2, c-Myc, and Klf4. iPS cells in this study possessed the immortal growth characteristics of self-renewing ES cells, expressed genes specific for ES cells, and generated embryoid bodies in vitro and teratomas in vivo. When iPS cells were injected into mouse blastocysts, they contributed to a variety of cell types in the embryo. However, although iPS cells selected in this way were pluripotent, they were not identical to ES cells. Unlike ES cells, chimeras made from iPS cells did not result in full-term pregnancies. Gene expression profiles of the iPS cells showed that they possessed a distinct gene expression signature that was different from that of ES cells. In addition, the epigenetic state of the iPS cells was somewhere between that found in somatic cells and that found in ES cells, suggesting that the reprogramming was incomplete.

These results were improved significantly by Wernig and Jaenisch in July 2007 [123]. Results from this study showed that DNA methylation, gene expression profiles, and the chromatin state of the reprogrammed cells were similar to those of ES cells. Teratomas induced by these cells contained differentiated cell types representing all three embryonic germ layers. Most importantly, the reprogrammed cells from this experiment were able to form viable chimeras and contribute to the germ line like ES cells, suggesting that these iPS cells were completely reprogrammed.

It has recently been shown that reprogramming of human cells is possible [124,125]. Yamanaka showed that retrovirus-mediated transfection of *OCT3/4, SOX2, KLF4,* and *c-MYC* generates human iPS cells that are similar to hES cells in terms of morphology, proliferation, gene expression, surface markers, and teratoma formation. Thompson's group showed that retroviral transduction of *OCT4, SOX2, NANOG,* and *LIN28* could generate pluripotent stem cells without introducing any oncogenes (c-MYC). Both studies showed that human iPS were similar but not identical to hES cells. However, despite these advances, a number of questions must be answered before iPS cells can be used in human therapies. One concern is that these cells contain three to six retroviral integrations, which may increase the risk of eventual tumorigenesis. Although this is an exciting phenomenon, our understanding of the mechanisms involved in reprogramming is still limited.

10.3   Tissue Engineering Strategies for Bladder Replacement

10.3.1   Biomaterial Matrices for Bladder Regeneration

Over the last few decades, several bladder wall substitutes have been attempted with both synthetic and organic materials. Synthetic materials that have been tried in experimental and clinical settings include polyvinyl sponges, Teflon, collagen matrices, Vicryl (PGA) matrices, and silicone. Most of these attempts have failed because of mechanical, structural, functional, or biocompatibility problems. Usually, permanent synthetic materials used for bladder reconstruction succumb to mechanical failure and urinary stone formation, and use of degradable materials leads to fibroblast deposition, scarring, graft contracture, and a reduced reservoir volume over time [78,126].

There has been a resurgence in the use of various collagen-based matrices for tissue regeneration. Non-seeded allogeneic acellular bladder matrices have served as scaffolds for the ingrowth of host bladder wall components. The matrices are prepared by mechanically and chemically removing all cellular components from bladder tissue [51,52,54,127,128]. The matrices serve as vehicles for partial bladder regeneration, and relevant antigenicity is not evident.

Cell-seeded allogeneic acellular bladder matrices have been used for bladder augmentation in dogs [52]. The regenerated bladder tissues contained a normal cellular organization consisting of urothelium and smooth muscle and exhibited a normal compliance. Biomaterials preloaded with cells before their implantation showed better tissue regeneration compared with biomaterials implanted with no cells, in which tissue regeneration depended on ingrowth of the surrounding tissue. The bladders showed a significant increase (100%) in capacity when augmented with scaffolds seeded with cells, compared to scaffolds without cells (30%). The acellular collagen matrices can be enhanced with growth factors to improve bladder regeneration [129].

SIS, a biodegradable, acellular, xenogeneic collagen-based tissue-matrix graft, was first described by Badylak and colleagues in the 1980s as an acellular matrix for tissue replacement in the vascular field [130]. It has been shown to promote regeneration of a variety of host tissues, including blood vessels and ligaments [131]. The matrix is derived from pig small intestine in which the mucosa is mechanically removed from the inner surface and the serosa and muscular layer are removed from the outer surface. Animal studies have shown that the non-seeded SIS matrix used for bladder augmentation is able to regenerate in vivo [132,133]. Histologically, the transitional layer was the same as that of the native bladder tissue, but, as with other non-seeded collagen matrices used experimentally, the muscle layer was not fully developed. A large amount of collagen was interspersed among a smaller number of muscle bundles. A computer-assisted image analysis demonstrated a decreased muscle-to-collagen ratio with loss of the normal architecture in the SIS-regenerated bladders. In vitro contractility studies performed on the SIS-regenerated dog bladders showed a decrease in maximal contractile response by 50% from those of normal bladder tissues. Expression of muscarinic, purinergic, and alpha-adrenergic receptors and functional cholinergic and purinergic innervation were demonstrated [133]. Cholinergic and purinergic innervation also occurred in rats [134].

Bladder augmentation using laparoscopic techniques was performed on minipigs with porcine bowel acellular tissue matrix, human placental membranes, or porcine SIS. At 12 weeks post-operatively the grafts had contracted to 70%, 65%, and 60% of their original sizes, respectively, and histologically the grafts showed predominantly only mucosal regeneration [135]. The same group evaluated the long-term results of laparoscopic hemicystectomy and bladder replacement with small intestinal submucosa (SIS) with ureteral reimplantation into the SIS material in minipigs. Histopathology studies after 1 year showed muscle at the graft periphery and center but it consisted of small fused bundles with significant fibrosis. Nerves were present at the graft periphery and center but they were decreased in number. Compared to primary bladder closure after hemi-cystectomy, no advantage in bladder capacity or compliance was documented [136]. More recently, bladder regeneration has been shown to be more reliable when the SIS was derived from the distal ileum [137].

In multiple studies using various materials as non-seeded grafts for cystoplasty, the urothelial layer was able to regenerate normally, but the muscle layer, although present, was not fully developed [52,54,127,133,138,139]. Studies involving acellular matrices that may provide the necessary environment to promote cell migration, growth, and differentiation are being conducted [140]. With continued bladder research in this area, these matrices may have a clinical role in bladder replacement in the future.

10.3.2 Regenerative Medicine for Bladder Using Cell Transplantation

Regenerative medicine with selective cell transplantation may provide a means to create functional new bladder segments [77]. The success of cell transplantation strategies for bladder reconstruction depends on the ability to use donor tissue efficiently and to provide the right conditions for long-term survival, differentiation, and growth. Various cell sources have been explored for bladder regeneration. Native cells are currently preferable due to their autologous source, wherein they can be used without rejection [71]. It has been shown experimentally that the bladder neck and trigone area has a higher propensity of urothelial progenitor cells [141], and these cells are localized in the basal region [142]. Amniotic fluid and bone marrow-derived stem cells can also be used in an autologous manner and have the potential to differentiate into bladder muscle [116,143] and urothelium [144]. Embryonic stem cells also have the potential to differentiate into bladder tissue [145].

Human urothelial and muscle cells can be expanded in vitro, seeded onto polymer scaffolds, and allowed to attach and form sheets of cells. The cell-polymer scaffold can then be implanted in vivo. Histologic analysis indicated that viable cells were able to self-assemble back into their respective tissue types, and would retain their native phenotype [67]. These experiments demonstrated, for the first time, that composite layered tissue-engineered structures could be created de novo. Before this study, only non-layered structures had been created in the field of regenerative medicine.

It has been well established for decades that portions of the bladder are able to regenerate generously over free grafts, most likely because the urothelium is associated with a high reparative capacity [146]. However, bladder muscle tissue is less likely to regenerate in a normal fashion. Both urothelial and muscle ingrowth are believed to be initiated at the edges of the injury, from the normal bladder tissue in toward the region of the free graft [147,148]. Usually, however, contracture or resorption of the graft has been evident. Inflammation in response to the matrix may contribute to the resorption of the free graft. As a result of this discovery, it was hypothesized that building the three-dimensional bladder constructs in vitro, before implantation, would facilitate the eventual terminal differentiation of the cells after implantation in vivo and would minimize the inflammatory response toward the matrix, thus avoiding graft contracture and shrinkage. The dog study described earlier supports this hypothesis and illustrates a major difference between matrices used with autologous cells (tissue-engineered matrices) and those used without cells [52]. Matrices that were seeded with cells and then used for bladder augmentation retained most of their preimplantation diameter, as opposed to matrices implanted without cells, in which significant graft contraction and shrinkage occurred. In addition, histological analysis demonstrated a marked paucity of muscle cells and a more aggressive inflammatory reaction in the matrices implanted without cells.

The results of these initial studies showed that the creation of artificial bladders may be achieved in vivo; however, it could not be determined whether the functional parameters noted were created by the augmented segment or by the remaining native bladder tissue. To better address this question, an animal model was designed in which subtotal cystectomies followed by replacement with a tissue-engineered organ were performed [85]. Cystectomy-only controls and animals that received bladder replacements made from non-seeded matrices maintained average capacities of 22% and 46% of preoperative values, respectively. However, an average bladder capacity of 95% of the original precystectomy volume was achieved in animals receiving cell-seeded tissue engineered bladder replacements. These findings were confirmed radiographically. The subtotal cystectomy reservoirs that were not reconstructed and the polymer-only reconstructed bladders showed a marked decrease in bladder compliance (10% and 42% total compliance). In contrast, the compliance of the cell-seeded tissue-engineered bladders showed almost no difference from preoperative values that were measured when the native bladder was present (106%). Histologically, the non-seeded bladder replacement scaffolds presented a pattern of normal urothelial cells with a thickened fibrotic submucosa and a thin layer of muscle fibers. The tissue-engineered bladders (scaffold + cells) showed a normal cellular organization, consisting of a trilayer of urothelium, submucosa, and muscle. Immunocytochemical analyses confirmed the muscle and urothelial phenotype. S-100 staining indicated the presence of neural structures [85]. These studies have been repeated by other investigators, and they obtained similar results using larger numbers of animals over the long-term [138,149]. Thus, the strategy of using biodegradable scaffolds seeded with cells can be pursued without concerns for local or systemic toxicity [150].

However, not all scaffold materials perform well if a large portion of the bladder must be replaced. In a study using SIS for subtotal bladder replacement in dogs, both the unseeded and cell seeded experimental groups showed graft shrinkage and poor results [151]. This confirms that the type of scaffold used in the construction of tissue-engineered bladders is critical for the success of these technologies. The use of bioreactors, which provide mechanical stimulation for the growing organ in vitro, has also been proposed as an important parameter for success [152]. Bioreactors provide can provide mechanical stimulation such as periodic stretching of the tissue, which has been shown to assist in in vitro muscle development, and exposure to flow conditions, which is important for the development of endothelial layers in blood vessels and hollow organs such as the bladder. In fact, Farhat and colleagues have developed bioreactor systems specifically for bladder development [153]. These systems provide simulated filling/emptying functions to the engineered tissue, and this may lead to a bladder construct with more functionality.

A clinical experience involving engineered bladder tissue for cystoplasty was conducted starting in 1998. A small pilot study of seven patients reported the use of either collagen scaffolds seeded with cells or a combined PGA-collagen scaffold seeded with cells for bladder replacement. These engineered tissues were implanted with or without omental coverage (Fig. 10.1). Patients reconstructed with engineered bladder tissue created with cell-seeded PGA-collagen scaffolds and omental coverage showed increased compliance, decreased end-filling pressures, increased capacities and longer dry periods over time (Fig. 10.2) [154]. It is clear from this experience that the engineered bladders continued to improve with time, mirroring their continued development. Although the experience is promising and shows that engineered tissues can be implanted safely, it is just a first step toward the goal of engineering fully functional bladders. This was a limited clinical experience, and the technology is not yet ready for wide dissemination, as further experimental and clinical studies are required.

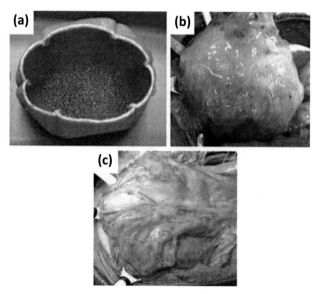

Figure 10.1 Construction of engineered bladder. (a) Scaffold material seeded with cells for use in bladder repair. (b) The seeded scaffold is anastamosed to native bladder with running 4-0 polyglycolic sutures. (c) Implant covered with fibrin glue and omentum.

In the past, an important area of concern in tissue engineering was the quality of the source of cells for regeneration. The concept of creating engineered constructs by obtaining cells for expansion from the diseased organ led investigators to consider whether or not the cell population derived and expanded from diseased tissue would be normal, with normal functional parameters. For example, would the cells obtained from a neuropathic bladder lead to the formation of normal bladder tissue or to the engineering of another neuropathic bladder? It has been shown that cultured neuropathic bladder smooth muscle cells possess different characteristics than normal smooth muscle cells in vitro, as demonstrated by growth assays, contractility, adherence tests, and microarray analysis [95,155,156]. However, when neuropathic smooth muscle cells were cultured in vitro, and seeded onto matrices and implanted in vivo, the tissue engineered constructs showed the same properties as the tissues engineered with normal cells [96]. Thus, it appears that genetically normal non-malignant progenitor cells are programmed to give rise to normal tissue, regardless of whether they exist in normal or diseased tissues [96,157,158]. Therefore, although the mechanisms for tissue self-assembly and regenerative medicine are not fully understood, it is known that the progenitor cells are able to "reset" their program for normal cell differentiation. The stem cell niche and its role in normal tissue regeneration remains a fertile area of ongoing investigation.

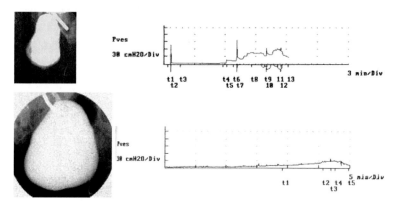

Figure 10.2 Cystograms and urodynamic studies of a patient before and after implantation of the tissue engineered bladder. (a) Preoperative results indicate an irregular-shaped bladder in the cystogram (left) and abnormal bladder pressures as the bladder is filled during urodynamic studies (right). (b) Postoperatively, findings are significantly improved.

10.4 Conclusions

From the above studies, it is evident that the use of cell-seeded matrices is superior to the use of non-seeded matrices for the creation of engineered bladder tissues. Although advances have been made with the engineering of bladder tissues, many challenges remain. Current research in many centers is aimed at the development of biologically active and "smart" biomaterials that may improve bladder tissue regeneration as well as regeneration of many other tissues in the body.

Acknowledgments

The author would like to thank Dr. Jennifer Olson for editorial assistance with this manuscript.

References

1. McDougal WS. Metabolic complications of urinary intestinal diversion. *Journal of Urology* 1992; **147**: 1199–1208.
2. Atala A, Bauer SB, Hendren WH, Retik AB. The effect of gastric augmentation on bladder function. *Journal of Urology* 1993; **149**: 1099–1102.
3. Kaefer M, Hendren WH, Bauer SB, Goldenblatt P, Peters CA, Atala A, Retik AB. Reservoir calculi: a comparison of reservoirs constructed from stomach and other enteric segments.. *Journal of Urology* 1998; **160**: 2187–2190.
4. Kaefer M, Tobin MS, Hendren WH, Bauer SB, Peters CA, Atala A, Colodny AH, Mandell J, Retik AB. Continent urinary diversion: the Children's Hospital experience. *Journal of Urology* 1997; **157**: 1394–1399.
5. Cartwright PC, Snow BW. Bladder autoaugmentation: partial detrusor excision to augment the bladder without use of bowel. *Journal of Urology* 1989; **142**: 1050–1053.
6. Cartwright PC, Snow BW. Bladder autoaugmentation: early clinical experience. *Journal of Urology* 1989; **142**: 505–508; discussion 520–521.
7. Bellinger MF. Ureterocystoplasty: a unique method for vesical augmentation in children. *Journal of Urology* 1993; **149**: 811–813.
8. Churchill BM, Aliabadi H, Landau EH, McLorie GA, Steckler RE, McKenna PH, Khoury AE. Ureteral bladder augmentation. *Journal of Urology* 1993; **150**: 716–720.
9. Adams MC, Brock JW, 3rd, Pope JCt, Rink RC. Ureterocystoplasty: is it necessary to detubularize the distal ureter? *Journal of Urology* 1998; **160**: 851–853.

10. Atala A, Peters CA, Retik AB, Mandell J. Endoscopic treatment of vesicoureteral reflux with a self-detachable balloon system. *Journal of Urology* 1992; **148**: 724–727.
11. Riehmann M, Gasser TC, Bruskewitz RC. The Hydroflex penile prosthesis: a test case for the introduction of new urological technology. *Journal of Urology* 1993; **149**: 1304–1307.
12. Levesque PE, Bauer SB, Atala A, Zurakowski D, Colodny A, Peters C, Retik AB. Ten-year experience with the artificial urinary sphincter in children. *Journal of Urology* 1996; **156**: 625–628.
13. Buckley JF, Scott R, Aitchison M. Periurethral microparticulate silicone injection for stress incontinence and vesicoureteric reflux. *Minimally Invasive Therapy* 1997; **1**: 72.
14. Atala A. Use of non-autologous substances in VUR and incontinence treatment. *Dial Pediatric Urology* 1994; **17**: 11–12
15. Alberts B, Bray D, Lewis JM. The extracellular matrix of animals, in *Molecular Biology of the Cell* (Alberts B, Bray D, Lewis JM, eds), New York, NY: Garland Publishing, 1994; 971–995.
16. Kim BS, Mooney DJ. Development of biocompatible synthetic extracellular matrices for tissue engineering. *Trends in Biotechnology* 1998; **16**: 224–230.
17. Ponder KP, Gupta S, Leland F, Darlington G, Finegold M, DeMayo J, Ledley FD, Chowdhury JR, Woo SL. Mouse hepatocytes migrate to liver parenchyma and function indefinitely after intrasplenic transplantation. *Proceedings of the National Academy of Sciences of the United States of America* 1991; **88**: 1217–1221.
18. Brittberg M, Lindahl A, Nilsson A, Ohlsson C, Isaksson O, Peterson L. Treatment of deep cartilage defects in the knee with autologous chondrocyte transplantation. *New England Journal of Medicine* 1994; **331**: 889–895.
19. Bergsma JE, Rozema FR, Bos RR, Boering G, de Bruijn WC, Pennings AJ. In vivo degradation and biocompatibility study of in vitro pre-degraded as-polymerized polyactide particles. *Biomaterials* 1995; **16**: 267–274.
20. Hynes RO. Integrins: versatility, modulation, and signaling in cell adhesion. *Cell* 1992; **69**: 11–25.
21. Deuel TF. Growth factors. In *Principles of Tissue Engineering* (Lanza R, Langer R, Chick WL, eds), New York, NY: Academic Press, 1997; 133–149.

22. Barrera DA, Zylstra E, Lansbury PT, Langer R. Synthesis and RGD peptide modification of a new biodegradable copolymer poly (lactic acid-co-lysine). *Journal of the American Chemical Society* 1993; **115**: 11010–11011.
23. Cook AD, Hrkach JS, Gao NN, Johnson IM, Pajvani UB, Cannizzaro SM, Langer R. Characterization and development of RGD-peptide-modified poly(lactic acid-co-lysine) as an interactive, resorbable biomaterial. *Journal of Biomedical Materials Research* 1997; **35**: 513–523.
24. Eberli D, Freitas Filho L, Atala A, Yoo JJ. Composite scaffolds for the engineering of hollow organs and tissues. *Methods (Duluth)* 2009; **47**: 109–115.
25. Atala A. Engineering tissues, organs and cells. *Journal of Tissue Engineering and Regenerative Medicine* 2007; **1**: 83–96.
26. Yoo JJ, Lee JE, Kim HJ, Kim SJ, Lim JH, Lee SJ, Lee JI, Lee YK, Lim BS, Rhee SH. Comparative in vitro and in vivo studies using a bioactive poly(epsilon-caprolactone)-organosiloxane nanohybrid containing calcium salt. *Journal of Biomedical Materials Research. Part B, Applied Biomaterials* 2007; **83**: 189–198.
27. Lee SJ, Van Dyke M, Atala A, Yoo JJ. Host cell mobilization for in situ tissue regeneration. *Rejuvenation Research* 2008; **11**: 747–756.
28. Choi JS, Lee SJ, Christ GJ, Atala A, Yoo JJ. The influence of electrospun aligned poly(epsilon-caprolactone)/collagen nanofiber meshes on the formation of self-aligned skeletal muscle myotubes. *Biomaterials* 2008; **29**: 2899–2906.
29. Lee SJ, Liu J, Oh SH, Soker S, Atala A, Yoo JJ. Development of a composite vascular scaffolding system that withstands physiological vascular conditions. *Biomaterials* 2008; **29**: 2891–2898.
30. Lee SJ, Oh SH, Liu J, Soker S, Atala A, Yoo JJ. The use of thermal treatments to enhance the mechanical properties of electrospun poly(epsilon-caprolactone) scaffolds. *Biomaterials* 2008; **29**: 1422–1430.
31. Lee SJ, Yoo JJ, Lim GJ, Atala A, Stitzel J. In vitro evaluation of electrospun nanofiber scaffolds for vascular graft application. *Journal of Biomedical Materials Research Part A* 2007; **83**: 999–1008.
32. Pariente JL, Kim BS, Atala A. In vitro biocompatibility assessment of naturally derived and synthetic biomaterials using normal human urothelial cells. *Journal of Biomedical Materials Research* 2001; **55**: 33–39.
33. Li ST. Biologic biomaterials: tissue derived biomaterials (collagen). in *The Biomedical Engineering Handbook* (JD B, Boca Raton, FL ed), CRS Press, 1995; 627–647.

34. Furthmayr H, Timpl R. Immunochemistry of collagens and procollagens. *International Review of Connective Tissue Research* 1976; **7**: 61–99.
35. Cen L, Liu W, Cui L, Zhang W, Cao Y. Collagen tissue engineering: development of novel biomaterials and applications. *Pediatr Res* 2008; **63**: 492–496.
36. Silver FH, Pins G. Cell growth on collagen: a review of tissue engineering using scaffolds containing extracellular matrix. *Journal of Long-Term Effects of Medical Implants* 1992; **2**: 67–80.
37. Sams AE, Nixon AJ. Chondrocyte-laden collagen scaffolds for resurfacing extensive articular cartilage defects. *Osteoarthritis & Cartilage* 1995; **3**: 47–59.
38. Yannas IV, Burke JF, Gordon PL, Huang C, Rubenstein RH. Design of an artificial skin. II. Control of chemical composition. *Journal of Biomedical Materials Research* 1980; **14**: 107–132.
39. Yannas IV, Burke JF. Design of an artificial skin. I. Basic design principles. *Journal of Biomedical Materials Research* 1980; **14**: 65–81.
40. Cavallaro JF, Kemp PD, Kraus KH. Collagen fabrics as biomaterials. *Biotechnology and Bioengineering* 1994; **43**: 781–791.
41. Smidsrod O, Skjak-Braek G. Alginate as immobilization matrix for cells. *Trends in Biotechnology* 1990; **8**: 71–78.
42. Rowley JA, Madlambayan G, Mooney DJ. Alginate hydrogels as synthetic extracellular matrix materials. *Biomaterials* 1999; **20**: 45–53.
43. Campbell PG, Weiss LE. Tissue engineering with the aid of inkjet printers. *Expert Opinion on Biological Therapy* 2007; **7**: 1123–1127.
44. Boland T, Xu T, Damon B, Cui X. Application of inkjet printing to tissue engineering. *Biotechnology Journal* 2006; **1**: 910–917.
45. Nakamura M, Kobayashi A, Takagi F, Watanabe A, Hiruma Y, Ohuchi K, Iwasaki Y, Horie M, Morita I, Takatani S. Biocompatible inkjet printing technique for designed seeding of individual living cells. *Tissue Engineering* 2005; **11**: 1658–1666.
46. Laflamme MA, Gold J, Xu C, Hassanipour M, Rosler E, Police S, Muskheli V, Murry CE. Formation of human myocardium in the rat heart from human embryonic stem cells. *American Journal of Pathology* 2005; **167**: 663–671.
47. Xu T, Rohozinski J, Zhao W, Moorefield EC, Atala A, Yoo JJ. Inkjet-mediated gene transfection into living cells combined with targeted delivery. *Tissue Engineering Part A* 2009; **15**: 95–101.

48. Ilkhanizadeh S, Teixeira AI, Hermanson O. Inkjet printing of macromolecules on hydrogels to steer neural stem cell differentiation. *Biomaterials* 2007; **28**: 3936–3943.
49. Roth EA, Xu T, Das M, Gregory C, Hickman JJ, Boland T. Inkjet printing for high-throughput cell patterning. *Biomaterials* 2004; **25**: 3707–3715.
50. Dahms SE, Piechota HJ, Dahiya R, Lue TF, Tanagho EA. Composition and biomechanical properties of the bladder acellular matrix graft: comparative analysis in rat, pig and human. *British Journal of Urology* 1998; **82**: 411–419.
51. Piechota HJ, Dahms SE, Nunes LS, Dahiya R, Lue TF, Tanagho EA. In vitro functional properties of the rat bladder regenerated by the bladder acellular matrix graft. *Journal of Urology* 1998; **159**: 1717–1724.
52. Yoo JJ, Meng J, Oberpenning F, Atala A. Bladder augmentation using allogenic bladder submucosa seeded with cells. *Urology* 1998; **51**: 221–225.
53. Chen F, Yoo JJ, Atala A. Acellular collagen matrix as a possible "off the shelf" biomaterial for urethral repair. *Urology* 1999; **54**: 407–410.
54. Probst M, Dahiya R, Carrier S, Tanagho EA. Reproduction of functional smooth muscle tissue and partial bladder replacement. *British Journal of Urology* 1997; **79**: 505–515.
55. Gilding D. Biodegradable Polymers. in *Biocompatibility of Clinical Implant Materials* (Williams D, ed), Boca Raton, FL: CRC Press, 1981; 209–232.
56. Freed LE, Vunjak-Novakovic G, Biron RJ, Eagles DB, Lesnoy DC, Barlow SK, Langer R. Biodegradable polymer scaffolds for tissue engineering. *Biotechnology (N Y)* 1994; **12**: 689–693.
57. Mikos AG, Lyman MD, Freed LE, Langer R. Wetting of poly(L-lactic acid) and poly(D,L-lactic-co-glycolic acid) foams for tissue culture. *Biomaterials* 1994; **15**: 55–58.
58. Harris LD, Kim BS, Mooney DJ. Open pore biodegradable matrices formed with gas foaming. *Journal of Biomedical Materials Research* 1998; **42**: 396–402.
59. Han D, Gouma PI. Electrospun bioscaffolds that mimic the topology of extracellular matrix. *Nanomedicine* 2006; **2**: 37–41.
60. Intveld PJA, Shen ZR, Takens GAJ. Glycine glycolic acid based copolymers. *Journal of Polymer Science Part A: Polymer Chemistry* 1994; **32**: 1063–1069.

61. Peppas NA, Langer R. New challenges in biomaterials. *Science* 1994; **263**: 1715–1720.
62. Boccaccini AR, Blaker JJ. Bioactive composite materials for tissue engineering scaffolds. *Expert Rev Med Devices* 2005; **2**: 303–317.
63. Harrison BS, Atala A. Carbon nanotube applications for tissue engineering. *Biomaterials* 2007; **28**: 344–353.
64. Harrington DA, Cheng EY, Guler MO, Lee LK, Donovan JL, Claussen RC, Stupp SI. Branched peptide-amphiphiles as self-assembling coatings for tissue engineering scaffolds. *Journal of Biomedical Materials Research Part A* 2006; **78**: 157–167.
65. Atala A, Vacanti JP, Peters CA, Mandell J, Retik AB, Freeman MR. Formation of urothelial structures in vivo from dissociated cells attached to biodegradable polymer scaffolds in vitro. *Journal of Urology* 1992; **148**: 658–662.
66. Atala A, Cima LG, Kim W, Paige KT, Vacanti JP, Retik AB, Vacanti CA. Injectable alginate seeded with chondrocytes as a potential treatment for vesicoureteral reflux. *Journal of Urology* 1993; **150**: 745–747.
67. Atala A, Freeman MR, Vacanti JP, Shepard J, Retik AB. Implantation in vivo and retrieval of artificial structures consisting of rabbit and human urothelium and human bladder muscle. *Journal of Urology* 1993; **150**: 608–612.
68. Atala A, Kim W, Paige KT, Vacanti CA, Retik AB. Endoscopic treatment of vesicoureteral reflux with a chondrocyte-alginate suspension. *Journal of Urology* 1994; **152**: 641–643; discussion 644.
69. Atala A. Tissue engineering, stem cells, and cloning for the regeneration of urologic organs. *Clinics in Plastic Surgery* 2003; **30**: 649–667.
70. Atala A. Recent applications of regenerative medicine to urologic structures and related tissues. *Current Opinion in Urology* 2006; **16**: 305–309.
71. Cilento BG, Freeman MR, Schneck FX, Retik AB, Atala A. Phenotypic and cytogenetic characterization of human bladder urothelia expanded in vitro. *Journal of Urology* 1994; **152**: 665–670.
72. Scriven SD, Booth C, Thomas DF, Trejdosiewicz LK, Southgate J. Reconstitution of human urothelium from monolayer cultures. *Journal of Urology* 1997; **158**: 1147–1152.

73. Liebert M, Hubbel A, Chung M, Wedemeyer G, Lomax MI, Hegeman A, Yuan TY, Brozovich M, Wheelock MJ, Grossman HB. Expression of mal is associated with urothelial differentiation in vitro: identification by differential display reverse-transcriptase polymerase chain reaction. *Differentiation* 1997; **61**: 177–185.

74. Puthenveettil JA, Burger MS, Reznikoff CA. Replicative senescence in human uroepithelial cells. *Advances in Experimental Medicine & Biology* 1999; 462: 83–91.

75. Atala A, Schlussel, RN, Retik, AB. Renal cell growth in vivo after attachment to biodegradable polymer scaffolds. *Journal of Urology* 1995; **153**: 4.

76. Atala A, Guzman L, Retik AB. A novel inert collagen matrix for hypospadias repair. *Journal of Urology* 1999; **162**: 1148–1151.

77. Atala A. Tissue engineering in the genitourinary system in *Tissue Engineering* (Atala A, Mooney DJ, eds), Boston, MA: Birkhauser Press, 1997; 149.

78. Atala A. Autologous cell transplantation for urologic reconstruction. *Journal of Urology* 1998; **159**: 2–3.

79. Yoo JJ, Atala A. A novel gene delivery system using urothelial tissue engineered neo-organs. *Journal of Urology* 1997; **158**: 1066–1070.

80. Fauza DO, Fishman SJ, Mehegan K, Atala A. Videofetoscopically assisted fetal tissue engineering: skin replacement. *Journal of Pediatric Surgery* 1998; **33**: 357–361.

81. Fauza DO, Fishman SJ, Mehegan K, Atala A. Videofetoscopically assisted fetal tissue engineering: bladder augmentation. *Journal of Pediatric Surgery* 1998; **33**: 7–12.

82. Machluf M, Atala A. Emerging concepts for tissue and organ transplantation. *Graft* 1998; **1**: 31–37.

83. Amiel GE, Atala A. Current and future modalities for functional renal replacement. *Urologic Clinics of North America* 1999; **26**: 235–246.

84. Kershen RT, Atala A. New advances in injectable therapies for the treatment of incontinence and vesicoureteral reflux. *Urologic Clinics of North America* 1999; **26**: 81–94.

85. Oberpenning F, Meng J, Yoo JJ, Atala A. De novo reconstitution of a functional mammalian urinary bladder by tissue engineering. *Nature Biotechnology* 1999; **17**: 149–155.

86. Park HJ, Yoo JJ, Kershen RT, Moreland R, Atala A. Reconstitution of human corporal smooth muscle and endothelial cells in vivo. *Journal of Urology* 1999; **162**: 1106–1109.

87. Liebert M, Wedemeyer G, Abruzzo LV, Kunkel SL, Hammerberg C, Cooper KD, Grossman HB. Stimulated urothelial cells produce cytokines and express an activated cell surface antigenic phenotype. *Seminars in Urology* 1991; **9**: 124–130.

88. Tobin MS, Freeman MR, Atala A. Maturational response of normal human urothelial cells in culture is dependent on extracellular matrix and serum additives. *Surgical Forum* 1994; **45**: 786.

89. Harriss DR. Smooth muscle cell culture: a new approach to the study of human detrusor physiology and pathophysiology. *British Journal of Urology* 1995; **75** Suppl 1: 18–26.

90. Freeman MR, Yoo JJ, Raab G, Soker S, Adam RM, Schneck FX, Renshaw AA, Klagsbrun M, Atala A. Heparin-binding EGF-like growth factor is an autocrine growth factor for human urothelial cells and is synthesized by epithelial and smooth muscle cells in the human bladder. *Journal of Clinical Investigation* 1997; **99**: 1028–1036.

91. Solomon LZ, Jennings AM, Sharpe P, Cooper AJ, Malone PS. Effects of short-chain fatty acids on primary urothelial cells in culture: implications for intravesical use in enterocystoplasties. *Journal of Laboratory & Clinical Medicine* 1998; **132**: 279–283.

92. Lobban ED, Smith BA, Hall GD, Harnden P, Roberts P, Selby PJ, Trejdosiewicz LK, Southgate J. Uroplakin gene expression by normal and neoplastic human urothelium. *American Journal of Pathology* 1998; **153**: 1957–1967.

93. Nguyen HT, Park JM, Peters CA, Adam RM, Orsola A, Atala A, Freeman MR. Cell-specific activation of the HB-EGF and ErbB1 genes by stretch in primary human bladder cells. *In vitro Cellular & Developmental Biology Animal* 1999; **35**: 371–375.

94. Rackley RR, Bandyopadhyay SK, Fazeli-Matin S, Shin MS, Appell R. Immunoregulatory potential of urothelium: characterization of NF-kappaB signal transduction. *Journal of Urology* 1999; **162**: 1812–1816.

95. Lin HK, Cowan R, Moore P, Zhang Y, Yang Q, Peterson JA, Jr., Tomasek JJ, Kropp BP, Cheng EY. Characterization of neuropathic bladder smooth muscle cells in culture. *Journal of Urology* 2004; **171**: 1348–1352.

96. Lai JY, Yoon CY, Yoo JJ, Wulf T, Atala A. Phenotypic and functional characterization of in vivo tissue engineered smooth muscle from normal and pathological bladders. *Journal of Urology* 2002; **168**: 1853–1857; discussion 1858.

97. Brivanlou AH, Gage FH, Jaenisch R, Jessell T, Melton D, Rossant J. Stem cells. Setting standards for human embryonic stem cells. *Science* 2003; **300**: 913–916.

98. Thomson JA, Itskovitz-Eldor J, Shapiro SS, Waknitz MA, Swiergiel JJ, Marshall VS, Jones JM. Embryonic stem cell lines derived from human blastocysts. [erratum appears in Science 1998 Dec 4;282(5395):1827]. *Science* 1998; **282**: 1145–1147.

99. Ballas CB, Zielske SP, Gerson SL. Adult bone marrow stem cells for cell and gene therapies: implications for greater use. *Journal of Cellular Biochemistry—Supplement* 2002; **38**: 20–28.

100. Jiao J, Chen DF. Induction of neurogenesis in nonconventional neurogenic regions of the adult central nervous system by niche astrocyte-produced signals. *Stem Cells* 2008; **26**: 1221–1230.

101. Taupin P. Therapeutic potential of adult neural stem cells. *Recent Patents CNS Drug Discovery* 2006; **1**: 299–303.

102. Jensen UB, Yan X, Triel C, Woo SH, Christensen R, Owens DM. A distinct population of clonogenic and multipotent murine follicular keratinocytes residing in the upper isthmus. *Journal of Cell Science* 2008; **121**: 609–617.

103. Crisan M, Casteilla L, Lehr L, Carmona M, Paoloni-Giacobino A, Yap S, Sun B, Leger B, Logar A, Penicaud L, Schrauwen P, Cameron-Smith D, Russell AP, Peault B, Giacobino JP. A reservoir of brown adipocyte progenitors in human skeletal muscle. *Stem Cells* 2008; **26**: 2425–2433.

104. Weiner LP. Definitions and criteria for stem cells. *Methods in Molecular Biology* 2008; **438**: 3–8.

105. Devine SM. Mesenchymal stem cells: will they have a role in the clinic? *Journal of Cellular Biochemistry—Supplement* 2002; **38**: 73–79.

106. Jiang Y, Jahagirdar BN, Reinhardt RL, Schwartz RE, Keene CD, Ortiz-Gonzalez XR, Reyes M, Lenvik T, Lund T, Blackstad M, Du J, Aldrich S, Lisberg A, Low WC, Largaespada DA, Verfaillie CM. Pluripotency of mesenchymal stem cells derived from adult marrow [erratum appears in *Nature*. 2007 June 14; 447(7146): 879–880]. *Nature* 2002; **418**: 41–49.

107. Caplan AI. Adult mesenchymal stem cells for tissue engineering versus regenerative medicine. *Journal of Cellular Physiology* 2007; **213**: 341–347.

108. da Silva Meirelles L, Caplan AI, Nardi NB. In search of the in vivo identity of mesenchymal stem cells. *Stem Cells* 2008; **26**: 2287–2299.

109. Duan X, Chang JH, Ge S, Faulkner RL, Kim JY, Kitabatake Y, Liu XB, Yang CH, Jordan JD, Ma DK, Liu CY, Ganesan S, Cheng HJ, Ming GL, Lu B, Song H. Disrupted-In-Schizophrenia 1 regulates integration of newly generated neurons in the adult brain. *Cell* 2007; **130**: 1146–1158.

110. Luttun A, Ross JJ, Verfaillie C, Aranguren X, Prosper F. Unit 22F.9: differentiation of multipotent adult progenitor cells into functional endothelial and smooth muscle cells in *Current Protocols in Immunology volume Supplement* 75. Hoboken, NJ: John Wiley and Sons, Inc., 2006.

111. Mimeault M, Batra SK. Recent progress on tissue-resident adult stem cell biology and their therapeutic implications. *Stem Cell Reviews* 2008; **4**: 27–49.

112. Ikeda E, Yagi K, Kojima M, Yagyuu T, Ohshima A, Sobajima S, Tadokoro M, Katsube Y, Isoda K, Kondoh M, Kawase M, Go MJ, Adachi H, Yokota Y, Kirita T, Ohgushi H. Multipotent cells from the human third molar: feasibility of cell-based therapy for liver disease. *Differentiation* 2008; **76**: 495–505.

113. Nolen-Walston RD, Kim CF, Mazan MR, Ingenito EP, Gruntman AM, Tsai L, Boston R, Woolfenden AE, Jacks T, Hoffman AM. Cellular kinetics and modeling of bronchioalveolar stem cell response during lung regeneration. *American Journal of Physiology—Lung Cellular & Molecular Physiology* 2008; **294**: L1158–L1165.

114. in 't Anker PS, Noort WA, Scherjon SA, Kleijburg-van der Keur C, Kruisselbrink AB, van Bezooijen RL, Beekhuizen W, Willemze R, Kanhai HH, Fibbe WE. Mesenchymal stem cells in human second-trimester bone marrow, liver, lung, and spleen exhibit a similar immunophenotype but a heterogeneous multilineage differentiation potential. *Haematologica* 2003; **88**: 845–852.

115. Hristov M, Zernecke A, Schober A, Weber C. Adult progenitor cells in vascular remodeling during atherosclerosis. *Biological Chemistry* 2008; **389**: 837–844.

116. De Coppi P, Bartsch G, Jr., Siddiqui MM, Xu T, Santos CC, Perin L, Mostoslavsky G, Serre AC, Snyder EY, Yoo JJ, Furth ME, Soker S, Atala A. Isolation of amniotic stem cell lines with potential for therapy. *Nature Biotechnology* 2007; **25**: 100–106.

117. Kolambkar YM, Peister A, Soker S, Atala A, Guldberg RE. Chondrogenic differentiation of amniotic fluid-derived stem cells. *Journal of Molecular Histology* 2007; **38**: 405–413.

118. Perin L, Giuliani S, Jin D, Sedrakyan S, Carraro G, Habibian R, Warburton D, Atala A, De Filippo RE. Renal differentiation of amniotic fluid stem cells. *Cell Prolif* 2007; **40**: 936–948.

119. Warburton D, Perin L, Defilippo R, Bellusci S, Shi W, Driscoll B. Stem/progenitor cells in lung development, injury repair, and regeneration. *Proceedings of the American Thoracic Society* 2008; **5**: 703–706.

120. De Coppi P, Callegari A, Chiavegato A, Gasparotto L, Piccoli M, Taiani J, Pozzobon M, Boldrin L, Okabe M, Cozzi E, Atala A, Gamba P, Sartore S. Amniotic fluid and bone marrow derived mesenchymal stem cells can be converted to smooth muscle cells in the cryo-injured rat bladder and prevent compensatory hypertrophy of surviving smooth muscle cells. *Journal of Urology* 2007; **177**: 369–376.

121. Hochedlinger K, Rideout WM, Kyba M, Daley GQ, Blelloch R, Jaenisch R. Nuclear transplantation, embryonic stem cells and the potential for cell therapy. *Hematology Journal* 2004; **5** Suppl 3: S114–S117.

122. Takahashi K, Yamanaka S. Induction of pluripotent stem cells from mouse embryonic and adult fibroblast cultures by defined factors *Cell* 2006; **126**: 663–676.

123. Wernig M, Meissner A, Foreman R, Brambrink T, Ku M, Hochedlinger K, Bernstein BE, Jaenisch R. In vitro reprogramming of fibroblasts into a pluripotent ES-cell-like state *Nature* 2007; **448**: 318–324.

124. Takahashi K, Tanabe K, Ohnuki M, Narita M, Ichisaka T, Tomoda K, Yamanaka S. Induction of pluripotent stem cells from adult human fibroblasts by defined factors. *Cell* 2007; **131**: 861–872.

125. Yu J, Vodyanik MA, Smuga-Otto K, Antosiewicz-Bourget J, Frane JL, Tian S, Nie J, Jonsdottir GA, Ruotti V, Stewart R, Slukvin II, Thomson JA. Induced pluripotent stem cell lines derived from human somatic cells. *Science* 2007: 1151526.

126. Atala A. Commentary on the replacement of urologic associated mucosa. *Journal of Urology* 1995; **156**: 338.

127. Sutherland RS, Baskin LS, Hayward SW, Cunha GR. Regeneration of bladder urothelium, smooth muscle, blood vessels and nerves into an acellular tissue matrix. *Journal of Urology* 1996; **156**: 571–577.

128. Wefer J, Sievert KD, Schlote N, Wefer AE, Nunes L, Dahiya R, Gleason CA, Tanagho EA. Time dependent smooth muscle regeneration and maturation in a bladder acellular matrix graft: histological studies and in vivo functional evaluation. *J Urol* 2001; **165**: 1755–1759.

129. Kikuno N, Kawamoto K, Hirata H, Vejdani K, Kawakami K, Fandel T, Nunes L, Urakami S, Shiina H, Igawa M, Tanagho E, Dahiya R. Nerve growth factor combined with vascular endothelial growth factor enhances regeneration of bladder acellular matrix graft in spinal cord injury-induced neurogenic rat bladder. *BJU Int* 2008; **103**(10): 1424–1428.

130. Badylak SF, Lantz GC, Coffey A, Geddes LA. Small intestinal submucosa as a large diameter vascular graft in the dog. *Journal of Surgical Research* 1989; **47**: 74–80.

131. Badylak SF. The extracellular matrix as a scaffold for tissue reconstruction. *Seminars in Cell & Developmental Biology* 2002; **13**: 377–383.

132. Kropp BP, Rippy MK, Badylak SF, Adams MC, Keating MA, Rink RC, Thor KB. Regenerative urinary bladder augmentation using small intestinal submucosa: urodynamic and histopathologic assessment in long-term canine bladder augmentations. *Journal of Urology* 1996; **155**: 2098–2104.

133. Kropp BP, Sawyer BD, Shannon HE, Rippy MK, Badylak SF, Adams MC, Keating MA, Rink RC, Thor KB. Characterization of small intestinal submucosa regenerated canine detrusor: assessment of reinnervation, in vitro compliance and contractility. *Journal of Urology* 1996; **156**: 599–607.

134. Vaught JD, Kropp BP, Sawyer BD, Rippy MK, Badylak SF, Shannon HE, Thor KB. Detrusor regeneration in the rat using porcine small intestinal submucosal grafts: functional innervation and receptor expression. *Journal of Urology* 1996; **155**: 374–378.

135. Portis AJ, Elbahnasy AM, Shalhav AL, Brewer A, Humphrey P, McDougall EM, Clayman RV. Laparoscopic augmentation cystoplasty with different biodegradable grafts in an animal model. *Journal of Urology* 2000; **164**: 1405–1411.

136. Landman J, Olweny E, Sundaram CP, Andreoni C, Collyer WC, Rehman J, Jerde TJ, Lin HK, Lee DI, Nunlist EH, Humphrey PA, Nakada SY, Clayman RV. Laparoscopic mid sagittal hemicystectomy and bladder reconstruction with small intestinal submucosa and reimplantation of ureter into small intestinal submucosa: 1-year followup. *Journal of Urology* 2004; **171**: 2450–2455.

137. Kropp BP, Cheng EY, Lin HK, Zhang Y. Reliable and reproducible bladder regeneration using unseeded distal small intestinal submucosa. *Journal of Urology* 2004; **172**: 1710–1713.

138. Jayo MJ, Jain D, Wagner BJ, Bertram TA. Early cellular and stromal responses in regeneration versus repair of a mammalian bladder using autologous cell and biodegradable scaffold technologies. *Journal of Urology* 2008; **180**: 392–397.

139. Zhang Y. Bladder reconstruction by tissue engineering—with or without cells? *Journal of Urology* 2008; **180**: 10–11.

140. Chun SY, Lim GJ, Kwon TG, Kwak EK, Kim BW, Atala A, Yoo JJ. Identification and characterization of bioactive factors in bladder submucosa matrix. *Biomaterials* 2007; **28**: 4251–4256.

141. Nguyen MM, Lieu DK, deGraffenried LA, Isseroff RR, Kurzrock EA. Urothelial progenitor cells: regional differences in the rat bladder. *Cell Proliferation* 2007; **40**: 157–165.

142. Kurzrock EA, Lieu DK, Degraffenried LA, Chan CW, Isseroff RR. Label-retaining cells of the bladder: candidate urothelial stem cells. *American Journal of Physiology—Renal Physiology* 2008; **294**: F1415–F1421.

143. Shukla D, Box GN, Edwards RA, Tyson DR. Bone marrow stem cells for urologic tissue engineering. *World Journal of Urology* 2008; **26**: 341–349.

144. Anumanthan G, Makari JH, Honea L, Thomas JC, Wills ML, Bhowmick NA, Adams MC, Hayward SW, Matusik RJ, Brock JW, 3rd, Pope JCt. Directed differentiation of bone marrow derived mesenchymal stem cells into bladder urothelium. *Journal of Urology* 2008; **180**: 1778–1783.

145. Oottamasathien S, Wang Y, Williams K, Franco OE, Wills ML, Thomas JC, Saba K, Sharif-Afshar AR, Makari JH, Bhowmick NA, DeMarco RT, Hipkens S, Magnuson M, Brock JW, 3rd, Hayward SW, Pope JCt, Matusik RJ. Directed differentiation of embryonic stem cells into bladder tissue. *Developmental Biology* 2007; **304**: 556–566.

146. de Boer WI, Schuller AG, Vermey M, van der Kwast TH. Expression of growth factors and receptors during specific phases in regenerating urothelium after acute injury in vivo. *American Journal of Pathology* 1994; **145**: 1199–1207.

147. Baker R, Kelly T, Tehan T, Putnam C, Beaugard E. Subtotal cystectomy and total bladder regeneration in treatment of bladder cancer. *Journal of the American Medical Association* 1958; **168**: 1178–1185.

148. Gorham SD, French DA, Shivas AA, Scott R. Some observations on the regeneration of smooth muscle in the repaired urinary bladder of the rabbit. *European Urology* 1989; **16**: 440–443.

149. Jayo MJ, Jain D, Ludlow JW, Payne R, Wagner BJ, McLorie G, Bertram TA. Long-term durability, tissue regeneration and neo-organ growth during skeletal maturation with a neo-bladder augmentation construct. *Regenerative Medicine* 2008; **3**: 671–682.

150. Kwon TG, Yoo JJ, Atala A. Local and systemic effects of a tissue engineered neobladder in a canine cystoplasty model. *Journal of Urology* 2008; **179**: 2035–2041.

151. Zhang Y, Frimberger D, Cheng EY, Lin HK, Kropp BP. Challenges in a larger bladder replacement with cell-seeded and unseeded small intestinal submucosa grafts in a subtotal cystectomy model. *BJU International* 2006; **98**: 1100–1105.

152. Farhat WA, Yeger H. Does mechanical stimulation have any role in urinary bladder tissue engineering? *World Journal of Urology* 2008; **26**: 301–305.

153. Farhat WA, Yeger H. Does mechanical stimulation have any role in urinary bladder tissue engineering? *World Journal of Urology* 2008; **26**: 301–305.

154. Atala A, Bauer SB, Soker S, Yoo JJ, Retik AB. Tissue-engineered autologous bladders for patients needing cystoplasty. *Lancet* 2006; **367**: 1241–1246.

155. Hipp J, Andersson KE, Kwon TG, Kwak EK, Yoo J, Atala A. Microarray analysis of exstrophic human bladder smooth muscle. *BJU International* 2008; **101**: 100–105.

156. Dozmorov MG, Kropp BP, Hurst RE, Cheng EY, Lin HK. Differentially expressed gene networks in cultured smooth muscle cells from normal and neuropathic bladder. *Journal of Smooth Muscle Research* 2007; **43**: 55–72.

157. Faris RA, Konkin T, Halpert G. Liver stem cells: a potential source of hepatocytes for the treatment of human liver disease. *Artificial Organs* 2001; **25**: 513–521.

158. Haller H, de Groot K, Bahlmann F, Elger M, Fliser D. Stem cells and progenitor cells in renal disease. *Kidney International* 2005; **68**: 1932–1936.

159. Lim F, Sun AM. Microencapsulated islets as bioartificial endocrine pancreas. *Science*. 1980; **210**(4472): 908–910.

Chapter 11

The Self-Assembling Process of Articular Cartilage and Self-Organization in Tissue Engineering

Pasha Hadidi, Rajalakshmanan Eswaramoorthy, Jerry C. Hu, and Kyriacos A. Athanasiou

Department of Biomedical Engineering, University of California, Davis, 1 Shields Avenue, Davis, CA 95616, USA

athanasiou@ucdavis.edu

11.1 Introduction

The classical tissue engineering paradigm incorporates cells, scaffolds, and soluble and/or mechanical signals. These three elements have formed the basis for much research in tissue engineering; yet problems associated with the use of scaffolds have led tissue engineers to consider alternate approaches. Thus, in recent years, scaffoldless methods have been used to engineer tissues as diverse as articular cartilage, fibrocartilage, vasculature, tendon, ligament, bone, liver, nerve, and the eye. Concurrently, these approaches have gained recognition within the field of tissue engineering for their ability to create tissues with appropriate mechanical, metabolic, and even electrical properties. Outside of scaffold-based and scaffoldless tissue engineering, several other approaches in tissue engineering and regenerative medicine exist, such as stem cell injections, growth factor treatments, and gene delivery [1–6]. These will not be discussed at length in this chapter.

Tissues engineered without a scaffold can exhibit generation of structure with or without exogenous forces. Following this, two distinct subsets within scaffoldless tissue engineering may be elucidated: self-organizing and self-assembling tissues. Significantly, both self-organization and the self-assembling process have resulted in the formation of robust tissues, as described below. However, there has been confusion, and, indeed, no definition in tissue engineering, concerning the terms "self-assembly" and "self-organization." Therefore, drawing from the definitions of self-assembly used in other fields, this chapter will define self-organization and the self-assembling process in tissue engineering.

This chapter will also delineate the self-assembling process as a novel tissue engineering technique with respect to underlying biological mechanisms and characteristics of self-assembling tissue, using articular cartilage as an example. We will seek to establish a framework for understanding the self-assembling process in articular cartilage, with the objective of comparing it to processes carried out in the engineering of various other tissues. To this end, biological mechanisms thought to underlie the self-assembling process will first be explained. Then, advances from the scientific literature will be used to give examples of the characteristics of self-organizing and self-assembling tissues. Finally, beneficial growth signals (soluble and mechanical) used in the synthesis of the various tissues described will be provided. Future directions for self-assembling and self-organizing tissues will conclude this chapter.

11.1.1 Scaffoldless versus Scaffold-Based Engineered Tissue

Although scaffolds have been used in tissue engineering to allow for cell adhesion, to give structure to developing tissue, and to provide biochemical cues, scaffoldless approaches eliminate certain limitations and design considerations intrinsic to scaffold use (Fig. 11.1). Thus, scaffoldless approaches have several advantages over traditional scaffold-based tissue engineering. For example, a primary concern associated with the use of scaffolds is harsh processing during scaffold formation or cell encapsulation. Seeding scaffolds with cells may involve exposure of the cells to toxic polymerizing chemicals, elevated temperatures, or shear (as in spinner flask seeding) [7]. Furthermore, studies have shown that cell attachment to exogenous materials can alter gene expression, induce changes in phenotype, and deter matrix synthesis [8–10]. Additionally, tissue engineers should attempt to prevent scaffolds themselves from interfering with the process of tissue generation. For example, encapsulating cells in hydrogels can limit cell-to-cell communication, which may detrimentally affect extracellular

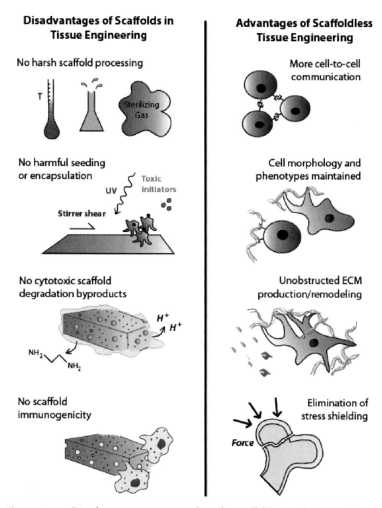

Figure 11.1 Disadvantages associated with scaffold use (left pane), and advantages of scaffoldless tissue engineering (right panel).

matrix (ECM) synthesis [11]. Additionally, scaffolds may create stress shielding effects that limit beneficial mechanotransduction [12]. Moreover, scaffold materials themselves may obstruct tissue formation or remodeling, since these processes are not necessarily coupled to scaffold degradation [13,14]. Finally, as with any implanted biomaterial, the use of an implanted scaffold raises concerns regarding immune response and the potential toxicity of degradation byproducts [15]. Thus, scaffoldless tissue generation using the self-assembling process and other similar techniques may overcome the need for exogenous scaffolds by providing a less harmful, more biomimetic microenvironment, which allows for greater ECM production and tissue remodeling. Therefore, scaffoldless tissue engineering comprises an exciting new area of research.

Scaffold-based tissue engineering is not without its own advantages. Many cell types are anchorage-dependent and require attachment to a substrate of specific stiffness for optimal viability and function [16,17]. Osteoblasts are a primary example of this within musculoskeletal tissues [18]. Another advantage of scaffold use in tissue engineering is the ability to incorporate signaling molecules within the scaffold. Multiple growth factors may be incorporated into a scaffold, which may degrade at varying rates and/or be spatially patterned to generate more complex tissues [19,20]. Finally, in certain applications such as vertebral fusion, implantation of a biomaterial scaffold may be preferable or even superior to implantation of tissue [21]. Cost, feasibility, and the need to adhere to FDA guidelines should also motivate decisions of whether to use scaffolds for a particular application or not [22]. For all of these reasons, some tissue engineering problems may be better suited to a scaffold-based approach. The focus of this chapter is the self-assembling process and self-organization within scaffoldless tissue engineering, however, and scaffold-based tissue engineering will not be discussed further here.

11.1.2 Scaffoldless Methods of Generating Tissue

Due to the concerns with scaffolds described previously, some researchers have pursued methods of generating tissue without exogenous scaffolds. Scaffoldless methods of generating tissue vary and, thus, present different characteristics, advantages, and disadvantages. Scaffoldless approaches range from pellet culture to aggregate culture to cell sheet engineering. New scaffoldless tissue generation techniques are continuously developed, but the examples detailed below have been selected to represent the more widespread and impactful techniques.

While pellet culture is one of the oldest and most straightforward methods of scaffoldless tissue generation [23,24], its relatively recent application to tissue engineering suffers from certain limitations. Pellet culture involves the suspension of cells in a conical tube followed by centrifugation to create a cell pellet. The pellet is then cultured in appropriate media without further agitation. This method is largely used in engineering cartilage [25,26], although other tissues generated include bone and liver [27,28]. In the case of cartilage, pellet culture may result in characteristic protein and/or gene expression for collagen II, glycosaminoglycans (GAGs), aggrecan, and Sox9 [25,26,29]. However, mechanical testing of this tissue, especially in tension, is technically difficult and rare, and thus translatability is limited. Additionally, the effect of organizing cells under large forces has not been thoroughly studied. Finally, implantation of pellet culture constructs may be difficult due to the small size of constructs generated.

Aggregate culture is similar to and slightly more versatile than pellet culture, but still holds drawbacks for the goal of tissue engineering. Like pellet culture, aggregate culture has been used for decades, including as a tool to study basic development [30,31]. Many cell types will aggregate under certain conditions in rotary culture, and most typically, an orbital shaker is used to agitate a cell suspension over a non-adherent coating, which is used to prevent settling and attachment to the bottom of the container. Aggregate culture has been used to generate bone, ligament, cartilage, retina, and pancreas micromasses, to varying degrees of success [32–36]. Aggregates often display appropriate differentiation markers, including collagens I and II in ligament and cartilage, respectively, the transcription factor Nrl in retina, and insulin in pancreas [32–36]. Aggregate culture has also been combined with other microscale technologies for tissue engineering. For example, polymer microspheres have been incorporated with mesenchymal stem cell (MSC) aggregates to facilitate chondrogenesis [37]. Magnetic microparticles have also been incorporated in aggregate cultures to direct spatial patterning under magnetic fields [38]. Despite these advances, aggregate culture tissue is seldom assessed for functional outcomes; sizes and shapes generated are not amenable to mechanical testing, for instance. Application is also limited for the same reasons, especially for load-bearing tissues.

Cell sheet engineering is a newer method of scaffoldless tissue engineering that involves monolayer culture [39–41]. This technique has shown promise in generating thin, two-dimensional tissues, and relatively homogeneous tissues, such as myocardium, but may fail in generating complex three-dimensional tissue organization or tissues with low cellularity such as cartilage. Cell sheet engineering works by growing a monolayer of cells, which is subsequently harvested as a whole sheet and applied for tissue engineering purposes. Multiple monolayers may be stacked to form cardiac tissue, or rolled sequentially into tubes to create engineered vasculature [41,42]. Tissue created by cell sheet engineering has been shown to be biologically active. Separate myocardial sheets will electrically couple and synchronize via the formation of gap junctions, and cell sheets assembled to form vasculature are responsive to relaxation and contraction stimuli [43–45]. Vascular cell sheet engineering can create functional blood vessels, which have been tested in human patients [46,47]. Cell sheet engineering has also been explored for the creation of cornea, bone, liver, and kidney tissues, but functional assessment of these tissues is scarce [48–51]. Other drawbacks of cell sheet engineering include multiple culture phases (monolayer, then stacked or rolled culture) that may increase culture time and/or complicate logistics, and potential dedifferentiation of cells while in monolayer.

Another form of scaffoldless tissue engineering that has received recent attention is bioprinting. Bioprinting takes advantage of developments in three-dimensional printing technology, and uses computer-aided seeding of high-density cell solutions in a precise pattern onto a dissolvable substrate, followed by the re-organization of these cells into higher order tissue-specific morphologies. This process has been used to create several tissues including skin, vasculature, and cartilage [52–54]. Several recent reviews have been given on bioprinting, and this form of self-organization will not be discussed further in this chapter [55–57].

11.1.3 Self-Organization and the Self-Assembling Process in Tissue Engineering

As described above, *scaffoldless tissue engineering* can be defined simply as the generation of tissue without the use of a scaffold. However, within scaffoldless tissue engineering, many approaches display self-organization. In this context, the term *self-organization in tissue engineering* refers to a subset of techniques within scaffoldless tissue engineering, which produce tissues that demonstrate native tissue-like organization by the use of external forces. Cell sheet engineering and bioprinting, as described above, are two types of self-organization in tissue engineering.

Self-organization may occur at different size scales (i.e., the cellular level or the tissue level) and/or at different time periods (i.e., hours or days) during tissue formation. At the cellular level, hepatocytes that are initially seeded onto collagen-coated surfaces may self-organize over the course of several hours into spheroids [58]. At the tissue level, previously seeded neurons and fibroblasts may self-organize over the course of several days into rod structures [59]. Self-organization may result in the formation of distinct structures found in native tissue, or recapitulate the gross morphology of native tissue. Within self-organizing tissues of the eye, specific structures and regions can form, such as the optic cup and distinct neurosensory tissues [60]. For tendon and ligament constructs, self-organization can recapitulate native gross morphology, resulting in cylindrical tissue constructs [61,62]. Therefore, self-organization within tissue engineering replicates the attributes of native tissue and manifests itself in a variety of scaffoldless approaches. The specific engineering techniques and resulting characteristics of these tissues will be detailed in the section on self-organization below.

Distinct from self-organization in tissue engineering, *the self-assembling process in tissue engineering* refers to a separate subset within scaffoldless tissue engineering. Thus, scaffoldless approaches within tissue engineering may be categorized as either self-organization or the self-assembling process (Fig. 11.2). Previously, the terms "self-assembly" and "self-organization" have been ascribed to various scaffoldless approaches without reference to a standard definition. Here, we give a set of criteria that defines the self-assembling process in tissue engineering based on underlying mechanisms, characteristics of scaffoldless and self-assembling tissue, and aims of the field of tissue engineering.

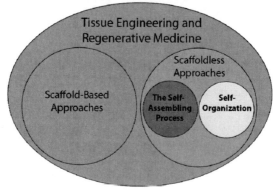

Figure 11.2 Subsets of tissue engineering and regenerative medicine. Approaches outside of scaffold-based and scaffoldless tissue engineering include stem cell therapies, growth factor treatments, and gene delivery. Scaffold-based and scaffoldless tissue engineering are two separate subsets of tissue engineering and regenerative medicine. Within scaffoldless tissue engineering, some approaches may be classified either as self-organization or the self-assembling process.

The self-assembling process in tissue engineering is similar to, but distinct from, self-assembly in other fields of research. Although the study of self-assembly originated in regard to molecules, self-assembly has also been deemed important for systems at larger scales, ranging up to galaxy formation [63,64]. Self-assembly with regard to biology represents one of the most fundamental processes underlying living organisms, involving protein folding as well as cell organization [64]. It is important to distinguish, however, that self-assembly in tissue engineering is distinct from molecular self-assembly or the self-assembly that occurs during embryogenesis. Indeed "self-assembly is not a formalized subject," and thus what constitutes self-assembly varies from field to field [64]. For this reason, it is important to define the self-assembling process and the similar term self-organization for use in the field of tissue engineering.

The self-assembling process in tissue engineering can be defined as *a scaffoldless technology which produces tissues that demonstrate spontaneous organization without external forces;* this occurs via the minimization of free energy through cell-to-cell interactions. The difference between the self-assembling process and self-organization is the input of external energy or force. External forces, such as high centrifugal accelerations or orbital shaking, are not present during the self-assembling process in tissue engineering, but they are present in various self-organization approaches. In the self-assembling process, the presence of a non-adherent substrate, in the absence of external forces, allows cells to organize themselves to minimize overall free energy via cell-to-cell interaction and/or cell sorting. Additionally, the characteristics of tissue produced via the self-assembling process are notable. Self-assembling tissue exhibits distinct phases of formation that resemble native tissue development. The tissue formed from the self-assembling process has functional properties approaching those of native tissue. Lastly, clinical application of self-assembling tissue is reasonable, as tissue constructs have appropriate sizes as well as native morphology.

In summary, the self-assembling process in tissue engineering refers to an approach that that minimizes free energy without the use of external forces or adherent substrates. Characteristics of self-assembling tissue include a set of distinct phases reminiscent of tissue development, clinically relevant tissue constructs with appropriate sizes and native morphology, and functional properties approaching those of native tissue. Although self-organizing tissues also employ scaffoldless approaches that display some of these characteristics, the self-assembling process in tissue engineering is distinct by following the minimization of free energy without external input.

11.2 Examples of Self-Organization in Tissue Engineering

As defined previously, *self-organization in tissue engineering* refers to engineered tissue which displays generation of distinct structures or gross morphology reminiscent of native tissue without exogenous scaffolds but with external force. The examples of self-organization in tissue engineering, described in this section, follow this definition. In addition, many of these self-organizing tissues display some degree of biomechanical, metabolic, or electrical properties (defined as functional properties). In contrast to the self-assembling process, all of these techniques use external forces, such as physical manipulation or thermal input, to direct cell position, after which cell-driven remodeling (e.g. tissue fusion) occurs. For these reasons, *self-organization in tissue engineering* is not synonymous with the *self-assembling process in tissue engineering*.

11.2.1 Tendon and Ligament

A pressing need for ligament and tendon tissue engineering exists, underscored by the more than 33 million soft tissue injuries in the United States each year [65]. Self-organizing tendons and ligaments recapitulate native tissue structure and morphology, although the process by which this occurs is uncharacterized. Several techniques exist for engineering ligament and tendon, but the most common method uses an adherent, protein-coated (usually laminin) sylgard culture plate, where self-organization of a seeded monolayer around two anchors leads to formation of a cylindrical tissue within 2 weeks [61,62]. The tensile forces imparted by the anchors are necessary to maintain a cylindrical construct. It is unclear if degradation of the initial laminin coat plays a role in this self-organization, and evaluation of cell-to-cell and cell-to-matrix interactions during this process has not been performed. Cadherin-11 has been implicated in development of tendon [66], but its expression during self-organization of these tissue constructs is unknown and should be investigated. However, ligament and tendon tissues engineered in this manner display morphologically relevant collagen fiber alignment, and ultrastructure similar to neo-natal tendon [61,62,67]. Furthermore, for comparison, a self-organization approach can create tendon-like tissue of up to 3 cm in length, while tissue generated with scaffoldless rotary culture has morphological deformities [68].

Self-organizing ligaments and tendons display notable functional properties. Mechanical testing of these tissues has produced tangent modulus values of 15–17 MPa, as well as abundant collagen I and III staining [61,62]. In addition, implantation of tendon or ligament constructs leads to functional maturation in vivo [67,69]. After 4 week subcutaneous implantation in rats, tendon constructs display an increase in tangent modulus over three orders of magnitude, as well as increases in collagen content and collagen fiber diameter over in vitro controls [67]. Similarly, interfacial bone–ligament–bone constructs implanted over 1–2 months in a rat model display significant increases in Young's modulus to 35 MPa, nearing neonatal tissue values [69]. Due to their interfacial nature and the lack of an intervening scaffold, self-organizing tendon and ligament have also been integrated with other tissues. Two examples are muscle and bone, where functional parameters such as isometric force and Young's modulus, respectively, have been found to be on the same order of magnitude as native tissue [69,70]. In conclusion, self-organizing tendon and ligament constructs should be further pursued, especially in terms of evaluating properties of interfacial constructs.

11.2.2 Liver

Up to 30 million individuals exhibit liver disease in the United States [71]. Liver tissue engineering aims to address this problem as well as to provide a solution for drug and toxicology screening. Self-organization for liver tissue engineering typically consists of seeding hepatocytes on a surface coated with a layer of collagen or glycoproteins. After a time period of several hours or days, the hepatocytes self-organize into spheroid structures [58,72]. Self-organization of hepatocyte spheroids appears to be dependent on actin function, as disruption by cytochalasin D has been reported [73]. It has also been shown that the size of these self-organizing spheroids is linearly correlated with initial cell seeding concentration [74].

Self-organization of liver tissue exhibits many characteristics of the self-assembling process. However, self-organization of liver tissue uses an initial adherent substrate for tissue formation. In addition to this, phases recapitulative of native liver development are not present. Therefore, this approach is classified as self-organization in tissue engineering. Self-organizing liver spheroids have been shown to display a rise and plateau in E-cadherin mRNA expression several days after cell seeding, which is similar to E-cadherin expression during hepatic plate development [75,76]. Self-organizing liver spheroids are also larger than micromasses generated using other scaffoldless techniques, and have reached sizes of up to 2.5 mm in diameter. Finally, self-organizing spheroids display several desirable structural/organizational features of developing liver tissue, such as bile canalicular formation, cell-to-cell communication, cuboidal hepatocyte morphology, and even sorting of liver progenitor cell subpopulations [76–78].

Self-organizing liver tissue displays several liver-specific metabolic functions. Spheroids containing both hepatocytes and hepatic stellate cells exhibit albumin secretion rates equivalent to those of freshly isolated hepatocytes and prolonged secretion of the oxidation enzyme cytochrome P-450 over several weeks [58]. Engineered tissue can also produce more α1-antitrypsin than individual hepatocytes on a per cell basis [48]. Functional urea production and bile excretion into canaliculi have also been reported [79,80]. Although these results bode well for the continued development of liver tissue, more work stands to be carried out evaluating these self-organizing tissues for a wider variety of metabolic functions.

11.2.3 Vascular

With 8 million patients suffering from peripheral arterial disease alone, self-organizing blood vessels have great clinical applicability [81]. Work on the underlying biological mechanisms of self-organizing vasculature is not prevalent, but these tissues display quantifiable functional properties. This method is achieved by high-density seeding of smooth muscle cells in annular agarose wells, similar to the ring-mold used in generating meniscus-shaped fibrocartilage [82–84]. After a culture period of 8 days, tissue rings form, which are then manually aligned on a silicone mandrel to fuse into a vascular tube [83]. Thus, the formation of the final tissue morphology follows exogenous physical manipulation.

Although this process uses non-adherent agarose as a substrate, little characterization of cell-to-cell interaction has been performed, and therefore the role of energy minimization in formation of this vasculature is unknown. Furthermore, the distinct layering of native blood vessels, composed of an inner endothelial lining, a medial smooth muscle cell layer, and an outer adventitia rich in ECM, is not present. Rather, these constructs are composed solely of a medial smooth muscle cell layer, and any distinct developmental phases during formation of these constructs are unspecified. However, constructs have been generated in this manner using both rat and human smooth muscle cells, increasing translatability [83]. Functional properties of these tissue constructs have also been assessed, and self-organizing vasculature has resulted in tissue with tensile moduli of up to 2 MPa [83]. Self-organizing vasculature represents an area for further research in tissue engineering.

11.2.4 Bone

In 2005, half a million bone grafts were performed in the United States, at an estimated cost of $2.5 billion [85]. To reduce the need for these grafts and develop technologies for other bone-related defects, tissue engineers are investigating self-organizing bone. Self-organization of bone starts with seeding bone marrow stromal cells onto a laminin-coated sylgard dish, where cells attach and form a monolayer. Similar to tendon and ligament, two anchors are used to impart tensile stress to the monolayer as it contracts and self-organizes into a cylindrical tissue several centimeters in length [86,87]. By comparison, scaffoldless bone culture on an orbital shaker does not form large, macroscopic tissue [88].

Bone tissue generated in this manner satisfies only some parts of the definition of the self-assembling process and displays some drawbacks in comparison to scaffold-based approaches. Self-organizing bone constructs have not been examined for cell-to-cell interactions, but since cadherin-11 is implicated in bone development [89], it represents one candidate for investigation. Self-organizing bone displays morphological properties similar to native tissue. Structures associated with these bone constructs include localization of osteocytes in lacunae, formation of lumen-containing structures similar to blood vessels, and development of cellular areas similar to bone marrow after implantation [51,86]. The developmental phases in the formation of these structures, if any, thus represent another area for further investigation. Self-organizing bone has also been assayed in terms of functional mechanical properties. Bone constructs with tangent modulus reaching 29 MPa and compressive strength surpassing 1.5 MPa after 6 weeks in culture have been reported [86,90]. These studies are encouraging, but it should be noted that values for mechanical properties of native bone are substantially higher, and that the compressive strength of recent composite scaffolds used in bone tissue engineering has been reported at up to 35 MPa [91]. Thus, more work, regarding functional mechanical properties (especially in compression), vascular morphology, and cadherins involved in generation of this bone tissue, needs to be pursued.

11.2.5 Optic and Nerve Tissues

Self-organization in engineering of tissues of the eye displays a highly coordinated process but has several barriers to applicability. Recently, tissue engineering resulting in self-organization of the complex tissues of the optic cup was described [60]. This approach began with culture of embryonic stem cells, which displayed early N-cadherin expression followed by sequential phases consistent with in vivo development [60]. When blocked with the ROCK inhibitor Y-27632, self-organization was attenuated, highlighting the role of the cytoskeleton in this process [92]. Some degree of native morphology is also apparent, with invagination of the optic cup and stratification of neurosensory tissue [60]. However, functional properties of photoreceptors and other relevant parts of the tissue require further investigation. The generation of tissues of a size that would be relevant to clinical application is also unclear. For comparison, scaffoldless cultures of optic retina and cornea using rotational culture and centrifugation, respectively, have also been pursued, but as of yet no functional properties of these tissues have been characterized [93,94].

Nerve tissue engineering is exciting for treatment of 15 million sufferers from Alzheimer's disease and other neurodegenerative disorders in the United States today [95]. Self-organization of nerves is accomplished by seeding fibroblasts on an adherent layer of laminin, with subsequent seeding of a layer of nerve cells. Contraction-inducing media is then introduced, and the two cell layers self-organize and roll into a cylindrical nerve with a fibroblast sheath [59,96]. Functional conduction velocities of these constructs have been measured at 12.5 m/s, equivalent to rat neo-natal sciatic nerve [59]. Furthermore, similar nerves have been engineered in conjunction with glial-like cells differentiated from adipose-derived stem cells, increasing the translational potential of this approach [96]. These tissues hold great regenerative potential and warrant continued investigation of functional properties, adhesion receptors involved in nerve self-organization, and unexplored phases of development.

11.3 Biological Mechanisms Underlying the Self-Assembling Process

The self-assembling process is achieved by the minimization of free energy aided by the use of a non-adherent mold, which prevents cell attachment and encourages cell-to-cell interaction [97,98]. Indeed, it has been shown that self-assembling chondrocytes upregulate N-cadherin early on in the process [99]. The high amount of cell-to-cell interaction, characteristic of the self-assembling process, will result in sorting of different cell subpopulations. Therefore, it is important to understand cell sorting and the underlying biological mechanisms responsible for cell sorting. Tissue fusion may also occur during the self-assembling process. Tissue fusion may be defined as the process by which two or more cell populations make contact and adhere [100]. This process may involve cell-to-cell or cell-to-ECM interactions and/or ECM production [100]. Recent articles [100,101] have addressed the topic of tissue fusion, so it will not be discussed here. Because it exhibits these underlying biological mechanisms, the self-assembling process is reminiscent of, though not exactly identical to, native tissue morphogenesis.

11.3.1 The Differential Adhesion Hypothesis and the Self-Assembling Process as an Energy-Driven Process

Early studies demonstrating that dissociated embryonic cells sort in vitro motivated investigation into what mechanism drove this behavior. One explanation, known as the differential adhesion hypothesis, advocated a thermodynamics-based mechanism [102, 103]. This hypothesis postulates that "cell segregation phenomena ... arise from tissue surface tensions that in turn arise from differences in intercellular adhesiveness" [104,105]. Subsequent work has revealed that tissue surface tension is directly correlated to the number of adhesion receptors expressed in a tissue [104]. Cadherins are homophilic cell-to-cell adhesion receptors that comprise a primary type of receptor studied in relation to cell sorting [104]. Thus, cell populations with similar cadherin expression levels and/or function will bind preferentially to one another, eventually resulting in the sorting of distinct cell populations within one continuous aggregate. Cell aggregates with the greatest intercellular adhesion (and thus the greatest tissue surface tension) will sort to the core of an aggregate, while cells with the least intercellular adhesion (and the least tissue surface tension) will sort to the periphery of an aggregate [106].

Mathematically, cells in an aggregate are organized in such a way as to decrease an aggregate's Gibbs free energy (G), according to the thermodynamic equation $\Delta G = \Delta H - T\Delta S$. To reduce free energy, total enthalpy (H) or entropy (S) of a system must decrease during cell sorting at constant temperature (T) and pressure. Minimization of free energy also results in minimization of surface tension (γ) of the aggregate, which is the derivative of free energy with respect to aggregate surface area (A), i.e., $\gamma = dG/dA$. It is important to realize that the intercellular adhesion and surface tension of any cell at a given instant in time does not change. However, the surface tension of the tissue as a whole depends on the intercellular adhesion of cells within the tissue and is especially dependent on cells comprising the boundary between the tissue and the environment [107].

Similar to its use in describing the sorting of embryonic cells, the differential adhesion hypothesis may be used to explain phenomena of the self-assembling process. Indeed, increased cadherin expression is seen during the initial phases of the process, although other proteins may also contribute to intracellular adhesion [99]. When cells are placed in high density into a non-adherent mold, cells are prevented from attaching to the substratum and express high levels of N-cadherin, thus minimizing their overall free energy by intercellular adhesion [97,98].

Even in the case of a homogeneous cell population, where no cell sorting occurs, the self-assembling process follows the minimization of free energy through intercellular adhesion [99]. Consider the presence of multiple aggregates, all composed of the same cell type. As separate aggregates, the sum of their surface areas is greater than the surface area of a single aggregate. By self-assembling into one single aggregate, a large decrease in surface area occurs. As per $\gamma = dG/dA$, to maintain a positive surface tension (γ), decreases in area (A) must be accompanied by decreases in free energy (G). Minimizing free energy therefore drives multiple aggregates to self-assemble into one continuous aggregate.

When two cell aggregates are combined during the self-assembling process, minimization of free energy also occurs through cell sorting. If large differences in surface tension and intercellular adhesiveness exist between these two cell aggregates, in order to minimize surface tension (γ) of the aggregate as a whole, the aggregate with the greatest intercellular adhesion will sort to the center of the self-assembling tissue. The aggregate with less intercellular adhesion will sort to the periphery of the self-assembling tissue. In cases where the surface tensions of the individual aggregates are approximately equal, other sorting patterns may manifest. In general, the self-assembling tissue will be organized such that intercellular adhesion is maximized in the center of the tissue, surface tension (γ) is minimized through the less adhesive cells comprising the boundary of the tissue, and surface free energy (G) is minimized since potential adhesiveness at the boundary of the tissue is reduced. As a reminder, it is important to note that this process occurs free of external forces and adherent substrates. Therefore, the differential adhesion hypothesis provides an energy-driven thermodynamic explanation of the biological mechanisms underlying the self-assembling process in tissue engineering.

11.3.2 Cell Contraction and the Cytoskeleton in Cell Sorting

Although the differential adhesion hypothesis emphasizes the function of intercellular adhesion in driving cell sorting, support also exists for other factors being involved [107–111]. Specifically, differences in cytoskeletal organization and/or contractility have been linked to cell sorting, and thus quantification of cortical cell tension, contractile function of a cell, or contact angle between cell membranes and surrounding media have been investigated [107,108]. In this model, for "the case of a cell... in contact with the medium, the interfacial tension is actually a surface tension" [109]. A cell with a highly organized, contractile cytoskeleton will have a greater surface tension with surrounding media, and given an aggregate with large enough cell-to-media surface tension, it will tend to be enveloped by another aggregate of cells with smaller cell-to-media surface tension [109,112]. Recent work has shown that cell cortical tension, which may be used as a "read-out" of cytoskeleton organization, may be necessary and sufficient for determining cell sorting, and that normal sorting was reversed by the use of a cytoskeleton-specific mutation [107]. Therefore, hypotheses labeled as "differential interfacial tension" or "differential surface contraction" emphasize that mechanical interactions among the cell membrane and cytoskeleton determine the cell sorting process [109,110].

It is important to note that the hypotheses of differential adhesion and differential tension/contraction may be related (Fig. 11.3). Clearly, cells with different interfacial or surface tensions due to cytoskeletal organization still require attachment or motility to achieve sorting. Indeed, some mathematical models of cell sorting have proposed that differences in cytoskeleton organization may be primarily relevant because of their effects on cell motility [113].

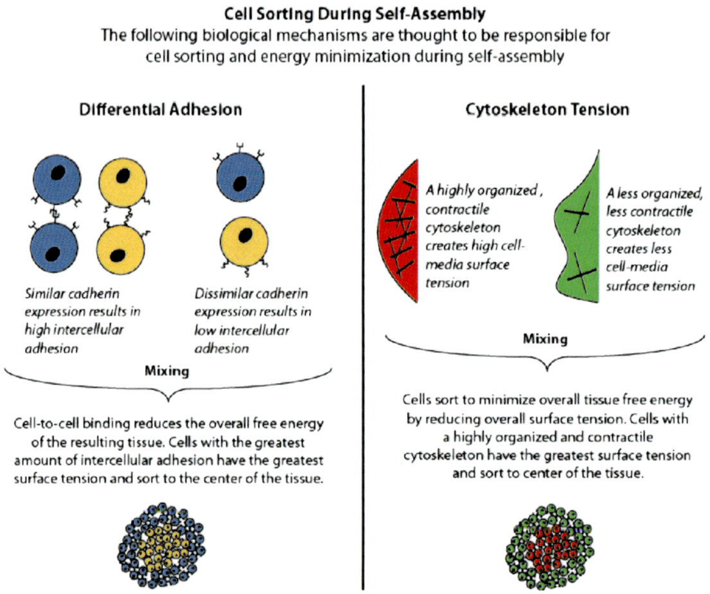

Cell Sorting During Self-Assembly
The following biological mechanisms are thought to be responsible for cell sorting and energy minimization during self-assembly

Differential Adhesion

Similar cadherin expression results in high intercellular adhesion

Dissimilar cadherin expression results in low intercellular adhesion

Mixing

Cell-to-cell binding reduces the overall free energy of the resulting tissue. Cells with the greatest amount of intercellular adhesion have the greatest surface tension and sort to the center of the tissue.

Cytoskeleton Tension

A highly organized, contractile cytoskeleton creates high cell-media surface tension

A less organized, less contractile cytoskeleton creates less cell-media surface tension

Mixing

Cells sort to minimize overall tissue free energy by reducing overall surface tension. Cells with a highly organized and contractile cytoskeleton have the greatest surface tension and sort to center of the tissue.

Figure 11.3 Biological mechanisms underlying the self-assembling process relating to cell sorting, as explained by the differential adhesion hypothesis and the differential interfacial tension hypothesis. These two mechanisms may work in conjunction. The differential adhesion hypothesis emphasizes that minimization of free energy is driven by differences in tissue surface tensions resulting from differences in intercellular adhesiveness. The differential interfacial tension hypothesis emphasizes that cell sorting is driven by differences in interfacial tension between cells due to mechanical interactions.

In addition, one recent study validates observations of both hypotheses, confirming that induced germ layer cells display differential binding affinity and cadherin expression, as well as different cell cortical tensions [107]. In conclusion, cell sorting and the self-assembling process in tissue engineering are thought to be influenced by both cell-to-cell adhesion receptors (which are necessary for intercellular binding and appear to promote cell sorting) and cytoskeleton organization (which is necessary for cell motility and also appears to promote cell sorting) [99,107,111].

11.4 The Self-Assembling Process in Tissue Engineering: Articular Cartilage and Fibrocartilage

In this section, examples of engineering articular cartilage and fibrocartilage will be used as a model to detail the self-assembling process. Articular cartilage is an avascular and almost acellular tissue, in which injury or trauma often leads to osteoarthritis or degradation of cartilage [114]. The meniscus is a fibrocartilaginous tissue that protects the underlying articular cartilage from excessive stresses through force distribution and shock absorption [115]. Meniscus tears may lead to meniscectomy, which over the long-term results in osteoarthritis [116]. Presently, osteoarthritis affects 27 million Americans [117]. Due to the characteristics described below, tissue engineering of cartilage and fibrocartilage using the self-assembling process represents a promising treatment for osteoarthritis. This is because the ultimate goal of tissue engineering is to synthesize neo-tissue in a manner similar to natural morphogenesis, resulting in tissue with correct morphology and dimensions, which displays functional properties approaching those of native tissue.

11.4.1 Distinct Phases of Self-Assembling Cartilage Reminiscent of Morphogenesis

During the self-assembling process of articular cartilage, there is a distinct set of phases that is recapitulative of native tissue formation and development (Fig. 11.4). The first two phases encompass tissue formation as part of minimization of free energy,

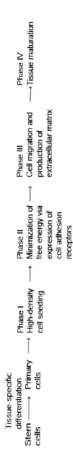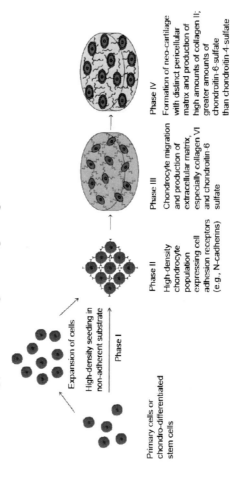

Figure 11.4 Various phases of the self-assembling process: cell seeding, cell recognition, matrix production, and tissue maturation. The distinct phases of the self-assembling process recapitulate the morphogenesis of native tissue.

as previously described in the biological mechanism section. As illustrated by articular cartilage, the first phase of the self-assembling process is the seeding of articular chondrocytes in high density into non-adherent agarose molds [118]. This promotes cell-to-cell interaction and/or cell sorting. Similar to articular cartilage, in fibrocartilage, high-density co-cultures of chondrocytes and fibrochondrocytes are seeded into meniscus-shaped non-adherent agarose molds to form meniscus-shaped tissue [82]. Alternatively, 2-hydroxyethyl methacrylate [119] and semi-permeable membranes [120] have also been used as non-adherent substrates. In the second phase of the self-assembling process, seeded chondrocytes express high levels of N-cadherin to minimize free energy, resulting in the formation of neo-tissue without the use of exogenous forces [99]. This is similar to the process of mesenchymal condensation, during which N-cadherin is highly expressed to enhance cell-to-cell interaction [121].

The third and fourth phases of the self-assembling process in articular cartilage recapitulate tissue development. In the third phase, chondrocytes migrate apart and secrete collagen VI and chondroitin-6-sulfate, similar to what is observed in morphogenesis [99]. Finally, in the fourth phase of development, collagen II and chondroitin-4-sulfate are secreted, and the secreted collagen VI localizes to form distinct areas of pericellular matrix surrounding cells. Production of collagen and relative levels of chondroitin-6-sulphate to chondroitin-4-sulphate in this phase also mimic those seen during native cartilage formation [99]. Therefore, the multiple phases of the self-assembling process mimic processes seen in native cartilage formation and development.

11.4.2 Native Tissue Dimensions and Morphology in Self-Assembling Cartilage

An important characteristic of the self-assembling process in tissue engineering is the recapitulation of native tissue dimensions and morphology. Articular cartilage constructs up to 3 mm thick, in various curvatures and sizes, can be generated. Similarly, both native gross and histological morphologies can be recapitulated. Chondrocytes rest in lacunae, surrounded by collagen type VI-rich pericellular and collagen type II rich-interterritorial matrices, and zonal arrangement can be seen with columnar cell arrangement in the center of self-assembling articular cartilage [122,123]. Self-assembling articular cartilage of clinically relevant sizes may provide a suitable treatment option for cartilage lesions.

Similarly, self-assembling meniscus tissue displays the semilunar, wedge-shaped gross morphology and circumferential collagen alignment seen in native menisci [82]. Since the geometry and structure of knee meniscus fibrocartilage is crucial for its loading functions [124], the wedge-shaped profile of self-assembling meniscus fibrocartilage can be used to recapitulate load distribution between the naturally incongruous curvatures of the femoral condyles and the tibial plateau [125]. Other fibrocartilages, such as those in the TMJ [126], will also require the engineering of tissues possessing specific dimensions, shapes, and zonal morphologies. The ability of the self-assembling process to create shape-specific tissues enhances the clinical applicability of this tissue engineering technique.

11.4.3 Near-Native Biomechanical Properties of Self-Assembling Cartilage

Self-assembling, engineered tissues display not only biomechanical properties approaching native tissue values, but also anisotropic properties that are critical to tissue function. As an example, the biomechanical properties of articular cartilage and fibrocartilage are conferred by ECM components and their interactions. Immature, self-assembling articular cartilage displays near-native levels of glycosaminoglycans and a corresponding compressive aggregate modulus of 280 kPa [127]; tensile stiffness, mostly conferred by collagen, can reach 2 MPa [122]. As another example, self-assembling fibrocartilage displays compressive instantaneous modulus of up to 800 kPa and tensile stiffness of up to 3 MPa [123,128]. Self-assembling fibrocartilage in a ring-shaped mold also displays a greater tensile modulus in the circumferential direction (226 kPa) than in the radial direction (67 kPa). This spontaneous formation of anisotropy is seldom seen in other forms of meniscus tissue engineering. In summary, the self-assembling process for articular cartilage mimics the biomechanical properties, gross morphology, and developmental phases of native tissue, and may be used as a model for other self-assembling tissues.

11.5 Signals Used to Engineer Self-Organizing and Self-Assembling Tissues

In the context of the tissue engineering paradigm, stimuli in tissue engineering can be broadly divided into soluble and mechanical stimuli. Both types of stimuli have been applied to self-organizing and self-assembling tissues to increase functional properties. Soluble stimuli dominate the literature for engineering liver and optic tissues, while both soluble and mechanical stimuli are used for engineering mechanically functional vasculature and musculoskeletal tissues.

11.5.1 Soluble Signals

Growth factors, small molecules, and enzymes have all been employed as stimuli for self-organizing and self-assembling tissues. As some of the most successful and potent stimuli in tissue engineering, growth factors have been used for liver, articular cartilage, and fibrocartilage tissues. Epidermal growth factor allows for the recapitulation of liver-specific functional properties when applied to self-organizing hepatocytes [73]. In response to TGF-β1, self-assembling articular cartilage and fibrocartilage develop near-native compressive properties [129]. Small molecules, such as ascorbic acid, have been used as supplements for self-organizing cornea, vasculature, tendon, and cartilaginous tissues to promote ECM production [97,130–132].

In addition to anabolic stimuli, agents that are expected to act directly on the ECM have been used. Ribose, used as a non-specific glycation agent, also strengthens self-assembling tissues [133]. Via collagen crosslinking, ribose treatment significantly improves cartilage compressive stiffness values by 40%, tensile stiffness by 44%, and tensile strength by 126% over untreated controls. In self-assembling constructs, ECM remodeling can be initiated by enzymes [134]. Chondroitinase-ABC (C-ABC), an enzyme that temporarily removes glycosaminoglycans, brings fibers within self-assembling cartilage into closer proximity to result in a denser collagen network, and thereby increases tensile modulus and ultimate tensile strength to 3.4 and 1.4 MPa, respectively. Since some of these soluble factors (e.g., ascorbic acid) are beneficial for multiple tissues, successes in one area of tissue engineering may borrow from soluble factors identified in other types of tissues. For example, growth factors that have been successful in liver tissue engineering may also improve the properties of self-organizing cornea and vasculature. Similarly, molecules and enzymes to induce collagen crosslinking and remodeling should be investigated in these two collagen-rich tissues.

11.5.2 Mechanical Signals

Mechanotransduction is a process in which cells convert mechanical forces into biochemical signals. Mechanically functional tissues such as ligament, bone, cartilage, and fibrocartilage all respond positively to mechanical stimuli [128,135–138]. An example where the effects of multiple mechanical stimuli have been demonstrated in tissue engineering is self-assembling articular cartilage. Exposing these constructs to 10 MPa of hydrostatic pressure at 1 Hz leads to greater collagen content over controls and retained glycosaminoglycans [135]. Other mechanical stimuli (shear, compression, and hydrostatic pressure) have also demonstrated beneficial effects for self-assembling articular cartilage or fibrocartilage, which is significant since the main function of this tissue is to bear and/or distribute load [128,136,137].

In recent years, investigations into the mechanisms of mechanotransduction have produced strong evidence implicating the involvement of ions and ion channels. As reviewed [139], hydrostatic pressure has been hypothesized to result in changes in streaming potential or altered protein conformation, and deformations of the cell membrane through shear or direct compression can stretch or activate ion channels. Inspired by this, chemical agents have been employed to duplicate mechanical loading. For instance, ouabain and ionomycin are ion channel regulators that increase collagen and glycosaminoglycan synthesis in self-assembling articular cartilage in a manner similar to hydrostatic pressure stimulus [140]. It is conceivable that similar agents may be identified for vascular tissues. The potential benefits of using such chemical equivalents to mechanical stimuli include better control and earlier application of the stimulus. Molecules that duplicate mechanical loading can be applied uniformly within self-organizing and self-assembling constructs before sufficient matrix has developed to bear load, thus shortening culture time before implantation.

The role of the mold in the self-assembling process is also expected to be significant insofar as the mechanical environment experienced by the cells is concerned. For example, the anti-adhesive properties of the walls of the mold may contribute to the mechanical forces experience by the growing neo-tissue [141]. Similarly, the roughness of the mold surface may affect the frictional forces experienced by the construct, resulting in altered mechanotransduction [142]. The shape of a mold can promote the generation of pre-stresses within self-assembling tissue [82]. For instance, a smooth ring-shaped 1% agarose mold increases the tensile properties and collagen content of fibrocartilage constructs, while the compressive modulus and total GAG are higher in smooth 2% agarose molds [142]. Additionally, collagen II production relative to collagen I production is significantly enhanced in smooth molds compared to rough molds [142]. Thus, selection of an appropriate mold is critical toward achieving enhanced functional properties.

11.5.3 Coordinated Soluble and Mechanical Signaling

Application of multiple stimuli is a promising approach to improve the functional properties of self-organizing and self-assembling tissues. For instance, combined application of ascorbic acid and TGF-β1 in self-organizing nerve constructs has resulted in near-native nerve conduction velocities [59]. TGF-β1 combined with hydrostatic pressure synergistically increases articular cartilage construct functional properties [127]. Likewise, combined treatment of catabolic (C-ABC) and anabolic (TGF-β1) agents with direct compression on anatomically shaped self-assembling meniscus constructs results in additive increases in collagen (4-fold), compressive stiffness (3-fold), and tensile strength (6-fold) [128]. The mechanisms for how additive and/or synergistic effects arise from combinations of stimuli are not yet completely understood. However, the benefits reaped by applying such regimens should encourage future studies in this area.

11.6 Conclusion and Future Directions

The self-assembling process in tissue engineering is defined as *the formation of tissue using a scaffoldless platform, where cells self-organize without external forces to minimize overall free energy.*

The self-assembling process in tissue engineering represents progress towards recapitulating native tissue morphogenesis. The mechanisms of free energy minimization and cell sorting underlying the self-assembling process are reminiscent of the processes that occur during native tissue formation. The phases of development exhibited during the self-assembling process also follow those of native tissue. Additionally, the large dimensions and correct morphologies of tissue generated are significant and important for clinical application. Lastly, the functional properties of self-assembling tissues attained thus far exemplify promising advances in tissue engineering.

The self-assembling process and self-organization are separate subsets within scaffoldless in tissue engineering. The rapid and growing adoption of scaffoldless techniques, such as the self-assembling process and self-organization, has led to alternate approaches of tissue engineering which avoid disadvantages of scaffolds and generate tissue with substantial biomechanical, metabolic, and electrical properties. Additionally, these approaches share advantages such as the encouragement of cell-to-cell interaction and the promotion of natural growth and/or remodeling. Because of these promising results, more research needs to be done in these areas.

Future investigations are necessary to enhance self-organization and the self-assembling process for wider use. As with all tissue engineering approaches, these scaffoldless techniques require a large number of cells to produce clinically applicable tissue constructs. However, isolation of large numbers of primary cells from a single donor is impractical. Therefore, stem cells represent a promising cell source for tissue engineering. Co-cultures may also reduce the number of primary cells necessary and provide other benefits. For instance, co-cultures have been used in cornea, liver, nerve, bone, and fibrocartilage tissue engineering, reducing the number of primary cells required and increasing functional properties [58,59,143,144]. Finally, although various soluble and mechanical stimuli have been used with success, identifying additional beneficial stimuli or combinations of stimuli is a long-term challenge. Work on the application of mechanical or electrical stimuli in appropriate tissues (i.e., bone and nerve, respectively) needs to be performed, especially with regard to temporal studies and treatment regimens.

Finally, many tissues exhibit zonal and/or regional variation. It is important to explore ways in which to engineer tissues with their native organization. Taken together, exploring these challenges and opportunities in tissue engineering will help pave the way towards effective clinical treatments.

Acknowledgments

We gratefully acknowledge support provided by the National Institutes of Health (R01AR053286, R01DE015038, R01DE019666, R01AR047839, and R01AR061496), the Arthritis Foundation, NFL Charities, and the Howard Hughes Medical Institute.

References

1. Krause K, Jaquet K, Schneider C, Haupt S, Lioznov MV, Otte KM, Kuck KH. Percutaneous intramyocardial stem cell injection in patients with acute myocardial infarction: first-in-man study. *Heart.* 2009; **95**: 1145–52.
2. Karp JM, Leng Teo GS. Mesenchymal stem cell homing: the devil is in the details. *Cell Stem Cell.* 2009; **4**: 206–216.
3. Horiguchi K, Hirano T, Ueki T, Hirakawa K, Fujimoto J. Treating liver cirrhosis in dogs with hepatocyte growth factor gene therapy via the hepatic artery. *J Hepatobiliary Pancreat Surg.* 2009; **16**: 171–177.
4. Ueki T, Kaneda Y, Tsutsui H, Nakanishi K, Sawa Y, Morishita R, Matsumoto K, Nakamura T, Takahashi H, Okamoto E, Fujimoto J. Hepatocyte growth factor gene therapy of liver cirrhosis in rats. *Nat Med.* 1999; **5**: 226–230.
5. Walsh AJ, Bradford DS, Lotz JC. In vivo growth factor treatment of degenerated intervertebral discs. *Spine* (Philadelphia, PA, 1976). 2004; **29**: 156–163.
6. Brown GL, Nanney LB, Griffen J, Cramer AB, Yancey JM, Curtsinger LJ, 3rd, Holtzin L, Schultz GS, Jurkiewicz MJ, Lynch JB. Enhancement of wound healing by topical treatment with epidermal growth factor. *N Engl J Med.* 1989; **321**: 76–79.
7. Vunjak-Novakovic G, Martin I, Obradovic B, Treppo S, Grodzinsky AJ, Langer R, Freed LE. Bioreactor cultivation conditions modulate the composition and mechanical properties of tissue-engineered cartilage. *J Orthop Res.* 1999; **17**: 130–138.

8. Meredith JC, Sormana JL, Keselowsky BG, Garcia AJ, Tona A, Karim A, Amis EJ. Combinatorial characterization of cell interactions with polymer surfaces. *J Biomed Mater Res A.* 2003; **66**: 483–490.

9. Yoon DM, Fisher JP. Chondrocyte signaling and artificial matrices for articular cartilage engineering. *Adv Exp Med Biol.* 2006; **585**: 67–86.

10. Barbero A, Grogan SP, Mainil-Varlet P, Martin I. Expansion on specific substrates regulates the phenotype and differentiation capacity of human articular chondrocytes. *J Cell Biochem.* 2006; **98**: 1140–1149.

11. Elder SH, Sanders SW, McCulley WR, Marr ML, Shim JW, Hasty KA. Chondrocyte response to cyclic hydrostatic pressure in alginate versus pellet culture. *J Orthop Res.* 2006; **24**: 740–747.

12. Bryant SJ, Anseth KS, Lee DA, Bader DL. Crosslinking density influences the morphology of chondrocytes photoencapsulated in PEG hydrogels during the application of compressive strain. *J Orthop Res.* 2004; **22**: 1143–1149.

13. Saeidi N, Guo X, Hutcheon AE, Sander EA, Bale SS, Melotti SA, Zieske JD, Trinkaus-Randall V, Ruberti JW. Disorganized collagen scaffold interferes with fibroblast mediated deposition of organized extracellular matrix in vitro. *Biotechnol Bioeng.* 2012; **109**: 2683–2698.

14. Ulrich TA, Lee TG, Shon HK, Moon DW, Kumar S. Microscale mechanisms of agarose-induced disruption of collagen remodeling. *Biomaterials.* 2011; **32**: 5633–5642.

15. Anderson JM. Biological responses to materials. *Ann Rev Mater Res.* 2001; **31**: 81–110.

16. Discher DE, Janmey P, Wang YL. Tissue cells feel and respond to the stiffness of their substrate. *Science.* 2005; **310**: 1139–1143.

17. Rosso F, Giordano A, Barbarisi M, Barbarisi A. From cell-ECM interactions to tissue engineering. *J Cell Physiol.* 2004; **199**: 174–180.

18. Burdick JA, Anseth KS. Photoencapsulation of osteoblasts in injectable RGD-modified PEG hydrogels for bone tissue engineering. *Biomaterials.* 2002; **23**: 4315–4323.

19. Richardson TP, Peters MC, Ennett AB, Mooney DJ. Polymeric system for dual growth factor delivery. *Nat Biotechnol.* 2001; **19**: 1029–1034.

20. Wang X, Wenk E, Zhang X, Meinel L, Vunjak-Novakovic G, Kaplan DL. Growth factor gradients via microsphere delivery in biopolymer scaffolds for osteochondral tissue engineering. *J Control Release.* 2009; **134**: 81–90.

21. Burkus JK, Heim SE, Gornet MF, Zdeblick TA. Is INFUSE bone graft superior to autograft bone? An integrated analysis of clinical trials using the LT-CAGE lumbar tapered fusion device. *J Spinal Disord Tech.* 2003; **16**: 113–122.

22. Hollister SJ, Murphy WL. Scaffold translation: barriers between concept and clinic. *Tissue Eng Part B Rev.* 2011; **17**: 459–474.

23. Holtzer H, Abbott J, Lash J, Holtzer S. The Loss of Phenotypic Traits by Differentiated Cells in Vitro, I. Dedifferentiation of Cartilage Cells. *Proc Natl Acad Sci U S A.* 1960; **46**: 1533–1542.

24. Manning WK, Bonner WM, Jr. Isolation and culture of chondrocytes from human adult articular cartilage. *Arthritis Rheum.* 1967; **10**: 235–239.

25. Mietsch A, Neidlinger-Wilke C, Schrezenmeier H, Mauer UM, Friemert B, Wilke HJ, Ignatius A. Evaluation of platelet-rich plasma and hydrostatic pressure regarding cell differentiation in nucleus pulposus tissue engineering. *J Tissue Eng Regen Med.* 2011; **7**: 244–252.

26. Matthies NF, Mulet-Sierra A, Jomha NM, Adesida AB. Matrix formation is enhanced in co-cultures of human meniscus cells with bone marrow stromal cells. *J Tissue Eng Regen Med.* 2012; doi: 10.1002/term.1489.

27. Gurkan UA, Kishore V, Condon KW, Bellido TM, Akkus O. A scaffold-free multicellular three-dimensional in vitro model of osteogenesis. *Calcif Tissue Int.* 2011; **88**: 388–401.

28. Ong SY, Dai H, Leong KW. Inducing hepatic differentiation of human mesenchymal stem cells in pellet culture. *Biomaterials.* 2006; **27**: 4087–4097.

29. Lee JM, Im GI. PTHrP isoforms have differing effect on chondrogenic differentiation and hypertrophy of mesenchymal stem cells. *Biochem Biophys Res Commun.* 2012; **421**: 819–824.

30. Castagnola P, Moro G, Descalzi-Cancedda F, Cancedda R. Type X collagen synthesis during in vitro development of chick embryo tibial chondrocytes. *J Cell Biol.* 1986; **102**: 2310–2317.

31. Tacchetti C, Quarto R, Nitsch L, Hartmann DJ, Cancedda R. In vitro morphogenesis of chick embryo hypertrophic cartilage. *J Cell Biol.* 1987; **105**: 999–1006.

32. Ferro F, Spelat R, D'Aurizio F, Falini G, De Pol I, Pandolfi M, Beltrami AP, Cesselli D, Beltrami CA, Ambesi Impiombato FS, Curcio F. Acellular bone colonization and aggregate culture conditions diversely influence murine periosteum mesenchymal stem cells differentiation potential in long-term in vitro osteo-inductive conditions. *Tissue Eng Part A.* 2012; **(13–14)**: 1509–1519.

33. Lim JJ, Scott L, Jr., Temenoff JS. Aggregation of bovine anterior cruciate ligament fibroblasts or marrow stromal cells promotes aggrecan production. *Biotechnol Bioeng.* 2011; **108**: 151–162.
34. Wolf F, Candrian C, Wendt D, Farhadi J, Heberer M, Martin I, Barbero A. Cartilage tissue engineering using pre-aggregated human articular chondrocytes. *Eur Cell Mater.* 2008; **16**: 92–99.
35. Dutt K, Cao Y. Engineering retina from human retinal progenitors (cell lines). *Tissue Eng Part A.* 2009; **15**: 1401–1413.
36. Matta SG, Wobken JD, Williams FG, Bauer GE. Pancreatic islet cell reaggregation systems: efficiency of cell reassociation and endocrine cell topography of rat islet-like aggregates. *Pancreas.* 1994; **9**: 439–449.
37. Solorio LD, Fu AS, Hernandez-Irizarry R, Alsberg E. Chondrogenic differentiation of human mesenchymal stem cell aggregates via controlled release of TGF-beta1 from incorporated polymer microspheres. *J Biomed Mater Res A.* 2010; **92**: 1139–1144.
38. Bratt-Leal AM, Kepple KL, Carpenedo RL, Cooke MT, McDevitt TC. Magnetic manipulation and spatial patterning of multi-cellular stem cell aggregates. *Integr Biol (Camb).* 2011; **3**: 1224–1232.
39. Kwon OH, Kikuchi A, Yamato M, Sakurai Y, Okano T. Rapid cell sheet detachment from poly(N-isopropylacrylamide)-grafted porous cell culture membranes. *J Biomed Mater Res.* 2000; **50**: 82–89.
40. Shimizu T, Yamato M, Isoi Y, Akutsu T, Setomaru T, Abe K, Kikuchi A, Umezu M, Okano T. Fabrication of pulsatile cardiac tissue grafts using a novel 3-dimensional cell sheet manipulation technique and temperature-responsive cell culture surfaces. *Circ Res.* 2002; **90**: e40.
41. L'Heureux N, Paquet S, Labbe R, Germain L, Auger FA. A completely biological tissue-engineered human blood vessel. *FASEB J.* 1998; **12**: 47–56.
42. Haraguchi Y, Shimizu T, Sasagawa T, Sekine H, Sakaguchi K, Kikuchi T, Sekine W, Sekiya S, Yamato M, Umezu M, Okano T. Fabrication of functional three-dimensional tissues by stacking cell sheets in vitro. *Nat Protoc.* 2012; **7**: 850–858.
43. L'Heureux N, Stoclet JC, Auger FA, Lagaud GJ, Germain L, Andriantsitohaina R. A human tissue-engineered vascular media: a new model for pharmacological studies of contractile responses. *FASEB J.* 2001; **15**: 515–524.
44. Haraguchi Y, Shimizu T, Yamato M, Okano T. Electrical interaction between cardiomyocyte sheets separated by non-cardiomyocyte sheets in heterogeneous tissues. *J Tissue Eng Regen Med.* 2010; **4**: 291–299.

45. Haraguchi Y, Shimizu T, Yamato M, Kikuchi A, Okano T. Electrical coupling of cardiomyocyte sheets occurs rapidly via functional gap junction formation. *Biomaterials*. 2006; **27**: 4765–4774.

46. McAllister TN, Maruszewski M, Garrido SA, Wystrychowski W, Dusserre N, Marini A, Zagalski K, Fiorillo A, Avila H, Manglano X, Antonelli J, Kocher A, Zembala M, Cierpka L, de la Fuente LM, L'Heureux N. Effectiveness of haemodialysis access with an autologous tissue-engineered vascular graft: a multicentre cohort study. *Lancet*. 2009; **373**: 1440–1446.

47. Wystrychowski W, Cierpka L, Zagalski K, Garrido S, Dusserre N, Radochonski S, McAllister TN, L'Heureux N. Case study: first implantation of a frozen, devitalized tissue-engineered vascular graft for urgent hemodialysis access. *J Vasc Access*. 2011; **12**: 67–70.

48. Ohashi K, Yokoyama T, Yamato M, Kuge H, Kanehiro H, Tsutsumi M, Amanuma T, Iwata H, Yang J, Okano T, Nakajima Y. Engineering functional two- and three-dimensional liver systems in vivo using hepatic tissue sheets. *Nat Med*. 2007; **13**: 880–885.

49. Kushida A, Yamato M, Kikuchi A, Okano T. Two-dimensional manipulation of differentiated Madin-Darby canine kidney (MDCK) cell sheets: the noninvasive harvest from temperature-responsive culture dishes and transfer to other surfaces. *J Biomed Mater Res*. 2001; **54**: 37–46.

50. Hayashida Y, Nishida K, Yamato M, Yang J, Sugiyama H, Watanabe K, Hori Y, Maeda N, Kikuchi A, Okano T, Tano Y. Transplantation of tissue-engineered epithelial cell sheets after excimer laser photoablation reduces postoperative corneal haze. *Invest Ophthalmol Vis Sci*. 2006; **47**: 552–557.

51. Pirraco RP, Obokata H, Iwata T, Marques AP, Tsuneda S, Yamato M, Reis RL, Okano T. Development of osteogenic cell sheets for bone tissue engineering applications. *Tissue Eng Part A*. 2011; **17**: 1507–1515.

52. Norotte C, Marga FS, Niklason LE, Forgacs G. Scaffold-free vascular tissue engineering using bioprinting. *Biomaterials*. 2009; **30**: 5910–5917.

53. Koch L, Deiwick A, Schlie S, Michael S, Gruene M, Coger V, Zychlinski D, Schambach A, Reimers K, Vogt PM, Chichkov B. Skin tissue generation by laser cell printing. *Biotechnol Bioeng*. 2012; **109**: 1855–1863.

54. Cui X, Breitenkamp K, Finn MG, Lotz M, D'Lima DD. Direct human cartilage repair using three-dimensional bioprinting technology. *Tissue Eng Part A*. 2012; **(11–12)**: 1304–1312.

55. Jakab K, Norotte C, Marga F, Murphy K, Vunjak-Novakovic G, Forgacs G. Tissue engineering by self-assembly and bio-printing of living cells. *Biofabrication*. 2010; **2**: 022001.
56. Mironov V, Reis N, Derby B. Review: bioprinting: a beginning. *Tissue Eng*. 2006; **12**: 631–634.
57. Marga F, Jakab K, Khatiwala C, Shepherd B, Dorfman S, Hubbard B, Colbert S, Gabor F. Toward engineering functional organ modules by additive manufacturing. *Biofabrication*. 2012; **4**: 022001.
58. Riccalton-Banks L, Liew C, Bhandari R, Fry J, Shakesheff K. Long-term culture of functional liver tissue: three-dimensional coculture of primary hepatocytes and stellate cells. *Tissue Eng*. 2003; **9**: 401–410.
59. Baltich J, Hatch-Vallier L, Adams AM, Arruda EM, Larkin LM. Development of a scaffoldless three-dimensional engineered nerve using a nerve-fibroblast co-culture. *In vitro Cell Dev Biol Anim*. 2010; **46**: 438–444.
60. Eiraku M, Takata N, Ishibashi H, Kawada M, Sakakura E, Okuda S, Sekiguchi K, Adachi T, Sasai Y. Self-organizing optic-cup morphogenesis in three-dimensional culture. *Nature*. 2011; **472**: 51–56.
61. Calve S, Dennis RG, Kosnik PE, 2nd, Baar K, Grosh K, Arruda EM. Engineering of functional tendon. *Tissue Eng*. 2004; **10**: 755–761.
62. Hairfield-Stein M, England C, Paek HJ, Gilbraith KB, Dennis R, Boland E, Kosnik P. Development of self-assembled, tissue-engineered ligament from bone marrow stromal cells. *Tissue Eng*. 2007; **13**: 703–710.
63. Whitesides GM, Boncheva M. Beyond molecules: self-assembly of mesoscopic and macroscopic components. *Proc Natl Acad Sci USA*. 2002; **99**: 4769–4774.
64. Whitesides GM, Grzybowski B. Self-assembly at all scales. *Science*. 2002; **295**: 2418–2421.
65. Butler DL, Awad HA. Perspectives on cell and collagen composites for tendon repair. *Clin Orthop Relat Res*. 1999: S324–S332.
66. Richardson SH, Starborg T, Lu Y, Humphries SM, Meadows RS, Kadler KE. Tendon development requires regulation of cell condensation and cell shape via cadherin-11-mediated cell-cell junctions. *Mol Cell Biol*. 2007; **27**: 6218–6228.
67. Calve S, Lytle IF, Grosh K, Brown DL, Arruda EM. Implantation increases tensile strength and collagen content of self-assembled tendon constructs. *J Appl Physiol*. 2010; **108**: 875–881.

68. de Wreede R, Ralphs JR. Deposition of collagenous matrices by tendon fibroblasts in vitro: a comparison of fibroblast behavior in pellet cultures and a novel three-dimensional long-term scaffoldless culture system. *Tissue Eng Part A.* 2009; **15**: 2707–2715.

69. Ma J, Goble K, Smietana M, Kostrominova T, Larkin L, Arruda EM. Morphological and functional characteristics of three-dimensional engineered bone–ligament–bone constructs following implantation. *J Biomech Eng.* 2009; **131**: 101017.

70. Larkin LM, Calve S, Kostrominova TY, Arruda EM. Structure and functional evaluation of tendon-skeletal muscle constructs engineered in vitro. *Tissue Eng.* 2006; **12**: 3149–3158.

71. Angulo P. Nonalcoholic fatty liver disease. *N Engl J Med.* 2002; **346**: 1221–1231.

72. Koide N, Sakaguchi K, Koide Y, Asano K, Kawaguchi M, Matsushima H, Takenami T, Shinji T, Mori M, Tsuji T. Formation of multicellular spheroids composed of adult rat hepatocytes in dishes with positively charged surfaces and under other nonadherent environments. *Exp Cell Res.* 1990; **186**: 227–235.

73. Tzanakakis ES, Hansen LK, Hu WS. The role of actin filaments and microtubules in hepatocyte spheroid self-assembly. *Cell Motil Cytoskeleton.* 2001; **48**: 175–189.

74. Torisawa YS, Takagi A, Nashimoto Y, Yasukawa T, Shiku H, Matsue T. A multicellular spheroid array to realize spheroid formation, culture, and viability assay on a chip. *Biomaterials.* 2007; **28**: 559–566.

75. Stamatoglou SC, Hughes RC. Cell adhesion molecules in liver function and pattern formation. *FASEB J.* 1994; **8**: 420–427.

76. Fukuda J, Sakai Y, Nakazawa K. Novel hepatocyte culture system developed using microfabrication and collagen/polyethylene glycol microcontact printing. *Biomaterials.* 2006; **27**: 1061–1070.

77. Landry J, Bernier D, Ouellet C, Goyette R, Marceau N. Spheroidal aggregate culture of rat liver cells: histotypic reorganization, biomatrix deposition, and maintenance of functional activities. *J Cell Biol.* 1985; **101**: 914–923.

78. Hansen LK, Hsiao CG, Friend JR, Wu FJ, Bridge GA, Remmel RP, Cerra FB, Hu WS. Enhanced morphology and function in hepatocyte spheroids: a model of tissue self-assembly. *Tissue Eng.* 1998; **4**: 65–74.

79. Meng Q, Wu D, Zhang G, Qiu H. Direct self-assembly of hepatocytes spheroids within hollow fibers in presence of collagen. *Biotechnol Lett.* 2006; **28**: 279–284.

80. Abu-Absi SF, Friend JR, Hansen LK, Hu WS. Structural polarity and functional bile canaliculi in rat hepatocyte spheroids. *Exp Cell Res.* 2002; **274**: 56–67.

81. Lloyd-Jones D, Adams RJ, Brown TM, Carnethon M, Dai S, De Simone G, Ferguson TB, Ford E, Furie K, Gillespie C, Go A, Greenlund K, Haase N, Hailpern S, Ho PM, Howard V, Kissela B, Kittner S, Lackland D, Lisabeth L, Marelli A, McDermott MM, Meigs J, Mozaffarian D, Mussolino M, Nichol G, Roger VL, Rosamond W, Sacco R, Sorlie P, Stafford R, Thom T, Wasserthiel-Smoller S, Wong ND, Wylie-Rosett J. Executive summary: heart disease and stroke statistics—2010 update: a report from the American Heart Association. *Circulation.* 2010; **121**: 948–954.

82. Aufderheide AC, Athanasiou KA. Assessment of a bovine co-culture, scaffold-free method for growing meniscus-shaped constructs. *Tissue Eng.* 2007; **13**: 2195–2205.

83. Gwyther TA, Hu JZ, Christakis AG, Skorinko JK, Shaw SM, Billiar KL, Rolle MW. Engineered vascular tissue fabricated from aggregated smooth muscle cells. *Cells Tissues Organs.* 2011; **194**: 13–24.

84. Gwyther TA, Hu JZ, Billiar KL, Rolle MW. Directed cellular self-assembly to fabricate cell-derived tissue rings for biomechanical analysis and tissue engineering. *J Vis Exp.* 2011: e3366.

85. Laurencin C, Khan Y, El-Amin SF. Bone graft substitutes. *Expert Rev Med Devices.* 2006; **3**: 49–57.

86. Syed-Picard FN, Larkin LM, Shaw CM, Arruda EM. Three-dimensional engineered bone from bone marrow stromal cells and their autogenous extracellular matrix. *Tissue Eng Part A.* 2009; **15**: 187–195.

87. Smietana MJ, Syed-Picard FN, Ma J, Kostrominova T, Arruda EM, Larkin LM. The effect of implantation on scaffoldless three-dimensional engineered bone constructs. *In vitro Cell Dev Biol Anim.* 2009; **45**: 512–522.

88. Hildebrandt C, Buth H, Thielecke H. A scaffold-free in vitro model for osteogenesis of human mesenchymal stem cells. *Tissue Cell.* 2011; **43**: 91–100.

89. Kawaguchi J, Azuma Y, Hoshi K, Kii I, Takeshita S, Ohta T, Ozawa H, Takeichi M, Chisaka O, Kudo A. Targeted disruption of cadherin-11 leads to a reduction in bone density in calvaria and long bone metaphyses. *J Bone Miner Res.* 2001; **16**: 1265–1271.

90. Ma D, Ren L, Liu Y, Chen F, Zhang J, Xue Z, Mao T. Engineering scaffold-free bone tissue using bone marrow stromal cell sheets. *J Orthop Res.* 2010; **28**: 697–702.

91. Eshraghi S, Das S. Micromechanical finite-element modeling and experimental characterization of the compressive mechanical properties of polycaprolactone-hydroxyapatite composite scaffolds prepared by selective laser sintering for bone tissue engineering. *Acta Biomater.* 2012; **8**: 3138–3143.

92. Kinoshita N, Sasai N, Misaki K, Yonemura S. Apical accumulation of Rho in the neural plate is important for neural plate cell shape change and neural tube formation. *Mol Biol Cell.* 2008; **19**: 2289–2299.

93. Rothermel A, Biedermann T, Weigel W, Kurz R, Ruffer M, Layer PG, Robitzki AA. Artificial design of three-dimensional retina-like tissue from dissociated cells of the mammalian retina by rotation-mediated cell aggregation. *Tissue Eng.* 2005; **11**: 1749–1756.

94. Zhang W, Xiao J, Li C, Wan P, Liu Y, Wu Z, Huang M, Wang X, Wang Z. Rapidly constructed scaffold-free cornea epithelial sheets for ocular surface reconstruction. *Tissue Eng Part C Methods.* 2011; **17**: 569–577.

95. Hebert LE, Scherr PA, Bienias JL, Bennett DA, Evans DA. Alzheimer disease in the US population: prevalence estimates using the 2000 census. *Arch Neurol.* 2003; **60**: 1119–1122.

96. Adams AM, Arruda EM, Larkin LM. Use of adipose-derived stem cells to fabricate scaffoldless tissue-engineered neural conduits in vitro. *Neuroscience.* 2012; **201**: 349–356.

97. Hu JC, Athanasiou KA. A self-assembling process in articular cartilage tissue engineering. *Tissue Eng.* 2006; **12**: 969–979.

98. Hoben GM, Hu JC, James RA, Athanasiou KA. Self-assembly of fibrochondrocytes and chondrocytes for tissue engineering of the knee meniscus. *Tissue Eng.* 2007; **13**: 939–946.

99. Ofek G, Revell CM, Hu JC, Allison DD, Grande-Allen KJ, Athanasiou KA. Matrix development in self-assembly of articular cartilage. *PLoS One.* 2008; **3**: e2795.

100. Perez-Pomares JM, Foty RA. Tissue fusion and cell sorting in embryonic development and disease: biomedical implications. *Bioessays.* 2006; **28**: 809–821.

101. Marga F, Neagu A, Kosztin I, Forgacs G. Developmental biology and tissue engineering. *Birth Defects Res C Embryo Today.* 2007; **81**: 320–328.

102. Steinberg MS. Mechanism of tissue reconstruction by dissociated cells. II. Time-course of events. *Science.* 1962; **137**: 762–763.

103. Steinberg MS. Differential adhesion in morphogenesis: a modern view. *Curr Opin Genet Dev.* 2007; **17**: 281–286.
104. Foty RA, Steinberg MS. The differential adhesion hypothesis: a direct evaluation. *Dev Biol.* 2005; **278**: 255–263.
105. Foty RA, Pfleger CM, Forgacs G, Steinberg MS. Surface tensions of embryonic tissues predict their mutual envelopment behavior. *Development.* 1996; **122**: 1611–1620.
106. Steinberg MS. Differential adhesion in morphogenesis: a modern view. *Curr Opin Genet Dev.* 2007; **17**: 281–286.
107. Krieg M, Arboleda-Estudillo Y, Puech PH, Kafer J, Graner F, Muller DJ, Heisenberg CP. Tensile forces govern germ-layer organization in zebrafish. *Nat Cell Biol.* 2008; **10**: 429–436.
108. Youssef J, Nurse AK, Freund LB, Morgan JR. Quantification of the forces driving self-assembly of three-dimensional microtissues. *Proc Natl Acad Sci USA.* 2011; **108**: 6993–6998.
109. Brodland GW. The differential interfacial tension hypothesis (DITH): a comprehensive theory for the self-rearrangement of embryonic cells and tissues. *J Biomech Eng.* 2002; **124**: 188–197.
110. Harris AK. Is Cell sorting caused by differences in the work of intercellular adhesion? A critique of the Steinberg hypothesis. *J Theor Biol.* 1976; **61**: 267–285.
111. Dean DM, Morgan JR. Cytoskeletal-mediated tension modulates the directed self-assembly of microtissues. *Tissue Eng Part A.* 2008; **14**: 1989–1997.
112. Brodland GW, Chen HH. The mechanics of heterotypic cell aggregates: insights from computer simulations. *J Biomech Eng.* 2000; **122**: 402–407.
113. Voss-Bohme A, Deutsch A. The cellular basis of cell sorting kinetics. *J Theor Biol.* 2010; **263**: 419–436.
114. Hunziker EB. Articular cartilage repair: basic science and clinical progress. A review of the current status and prospects. *Osteoarthritis Cartilage.* 2002; **10**: 432–463.
115. Makris EA, Hadidi P, Athanasiou KA. The knee meniscus: structure-function, pathophysiology, current repair techniques, and prospects for regeneration. *Biomaterials.* 2011; **32**: 7411–7431.
116. Fairbank TJ. Knee joint changes after meniscectomy. *J Bone Joint Surg Br.* 1948; **30B**: 664–670.

117. McNickle AG, Provencher MT, Cole BJ. Overview of existing cartilage repair technology. *Sports Med Arthrosc.* 2008; **16**: 196–201.
118. Hu JC, Athanasiou KA. A self-assembling process in articular cartilage tissue engineering. *Tissue Eng.* 2006; **12**: 969–979.
119. Novotny JE, Turka CM, Jeong C, Wheaton AJ, Li C, Presedo A, Richardson DW, Reddy R, Dodge GR. Biomechanical and magnetic resonance characteristics of a cartilage-like equivalent generated in a suspension culture. *Tissue Eng.* 2006; **12**: 2755–2764.
120. Brehm W, Aklin B, Yamashita T, Rieser F, Trub T, Jakob RP, Mainil-Varlet P. Repair of superficial osteochondral defects with an autologous scaffold-free cartilage construct in a caprine model: implantation method and short-term results. *Osteoarthritis Cartilage.* 2006; **14**: 1214–1226.
121. DeLise AM, Tuan RS. Alterations in the spatiotemporal expression pattern and function of N-cadherin inhibit cellular condensation and chondrogenesis of limb mesenchymal cells in vitro. *J Cell Biochem.* 2002; **87**: 342–359.
122. Responte DJ, Arzi B, Natoli RM, Hu JC, Athanasiou KA. Mechanisms underlying the synergistic enhancement of self-assembled neocartilage treated with chondroitinase-ABC and TGF-beta1. *Biomaterials.* 2012; **33**: 3187–3194.
123. Huey DJ, Athanasiou KA. Maturational growth of self-assembled, functional menisci as a result of TGF-beta1 and enzymatic chondroitinase-ABC stimulation. *Biomaterials.* 2011; **32**: 2052–2058.
124. Haut Donahue TL, Hull ML, Rashid MM, Jacobs CR. The sensitivity of tibiofemoral contact pressure to the size and shape of the lateral and medial menisci. *J Orthop Res.* 2004; **22**: 807–814.
125. Kurosawa H, Fukubayashi T, Nakajima H. Load-bearing mode of the knee joint: physical behavior of the knee joint with or without menisci. *Clin Orthop Relat Res.* 1980; **149**: 283–290.
126. Donzelli PS, Gallo LM, Spilker RL, Palla S. Biphasic finite element simulation of the TMJ disc from in vivo kinematic and geometric measurements. *J Biomech.* 2004; **37**: 1787–1791.
127. Elder BD, Athanasiou KA. Synergistic and additive effects of hydrostatic pressure and growth factors on tissue formation. *PLoS One.* 2008; **3**: e2341.
128. Huey DJ, Athanasiou KA. Tension-compression loading with chemical stimulation results in additive increases to functional properties of anatomic meniscal constructs. *PLoS One.* 2011; **6**: e27857.

129. Elder BD, Athanasiou KA. Systematic assessment of growth factor treatment on biochemical and biomechanical properties of engineered articular cartilage constructs. *Osteoarthritis Cartilage.* 2008; **17**: 114–123.

130. Proulx S, d'Arc Uwamaliya J, Carrier P, Deschambeault A, Audet C, Giasson CJ, Guerin SL, Auger FA, Germain L. Reconstruction of a human cornea by the self-assembly approach of tissue engineering using the three native cell types. *Mol Vis.* 2010; **16**: 2192–2201.

131. Kelm JM, Lorber V, Snedeker JG, Schmidt D, Broggini-Tenzer A, Weisstanner M, Odermatt B, Mol A, Zund G, Hoerstrup SP. A novel concept for scaffold-free vessel tissue engineering: self-assembly of microtissue building blocks. *J Biotechnol.* 2010; **148**: 46–55.

132. Paxton JZ, Grover LM, Baar K. Engineering an in vitro model of a functional ligament from bone to bone. *Tissue Eng Part A.* 2010; **16**: 3515–3525.

133. Eleswarapu SV, Chen JA, Athanasiou KA. Temporal assessment of ribose treatment on self-assembled articular cartilage constructs. *Biochem Biophys Res Commun.* 2011; **414**: 431–436.

134. Natoli RM, Responte DJ, Lu BY, Athanasiou KA. Effects of multiple chondroitinase ABC applications on tissue engineered articular cartilage. *J Orthop Res.* 2009; **27**: 949–956.

135. Hu JC, Athanasiou KA. The effects of intermittent hydrostatic pressure on self-assembled articular cartilage constructs. *Tissue Eng.* 2006; **12**: 1337–1344.

136. Elder BD, Athanasiou KA. Hydrostatic pressure in articular cartilage tissue engineering: from chondrocytes to tissue regeneration. *Tissue Eng Part B Rev.* 2009; **15**: 43–53.

137. Hoenig E, Winkler T, Mielke G, Paetzold H, Schuettler D, Goepfert C, Machens HG, Morlock MM, Schilling AF. High amplitude direct compressive strain enhances mechanical properties of scaffold-free tissue-engineered cartilage. *Tissue Eng Part A* 2011; **17**: 1401–1411.

138. Brindley D, Moorthy K, Lee JH, Mason C, Kim HW, Wall I. Bioprocess forces and their impact on cell behavior: implications for bone regeneration therapy. *J Tissue Eng.* 2011; 2011: 620247.

139. Wilkins RJ, Browning JA, Urban JPG. Chondrocyte regulation by mechanical load. *Biorheology.* 2000; **37**: 67–74.

140. Natoli RM, Skaalure S, Bijlani S, Chen KX, Hu J, Athanasiou KA. Intracellular $Na^{(+)}$ and $Ca^{(2+)}$ modulation increases the tensile properties of developing engineered articular cartilage. *Arthritis Rheum.* 2010; **62**: 1097–1107.

141. Elder BD, Athanasiou KA. Effects of confinement on the mechanical properties of self-assembled articular cartilage constructs in the direction orthogonal to the confinement surface. *J Orthop Res.* 2008; **26**: 238–246.

142. Gunja NJ, Huey DJ, James RA, Athanasiou KA. Effects of agarose mould compliance and surface roughness on self-assembled meniscus-shaped constructs. *J Tissue Eng Regen Med.* 2009; **3**: 521–530.

143. Hoben GM, Willard VP, Athanasiou KA. Fibrochondrogenesis of hESCs: growth factor combinations and cocultures. *Stem Cells Dev.* 2009; **18**: 283–292.

144. Carrier P, Deschambeault A, Audet C, Talbot M, Gauvin R, Giasson CJ, Auger FA, Guerin SL, Germain L. Impact of cell source on human cornea reconstructed by tissue engineering. *Invest Ophthalmol Vis Sci.* 2009; **50**: 2645–2652.

Chapter 12

Environmental Factors in Cartilage Tissue Engineering

Yueh-Hsun Yang and Gilda A. Barabino

*The Wallace H. Coulter Department of Biomedical Engineering,
Georgia Institute of Technology and Emory University,
313 Ferst Dr., Atlanta, GA 30332, USA*

barabino@gatech.edu

The limited ability of articular cartilage for self-repair of defects due to injury or disease persists as a challenge for orthopedic medicine. Tissue engineering approaches combining cells, bioactive molecules and biocompatible/biodegradable scaffolds in scalable bioreactors for regeneration of functional cartilage tissues hold promise. Successful creation of tissue substitutes requires a thorough understanding of environmental factors that regulate cellular behavior and tissue formation. In this review, we focus on the influence of microenvironmental stimuli on cultivation of neocartilage within bioreactors and on stem cell differentiation. Exploiting the synergy between cells, biochemical signals, biophysical cues, and mechanical forces to optimize the correct combination of parameters that mimic the native microenvironment is an important step toward the development of clinically relevant cartilage tissue replacements.

Tissue and Organ Regeneration: Advances in Micro- and Nanotechnology
Edited by Lijie Grace Zhang, Ali Khademhosseini, and Thomas J. Webster
Copyright © 2014 Pan Stanford Publishing Pte. Ltd.
ISBN 978-981-4411-67-7 (Hardcover), 978-981-4411-68-4 (eBook)
www.panstanford.com

12.1 Articular Cartilage

12.1.1 Structure and Function

Articular cartilage is a lubricant substrate that serves as a cushion between the bones of diarthrodial joints. The main function of articular cartilage is to provide a smooth medium for force transfer between long bones; therefore, its tough but resilient structure is designed to endure constant cyclic loading and to further protect the underlying bones. Structurally, articular cartilage has no nerves and blood vessels and consists of 65–80 wt.% of water, 10–20 wt.% of collagen fibrils and 5–10 wt.% of proteoglycans [93]. Very few cells, called articular chondrocytes, reside in the cartilage tissue and secrete a matrix primary of collagen and proteoglycan. Type II collagen, a triple helix made of three identical polypeptide chains, contributes about 95% of the total collagen content within articular cartilage [29]. These collagen fibrils form a highly cross-linked network to establish a well-organized extracellular architec-ture and thereby grant cartilage tensile strength (20 MPa). Aggrecan containing branched negatively charged glycosamino-glycans (GAG) is the predominant proteoglycan in articular cartilage and is encapsulated in the collagen mesh. As a result, the trapped negatively charged components create a repelling force and recruit massive water molecules, which generates a high swelling pressure against external compressive loading (0.5–1 MPa). The shear capability (10 MPa) of articular cartilage is attributed to a combination of both solid and fluid constituents. Taken together, the mechanical behavior of articular cartilage is modulated by three major factors: (1) elasticity of the solid matrix, (2) swelling property of the ionic elements, and (3) solid–fluid interactions.

At rest, the synovial fluid transmits hydrostatic pressure to the interstitial water within the cartilage matrix. During normal ambulation, articular cartilage undergoes direct compression thousands of times each day without causing damage. Under a loading period, deformation of cartilage results in changes in environmental conditions experienced by chondrocytes, such as matrix organization, tissue permeability, and water content within the tissue [61]. When cartilage is compressed, water molecules tend to escape from the tissue, yet they cannot instantly leave the tissue due to the reduced permeability such that the interstitial fluid absorbs the majority of mechanical energy and becomes pressurized. As the fluid eventually exits the matrix into the synovial cavity, the gaps in the collagen network shrink and GAG molecules are thereby in closer proximity, producing stronger resistance against compression. The movement of the interstitial fluid precipitates several events. For instance, transient fluid flow generates shear stress that not only directly acts on cells but activates some latent bioactive agents such as transforming growth factor-β (TGF-β) [1]. The release of the fluid also enhances the efficiency of the removal of waste produced by chondrocytes and fresh nutrients can be brought back to the tissue as cartilage is relaxed. As a result, this complex mechanism supports the development of articular cartilage and maintains its functionality. Conversely, immobilization of diarthrodial joints can accelerate the deterioration of articular cartilage [78].

12.1.2 Degeneration and Repair

The degeneration of articular cartilage is one of the most frequent causes of pain and disability in middle-aged and older people. Among the over 100 different types of common degenerative conditions, the most commonly reported cause of cartilage degeneration is osteoarthritis (OA), where the cartilaginous layers covering the ends of the bones gradually wear away, which increases the friction coefficient of the articular surface. Moreover, in the event that an injury compromises the articular surface, a degenerative condition coined post-traumatic osteoarthritis (PTOA) may soon follow, which if allowed to progress persistently could lead to chronic, debilitating pain and swelling. Post-traumatic osteoarthritis results in an estimated cost of $13.5 billion per year in work loss and direct medical costs in the United States alone [15]. Because self-repair of articular cartilage is limited and the damaged tissue is usually reconstructed with fibro-cartilage, which exhibits weaker mechanical strength than articular cartilage, the injury site becomes a nucleating center for the progressive degeneration of the articular surface by altering the native loading state of the joint. The subsequent abnormal wear on the articular surface as a result of this altered loading state, becomes accelerated and ultimately leads to end-stage OA. Post-traumatic osteoarthritis can occur as soon as three months after a severe injury and despite advances in surgical treatment and rehabilitation of injured joints, the risk of PTOA has not decreased in the last 50 years [15]. Thus, new therapeutic approaches aimed at regenerating articular cartilage with respect to biological and mechanical function are sought which might prevent the onset of PTOA, and mitigate future physical and medical costs associated with end-stage OA.

Current strategies for cartilage repair include cell-based therapies, tissue graft implantation and subchondral shaving, and while there has been some success in short-term treatment of tissue lesions, long-term cartilage restoration remains elusive [118,157]. While cell therapies and transplantation are commonly used to restore small cartilage lesions, these approaches are unable to replicate intact native cartilage. Chondrocytes are the most common cell source for cartilage repair, yet the obtainment of healthy autologous chondrocytes from patients requires invasive surgery, which may cause donor site morbidity and the use of allogeneic chondrocytes may yield rejection responses of the host. In addition, harvested chondrocytes may also experience phenotypic changes during in vitro two-dimensional expansion before being transplanted to the damaged sites [31]. To overcome these obstacles and provide alternative therapeutic strategies, tissue engineering has emerged as a promising approach.

12.1.3 Cartilage Tissue Engineering

The production of tissue-engineered cartilage typically involves cultivation of primary chondrocytes on three-dimensional biodegradable polymer scaffolds or naturally derived hydrogels within the controlled environment of bioreactor culture systems [11,30] (Fig. 12.1). In order to be clinically relevant, cartilage substitutes must meet specific functional criteria related to their mechanical properties, biochemical composition, tissue ultrastructure, immunological compatibility, and integration capability. However, all of these properties of engineered cartilage are still inferior to those of native tissues. An explanation for this gap is that cultured chondrocytes undergo a process of rapid in vitro hypertrophic maturation such that tissue development is impeded [13]. In vitro, harvested chondrocytes may only have a limited lifespan and potential to develop into mature articular cartilage tissues when exposed to culture conditions. Researchers seek to develop novel biomaterials and bioreactor systems in order to improve current tissue engineering strategies that can maximize the efficacy of chondrocytes within their restricted lifetime.

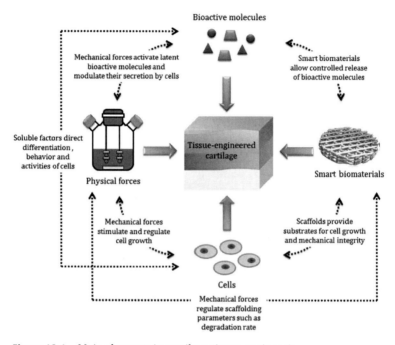

Figure 12.1 Main elements in cartilage tissue engineering.

Biodegradable scaffolds are used in tissue engineering strategies to provide three-dimensional substrates and appropriate microenvironments for cell growth and tissue regeneration. These scaffolds need to mimic the natural environment of cells and are fabricated to meet the requirements for cell survival, matrix biosynthesis, mechanical integrity, and integration capacity with host tissues. Smart biomaterials, those that have capacity to present localized bioactive molecules and that respond to environmental cues and cellular signals, are the best candidates for tissue engineering. Among these smart biomaterials are hydrogels and synthetic meshes. Hydrogels are formed by gelation of polymers dissolved in a liquid medium, usually water. Depending on the mechanism of cross-linking, the network structure of hydrogels can be physically or chemically bonded. Hydrogels that are utilized in cartilage repair are commonly composed of agarose [20,46,72,107,109,147], alginate [21,80,112,134], fibrin [72,120,132,134], collagen [64,89,136,175], hyaluronic acid [28,46,80,98], or self-assembling peptides such as KLD-12 [85,88] and Puramatrix [46]. Although hydrogels yield more homogeneous distribution of encapsulated cells and have high flexibility in size and shape, they are usually less porous and exhibit inferior mechanical properties in comparison with meshed scaffolds [27]. Meshed synthetic scaffolds such as polyglycolic acid (PGA) [49, 121,171], poly-L-lactic acid (PLA) [99,115], and polycaprolactone (PCL) [94,144] may be preferred in the fabrication of tissue replacements because of their tunable biomechanical properties that can be modified using techniques like soft lithography [163], UV polymerization [81], and electrospinning [26,95]. A meshed poly(ethylene oxide) terephthalate/poly(butylene) terephthalate scaffold has been recently fabricated to possess mechanical strength comparable to the level of native cartilage [114]. Electrospinning is a novel approach to the manufacture of nanofibrous scaffolds. This type of scaffold provides three-dimensional architecture that mimics the network of fibrillar extracellular matrix (ECM) components in nanoscale and has high porosities and surface-area-to-volume ratios that are suitable for cell adhesion and proliferation [26,95]. More important, electrospun scaffolds can be engineered to consist of highly aligned nanofibers that will be useful for regeneration of specific tissue types, for example, tendon or superficial and deep zones of articular cartilage [75,94].

12.2 Environmental Stimuli

Microenvironments define the immediate surroundings of a cell, which encompass essential elements that mediate cellular activities and further tissue formation. These elements include, but are not limited to, soluble molecules, ECM components bound to the cell and adjacent cells. Therefore, the development of functional tissue replacements requires a thorough understanding of the roles environmental factors play in native and culture environments. Among these factors, biochemical agents are thought to be involved in cell-to-cell communication and signaling, in which extracellular biomolecules, such as growth factors, cytokines and chemokines, transmit chemical signals directly to individual cells and activate a series of chain reactions inside the cells that give rise to particular transcription factors in response to external stimulation and changes in environmental conditions. It is also believed that mechanical stimuli present in the physiological or culture environments can significantly influence cell shape, orientation, apoptosis, gene expression, secretion of signaling molecules as well as synthesis and degradation of ECM components by cells though the mechanisms that transduce mechanical cues into chemical signals that trigger cellular responses are still not fully understood [61]. It has been reported that there may be several regulatory pathways by which cells can respond to mechanical forces, including crosstalk between chemo- and mechano-signaling mediators [32,34] and possible mechanisms that alter cellular activities in transcription [69,150,160], translation and post-translational modifications [84,149]. In the fabrication of tissue-engineered constructs, in order to compensate for low functional properties of engineered tissues derived from static cultures, bioreactor systems have been designed to impart mechanical loading to foster the growth and development of different types of tissues, such as cardiovascular and musculo-skeletal tissues [11]. Bioreactors do their part by providing a well-defined environment to control biochemical and mechanical stimuli. There are several bioreactor approaches that have been utilized in cartilage tissue engineering applications, for example, systems that deliver compressive loading, shear deformation, hydrostatic pressure or hydrodynamic forces [30]. The role of biophysical, biochemical and mechanical environmental factors in cartilage tissue engineering will be briefed in this section.

12.2.1 Mechanical Forces

12.2.1.1 Deformational loading

Ex vivo compression, in both confined and unconfined fashions (Fig. 12.2a), at certain amplitudes and frequencies has been considered to be capable of replicating joint activities and thereby stimulating chondrocyte and cartilage growth [59,84,138,139,155]. However, such loading has been shown to possibly reduce the efficiency at which the produced ECM components are encapsulated in the tissue network as a result of frequent flow movement that increases the release of those molecules into the surroundings

[59,139]. Given the fact that stimulatory effects of compressive loading on protein synthesis can last for hours [59,138], tissue constructs are usually exposed to intermittent compression in long-term experiments in order to maximize the retention of ECM components within engineered tissues [35,86,107,167]. Studies have demonstrated that dynamic compression can enhance gene expression of aggrecan by cultured chondrocytes [160] and influence chondrocyte-specific biosynthetic pathways [84], resulting in improved biochemical and mechanical properties of cell-laden agarose [107] and self-assembling peptide [86] hydrogels. These dynamically loaded samples can achieve at least 50% greater ECM deposition and mechanical strength than static tissue constructs [86,107,167].

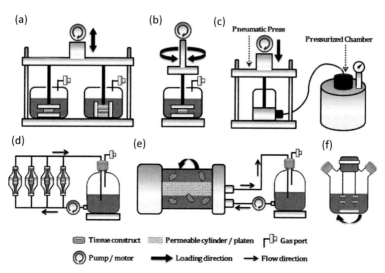

Figure 12.2 Bioreactor systems in cartilage tissue engineering. (a) Confined and unconfined compressive loading. (b) Shear deformation. (c) Hydrostatic pressure. (d) Direct perfusion. (e) Rotating vessel. (f) Spinner flask.

Dynamic compression yields a culture condition as complex as the natural environment within the synovial capsule. Under dynamic compressive loading, cells or tissues experience not only volumetric deformation, but also gradients in osmotic stress, hydrostatic pressure, hydrodynamic forces, electric field stimulation and more [61]. This complexity increases the difficulty in isolating the effects of a single environmental factor on the development of tissue-engineered cartilage. Therefore, the design of bioreactors has shifted to systems that only emulate one of many conditions that take place in the knee or other joints. For example, using parallel impermeable platens (Fig. 12.2b), sinusoidal shear deformation has been successfully applied to cartilage explants in a range of 0.5–6% strain amplitude at 0.1 Hz without introducing significant interstitial fluid flow [76]. The shear-loaded cartilage tissues exhibited 35% and 25% greater protein and proteoglycan synthesis, respectively, than the non-loaded samples in a 24 h loading period. This enhancement of tissue properties, however, was independent of amplitude and frequency of applied shear deformation. Similar shear instruments have also been utilized in the long-term cultivation of chondrocyte-seeded substrates. The intermittent dynamic shear deformation resulted in engineered cartilage with a sixfold higher stiffness than the static controls [166].

12.2.1.2 Hydrostatic pressure

Bioreactor systems that simulate physiological levels of hydrostatic pressure in diarthrodial joints have been fabricated in the laboratory by compressing a gas or liquid phase that transmits load through culture media to cells (Fig. 12.2c) [42]. Hydrostatic pressure in the physiological range of 7 to 10 MPa is preferred in this type of application because loading at such levels stimulates tissue constructs without causing evident deformation of samples and thus maintains the integrity of matrix architecture [30,63]. A study in which the effects of the loading profile of hydrostatic pressure at 10 MPa on articular chondrocytes was evaluated in a 4 h loading period demonstrated that, relative to the non-loaded cells, intermittent pressure applied at 1 Hz was found to increase aggrecan and type II collagen mRNA signals by 31% and 36%, respectively, whereas constant pressure did not influence mRNA expression [149]. A follow-up experiment was conducted to investigate the time-dependent effects of intermittent hydrostatic pressure loaded at 10 MPa and 1 Hz for up to 24 h. A biphasic behavior was detected in mRNA expression of type II collagen by loaded chondrocytes with a peak value at the 4 h period while aggrecan signals continuously increased with the loading period [150]. Intermittent hydrostatic pressure was also applied to grow tissue-engineered cartilage and was shown to positively regulate functional maturation of neocartilage [42].

12.2.1.3 Laminar flow

In addition to direct deformation and hydrostatic pressure, fluid flow also plays a key role in the development of both native and engineered cartilage. In vivo, joint movement during normal walking or exercise not only alters pericellular concentrations of cytokines, growth factors, enzymes and more other molecules, driving protein or ion flux in and out of the cartilage tissue, but also forces the exchange of substances between the interstitial fluid within cartilage and the surrounding synovial fluid. Because of the avascular nature of articular cartilage, nutrient delivery to and waste removal from chondrocytes largely rely on this flow-enabled exchange. The individual contributions of diffusion and convection to the transport of neutral and charged proteins within articular cartilage have been examined [54,55]. These studies suggest that when cartilage is stimulated by fluid flowing at a velocity of 1 μm/s (flow velocity within articular cartilage at normal walking frequencies [70]), the efficiency of mass transfer of solutes is tremendously enhanced. Fluid flow bioreactors can be divided into two major categories based on flow profiles, i.e., laminar or turbulent flow [40,43,106,128,164,165].

Among the reactors that generate laminar flow, direct perfusion systems (Fig. 12.2d) push culture media through cell-seeded scaffolds such that cells within constructs can directly sense hydrodynamic shear stress as fluid flows through the pores. In order to achieve uniform medium flow, constructs have to tightly fit in the perfusion chamber and no gaps between samples and the chamber wall are allowed. Cells under perfusion stimulation become aligned in the direction of the flow, which makes it possible to engineer a tissue with specific cell orientations [40,128]. Although it has been demonstrated that perfusion flows at both low (1 μm/s) [128] and high (11 μm/s) [40] velocities significantly increased ECM production of tissue-engineered cartilage, denser matrix deposition occurred near the surface facing the oncoming flow. As a result, the nonhomogeneous matrix distribution along the thickness of constructs affects overall mechanical properties of engineered cartilage. This "one-side effect," however, can be overcome by reversing medium flow periodically during the cultivation [30].

Another representative system that employs laminar flow is the rotating vessel bioreactor (Fig. 12.2e), which utilizes fluid flow and gravity to apply a relatively low level of shear stress to cells or tissue constructs suspended in culture [43,106,165]. Remarkably, a research group has shown that chondrocyte-seeded PGA scaffolds cultivated within a rotating vessel bioreactor were able to develop into robust tissues with equilibrium moduli and GAG contents similar to or better than native cartilage after seven months in culture [106]. Nevertheless, a major concern with this type of bioreactor is that the path of the suspended constructs within flow is unpredictable such that it is difficult to build a simulation model to optimize the bioprocessing conditions [30]. A hybrid bioreactor combining perfusion and rotating vessel systems was designed, in which cartilage constructs are mounted in the perfusion chamber while the outer wall of the reactor simultaneously spins during the cultivation [47]. A computational fluid dynamics (CFD) model was established to define this unique hydrodynamic environment. Experimentally, the hybrid bioreactor further improved chondrocyte doubling rate and collagen accumulation within engineered tissues in comparison with the system without the perfusion flow. This evidence suggests that the development of tissue-engineered cartilage can possibly benefit from enhanced hydrodynamic shear stress, such as that introduced by turbulent flow.

12.2.1.4 Turbulent flow

Turbulent flow-induced shear environments can be established within a simple mechanically stirred bioreactor system equipped with an impeller or stir bar and referred to as a spinner flask (Fig. 12.2f). Under mixing, oxygen and nutrients can be efficiently delivered to cells seeded within and/or on the scaffolds. Vunjak-Novakovic et al. have suggested that mechanically stirred bioreactors can yield the best cell attachment efficiency to meshed synthetic scaffolds during the cell seeding process [164]. The induced hydrodynamic shear stress possesses the potential to regulate matrix architecture. Figure 12.3 demonstrates that the orientation of newly synthesized collagen fibrils is in the same direction as fluid flow at the periphery of engineered tissues, which is in direct contact with the flow, but is disorderly in the interior of constructs. Furthermore, cultured cells can also be damaged when exposed to extremely high agitation rates (150–300 rpm) [125]. Therefore, it is important to find a balance between hydrodynamic parameters and cell/tissue growth.

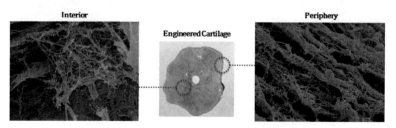

Figure 12.3 Orientation of collagen fibrils in tissue-engineered cartilage under turbulent flow. Scanning electron microscopic images: 6500×.

A wavy-walled bioreactor system (WWB) (Fig. 12.4) designed in our laboratory is an alternative version of the conventional spinner flask whose circular glass wall is modified into a sinusoidal curve:

$$r = R_{avg} + A\sin(N\theta),$$

where R_{avg} is the average internal radius of the bioreactor (3.35 cm), A is the magnitude of peak amplitude at the node (0.45 cm), N is the number of lobes in the WWB (6), and r and θ are the cylindrical coordinates. The unique hydrodynamic culture environment within the WWB has been characterized using CFD simulation (Fig. 12.5) which was further validated by particle image velocimetry (PIV) methods [8,9]. This characterization suggests that three hydrodynamic parameters (1) the average shear stress, (2) axial, and (3) tangential fluid velocities on the control volume surface created around tissue constructs explain more than 99.9% of the variability of the hydrodynamic environment. In comparison with the spinner flask, the WWB yields a higher axial velocity, but lower shear stress applied to the construct surface. These conditions lead to enhanced chondrocyte aggregation [16], increased cell seeding efficiency [18], and improved cell proliferation and ECM deposition within engineered cartilage [17,19].

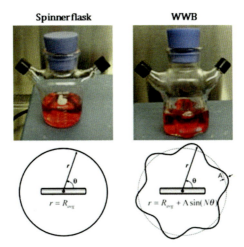

Figure 12.4 Configuration of spinner flask and wavy-walled bioreactor (WWB).

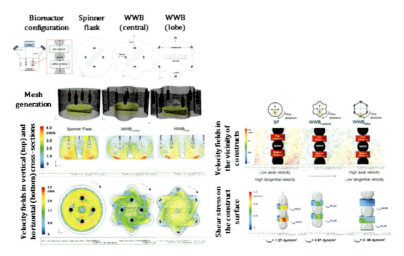

Figure 12.5 Computational fluid dynamics modeling for spinner flask and WWB at 50 rpm. Modified from Bilgen and Barabino [9].

12.2.3 Biochemical Signals

Extracellular biochemical signals are required to both initiate a series of biological reactions associated with specific cellular activities in response to external stimulation and provide essential elements for regulation of cell growth and tissue development. In vitro, nutrients assimilated by cells mainly originate from the constituents present in culture media.

12.2.3.1 Fetal bovine serum

Fetal bovine serum (FBS) is a typical medium supplement in the cultivation of mammalian cells because it is composed of rich growth factors, such as TGF-β, and cytokines, such as interleukin-6 (IL-6). Although culture media supplemented with high serum contents (10–20% v/v) have been extensively utilized to grow different types of cells and tissues, contradictory reports on the effects of serum have been documented. These variations may result from highly undefined serum composition and varied concentrations of its constituents when extracted from different donor herds, thereby introducing unpredictable experimental outcomes. For instance, while high serum levels have been shown to increase cell doubling rate [57] and to effectively support in vitro development of engineered tissues [49,107], serum has also been shown to interfere with particular cellular activities and with the function of exogenous growth factors. Specifically, chondrocyte proliferation [104] and cartilage matrix production [57] in serum-containing conditions were compromised in comparison with serum-starved cultures supplemented with basic fibroblast growth factor (FGF-2) and TGF-β, respectively. It has also been demonstrated that embryonic bodies in culture with FBS had less capability to differentiate into functional neuronal cells [178], whereas serum-free media were shown to induce massive neural differentiation of embryonic carcinoma cells [123]. Moreover, serum-containing cultures failed to support the differentiation of porcine stromal vascular cells into adipocytes as indicated by reduced glycerol-3-phosphate dehydrogenase (GPDH) activities while the addition of insulin and hydrocortisone to serum-free media facilitated adipose differentiation [156]. Recent studies also indicated that the presence of serum components led to chondrocyte dedifferentiation [97] and inhibited the activity of TGF-β1 in chondrogenesis of synoviocyte pellet cultures [10]. Thus, there is a need to reduce the dependency on serum while retaining its beneficial effects in the preparation of chemically defined culture media for cell and tissue engineering.

Bioactive molecules within serum are transported between cell culture medium and cells and as such are important mediators in the soluble local environment of developing tissues.

12.2.3.2 Growth factors: insulin-like growth factor-1 (IGF-1) and transforming growth factor-β (TGF-β)

Incorporation of exogenous growth factors, such as insulin-like growth factor-1 (IGF-1) [33,76,108,137,169], TGF-β [12,33,41,43, 57,103,108,129,169], FGF-2 [105,137] and others, into tissue engineering strategies is a vital step in the generation of engineered tissues. Among these bioactive agents, IGF-1 and TGF-β molecules are two of the common stimulating factors in cartilage biology [27]. In articular cartilage, IGF-1 is one of the main anabolic growth factors responsible for cartilage homeostasis and balancing matrix synthesis and degradation by chondrocytes. IGF-1 has the potential to maintain the viability of native cartilage [137], to stimulate gene expression of both aggrecan and type II collagen by chondrocytes [33,169] and subsequent biosynthesis of associated protein molecules [76], and to enhance stiffness of engineered cartilage [108].

The TGF-β family is a more complex group that consists of at least three isoforms, TGF-β1, -β2, and -β3, which are associated with chondrocyte activities. The major functions of TGF-β molecules are to induce ECM deposition and inhibit protease production by cells. Although these isoforms have a high degree of similarity (65–80%) in their structure [38] and most studies have reported an overall stimulatory effect of TGF-β on chondrocyte proliferation and cartilage maturation [12,33,41,43,57,103,108,129,169], they may still serve different biological roles. For instance, it has been found that the distribution of these three isoforms in the pathological joint is quite discrete. Specifically, abundant TGF-β1 was localized in the superficial chondrocytes of osteophyte cartilage [159] while TGF-β2 was present within lining layer and pannus over the joint surface and TGF-β3 was only observed in the scatter cells within the deeper layers of the synovia in an arthritic mouse model [116]. Moreover, in fracture healing, TGF-β1 was expressed in early callus and the expression further increased during chondrogenesis and endochondral ossification whereas no stable trend was detected in both TGF-β2 and -β3 expression throughout the healing process [135]. Nevertheless, the total expression of TGF-β isoforms in mRNA level was found to increase in the early phase of osteoarthritic cartilage [161]. This evidence substantiates their functional roles in cartilage regeneration mechanisms.

Delivery of exogenous growth factors to cultured cells is mostly through the direct addition of bulk molecules to culture media [12,33,41,43,76,105,108,129,137,169]. This method requires excess additives to increase the probability of cells capturing these molecules and continuous supplementation is usually applied, which makes this strategy less economic. Alternatively, growth factors can be embedded in microparticles or scaffolding materials such as hydrogels for local distribution [14,37,67,68,96,126,127,151]. When loaded microparticles are further encapsulated into scaffolds, it largely reduces the burst release of incorporated molecules [27,37]. In this fashion, the release of growth factors is based on loading density, diffusivity and properties of biomaterials, such as the size of microparticles and degradation rate of hydrogels [27]. Several studies have demonstrated that constructs loaded with TGF-β and/or IGF-1 microcarriers exhibited a higher level of chondrogenesis than the non-loaded ones [14,68,126,127,151]. A novel approach utilizing layer-by-layer (LbL) techniques to incorporate proteins into meshed biodegradable scaffolds has been developed. In this system, single or multiple growth factors are coated onto the surface of scaffolds based on electrostatic properties of biomolecules in a water-based, room temperature environment [100–102,143,148,168] to avoid the use of solvents, heat or other severe conditions that are necessary in the traditional polymer encapsulation process and may denature the encapsulated proteins [53]. The controlled release of growth factors in LbL vehicles can be modulated by simply adjusting the architecture of the nanolayered film and the number of incorporated growth factor layers [100,101,168]. BMP-2/VEGF-loaded LbL scaffolds have been shown to successfully simulate in vivo conditions of molecule release and recruit progenitor cells at the implant site to foster in situ development of regenerating bone [102,143]. To our best knowledge, however, this technique has not been extensively utilized in cartilage repair.

12.3 Interplay between Mechanical and Biochemical Stimuli

Certain bioactive molecules, such as IGF-1 [12,76,108,129] and TGF-β [12,43,108,129], are thought to be shear-responsive, i.e., capable of interacting synergistically with mechanical forces to further accelerate functional maturation of engineered tissues. Differential responses to varying levels of shear or other mechanical stimuli have been observed. For example, Gooch and coworkers showed that engineered cartilage stimulated by exogenous IGF-1 exhibited increased ECM deposition when they were cultivated under laminar flow induced within a rotating vessel reactor, but not in a spinner flask that imparts turbulent flow [58]. Several groups have also reported that the pathways of TGF-β and IGF-1 are sensitive to shear stress, resulting in enhanced cell proliferation [103], cell biosynthesis [76] and tissue remodeling [122], and that the production of these shear-responsive factors by cells increases under fluid shear stress [79,117,122,141]. In addition, TGF-β, in particular, is synthesized in a latent form by cells, which can be activated when exposed to shear conditions, and the activation largely depends on the magnitude of applied shear stress [1]. These findings speak to the complexity of fluid shear stress in the modulation of not only tissue properties and morphology but also synthesis, activation and function of certain growth factors. Thus, thorough strategies are needed in order to set the stage for the use of exogenous growth factors for the cultivation of cartilage tissue constructs in a high-shear hydrodynamic environment. To better understand the role of biochemical cues in the local environment of developing constructs, we evaluated a low-serum culture medium for hydrodynamic cultivation of tissue-engineered cartilage within a WWB, as described in the following section.

12.3.1 Low Serum Effects on Cultivation of Neocartilage

We recently reported a study in which chondrocyte-laden PGA scaffolds were cultivated in the presence or absence of fluid flow-induced shear stress in medium containing FBS either partially or completely replaced by insulin–transferrin–selenium (ITS), a potential serum substitute (see reference [171] for further details). Insulin–transferring–selenium is a commercially available media supplement and its components are associated with essential cellular activities, such as cell proliferation and protein synthesis [111,145,146,162]. The standard concentration of ITS added to culture media (1%, v/v, 10 μg/mL insulin, 5.5 μg/mL transferrin, and 5 μg/mL selenium) is based on the concentration of insulin previously found to stimulate proteoglycan synthesis in cultured cartilage [87,111].

Briefly, tissue constructs were formed by seeding freshly isolated chondrocytes onto PGA meshed scaffolds at an initial density of 5 million live cells per construct. The cell/PGA complexes were then cultured with reduced serum content (0%, 0.2%, or 2% FBS, v/v) plus 1% ITS for 4 weeks either statically or dynamically. Tissue constructs were harvested at specific time points for evaluation and compared with those cultivated with typical high-serum media (10% FBS). The results demonstrated that, under static conditions, the serum-free (0% FBS) and low-serum (0.2% or 2% FBS) ITS-supplemented groups resulted in constructs with tissue properties similar to the high-serum constructs (Fig. 12.6a), suggesting that ITS is a potential substitute for FBS in the static chondrocyte/PGA culture system and that serum is not a requirement. This is in agreement with other studies in which serum-free ITS media were able to support the cultivation of cartilage explants [6] or chondrocytes encapsulated in self-assembling peptide hydrogels [87] in the absence of mechanical loading.

Conversely, ITS alone was not sufficient to foster hydrodynamic development of engineered cartilage (Fig. 12.6a), yielding fragile constructs that could be damaged by applied shear forces. When cultivated with low-serum ITS media, hydrodynamic constructs achieved at least 79% and 78% of the high-serum values in collagen and GAG contents, respectively. This implies that some critical components present in serum exhibit increased activities in response to fluid shear stress and further facilitate mechanical-stimuli-induced cell proliferation and ECM production. Such shear-responsive signals associated with chondrocyte metabolic activities include TGF-β [103,117,122], IGF-I [76], IL-6 [113] and matrix metalloproteinase (MMPs) [174]. In particular, the 2% FBS + 1% ITS constructs exhibited biomechanical and biochemical properties that were not significantly different from those of the high-serum constructs. This is in agreement with a previous study carried out by Kelly et al., where dynamic compressive loading was applied to chondrocyte-laden agarose gels cultivated with 2% FBS + 1% ITS [82]. Both studies suggest that, in the presence of mechanical forces, the biochemical stimuli in the 2% FBS + 1% ITS group are not compromised relative to the high-serum condition and thus this combination of FBS and ITS can substitute for traditional high-serum media. To further substantiate the requirement for ITS in the low-serum dynamic cultivation of tissue-engineered cartilage, constructs were cultivated with 2% FBS supplemented with or without ITS. The results revealed that functional properties of low-serum constructs grown without ITS were at a lower level than that achieved in the presence of ITS, suggesting that ITS is a required element in the low-serum cultivation of neocartilage [82,171].

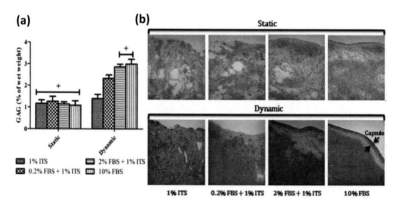

Figure 12.6 Serum effects on 28-day cultivation of tissue-engineered cartilage within the WWB in the absence (static) or presence (dynamic) of fluid shear stress. (a) GAG content. +Non-significance; $p > 0.05$; $n = 6$. (b) GAG histochemistry. GAG: pink/red; cytoplasm: green; 10×. Modified from Yang and Barabino [171].

A fibrous outer capsule, which is characterized by increased cell density and decreased (virtually none) GAG deposition, was not observed in both static and hydrodynamic groups when engineered tissues were cultured with FBS concentration equal to or less than 0.2% (Fig. 12.6b). This indicates that reduced serum content may suppress the formation of the fibrous cell outgrowth that is often seen in high-serum cultures [82,85,87], especially at the outer edge of engineered tissues in which cells have easy access to a sufficient concentration of serum constituents that facilitate fibrosis, such as TGF-β and platelet-derived growth factor (PDGF) [73,82,99]. Therefore, the elimination of a fibrous capsule as FBS concentration decreased from 2% to 0.2% or lower implied that the concentration of these molecules did not reach the level required for capsule formation. Notably, the fibrous capsule is more evident and organized in hydrodynamic constructs than in those cultured under static conditions or dynamic compressive loading [82,165,171]. One possible explanation is that some of the fibrotic mechanisms are also up-regulated by fluid shear stress [73,103]; as a result, the level of fibrosis is not promoted in the absence of hydrodynamic stimuli, resulting in a less apparent fibrous capsule. The presence and analysis of the fibrous capsule provide additional insights into the combined role of biochemical and mechanical factors in the development of engineered tissues.

12.3.2 Continuous versus Transient Exposure of Engineered Cartilage to Growth Factors

To further clarify the interplay between turbulent flow-induced shear forces and growth factors, we evaluated the development of tissue-engineered cartilage in response to continuous or transient growth factor supplementation using a low-serum ITS (2% FBS + 1% ITS) culture medium and IGF-1 as a model bioactive molecule.

Chondrocyte-seeded constructs were cultivated for 4 weeks with the 2% FBS + 1% ITS medium (basal medium) in the WWB with or without fluid agitation and the basal medium was further supplemented with 100 ng/mL IGF-1 either for the first two weeks of the culture (transient group) or throughout the whole 4 week cultivation (continuous group). The concentration of IGF-1 used here was determined from its most commonly reported range of effective doses for the cultivation of engineered cartilage, which is 100–300 ng/mL [12,58,76,108,129], and a minimal dose was employed. After 4 weeks in culture, harvested static and hydrodynamic constructs exhibited differential responses to added IGF-1 molecules. In static cultures (Fig. 12.7a), the presence of exogenous IGF-1 seemed to be ineffective in the first two weeks of the tissue development because comparable construct properties between IGF-1 treated and untreated groups were detected. By day 28, however, the continuous IGF-1 group resulted in samples with elevated cell proliferation and matrix deposition while the transient group yielded constructs with almost identical properties in comparison with the untreated controls. This outcome suggests that the continuous addition of IGF-1 to the basal medium is required to support static cultivation of chondrocyte/PGA constructs and that the stimulatory effects of IGF-1 on cartilage development can be impeded if the supplementation is removed from the culture.

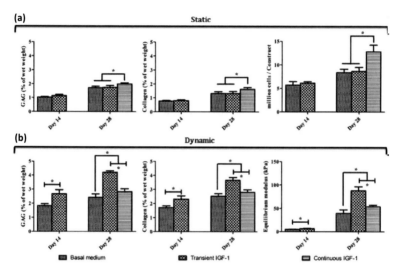

Figure 12.7 Effects of transient versus continuous exposure to 100 ng/mL IGF-1 on cartilage development. (a) From left to right: GAG, collagen and cell contents of static constructs. (b) From left to right: GAG content, collagen content and equilibrium modulus of dynamic constructs. *Significance; $p < 0.05$; $n = 4$–7. Modified from Yang and Barabino [173].

When engineered cartilage was cultivated under fluid agitation (Fig. 12.7b), IGF-1 could be effective in promoting neocartilage development as early as 2 weeks in culture, yielding stronger biomechanical and biochemical tissue properties than the untreated control group. In comparison with the results of the static experiment, this evidence substantiates that signals derived from IGF-1 are sensitive to shear stress [76] and its stimulatory function in cell/tissue growth can further be enhanced by hydrodynamic forces [79]. Although both continuous and transient IGF-1 treated groups improved construct quality at the end of the 4 week dynamic cultivation, the continuous IGF-1 constructs only exhibited slightly better properties than the untreated samples, but were significantly inferior to the transient IGF-1 cultures. This implies that the prolonged exposure to IGF-1 may limit the development of chondrocyte/PGA constructs stimulated by turbulent fluid flow.

In contrast to the study reported by Gooch and colleagues [58], in which IGF-1 (only continuous treatment was applied) was found to have no beneficial effects on engineered cartilage cultured within a spinner flask regardless of flow conditions, our results demonstrated that the addition of IGF-1 promoted construct development in the WWB cultivation both with and without fluid agitation. In these two studies, the scaffold type, cell source and cell seeding density were identical; therefore, this divergent outcome can be attributed to the use of culture media containing different serum concentrations (10% and 2% FBS in Gooch's and our studies, respectively). It may be that some of serum constituents, such as IGF binding proteins [51], neutralize exogenous IGF-1 molecules. We found that IGF-1 in combination with low-serum culture media is more suitable for both static and hydrodynamic cultivation of chondrocyte-seeded PGA scaffolds.

When the IGF-1 supplementation was interrupted after 2 weeks in hydrodynamic culture, functional properties of tissue constructs were further enhanced thereafter. This beneficial effect due to the transient exposure to growth factors is partially consistent with the work performed by Byers et al. [20], in which chondrocytes were encapsulated in agarose hydrogels and cultivated with a serum-starved medium supplemented with TGF-β3 for up to 8 weeks. When engineered constructs were exposed to TGF-β3 for the first two or four weeks of the cultivation, a similar 2 week delay prior to the drastic tissue growth was detected, suggesting that cultured cells require substantial time to adapt themselves to signaling cascades resulting from growth factor removal from the surrounding environment before exhibiting stronger potential for matrix synthesis. However, the temporal effect of exposure to growth factors in the Byers' study was observed in a culture system without any mechanical stimulation. This evidence reveals that the beneficial effects of transient growth factor exposure are largely dependent on the type of growth factors and their interaction with other environmental factors, for example, the use of serum, scaffolding materials or physical forces, which may need to be reviewed on a case-by-case basis. Furthermore, in the Byers' work, the transient growth factor treatment was shown to only facilitate construct development in mechanical strength and GAG production, but not in collagen deposition. In comparison with our study, it substantiates that IGF-1 may have higher potency in collagen synthesis than TGF-β3 and the synthesis mechanism is likely further promoted by fluid shear stress.

12.4 Multipotent Mesenchymal Stem Cells

Mesenchymal stem cells (MSCs) that were first identified in bone marrow, spleen and thymus of adult mice by Friedenstein et al. in 1976 by examining their clonogenic potential and were referred to as colony-forming unit-fibroblasts (CFU-f) [50] are uncommitted, multipotent progenitor cells that possess the ability to differentiate into various mesenchymal lineages, such as chondrocytes, osteoblasts, adipocytes, myocytes, cardiomyocytes, and tendon cells [23]. Thus, MSCs are attractive for repair and regeneration of tissue or organ defects due to their multipotency and expandable lifespan. Although MSCs can be derived from bone marrow [92,176], adipose tissues [5,176], synovial membrane [176], umbilical cord blood [39,179], skeletal muscle [140,177] or pancreas [71], MSCs isolated from different origins may have differential differentiation capacity even if cultured in exactly the same environment. For example, a study reported by Sakaguchi and coworkers demonstrated that, among human MSCs isolated from bone marrow, synovium, periosteum, skeletal muscle, and adipose tissues, bone marrow derived cells exhibited the highest osteogenic potential whereas synovium derived cells were predominant in chondrogenesis and adipogenesis [140]. A similar experiment was carried out in rats by Yoshimura et al., in which evident osteogenesis was detected in periosteum and muscle derived MSCs while synovium derived cells still had stronger potential for chondrogenesis and adipogenesis [176]. This evidence suggests that the plasticity of MSCs is also species-dependent. However, bone marrow is still by far the best characterized source of MSCs due to a less invasive isolation procedure.

In the case of cartilage regeneration, transplantation of MSCs into rabbit [89] or porcine [152] defective knee joints to restore cartilage function have met with some success, yet the use of MSCs for cartilage repair is still at the preclinical and phase-I stages and no comparative clinical studies have been reported [90]. On the other hand, given the tendency of articular chondrocytes to lose the chondrocyte phenotype during monolayer expansion, investigators have turned to MSCs as an alternative cell source for cartilage tissue engineering. While promising, MSCs offer their own challenges and their widespread use is limited due to the need to precisely control their differentiation into a desired cell lineage through manipulation of environmental factors.

12.4.1 Driving Forces of MSC Chondrogenic Differentiation

In vitro, several biochemical signals, such as TGF-β, IGF-1, FGF-2, and bone morphogenetic proteins (BMPs), have been investigated for their ability to direct MSC differentiation into the chondrogenic lineage [65]. Among these candidates, TGF-β (TGF-β1, -β2, and -β3) seems to be most effective and widely utilized in the induction of MSC chondrogenesis [39,46,109,119,124,130,131,154]. In addition to TGF-β, IGF-1 [2,56], BMP-2 [2,56,153,154], BMP-4 [153] or BMP-7 [83,170] alone is capable of driving MSC chondrogenic differentiation in vitro and exposure of MSCs to multiple inductive biomolecules results in a higher level of chondrogenesis [2,56,74,83,153,154,170]. Recently, a medium cocktail consisting of TGF-β1, IGF-1 and FGF-2 was formulated and shown to successfully produce more robust chondrogenesis of synovium-derived MSCs compared with TGF-β1 alone [130,131]. Taken together, this evidence confirms that a single inductive molecule may have a limited potential to trigger specific differentiation pathways due to the complex crosstalk between chemical signals during differentiation, and that the synergy between these cues is required to finalize cell fate [3,91].

In addition, the most straightforward and common way to deliver soluble factors to cultured MSCs is through direct addition of bulk molecules to culture media [46,109,130,131]. These traditional protocols, however, produce cells with typical features of hypertrophic chondrocytes which express a relatively significant level of type X collagen, instead of type II, [3,133] and alkaline phosphatase that facilitates endochondral bone formation [36,133,152]. A recent study reported by Macdonald et al. suggests that a bulk and quick release of inductive molecules may yield compromised and unstable cell differentiation and that a gradual delivery of those biomolecules to target cells can more closely replicate in vivo conditions [102]. Thus, it makes sense to identify delivery of soluble agents to cells in a gradual fashion. Such approaches include gene therapy [2,56,124,153,154] and development of polymeric vehicles for molecule release [39,102,143]. Interestingly, when primary MSCs were infected with IGF-1-encoded adenoviral vectors, Gelse and colleagues showed that rat cells underwent chondrogenic differentiation [56], while Steinert et al. demonstrated that chondrogenesis could not be induced in bovine cells [154]. These findings suggest that the role of IGF-1 in MSC chondrogenic differentiation may depend on animal species.

Besides soluble factors, there is currently limited evidence that microenvironmental physical cues are also capable of inducing certain MSC differentiation [62]. A study reported by McBeath et al. demonstrated that MSC differentiation could be manipulated by control of cell shape using a micropatterning technique [110]. Specifically, when human MSCs were cultivated on the surface of polydimethylsiloxane substrates coated with large areas of fibronectin that enhanced cell spreading, they experienced strong cytoskeletal tension and tended to differentiate into osteoblasts. Conversely, adipogenic commitment occurred when cells were on small islands of fibronectin and remained round. In addition, Engler and coworkers cultured human MSCs on the surface of collagen-modified polyacrylamide hydrogels with the tissue-level elasticity ranged from 0.1 to 40 kPa [44]. Cells exhibited the neurogenic, myogenic, and osteogenic potential when being grown on the soft, intermediate, and stiff substrates, respectively, in the absence of exogenous inductive molecules. Committed cells could be reprogrammed by the addition of soluble inducers during the first week of the cultivation whereas phenotype commitment was irreversible in longer cultures. When nonmuscle myosin II was inhibited, MSCs lost the ability to respond matrix stiffness and were not able to differentiate. These studies substantiate that MSCs can secrete various soluble factors in response to the microenvironment that alters cellular mechanics and further commit to specialized cell lineages through autocrine signaling. However, such mechanisms have not been validated in MSC chondrogenic differentiation.

12.4.2 Coculture-Enabled MSC Chondrogenesis

Another possible strategy to direct differentiation of stem cells is to coculture them with specialized cells. Given that cultured chondrocytes possess the ability to gradually secrete a variety of protein molecules including TGF-β [22,25], IGF-1 [52,142], BMP-2 [45,60] and FGF-2 [66], they can be an effective and economic source of an endogenous growth factor cocktail for directing MSC chondrogenesis. As a result, several studies involving cocultivation of MSCs with chondrocytes at different stages have been conducted [4,7,24,48,112,158]. In most of these experiments, MSCs and chondrocytes were mixed in monolayers [24], cell pellets [48,158] or different types of three-dimensional substrates [7,112] such that the two cell populations were in close proximity or had direct physical contact. For example, Bian and colleagues demonstrated that, when stimulated by TGF-β3, human MSCs (derived from a cell line) co-encapsulated with human osteoarthritic chondrocytes in hyaluronic acid hydrogels yielded engineered cartilage constructs with superior tissue properties in comparison with those seeded with MSCs alone. Suppressive gene expression of type X collagen was identified in the chondrocyte/MSC coculture, indicating that the cocultivated constructs exhibited a lower level of hypertrophic potential than the MSC samples. It is confirmed by Fischer et al. who suggest that osteoarthritic chondrocytes can release parathyroid hormone-related protein that may stabilize the phenotype of and reduce hypertrophy of chondrocyte-like cells differentiated from MSCs that are stimulated by exogenous inductive molecules [48]. The main benefit of these direct contact coculture systems is to allow intimate interactions between the two cell types, which results in a more efficient transduction of paracrine signals. However, there are concerns that, in these studies, data collected in characterization assays represent the summation of signals derived from both cell types and not solely from a pure MSC product, making it difficult to distinguish the origin of detected chondrogenic signals. Although additional separation processes, such as fluorescence-activated or magnetic-affinity cell sorting, can be utilized to isolate the MSC population, such techniques require intense skill and are costly and time-consuming. Another concern is that direct cell–cell contact can cause a strong risk of transmission of pathogens [65]. These obstacles, if left unaddressed, limit the potential of such coculture approaches for further tissue engineering or clinical applications.

In contrast to the chondrocyte/MSC coculture systems providing intimate cell–cell contact, a recent study reported by Aung and coworkers demonstrated that human osteoarthritic chondrocytes could trigger chondrogenesis of human MSCs, p7043L cell line, encapsulated in poly(ethylene-glycol) diacrylate gels, even without direct physical interactions and exogenous soluble inducers [4]. A cocultivation model utilizing bovine articular chondrocytes and bone marrow–derived MSCs was developed in our laboratory. Juvenile primary cells were employed here such that the development of this in vitro chondrocyte/MSC coculture system can help us further understand in vivo paracrine regulation of articular chondrocytes and bone marrow MSCs in MSC differentiation during skeletal development. In this coculture system, chondrocyte pellets and MSC monolayer were separated by a 0.4 µm transmembrane and cocultivated at a cell number ratio of 63:1 chondrocyte/MSC in a static, serum-free, growth factor-free environment. The coculture group was compared with the groups consisting of either monolayer MSCs (MSC control) or chondrocyte pellets (chondrocyte control) (Fig. 12.8a). After 15 days in culture, cells harvested from monolayer in the coculture group tended to lose the ability to secrete mesenchymal surface markers, CD166 and CD44 [77] (Fig. 12.8c), and had a chondrocyte-similar gene expression profile with a relatively inferior hypertrophic phenotype to the chondrocyte control (Fig. 12.8b). These MSC-differentiated cells also reproduced chondrocyte-like clusters when re-plated two-dimensionally after the coculture induction process (Fig. 12.8d). This evidence suggests that our in vitro chondrocyte/MSC model successfully emulates in vivo conditions and that juvenile chondrocytes can readily drive chondrogenic differentiation of bone marrow MSCs. In combination with the LbL nanolayer techniques [100–102,143,148,168], the specific individual or combined effects of chondrocyte-secreted paracrine factors on MSC chondrogenic differentiation can be determined. Incorporation of MSCs into scaffolds coated with LbL-enabled growth factor layers will further improve current protocols for the design of engineered constructs that promote in situ MSC chondrogenesis toward in vivo regeneration of articular cartilage.

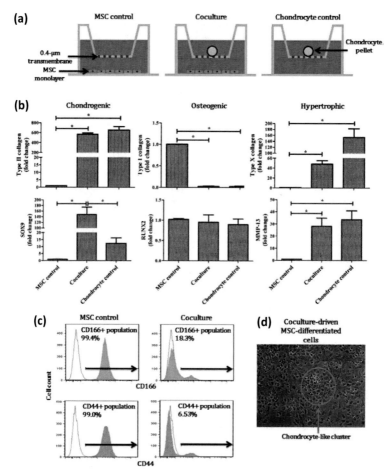

Figure 12.8   Coculture-driven MSC chondrogenic differentiation. (a) Culture groups. (b) mRNA expression of chondrogenic (collagen II, *SOX9*), osteogenic (collagen I, *RUNX2*) and hypertrophic (collagen X, MMP-13) markers in harvested monolayer cells (MSC control and coculture groups) or pellets (chondrocyte control). *Significance; $p < 0.05$; $n = 6$. (c) Flow cytometry analysis of mesenchymal surface markers, CD166 and CD44, in harvested monolayer cells. (d) Formation of chondrocyte-like clusters by coculture-driven MSC-differentiated cells; 10×. Modified from Yang et al. [172].

12.5 Conclusions and Future Directions

Restoration of cartilage defects due to injury or disease has not been achieved. Cartilage tissue engineering holds great potential to produce functional cartilage tissue replacements that are suitable for clinical implantation, yet hurdles like inferior properties of engineered tissues, insufficient or uncontrolled differentiation of stem cells, degradation of implants, and compromised integration of regenerating and adjacent native tissues exist. Much work still needs to be done in order to fully understand the role of individual environmental factors in and their synergistic effects on cartilage development and repair. Immediate steps to further our understanding of the field of cartilage tissue engineering and regeneration include (1) developing bioreactor systems that maximize the efficacy of cultured cells, (2) fabricating biocompatible scaffolding materials that mimic properties and ultrastructure of native cartilage and stabilize incorporated cells, (3) designing naturally derived or synthetic vehicles for controlled release and efficient delivery of multiple growth factors, (4) extending skills for cell sourcing and preservation, (5) controlling and understanding desired differentiation of stem cells, (6) stabilizing the phenotype of cells or tissue substitutes implanted in vivo, (7) discovering new techniques that ameliorate tissue integration and (8) establishing computation models which optimize all of the addressed factors and parameters that best describe bioprocessing conditions with respect to cartilage repair. Meeting these future needs through an optimal combination of microenvironmental parameters will enable the development of engineered replacement tissues suitable for the reinstatement of degenerative articular cartilage.

References

1. Ahamed, J., Burg, N., Yoshinaga, K., Janczak, C. A., Rifkin, D. B., and Coller, B. S. (2008). In vitro and in vivo evidence for shear-induced activation of latent transforming growth factor-β1, *Blood*, **112**, 3650–3660.

2. An, C., Cheng, Y., Yuan, Q., and Li, J. (2010). IGF-1 and BMP-2 induces differentiation of adipose-derived mesenchymal stem cells into chondrocytes-like cells, *Ann. Biomed. Eng.*, **38**, 1647–1654.

3. Augello, A., and De Bari, C. (2010). The regulation of differentiation in mesenchymal stem cells, *Hum. Gene Ther.*, **21**, 1226–1238.
4. Aung, A., Gupta, G., Majid, G., and Varghese, S. (2011). Osteoarthritic chondrocyte-secreted morphogens induce chondrogenic differentiation of human mesenchymal stem cells, *Arthritis Rheum.*, **63**, 148–158.
5. Awad, H. A., Halvorsen, Y.-D. C., Gimble, J. M., and Guilak, F. (2003). Effects of TGF-β1 and dexamethasone on the growth and chondrogenic differentiation of adipose-derived stromal cells, *Tissue Eng.*, **9**, 1301–1312.
6. Bian, L., Lima, E. G., Angione, S. L., Ng, K. W., Williams, D. Y., Xu, D., Stoker, A. M., Cook, J. L., Ateshian, G. A., and Hung, C. T. (2008). Mechanical and biochemical characterization of cartilage explants in serum-free culture, *J. Biomech.*, **41**, 1153–1159.
7. Bian, L., Zhai, D. Y., Mauck, R. L., and Burdick, J. A. (2011). Coculture of human mesenchymal stem cells and articular chondrocytes reduces hypertrophy and enhances functional properties of engineered cartilage, *Tissue Eng. Part A*, **17**, 1137–1145.
8. Bilgen, B., Sucosky, P., Neitzel, P. G., and Barabino, G. A. (2006). Flow characterization of a wavy-walled bioreactor for cartilage tissue engineering, *Biotechnol. Bioeng.*, **95**, 1009–1022.
9. Bilgen, B., and Barabino, G. A. (2007). Location of scaffolds in bioreactors modulates the hydrodynamic environment experienced by engineered tissues, *Biotechnol. Bioeng.*, **98**, 282–294.
10. Bilgen, B., Orsini, E., Aaron, R. K., and Ciombor, D. M. (2007). Fetal bovine serum suppresses transforming growth factor-β1-induced chondrogenesis in synoviocyte pellet cultures while dexamethasone and dynamic stimuli are beneficial, *J. Tissue Eng. Regen. Med.*, **1**, 436–442.
11. Bilodeau, K., and Mantovani, D. (2006). Bioreactors for tissue engineering: focus on mechanical constraints. A comparative review, *Tissue Eng.*, **12**, 2367–2383.
12. Blunk, T., Sieminski, A. L., Gooch, K. J., Courter, D. L., Hollander, A. P., Nahir, A. M., Langer, R., Vunjak-Novakovic, G., and Freed, L. E. (2002). Differential effects of growth factors on tissue-engineered cartilage, *Tissue Eng.*, **8**, 73–84.
13. Böhme, K., Winterhalter, K. H., and Bruckner, P. (1995). Terminal differentiation of chondrocytes in culture is a spontaneous process and is arrested by transforming growth factor-β2 and basic fibroblast growth factor in synergy, *Exp. Cell Res.*, **216**, 191–198.

14. Bouffi, C., Thomas, O., Bony, C., Giteau, A., Venier-Julienne, M.-C., Jorgensen, C., Montero-Menei, C., and Noël, D. (2010). The role of pharmacologically active microcarriers releasing TGF-β3 in cartilage formation in vivo by mesenchymal stem cells, *Biomaterials*, **31**, 6485–6493.
15. Brown, T. D., Johnston, R. C., Saltzman, C. L., Marsh, J. L., and Buckwalter, J. A. (2006). Posttraumatic osteoarthritis: a first estimate of incidence, prevalence, and burden of disease, *J. Orthop. Trauma*, **20**, 739–744.
16. Bueno, E. M., Bilgen, B., Carrier, R. L., and Barabino, G. A. (2004). Increased rate of chondrocyte aggregation in a wavy-walled bioreactor, *Biotechnol. Bioeng.*, **88**, 767–777.
17. Bueno, E. M., Bilgen, B., and Barabino, G. A. (2005). Wavy-walled bioreactor supports increased cell proliferation and matrix deposition in engineered cartilage constructs, *Tissue Eng.*, **11**, 1699–1709.
18. Bueno, E. M., Laevsky, G., and Barabino, G. A. (2007). Enhancing cell seeding of scaffolds in tissue engineering through manipulation of hydrodynamic parameters, *J. Biotechnol.*, **129**, 516–531.
19. Bueno, E. M., Bilgen, B., and Barabino, G. A. (2009). Hydrodynamic parameters modulate biochemical, histological, and mechanical properties of engineered cartilage, *Tissue Eng. Part A*, **15**, 773–785.
20. Byers, B. A., Mauck, R. L., Chiang, I. E., and Tuan, R. S. (2008). Transient exposure to transforming growth factor β3 under serum-free conditions enhances the biomechanical and biochemical maturation of tissue-engineered cartilage, *Tissue Eng. Part A*, **14**, 1821–1834.
21. Caterson, E. J., Nesti, L. J., Li, W.-J., Danielson, K. G., Albert, T. J., Vaccaro, A. R., and Tuan, R. S. (2001). Three-dimensional cartilage formation by bone marrow-derived cells seeded in polylactide/alginate amalgam, *J. Biomed. Mater. Res.*, **57**, 394–403.
22. Chang, S. C., Hoang, B., Thomas, J. T., Vukicevic, S., Luyten, F. P., Ryba, N. J., Kozak, C. A., Reddi, A. H., and Moos, M. (1994). Cartilage-derived morphogenetic proteins. New members of the transforming growth factor-β superfamily predominantly expressed in long bones during human embryonic development, *J. Biol. Chem.*, **269**, 28227–28234.
23. Chen, F. H., Rousche, K. T., and Tuan, R. S. (2006). Technology insight: adult stem cells in cartilage regeneration and tissue engineering, *Nat. Clin. Pract. Rheum.*, **2**, 373–382.
24. Chen, W.-H., Lai, M.-T., Wu, A. T. H., Wu, C.-C., Gelovani, J. G., Lin, C.-T., Hung, S.-C., Chiu, W.-T., and Deng, W.-P. (2009). In vitro stage-specific chondrogenesis of mesenchymal stem cells committed to chondrocytes, *Arthritis Rheum.*, **60**, 450–459.

25. Cheung, W.-H., Lee, K.-M., Fung, K.-P., Lui, P.-Y. P., and Leung, K.-S. (2001). TGF-β1 is the factor secreted by proliferative chondrocytes to inhibit neo-angiogenesis, *J. Cell. Biochem.*, **81**, 79–88.
26. Chiu, J. B., Luu, Y. K., Fang, D., Hsiao, B. S., Chu, B., and Hadjiargyrou, M. (2005). Electrospun nanofibrous scaffolds for biomedical applications, *J. Biomed. Nanotechnol.*, **1**, 115–132.
27. Chung, C., and Burdick, J. A. (2008). Influence of three-dimensional hyaluronic acid microenvironments on mesenchymal stem cell chondrogenesis, *Tissue Eng. Part A*, **15**, 243–254.
28. Chung, C., and Burdick, J. A. (2008). Engineering cartilage tissue, *Adv. Drug Deliver. Rev.*, **60**, 243–262.
29. Cole, B. J., and Malek, M. M. (2004). *Articular Cartilage Lesions: a Practical Guide to Assessment and Treatment*. (Springer, New York).
30. Darling, E. M., and Athanasiou, K. A. (2003). Articular cartilage bioreactors and bioprocesses, *Tissue Eng.*, **9**, 9–26.
31. Darling, E. M., and Athanasiou, K. A. (2005). Rapid phenotypic changes in passaged articular chondrocyte subpopulations, *J. Orthop. Res.*, **23**, 425–432.
32. Das, P., Schurman, D. J., and Smith, R. L. (1997). Nitric oxide and g proteins mediate the response of bovine articular chondrocytes to fluid-induced shear, *J. Orthop. Res.*, **15**, 87–93.
33. Davies, L. C., Blain, E. J., Gilbert, S. J., Caterson, B., and Duance, V. C. (2008). The potential of insulin-like growth factor-1 and transforming growth factor-β1 for promoting "adult" articular cartilage repair: an in vitro study, *Tissue Eng. Part A*, **14**, 1251–1261.
34. Davies, P. F. (1995). Flow-mediated endothelial mechanotransduction, *Physiol. Rev.*, **75**, 519–560.
35. Davisson, T., Kunig, S., Chen, A., Sah, R., and Ratcliffe, A. (2002). Static and dynamic compression modulate matrix metabolism in tissue engineered cartilage, *J. Orthop. Res.*, **20**, 842–848.
36. De Bari, C., Dell'accio, F., and Luyten, F. P. (2004). Failure of in vitro-differentiated mesenchymal stem cells from the synovial membrane to form ectopic stable cartilage in vivo, *Arthritis Rheum.*, **50**, 142–150.
37. Defail, A. J., Chu, C. R., Izzo, N., and Marra, K. G. (2006). Controlled release of bioactive TGF-β1 from microspheres embedded within biodegradable hydrogels, *Biomaterials*, **27**, 1579–1585.
38. Derynck, R., Lindquist, P. B., Lee, A., Wen, D., Tamm, J., Graycar, J. L., Rhee, L., Mason, A. J., Miller, D. A., Coffey, R. J., Moses, H. L., and Chen,

E. Y. (1988). A new type of transforming growth factor-β, TGF-β3, *EMBO J.*, **7**, 3737–3743.

39. Diao, H., Wang, J., Shen, C., Xia, S., Guo, T., Dong, L., Zhang, C., Chen, J., Zhao, J., and Zhang, J. (2009). Improved cartilage regeneration utilizing mesenchymal stem cells in TGF-β1 gene–activated scaffolds, *Tissue Eng. Part A*, **15**, 2687–2698.

40. Dunkelman, N. S., Zimber, M. P., Lebaron, R. G., Pavelec, R., Kwan, M., and Purchio, A. F. (1995). Cartilage production by rabbit articular chondrocytes on polyglycolic acid scaffolds in a closed bioreactor system, *Biotechnol. Bioeng.*, **46**, 299–305.

41. Duraine, G., Neu, C. P., Chan, S. M. T., Komvopoulos, K., June, R. K., and Reddi, H. A. (2009). Regulation of the friction coefficient of articular cartilage by transforming growth factor-β1 and interleukin-1β, *J. Orthop. Res.*, **27**, 249–256.

42. Elder, B. D., and Athanasiou, K. A. (2009). Hydrostatic pressure in articular cartilage tissue engineering: from chondrocytes to tissue regeneration, *Tissue Eng. Part B: Rev.*, **15**, 43–53.

43. Emin, N., Koç, A., Durkut, S., Elçin, A. E., and Elçin, Y. M. (2008). Engineering of rat articular cartilage on porous sponges: effects of TGF-β1 and microgravity bioreactor culture, *Artif. Cells Blood Substit. Biotechnol.*, **36**, 123–137.

44. Engler, A. J., Sen, S., Sweeney, H. L., and Discher, D. E. (2006). Matrix elasticity directs stem cell lineage specification, *Cell*, **126**, 677–689.

45. Erickson, D. M., Harris, S. E., Dean, D. D., Harris, M. A., Wozney, J. M., Boyan, B. D., and Schwartz, Z. (1997). Recombinant bone morphogenetic protein (BMP)-2 regulates costochondral growth plate chondrocytes and induces expression of BMP-2 and BMP-4 in a cell maturation-dependent manner, *J. Orthop. Res.*, **15**, 371–380.

46. Erickson, I. E., Huang, A. H., Chung, C., Li, R. T., Burdick, J. A., and Mauck, R. L. (2009). Differential maturation and structure–function relationships in mesenchymal stem cell- and chondrocyte-seeded hydrogels, *Tissue Eng. Part A*, **15**, 1041–1052.

47. Farooque, T. M. (2008). *Biochemical and Mechanical Stimuli for Improved Material Properties and Preservation of Tissue-Engineered Cartilage.* (Georgia Institute of Technology, Atlanta).

48. Fischer, J., Dickhut, A., Rickert, M., and Richter, W. (2010). Human articular chondrocytes secrete parathyroid hormone–related protein and inhibit hypertrophy of mesenchymal stem cells in coculture during chondrogenesis, *Arthritis Rheum.*, **62**, 2696–2706.

49. Freed, L. E., Marquis, J. C., Nohria, A., Emmanual, J., Mikos, A. G., and Langer, R. (1993). Neocartilage formation in vitro and in vivo using cells cultured on synthetic biodegradable polymers, *J. Biomed. Mater. Res.*, **27**, 11–23.

50. Friedenstein, A. J., Gorskaja, J. F., and Kulagina, N. N. (1976). Fibroblast precursors in normal and irradiated mouse hematopoietic organs, *Exp. Hematol.*, **4**, 267–274.

51. Friedrich, N., Haring, R., Nauck, M., Lüdemann, J., Rosskopf, D., Spilcke-Liss, E., Felix, S. B., Dörr, M., Brabant, G., Völzke, H., and Wallaschofski, H. (2009). Mortality and serum insulin-like growth factor (IGF)-1 and IGF binding protein 3 concentrations, *J. Clin. Endocrinol. Metab.*, **94**, 1732–1739.

52. Froger-Gaillard, B., Hossenlopp, P., Adolphe, M., and Binoux, M. (1989). Production of insulin-like growth factors and their binding proteins by rabbit articular chondrocytes: relationships with cell multiplication, *Endocrinology*, **124**, 2365–2372.

53. Fu, K., Pack, D. W., Klibanov, A. M., and Langer, R. (2000). Visual evidence of acidic environment within degrading poly(lactic-co-glycolic acid) (PLGA) microspheres, *Pharm. Res.*, **17**, 100–106.

54. Garcia, A. M., Frank, E. H., Grimshaw, P. E., and Grodzinsky, A. J. (1996). Contributions of fluid convection and electrical migration to transport in cartilage: relevance to loading, *Arch. Biochem. Biophys.*, **333**, 317–325.

55. Garcia, A. M., Lark, M. W., Trippel, S. B., and Grodzinsky, A. J. (1998). Transport of tissue inhibitor of metalloproteinases-1 through cartilage: contributions of fluid flow and electrical migration, *J. Orthop. Res.*, **16**, 734–742.

56. Gelse, K., Von Der Mark, K., Aigner, T., Park, J., and Schneider, H. (2003). Articular cartilage repair by gene therapy using growth factor-producing mesenchymal cells, *Arthritis Rheum.*, **48**, 430–441.

57. Glowacki, J., Yates, K. E., Maclean, R., and Mizuno, S. (2005). In vitro engineering of cartilage: effects of serum substitutes, TGF-β, and IL-1α, *Orthod. Craniofac. Res.*, **8**, 200–208.

58. Gooch, K. J., Blunk, T., Courter, D. L., Sieminski, A. L., Bursac, P. M., Vunjak-Novakovic, G., and Freed, L. E. (2001). Insulin-like growth factor-1 and mechanical environment interact to modulate engineered cartilage development, *Biochem. Biophys. Res. Commun.*, **286**, 909–915.

59. Gray, M. L., Pizzanelli, A. M., Lee, R. C., Grodzinsky, A. J., and Swann, D. A. (1989). Kinetics of the chondrocyte biosynthetic response to

compressive load and release, *Biochim. Biophys. Acta (BBA)—Gen. Subj.*, **991**, 415–425.

60. Grimsrud, C. D., Romano, P. R., D'souza, M., Puzas, J. E., Schwarz, E. M., Reynolds, P. R., Roiser, R. N., and O'keefe, R. J. (2001). BMP signaling stimulates chondrocyte maturation and the expression of indian hedgehog, *J. Orthop. Res.*, **19**, 18–25.

61. Grodzinsky, A. J., Levenston, M. E., Jin, M., and Frank, E. H. (2000). Cartilage tissue remodeling in response to mechanical forces, *Annu. Rev. Biomed. Eng.*, **2**, 691–713.

62. Guilak, F., Cohen, D. M., Estes, B. T., Gimble, J. M., Liedtke, W., and Chen, C. S. (2009). Control of stem cell fate by physical interactions with the extracellular matrix, *Cell Stem Cell*, **5**, 17–26.

63. Hall, A., Horwitz, E., and Wilkins, R. (1996). The cellular physiology of articular cartilage, *Exp. Physiol.*, **81**, 535–545.

64. Hannouche, D., Terai, H., Fuchs, J. R., Terada, S., Zand, S., Nasseri, B. A., Petite, H., Sedel, L., and Vacanti, J. P. (2007). Engineering of implantable cartilaginous structures from bone marrow–derived mesenchymal stem cells, *Tissue Eng.*, **13**, 87–99.

65. Heng, B. C., Cao, T., and Lee, E. H. (2004). Directing stem cell differentiation into the chondrogenic lineage in vitro, *Stem Cells*, **22**, 1152–1167.

66. Hill, D. J., Logan, A., Ong, M., De Sousa, D., and Gonzalez, A. M. (1992). Basic fibroblast growth factor is synthesized and released by isolated ovine fetal growth plate chondrocytes: potential role as an autocrine mitogen, *Growth Factors*, **6**, 277–294.

67. Holland, T. A., Tabata, Y., and Mikos, A. G. (2005). Dual growth factor delivery from degradable oligo(poly(ethylene glycol) fumarate) hydrogel scaffolds for cartilage tissue engineering, *J. Control. Release*, **101**, 111–125.

68. Holland, T. A., Bodde, E. W. H., Cuijpers, V. M. J. I., Baggett, L. S., Tabata, Y., Mikos, A. G., and Jansen, J. A. (2007). Degradable hydrogel scaffolds for in vivo delivery of single and dual growth factors in cartilage repair, *Osteoarthr. Cartilage*, **15**, 187–197.

69. Holmvall, K., Camper, L., Johansson, S., Kimura, J. H., and Lundgren-Åkerlund, E. (1995). Chondrocyte and chondrosarcoma cell integrins with affinity for collagen type II and their response to mechanical stress, *Exp. Cell Res.*, **221**, 496–503.

70. Hou, J. S., Mow, V. C., Lai, W. M., and Holmes, M. H. (1992). An analysis of the squeeze-film lubrication mechanism for articular cartilage, *J. Biomech.*, **25**, 247–259.

71. Hu, Y., Liao, L., Wang, Q., Ma, L., Ma, G., Jiang, X., and Zhao, R. C. (2003). Isolation and identification of mesenchymal stem cells from human fetal pancreas, *J. Lab clin. Med.*, **141**, 342–349.
72. Hunter, C. J., and Levenston, M. E. (2004). Maturation and integration of tissue-engineered cartilages within an in vitro defect repair model, *Tissue Eng.*, **10**, 736–746.
73. Ignotz, R. A., and Massagué, J. (1986). Transforming growth factor-β stimulates the expression of fibronectin and collagen and their incorporation into the extracellular matrix, *J. Biol. Chem.*, **261**, 4337–4345.
74. Indrawattana, N., Chen, G., Tadokoro, M., Shann, L. H., Ohgushi, H., Tateishi, T., Tanaka, J., and Bunyaratvej, A. (2004). Growth factor combination for chondrogenic induction from human mesenchymal stem cell, *Biochem. Biophys. Res. Commun.*, **320**, 914–919.
75. Janjanin, S., Li, W.-J., Morgan, M. T., Shanti, R. M., and Tuan, R. S. (2008). Mold-shaped, nanofiber scaffold-based cartilage engineering using human mesenchymal stem cells and bioreactor, *J. Surg. Res.*, **149**, 47–56.
76. Jin, M., Emkey, G. R., Siparsky, P., Trippel, S. B., and Grodzinsky, A. J. (2003). Combined effects of dynamic tissue shear deformation and insulin-like growth factor-1 on chondrocyte biosynthesis in cartilage explants, *Arch. Biochem. Biophys.*, **414**, 223–231.
77. Jones, E. A., Crawford, A., English, A., Henshaw, K., Mundy, J., Corscadden, D., Chapman, T., Emery, P., Hatton, P., and Mcgonagle, D. (2008). Synovial fluid mesenchymal stem cells in health and early osteoarthritis: detection and functional evaluation at the single-cell level, *Arthritis Rheum.*, **58**, 1731–1740.
78. Jurvelin, J., Kiviranta, I., Tammi, M., and Helminen, J. H. (1986). Softening of canine articular cartilage after immobilization of the knee joint, *Clin. Orthop. Relat. Res.*, 246–252.
79. Kapur, S., Mohan, S., Baylink, D. J., and Lau, K.-H. W. (2005). Fluid shear stress synergizes with insulin-like growth factor-1 (IGF-1) on osteoblast proliferation through integrin-dependent activation of IGF-1 mitogenic signaling pathway, *J. Biol. Chem.*, **280**, 20163–20170.
80. Kavalkovich, K., Boynton, R., Mary Murphy, J., and Barry, F. (2002). Chondrogenic differentiation of human mesenchymal stem cells within an alginate layer culture system, *In vitro Cell Dev Biol—Animal*, **38**, 457–466.

81. Ke, Y., Wang, Y. J., Ren, L., Zhao, Q. C., and Huang, W. (2010). Modified PHBV scaffolds by in situ UV polymerization: structural characteristic, mechanical properties and bone mesenchymal stem cell compatibility, *Acta Biomater.*, **6**, 1329–1336.
82. Kelly, T.-A. N., Fisher, M. B., Oswald, E. S., Tai, T., Mauck, R. L., Ateshian, G. A., and Hung, C. T. (2008). Low-serum media and dynamic deformational loading in tissue engineering of articular cartilage, *Ann. Biomed. Eng.*, **36**, 769–779.
83. Kim, H.-J., and Im, G.-I. (2008). Combination of transforming growth factor-β2 and bone morphogenetic protein 7 enhances chondrogenesis from adipose tissue-derived mesenchymal stem cells, *Tissue Eng. Part A*, **15**, 1543–1551.
84. Kim, Y.-J., Grodzinsky, A. J., and Plaas, A. H. K. (1996). Compression of cartilage results in differential effects on biosynthetic pathways for aggrecan, link protein, and hyaluronan, *Arch. Biochem. Biophys.*, **328**, 331–340.
85. Kisiday, J., Jin, M., Kurz, B., Hung, H., Semino, C., Zhang, S., and Grodzinsky, A. J. (2002). Self-assembling peptide hydrogel fosters chondrocyte extracellular matrix production and cell division: implications for cartilage tissue repair, *Proc. Natl. Acad. Sci. U. S. A.*, **99**, 9996–10001.
86. Kisiday, J. D., Jin, M., Dimicco, M. A., Kurz, B., and Grodzinsky, A. J. (2004). Effects of dynamic compressive loading on chondrocyte biosynthesis in self-assembling peptide scaffolds, *J. Biomech.*, **37**, 595–604.
87. Kisiday, J. D., Kurz, B., Dimicco, M. A., and Grodzinsky, A. J. (2005). Evaluation of medium supplemented with insulin–transferrin–selenium for culture of primary bovine calf chondrocytes in three-dimensional hydrogel scaffolds, *Tissue Eng.*, **11**, 141–151.
88. Kisiday, J. D., Kopesky, P. W., Evans, C. H., Grodzinsky, A. J., Mcilwraith, C. W., and Frisbie, D. D. (2008). Evaluation of adult equine bone marrow- and adipose-derived progenitor cell chondrogenesis in hydrogel cultures, *J. Orthop. Res.*, **26**, 322–331.
89. Koga, H., Muneta, T., Nagase, T., Nimura, A., Ju, Y.-J., Mochizuki, T., and Sekiya, I. (2008). Comparison of mesenchymal tissues-derived stem cells for in vivo chondrogenesis: suitable conditions for cell therapy of cartilage defects in rabbit, *Cell Tissue Res.*, **333**, 207–215.
90. Koga, H., Engebretsen, L., Brinchmann, J., Muneta, T., and Sekiya, I. (2009). Mesenchymal stem cell-based therapy for cartilage repair: a review, *Knee Surg. Sports Traumatol. Arthrosc.*, **17**, 1289–1297.

91. Kolf, C. M., Cho, E., and Tuan, R. S. (2007). Mesenchymal stromal cells. Biology of adult mesenchymal stem cells: regulation of niche, self-renewal and differentiation, *Arthritis Res. Ther.*, **9**, 204–213.
92. Kopen, G. C. (1999). *Murine Bone Marrow Stromal Cells: Isolation, Characterization, and Differentiation* (MCP Hahnemann University, Pennsylvania).
93. Kuettner, K. E. (1992). Biochemistry of articular cartilage in health and disease, *Clin. Biochem.*, **25**, 155–163.
94. Li, W.-J., Danielson, K. G., Alexander, P. G., and Tuan, R. S. (2003). Biological response of chondrocytes cultured in three-dimensional nanofibrous poly(ε-caprolactone) scaffolds, *J. Biomed. Mater. Res. A*, **67A**, 1105–1114.
95. Liang, D., Hsiao, B. S., and Chu, B. (2007). Functional electrospun nanofibrous scaffolds for biomedical applications, *Adv. Drug Deliver. Rev.*, **59**, 1392–1412.
96. Lim, S., Oh, S., Lee, H., Yuk, S., Im, G., and Lee, J. (2010). Dual growth factor-releasing nanoparticle/hydrogel system for cartilage tissue engineering, *J Mater Sci Mater Med*, **21**, 2593–2600.
97. Lin, Z., Willers, C., Xu, J., and Zheng, M.-H. (2006). The chondrocyte: biology and clinical application, *Tissue Eng.*, **12**, 1971–1984.
98. Liu, Y., Shu, X. Z., and Prestwich, G. D. (2006). Osteochondral defect repair with autologous bone marrow–derived mesenchymal stem cells in an injectable, in situ, cross-linked synthetic extracellular matrix, *Tissue Eng.*, **12**, 3405–3416.
99. Lohmann, C. H., Schwartz, Z., Niederauer, G. G., Carnes, D. L., Dean, D. D., and Boyan, B. D. (2000). Pretreatment with platelet derived growth factor-BB modulates the ability of costochondral resting zone chondrocytes incorporated into PLA/PGA scaffolds to form new cartilage in vivo, *Biomaterials*, **21**, 49–61.
100. Macdonald, M., Rodriguez, N. M., Smith, R., and Hammond, P. T. (2008). Release of a model protein from biodegradable self assembled films for surface delivery applications, *J. Control. Release*, **131**, 228–234.
101. Macdonald, M. L., Rodriguez, N. M., Shah, N. J., and Hammond, P. T. (2010). Characterization of tunable FGF-2 releasing polyelectrolyte multilayers, *Biomacromolecules*, **11**, 2053–2059.
102. Macdonald, M. L., Samuel, R. E., Shah, N. J., Padera, R. F., Beben, Y. M., and Hammond, P. T. (2011). Tissue integration of growth factor-eluting layer-by-layer polyelectrolyte multilayer coated implants, *Biomaterials*, **32**, 1446–1453.

103. Malaviya, P., and Nerem, R. M. (2002). Fluid-induced shear stress stimulates chondrocyte proliferation partially mediated via transforming growth factor-β1, *Tissue Eng.*, **8**, 581–590.
104. Mandl, E. W., Van Der Veen, S. W., Verhaar, J. A. N., and Van Osch, G. J. V. M. (2002). Serum-free medium supplemented with high-concentration fibroblast growth factor-2 for cell expansion culture of human ear chondrocytes promotes redifferentiation capacity, *Tissue Eng.*, **8**, 573–580.
105. Martin, I., Vunjak-Novakovic, G., Yang, J., Langer, R., and Freed, L. E. (1999). Mammalian chondrocytes expanded in the presence of fibroblast growth factor 2 maintain the ability to differentiate and regenerate three-dimensional cartilaginous tissue, *Exp. Cell Res.*, **253**, 681–688.
106. Martin, I., Obradovic, B., Treppo, S., Grodzinsky, A. J., Langer, R., Freed, L. E., and Vunjak-Novakovic, G. (2000). Modulation of the mechanical properties of tissue engineered cartilage, *Biorheology*, **37**, 141–147.
107. Mauck, R. L., Soltz, M. A., Wang, C. C. B., Wong, D. D., Chao, P.-H. G., Valhmu, W. B., Hung, C. T., and Ateshian, G. A. (2000). Functional tissue engineering of articular cartilage through dynamic loading of chondrocyte-seeded agarose gels, *J. Biomech. Eng.*, **122**, 252–260.
108. Mauck, R. L., Nicoll, S. B., Seyhan, S. L., Ateshian, G. A., and Hung, C. T. (2003). Synergistic action of growth factors and dynamic loading for articular cartilage tissue engineering, *Tissue Eng.*, **9**, 597–611.
109. Mauck, R. L., Yuan, X., and Tuan, R. S. (2006). Chondrogenic differentiation and functional maturation of bovine mesenchymal stem cells in long-term agarose culture, *Osteoarthr. Cartilage*, **14**, 179–189.
110. Mcbeath, R., Pirone, D. M., Nelson, C. M., Bhadriraju, K., and Chen, C. S. (2004). Cell shape, cytoskeletal tension, and rhoa regulate stem cell lineage commitment, *Dev. Cell*, **6**, 483–495.
111. Mcquillan, D. J., Handley, C. J., Campbell, M. A., Bolis, S., Milway, V. E., and Herington, A. C. (1986). Stimulation of proteoglycan biosynthesis by serum and insulin-like growth factor-1 in cultured bovine articular cartilage, *Biochem. J.*, **240**, 423–430.
112. Mo, X.-T., Guo, S.-C., Xie, H.-Q., Deng, L., Zhi, W., Xiang, Z., Li, X.-Q., and Yang, Z.-M. (2009). Variations in the ratios of co-cultured mesenchymal stem cells and chondrocytes regulate the expression of cartilaginous and osseous phenotype in alginate constructs, *Bone*, **45**, 42–51.
113. Mohtai, M., Gupta, M. K., Donlon, B., Ellison, B., Cooke, J., Gibbons, G., Schurman, D. J., and Smith, R. L. (1996). Expression of interleukin-6

in osteoarthritic chondrocytes and effects of fluid-induced shear on this expression in normal human chondrocytes in vitro, *J. Orthop. Res.*, **14**, 67–73.

114. Moroni, L., De Wijn, J. R., and Van Blitterswijk, C. A. (2006). 3D fiber-deposited scaffolds for tissue engineering: influence of pores geometry and architecture on dynamic mechanical properties, *Biomaterials*, **27**, 974–985.

115. Moyer, H. R., Wang, Y., Farooque, T., Wick, T., Singh, K. A., Xie, L., Guldberg, R. E., Williams, J. K., Boyan, B. D., and Schwartz, Z. (2010). A new animal model for assessing cartilage repair and regeneration at a nonarticular site, *Tissue Eng. Part A*, **16**, 2321–2330.

116. MüSsener, Å., Litton, M. J., Lindroos, E., and Klareskog, L. (1997). Cytokine production in synovial tissue of mice with collagen-induced arthritis (CIA), *Clin. Exp. Immunol.*, **107**, 485–493.

117. Negishi, M., Lu, D., Zhang, Y.-Q., Sawada, Y., Sasaki, T., Kayo, T., Ando, J., Izumi, T., Kurabayashi, M., Kojima, I., Masuda, H., and Takeuchi, T. (2001). Upregulatory expression of furin and transforming growth factor-β by fluid shear stress in vascular endothelial cells, *Arterioscler. Thromb. Vasc. Biol.*, **21**, 785–790.

118. Nerem, R. M., and Sambanis, A. (1995). Tissue engineering: from biology to biological substitutes, *Tissue Eng.*, **1**, 3–13.

119. Ng, F., Boucher, S., Koh, S., Sastry, K. S. R., Chase, L., Lakshmipathy, U., Choong, C., Yang, Z., Vemuri, M. C., Rao, M. S., and Tanavde, V. (2008). PDGF, TGF-β, and FGF signaling is important for differentiation and growth of mesenchymal stem cells (MSCs): transcriptional profiling can identify markers and signaling pathways important in differentiation of MSCs into adipogenic, chondrogenic, and osteogenic lineages, *Blood*, **112**, 295–307.

120. Nixon, A. J., Fortier, L. A., Williams, J., and Mohammed, H. (1999). Enhanced repair of extensive articular defects by insulin-like growth factor-1-laden fibrin composites, *J. Orthop. Res.*, **17**, 475–487.

121. Obradovic, B., Martin, I., Padera, R. F., Treppo, S., Freed, L. E., and Vunjak-Navakovic, G. (2001). Integration of engineered cartilage, *J. Orthop. Res.*, **19**, 1089–1097.

122. Ohno, M., Cooke, J. P., Dzau, V. J., and Gibbons, G. H. (1995). Fluid shear stress induces endothelial transforming growth factor β1 transcription and production. Modulation by potassium channel blockade, *J. Clin. Invest.*, **95**, 1363–1369.

123. Pacherník, J., Bryja, V., Ešner, M., Kubala, L., Dvořák, P., and Hampl, A. (2005). Neural differentiation of pluripotent mouse embryonal

carcinoma cells by retinoic acid: inhibitory effect of serum, *Physiol. Res.*, **54**, 115–122.

124. Pagnotto, M. R., Wang, Z., Karpie, J. C., Ferretti, M., Xiao, X., and Chu, C. R. (2007). Adeno-associated viral gene transfer of transforming growth factor-β1 to human mesenchymal stem cells improves cartilage repair, *Gene Ther.*, **14**, 804–813.

125. Papoutsakis, E. T. (1991). Fluid-mechanical damage of animal cells in bioreactors, *Trends Biotechnol.*, **9**, 427–437.

126. Park, H., Temenoff, J. S., Holland, T. A., Tabata, Y., and Mikos, A. G. (2005). Delivery of TGF-β1 and chondrocytes via injectable, biodegradable hydrogels for cartilage tissue engineering applications, *Biomaterials*, **26**, 7095–7103.

127. Park, H., Temenoff, J. S., Tabata, Y., Caplan, A. I., and Mikos, A. G. (2007). Injectable biodegradable hydrogel composites for rabbit marrow mesenchymal stem cell and growth factor delivery for cartilage tissue engineering, *Biomaterials*, **28**, 3217–3227.

128. Pazzano, D., Mercier, K. A., Moran, J. M., Fong, S. S., Dibiasio, D. D., Rulfs, J. X., Kohles, S. S., and Bonassar, L. J. (2000). Comparison of chondrogensis in static and perfused bioreactor culture, *Biotechnol. Prog.*, **16**, 893–896.

129. Pei, M., Seidel, J., Vunjak-Novakovic, G., and Freed, L. E. (2002). Growth factors for sequential cellular de- and re-differentiation in tissue engineering, *Biochem. Biophys. Res. Commun.*, **294**, 149–154.

130. Pei, M., He, F., Kish, V., and Vunjak-Novakovic, G. (2008). Engineering of functional cartilage tissue using stem cells from synovial lining: a preliminary study, *Clin. Orthop. Relat. Res.*, **466**, 1880–1889.

131. Pei, M., He, F., and Vunjak-Novakovic, G. (2008). Synovium-derived stem cell-based chondrogenesis, *Differentiation*, **76**, 1044–1056.

132. Pelaez, D., Charles Huang, C.-Y., and Cheung, H. S. (2008). Cyclic compression maintains viability and induces chondrogenesis of human mesenchymal stem cells in fibrin gel scaffolds, *Stem Cells Dev.*, **18**, 93–102.

133. Pelttari, K., Winter, A., Steck, E., Goetzke, K., Hennig, T., Ochs, B. G., Aigner, T., and Richter, W. (2006). Premature induction of hypertrophy during in vitro chondrogenesis of human mesenchymal stem cells correlates with calcification and vascular invasion after ectopic transplantation in scid mice, *Arthritis Rheum.*, **54**, 3254–3266.

134. Perka, C., Schultz, O., Spitzer, R. S., and Lindenhayn, K. (2000). The influence of transforming growth factor β1 on mesenchymal cell repair of full-thickness cartilage defects, *J. Biomed. Mater. Res.*, **52**, 543–552.

135. Rosier, R. N., O'keefe, R. J., and Hicks, D. G. (1998). The potential role of transforming growth factor β in fracture healing, *Clin. Orthop. Relat. Res.*, **355**, S294–S300.

136. Roy, R., Boskey, A. L., and Bonassar, L. J. (2008). Non-enzymatic glycation of chondrocyte-seeded collagen gels for cartilage tissue engineering, *J. Orthop. Res.*, **26**, 1434–1439.

137. Sah, R. L., Trippel, S. B., and Grodzinsky, A. J. (1996). Differential effects of serum, insulin-like growth factor-1, and fibroblast growth factor-2 on the maintenance of cartilage physical properties during long-term culture, *J. Orthop. Res.*, **14**, 44–52.

138. Sah, R. L. Y., Kim, Y.-J., Doong, J.-Y. H., Grodzinsky, A. J., Plass, A. H. K., and Sandy, J. D. (1989). Biosynthetic response of cartilage explants to dynamic compression, *J. Orthop. Res.*, **7**, 619–636.

139. Sah, R. L. Y., Doong, J.-Y. H., Grodzinsky, A. J., Plaas, A. H. K., and Sandy, J. D. (1991). Effects of compression on the loss of newly synthesized proteoglycans and proteins from cartilage explants, *Arch. Biochem. Biophys.*, **286**, 20–29.

140. Sakaguchi, Y., Sekiya, I., Yagishita, K., and Muneta, T. (2005). Comparison of human stem cells derived from various mesenchymal tissues: superiority of synovium as a cell source, *Arthritis Rheum.*, **52**, 2521–2529.

141. Sakai, K., Mohtai, M., and Iwamoto, Y. (1998). Fluid shear stress increases transforming growth factor β1 expression in human osteoblast-like cells: modulation by cation channel blockades, *Calcif. Tissue Int.*, **63**, 515–520.

142. Schlechter, N. L., Russell, S. M., Spencer, E. M., and Nicoll, C. S. (1986). Evidence suggesting that the direct growth-promoting effect of growth hormone on cartilage in vivo is mediated by local production of somatomedin, *Proc. Natl. Acad. Sci. U. S. A.*, **83**, 7932–7934.

143. Shah, N. J., Macdonald, M. L., Beben, Y. M., Padera, R. F., Samuel, R. E., and Hammond, P. T. (2011). Tunable dual growth factor delivery from polyelectrolyte multilayer films, *Biomaterials*, **32**, 6183–6193.

144. Shao, X., Goh, J. C. H., Hutmacher, D. W., Lee, E. H., and Zigang, G. (2006). Repair of large articular osteochondral defects using hybrid scaffolds and bone marrow-derived mesenchymal stem cells in a rabbit model, *Tissue Eng.*, **12**, 1539–1551.

145. Shapiro, L. E., and Wagner, N. (1988). Growth of H-35 rat hepatoma cells in unsupplemented serum-free media: effect of transferrin, insulin and cell density, *In vitro Cell. Dev. Biol. Anim.*, **24**, 299–303.

146. Shapiro, L. E., and Wagner, N. (1989). Transferrin is an autocrine growth factor secreted by reuber H-35 cells in serum-free culture *In vitro Cell. Dev. Biol. Anim.*, **25**, 650–654.

147. Sheehy, E. J., Buckley, C. T., and Kelly, D. J. (2011). Chondrocytes and bone marrow-derived mesenchymal stem cells undergoing chondrogenesis in agarose hydrogels of solid and channelled architectures respond differentially to dynamic culture conditions, *J. Tissue Eng. Regen. Med.*, **5**, 747–758.

148. Shukla, A., Fleming, K. E., Chuang, H. F., Chau, T. M., Loose, C. R., Stephanopoulos, G. N., and Hammond, P. T. (2010). Controlling the release of peptide antimicrobial agents from surfaces, *Biomaterials*, **31**, 2348–2357.

149. Smith, R. L., Rusk, S. F., Ellison, B. E., Wessells, P., Tsuchiya, K., Carter, D. R., Caler, W. E., Sandell, L. J., and Schurman, D. J. (1996). In vitro stimulation of articular chondrocyte mRNA and extracellular matrix synthesis by hydrostatic pressure, *J. Orthop. Res.*, **14**, 53–60.

150. Smith, R. L., Trindade, M. C. D., Shida, J., Kajiyama, G., Vu, T., Hoffman, A. R., Mch, Goodman, S. B., Schurman, D. J., and Carter, D. R. (2000). Time-dependent effects of intermittent hydrostatic pressure on articular chondrocyte type II collagen and aggrecan mRNA expression, *J. Rehabil. Res. Dev.*, **37**, 153–161.

151. Spiller, K. L., Liu, Y., Holloway, J. L., Maher, S. A., Cao, Y., Liu, W., Zhou, G., and Lowman, A. M. (2012). A novel method for the direct fabrication of growth factor-loaded microspheres within porous nondegradable hydrogels: controlled release for cartilage tissue engineering, *J. Control. Release*, **157**, 39–45.

152. Steck, E., Fischer, J., Lorenz, H., Gotterbarm, T., Jung, M., and Richter, W. (2009). Mesenchymal stem cell differentiation in an experimental cartilage defect: restriction of hypertrophy to bone-close neocartilage, *Stem Cells Dev.*, **18**, 969–978.

153. Steinert, A., Weber, M., Dimmler, A., Julius, C., Schütze, N., Nöth, U., Cramer, H., Eulert, J., Zimmermann, U., and Hendrich, C. (2003). Chondrogenic differentiation of mesenchymal progenitor cells encapsulated in ultrahigh-viscosity alginate, *J. Orthop. Res.*, **21**, 1090–1097.

154. Steinert, A. F., Palmer, G. D., Pilapil, C., Nöth, U., Evans, C. H., and Ghivizzani, S. C. (2008). Enhanced in vitro chondrogenesis of primary mesenchymal stem cells by combined gene transfer, *Tissue Eng. Part A*, **15**, 1127–1139.

155. Steinmeyer, J., and Knue, S. (1997). The proteoglycan metabolism of mature bovine articular cartilage explants superimposed to continuously applied cyclic mechanical loading, *Biochem. Biophys. Res. Commun.*, **240**, 216–221.

156. Suryawan, A., and Hu, C. Y. (1993). Effect of serum on differentiation of porcine adipose stromal-vascular cells in primary culture, *Comp. Biochem. Physiol. Comp. Physiol.*, **105**, 485–492.

157. Temenoff, J. S., and Mikos, A. G. (2000). Review: Tissue engineering for regeneration of articular cartilage, *Biomaterials*, **21**, 431–440.

158. Tsuchiya, K., Chen, G., Ushida, T., Matsuno, T., and Tateishi, T. (2004). The effect of coculture of chondrocytes with mesenchymal stem cells on their cartilaginous phenotype in vitro, *Mater. Sci. Eng. C*, **24**, 391–396.

159. Uchino, M., Izumi, T., Tominaga, T., Wakita, R., Minehara, H., Sekiguchi, M., and Itoman, M. (2000). Growth factor expression in the osteophytes of the human femoral head in osteoarthritis, *Clin. Orthop. Relat. Res.*, **377**, 119–125.

160. Valhmu, W. B., Stazzone, E. J., Bachrach, N. M., Saed-Nejad, F., Fischer, S. G., Mow, V. C., and Ratcliffe, A. (1998). Load-controlled compression of articular cartilage induces a transient stimulation of aggrecan gene expression, *Arch. Biochem. Biophys.*, **353**, 29–36.

161. van der Kraan, P. M., Glansbeek, H. L., Vitters, E. L., and van den Berg, W. B. (1997). Early elevation of transforming growth factor-β, decorin, and biglycan mRNA levels during cartilage matrix restoration after mild proteoglycan depletion, *J. Rheumatol.*, **24**, 543–549.

162. Venkateswaran, V., Klotz, L. H., and Fleshner, N. E. (2002). Selenium modulation of cell proliferation and cell cycle biomarkers in human prostate carcinoma cell lines, *Cancer Res.*, **62**, 2540–2545.

163. Vozzi, G., Flaim, C., Ahluwalia, A., and Bhatia, S. (2003). Fabrication of PLGA scaffolds using soft lithography and microsyringe deposition, *Biomaterials*, **24**, 2533–2540.

164. Vunjak-Novakovic, G., Obradovic, B., Martin, I., Bursac, P. M., Langer, R., and Freed, L. E. (1998). Dynamic cell seeding of polymer scaffolds for cartilage tissue engineering, *Biotechnol. Prog.*, **14**, 193–202.

165. Vunjak-Novakovic, G., Martin, I., Obradovic, B., Treppo, S., Grodzinsky, A. J., Langer, R., and Freed, L. E. (1999). Bioreactor cultivation conditions modulate the composition and mechanical properties of tissue-engineered cartilage, *J. Orthop. Res.*, **17**, 130–138.

166. Waldman, S. D., Spiteri, C. G., Grynpas, M. D., Pilliar, R. M., and Kandel, R. A. (2003). Long-term intermittent shear deformation improves the quality of cartilaginous tissue formed in vitro, *J. Orthop. Res.*, **21**, 590–596.
167. Waldman, S. D., Spiteri, C. G., Grynpas, M. D., Pilliar, R. M., and Kandel, R. A. (2004). Long-term intermittent compressive stimulation improves the composition and mechanical properties of tissue-engineered cartilage, *Tissue Eng.*, **10**, 1323–1331.
168. Wood, K. C., Chuang, H. F., Batten, R. D., Lynn, D. M., and Hammond, P. T. (2006). Controlling interlayer diffusion to achieve sustained, multiagent delivery from layer-by-layer thin films, *Proc. Natl. Acad. Sci. U. S. A.*, **103**, 10207–10212.
169. Yaeger, P. C., Masi, T. L., De Ortiz, J. L. B., Binette, F., Tubo, R., and Mcpherson, J. M. (1997). Synergistic action of transforming growth factor-β and insulin-like growth factor-1 induces expression of type II collagen and aggrecan genes in adult human articular chondrocytes, *Exp. Cell Res.*, **237**, 318–325.
170. Yamane, S., and Reddi, A. H. (2008). Induction of chondrogenesis and superficial zone protein accumulation in synovial side population cells by BMP-7 and TGF-β1, *J. Orthop. Res.*, **26**, 485–492.
171. Yang, Y.-H., and Barabino, G. A. (2011). Requirement for serum in medium supplemented with insulin-transferrin-selenium for hydrodynamic cultivation of engineered cartilage, *Tissue Eng. Part A*, **17**, 2025–2035.
172. Yang, Y.-H., Lee, A. J., and Barabino, G. A. (2012). Coculture-driven mesenchymal stem cell-differentiated articular chondrocyte-like cells support neocartilage development, *Stem Cells Transl. Med.*, **1**, 843–854.
173. Yang, Y.-H., and Barabino, G. A. (2013). Differential morphology and homogeneity of tissue-engineered cartilage in hydrodynamic cultivation with transient exposure to insulin-like growth factor-1 and transforming growth factor-β1, *Tissue Eng. Part A*, **19**, 2349–2360.
174. Yokota, H., Goldring, M. B., and Sun, H. B. (2003). CITED2-mediated regulation of MMP-1 and MMP-13 in human chondrocytes under flow shear, *J. Biol. Chem.*, **278**, 47275–47280.
175. Yokoyama, A., Sekiya, I., Miyazaki, K., Ichinose, S., Hata, Y., and Muneta, T. (2005). In vitro cartilage formation of composites of synovium-

derived mesenchymal stem cells with collagen gel, *Cell Tissue Res.*, **322**, 289–298.

176. Yoshimura, H., Muneta, T., Nimura, A., Yokoyama, A., Koga, H., and Sekiya, I. (2007). Comparison of rat mesenchymal stem cells derived from bone marrow, synovium, periosteum, adipose tissue, and muscle, *Cell Tissue Res.*, **327**, 449–462.

177. Young, H. E., Mancini, M. L., Wright, R. P., Smith, J. C., Black, A. C., Reagan, C. R., and Lucas, P. A. (1995). Mesenchymal stem cells reside within the connective tissues of many organs, *Dev. Dyn.*, **202**, 137–144.

178. Zhang, E., Li, X., Zhang, S., Chen, L., and Zheng, X. (2005). Cell cycle synchronization of embryonic stem cells: effect of serum deprivation on the differentiation of embryonic bodies in vitro, *Biochem. Biophys. Res. Commun.*, **333**, 1171–1177.

179. Zucconi, E., Vieira, N. M., Bueno, D. F., Secco, M., Jazedje, T., Ambrosio, C. E., Passos-Bueno, M. R., Miglino, M. A., and Zatz, M. (2010). Mesenchymal stem cells derived from canine umbilical cord vein: a novel source for cell therapy studies, *Stem Cells Dev.*, **19**, 395–402.

Chapter 13

Bone Regenerative Engineering: The Influence of Micro- and Nano-Dimension

Roshan James, Meng Deng, Sangamesh G. Kumbar, and Cato T. Laurencin

Institute for Regenerative Engineering, The Raymond and Beverly Sackler Center For Biomedical, Biological, Engineering and Physical Sciences, Department of Orthopaedic Surgery, and Chemical, Materials and Biomolecular Engineering, The University of Connecticut Health Center, 263 Farmington Avenue, Farmington, CT 06030, USA

Laurencin@uchc.edu

13.1 Introduction

Health care issues arising from tissue loss or organ failure are among the most devastating and costliest world over [1]. More than 33 million musculoskeletal injuries are reported annually in the United States alone. Fractures comprise approximately 6.5 million annually and more than 1,300,000 of these individual cases in 2003 required application of a bone graft material [2–4]. Fractures of the hip, ankle, tibia, and fibula occur most frequently, and in general men experience more fractures than women. The total number of hip replacements increased 33% to 152,000 cases in the year 2000 as compared to the year 1990 in the United States alone, and it is expected to increase to about 272,000 by the year 2030 [5]. The currently available therapeutic options to treat bone tissue loss include transplantation of autografts/allografts, delivery

---

Tissue and Organ Regeneration: Advances in Micro- and Nanotechnology
Edited by Lijie Grace Zhang, Ali Khademhosseini, and Thomas J. Webster
Copyright © 2014 Pan Stanford Publishing Pte. Ltd.
ISBN 978-981-4411-67-7 (Hardcover), 978-981-4411-68-4 (eBook)
www.panstanford.com

of stimulatory molecules, and implantation of tissue replacements which are composed of metal, polymer, and ceramic alone or in combination [6]. However, each approach offers unique advantages and a number of limitations. For example, autografts and allografts are often associated with the limited availability and risks of immune rejection, respectively. Thus, there is a large need for synthetic grafts for fracture repair, and there are significant opportunities to improve the existing graft material. The tissue engineering (TE) approach has emerged as a promising strategy that provides viable tissue substitutes and eliminates many of the limitations that exist in current therapies.

Tissue engineering can be defined as the application of biological, chemical, and engineering principles toward the repair, restoration or regeneration of tissues using cells, factors, and biomaterials alone or in combination [7]. The classic paradigm for in vitro tissue engineering of bone involves the isolation and culture of donor osteoblasts or osteoprogenitor cells within three-dimensional (3D) biomaterials as scaffolds under conditions that support tissue growth of new bone. By combining appropriately engineered biomaterials, cells, and cell culture conditions, strategies may ultimately be found to produce synthetic bone grafts capable of providing bony repair [7,8]. Biodegradable scaffolds play a crucial role in the TE approach [2,5,9–16]. During regeneration, the biodegradable scaffold provides structural and mechanical support to the damaged tissues, degrades in a controlled manner into biocompatible by-products, and presents an interconnected porous structure to accommodate cell infiltration and vascularization, and promote extracellular matrix (ECM) synthesis [8,17,18]. Additionally, the delivery of donor osteoblasts or progenitor populations on the scaffold contributes to the tissue formation capacity, and addition of growth factors will provide added benefit to accelerate cell differentiation. The regeneration efficacy of a 3D scaffold is largely dependent on its nature, composition, topography and structural properties.

Biocompatible materials, including biodegradable polymers and composites have been fabricated using various techniques into 3D scaffolds that mimic the architecture of natural ECM and have inductive capacity to modulate the regenerative process [19]. The intersection of advanced biomaterials engineering, advances in stem cell science and developmental biology over the past 10 years has led to the emergence of a new field "Regenerative Engineering," defined as "the integration of tissue engineering with advanced materials science, stem cell science and developmental biology toward the regeneration of complex tissues, organs, or organ systems" (Fig. 13.1) [20,21]. Regenerative engineering has elements of tissue engineering but is distinct in recognizing the robust new technologies that have come to the fore in the design of solutions for the regeneration of tissues.

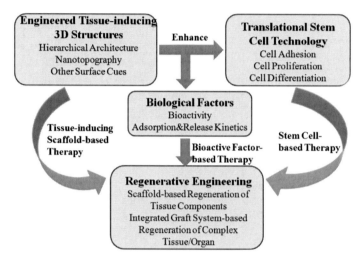

Figure 13.1 Schematics of regenerative engineering approach to create complex functional tissues and organs [21]. Reprinted from *IEEE Transactions on NanoBioscience*, **11**(1), Meng et al., Nanostructured polymeric scaffolds for orthopaedic regenerative engineering, 3–14, 2012, with permission from IEEE.

13.2 Understanding Native Bone

Bone is a highly specialized organ that constitutes the rigid skeleton found in all vertebrates [41,42]. The primary bone structural functions are to support the organs and tissues of the body, act as a lever system to enable movement, and protect the internal organs from shock and injury. Physiological functions include hematopoiesis, the formation of blood cells, a source of stem cells, and actions centered around being an ion reservoir for calcium, phosphate, sodium, potassium, zinc and magnesium. In addition, bone matrix maintains growth factors that are released as required, buffers against extreme pH changes, and is involved in endocrine signaling. Bone is a very dynamic organ undergoing constant self-remodeling and has within itself the unique ability to repair/regenerate to a certain extent following injury.

13.2.1 Hierarchical Organization of Bone

Microscopically, bone is differentiated into two phenotypes that are described as woven and lamellar bone [42,43]. Woven bone is characteristic of the fetal development stage, and present in young children (primary bone) and at tendon/ligament insertion sites. It is composed of randomly oriented and disorganized collagen fibers and populated randomly by osteocytes. It has been observed in the callus stage of the fracture healing process, and it resorbed and replaced by lamellar bone within duration of few weeks. Lamellar bone also known as mature or secondary bone tissue is composed of collagen fibers oriented in lamellae or sheets and arises from the remodeling of primary bone tissue.

At the macroscopic level, mature bone is differentiated into cortical and spongy bones, which vary in density (Fig. 13.2) [42–44]. Compact or cortical bones appear as solid masses, whereas trabecular bones are sponge-like where free spaces are filled with bone marrow. The lamellar bones are organized with porosity varying from macro- to nano-dimension allowing transport of nutrients, oxygen, and body fluids. Compact bone is composed of osteon units that are cemented to another, but separated by interstitial and circumferential lamellae. Each osteon comprises of a longitudinal central canal (Haversian canal), surrounded by 20–30 concentric lamellae of deposited collagen fibers, and osteocytes are buried within these lamellae. Volkmann's canals connect each Haversian canal to each other, and to the blood supply and the bone marrow cavity. In comparison, spongy bone is porous and has a higher concentration of blood vessels. Here the lamellae are arranged in parallel and are mainly involved in mineral homeostasis. The compact bone functions mechanically in tension, compression, and torsion, whereas spongy bone functions mainly in compression. The mechanical properties of cancellous and cortical bone are listed in Table 13.1.

Understanding Native Bon | 459

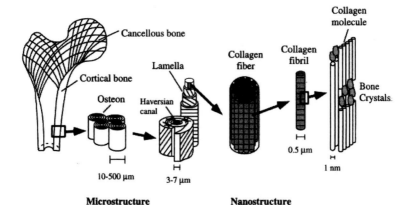

Figure 13.2 Hierarchical structural organization of bone where the macrostructure is composed of (a) cortical and cancellous bone, which is composed of (b) osteons with Haversian systems and (c) lamellae. This microstructure is composed of (d) collagen fibers made up of nano-diameter collagen fibrils. The smallest structural unit in bone is (e) bone mineral crystals, collagen molecules, and non-collagenous proteins. Reprinted from *Medical Engineering & Physics*, **20**(2), Rho et al., Mechanical properties and the hierarchical structure of bone, 92–102, 1998, with permission from Elsevier [44].

Table 13.1 Bone biomechanical properties

Properties	Measurements	
	Cortical bone	Cancellous bone
Young's modulus (GPa)	14–20	0.05–0.5
Tensile strength (MPa)	50–150	10–20
Compressive strength (MPa)	170–193	7–10
Fracture toughness (MPa m$^{1/2}$)	2–12	0.1
Strain to failure	1–3	5–7
Density (g/cm^3)	18–22	0.1–1.0
Apparent density (g/cm^3)	1.8–2.0	0.1–1.0
Surface/bone volume (mm^2/mm^3)	2.5	20
Total bone volume (mm^3)	1.4×10^6	0.35×10^6
Total internal surface	3.5×10^6	7.0×10^6

Source: Reprinted from *Composites Science and Technology*, **65**(15–16), Murugan et al., Development of nanocomposites for bone grafting, 2385–2406, 2005, with permission from Elsevier [45].

These hierarchical structures are unique to bone tissue, and their different length scales play a significant role in maintaining the chemical, mechanical, and biological properties of bone [44,46]. The structural hierarchy of bone architecture includes five levels on the basis of the length scales discussed earlier: (1) the macrostructures of cortical bone and trabecular bone; (2) the microstructures (10–500 µm) of the osteons and trabeculae; (3) the submicro-structures (1–10 µm) of bone lamella [47]; (4) the nanostructures (from a few hundred nanometers to 1 µm) of collagen fibrils; and (5) the subnanostructures (below a few hundred nanometers) of collagen molecules, bone crystals and non-collagenous organic proteins.

Collagens (i.e., type I collagen) constitute the major structural protein of the bone ECM [41,48]. Collagens secreted by the osteoblasts self-assemble into fibrils having a specific tertiary structure. The tertiary structure includes a 67 nm periodicity and 40 nm gaps between the collagen molecules [44]. Collagen chain is characterized by the highly organized fibrils forming a continuous triple helix, consisting of three intertwining helical polypeptides [49]. The organized fibrils possess high tensile strength. Type I collagen fibrils form the fiber bundles in tendons, whereas in bone they are present as a concentric network of fibrils encapsulating hydroxyapatite (HA) crystals in the gaps between collagen molecules. The inorganic mineral HA comprises 60% of bone, and 33% is comprised of an organic matrix, comprising of 20% type I collagen and 3% noncollagenous proteins (Table 13.2) [45,50]. The inorganic phase is primarily composed of HA $(Ca_{10}(PO_4)_6(OH)_2)$. At the nanoscale, plate-like apatite crystals form discretely and discontinuously with a specific crystalline orientation within the collagen fibrils [51–53]. These two major phases interact to form a bone composite with other components such as minerals, water, lipids, vascular elements, and cells. The collagen fibers present in bone provides the structural frame onto which inorganic HA are embedded thus strengthening the collagen framework [42]. The HA crystal plates are in the dimension of 50 nm × 25 nm (length × width). Several other components such as HPO_4^{2-}, Na^+, Mg^{2+}, citrate, carbonate, K^+ are also present in the bone apatite, which is characterized to be nanocrystalline HA without hydroxyl groups [54]. The presence of non-collagenous proteins such as osteocalcin, osteopontin, sialoprotein, and osteonectin may contribute to the regulation of crystal size, orientation, and mineral deposition by binding calcium or helping release phosphate. Thus, collagen fibers are important constituents and form structures that contribute to the outstanding properties of bone. They are further reinforced by the impregnated mineral HA.

Table 13.2 Composition of bone

Inorganic phase	wt%	Organic phase	wt%
Hydroxyapatite	~60	Collagen	~20
Carbonate	~4	Water	~9
Citrate	~0.9	Non-collagenous proteins (osteocalcin, osteonectin, osteopontin, thrombospondin, morphogenetic proteins, sialoprotein, serum proteins)	~3
Sodium	~0.7		
Magnesium	~0.5		
Other traces: Cl^-, F^-, K^+ Sr^{2+}, Pb^{2+}, Zn^{2+}, Cu^{2+}, Fe^{2+}		Other traces: Polysaccharides, lipids, cytokines	
		Primary bone cells: osteoblasts, osteocytes, osteoclasts	

Source: Reprinted from *Composites Science and Technology*, **65**(15–16), Murugan et al., Development of nanocomposites for bone grafting, 2385–2406, 2005, with permission from Elsevier [45].

13.2.2 Biology of Bone

Formation and the maintenance of bone tissue is the result of highly organized and coordinated multi-cellular actions. Three distinctly different cell types are present in bone tissue namely, osteoblasts, osteoclast, and osteocytes which account for about 90% of all cells in the adult skeleton. In addition, osteoprogenitor cells and bone-lining cells are associated with bone function. During vertebrate embryo development, cells derived from the neural crest are responsible for the development of the craniofacial skeleton [55]. Sclerotome cells, which are of mesodermal origin, give rise to the axial skeleton, and the lateral mesoderm gives rise to the limb bud and eventually development of the long bone. The mesenchymal cells during morphogenesis undergo either direct differentiating into osteoblasts, which proceed to form bone, or differentiation proceeds via chondrocytes, which form a cartilaginous template that later ossify in a process known as endochondral ossification. These progenitors are termed osteoprogenitor cells or bone-precursor cells.

Functionally, osteoblasts are the cells within bone responsible for deposition of the new ECM. These cells are derived from the progenitor population, appear cuboidal in shape, and are located at the bone surface in a monolayer [42,43,56]. Osteoblasts are highly anchorage dependent, and start by secreting collagen and then coat them with non-collagenous proteins, which have the ability to bind minerals such as calcium and phosphate, and thus regulate mineralization. The osteoblasts maintain cellular function, and respond to stimuli facilitated by cell–matrix and cell–cell communications conducted via a variety of transmembranous proteins and specific receptors [57,58]. As the newly formed bone mineralizes, some osteoblasts become enclosed in their own calcified matrix, and will change phenotype developing into osteocytes or mature osteoblasts.

Osteocytes are the most abundant cells in bone, and remain connected with other osteocytes and with the bone-lining cells present at the bone's surface allowing for intercellular communication which is responsible for the spatial and temporal recruitment of cells that form and resorb bone, and allow the transport of minerals between bone and blood [42,59]. Osteoclasts are found at the surface of the bone and their responsibility is to resorb fully mineralized bone [42,60,61]. They originate from hematopoietic stem cells, and are highly specialized as they release acids and enzymes to dissolve the minerals and collagens present in mature bone. The dissolved minerals recycle back into the blood, and their transportation in and out of the bone is regulated by the bone-lining cells.

All these cellular processes regulated by the various distinct cell types must be in equilibrium to coordinate the processes of bone formation and resorption. This crosstalk will ensure formation of healthy bone, its maintenance, and renewal as necessary. The process termed bone modeling, is necessary for development of normal bone architecture, to maintain bones biomechanically and metabolically adequate, and to repair micro-damage. These processes occur naturally throughout the life of the tissue and quite simply are described as shaping and repairing processes.

13.3 Bone Grafts

Although bone itself can help restore and repair minor fractures, its regenerative capacity is limited especially in the case of fracture non-unions (up to 10% of the fractures) and large mass of bone loss associated with osteoporosis, osteosarcoma, and revision total joint replacements [62–64]. The patients will experience major dysfunction and severe pain if no treatment is undertaken.

13.3.1 Autografts

Autografts and allografts as well as a variety of bone graft substitutes are used for surgical treatment [63,65,66]. Autografts constitute about 58% of the bone substitutes, and are typically tissues harvested from the patient's own iliac crest. They are considered the gold standard for bone repair since they possess all the properties necessary for new bone growth. Upon implantation, the grafts are able to support the attachment and migration of new osteoblasts and osteoprogenitor cells (osteoconductivity), in situ mineralization of the collagen matrix produced by osteoblasts to form new bone (osteogenicity), the recruitment and differentiation of stem cells or osteoprogenitor cells into osteoblasts (osteoinductivity), and formation of intimate bonding between the newly formed mineralized tissues and surrounding bone tissues (osteointegrativity). However, they are limited in availability and often associated with donor-site morbidity and increased operative blood loss particularly when a large graft is required [67].

13.3.2 Allografts

Allografts are tissues obtained from banked freeze-dried bones of human cadavers and represent about ~34% of the bone substitutes. They are osteoconductive and have fewer limitations on supply [63]. However, allografts are usually not osteoinductive or osteogenic and are associated with risks of immunological reaction or disease transmission. Furthermore, they possess insufficient mechanical properties for load-bearing bone applications. Studies have shown the failure rate of allografts is between 25% and 35% [68,69].

13.3.3 Bone Graft Substitutes

As alternatives to the autografts and allografts a variety of bone graft substitutes have been developed. Following a market survey conducted by Medtech Insight, they reported that biomaterial sales for orthopedic use was found to exceed 980 million dollars in 2001 in the USA, and was 1.16 billion dollars in 2002 [70]. Sales of bone graft and bone graft substitutes in US alone were 1.5 billion dollars in 2009 [71]. The number of bone graft procedures has increased worldwide, and in 2000, 15% of all bone graft surgeries conducted in the world used synthetic bone grafts. The success in developing synthetic bone substitutes is governed by a strong understanding of the composition of bone, its architecture, and its organization into the bone matrix [63]. On the basis of material composition, they can be classified as allograft-based, factor-based, cell-based, ceramic-based, and polymer-based bone graft substitutes [6,63,65]. They have been developed for repair due to unlimited supply, ease of sterilization and storage. However, each suffers from a number of disadvantages. Human derived allograft-based bone graft substitutes can be potentially associated with immunogenicity and disease transmission. Factor- and cell-based bone graft substitutes often need additional structural support. Ceramic-based bone graft substitutes are brittle and possess inappropriate mechanical properties for use in load-bearing sites.

13.4 Design Considerations for Bone Graft Substitutes

The primary requirement of any engineered implant material or scaffold is related to their biocompatibility aspects in vivo [64]. The grafts need to be sterile, free of pyrogens, and biocompatible with tissues and body fluids. Furthermore, to repair bone defects the scaffold must be designed to be load-bearing and maintain the structure of the defect and restore bone function. Ideally the scaffold will satisfy a number of design criteria:

(i) Host–graft interaction after implantation. When the grafts are covered with body fluids, proteins adsorb onto it modifying the implant surface and thus regulating the host response, attachment of cells and their functions [72–74]. The implant should ideally have no adverse immune response, which is an important regulator of integration with the host tissue.

(ii) Degradation is modulated strongly by the local environment. The degradation by-products of the graft may direct local and systemic immune response, which significantly affects the implant–host integration in the long-term. Depending on the graft materials, various mechanisms such as corrosion, resorption, hydrolysis, and enzymatic reactions are involved during in vivo degradation [75–77]. Biodegradable polymers should form non-toxic degradation products that are metabolized and excreted by the body, and exhibit controlled degradation kinetics to match the rate of bone healing process so that the newly formed tissue compensates the mechanical and mass loss of the degraded matrices [78,79].

(iii) The locally activated immune response immediately following injury and graft implantation are directed toward establishing wound continuity. These responses will modulate repair and regeneration events at all stages of healing to restore function. Complete regeneration and functional restoration may be achieved when the bone graft is well integrated with the host, remodeled and replaced with native bone tissue at similar rates of graft degradation [80]. Factors such as porosity, adhesiveness, mechanical strength, and osteogenic characteristics, and chemical and mechanical cues modulate the rates of remodeling and replacement of the implanted bone grafts with competent new bone tissue.

(iv) Porosity is the percentage of void space within a solid object, and macroporosity (pore size > 50 µm) in bone grafts support the ingrowth of new bone and vasculature [81–83]. The interconnected pore spaces enable the transport of oxygen and nutrients, and surface roughness promotes cellular adhesion, proliferation, and differentiation of anchorage-dependent cells. To improve the ability of bone grafts to support cell attachment and proliferation; ECM components especially cell adhesion receptors such as integrins may be incorporated by chemical or physical means to improve the cell–biomaterial interactions.

(v) Bone graft substitutes should have adequate mechanical properties to support the native forces usually experienced under loading. This is most critical to protect the tissues and transmit the compressive and tensile force and mechanical cues across the defect to the regenerative cells. The degradation profile of the implanted graft should allow the mechanical load to be supported and gradually transferred to the new tissue being formed within the implant.

Bone graft materials can be further selected or classified based on their bone forming abilities in vivo, namely osteoconductive, osteoinductive, and osteogenic properties. Osteoconductive materials function to provide a skeletal framework that promotes infiltration of cells and regeneration of new bone tissue, with autogeneic and allogeneic bone, hydroxyapatite, and collagen being excellent examples of osteoconductive materials [14,84–88]. Graft materials capable of inducing differentiation of stromal cell population into osteogenic lineage or phenotype are known as osteoinductive [15,89]. Demineralized bone (DBM) is found to promote formation of new bone when applied to defect sites, and it was discovered that proteins sequestered within the DBM matrix possessed this osteoinductive property, and were named bone morphogenetic proteins (BMPs). Recombinant BMP-2 is non-immunogenic and high osteoinductive but has a short half-life in vivo and thus requires a carrier system to effectively deliver active and controlled doses [90,91]. Combining such novel composite grafts with bone marrow aspirates (BMA) will additionally deliver osteogenic stromal cells harvested from the patient [16,92]. This tissue engineering approach will yield an osteogenic graft, which may deliver significantly improved treatment options to repair critical-sized bone defects. Biomaterials including synthetic biodegradable polymers and composites have shown great promise in a regenerative engineering approach [9–11,18,19,93,94]. Tremendous efforts have been focused on the development of biodegradable biomaterials and their fabrication into appropriate 3D constructs that mimic the architecture of native tissue [93].

13.5 Regeneration Using Surface Topography and Scaffold Architecture

The nature of the bone–implant interface is determined by many factors resulting in different cellular responses to the implant system both in experimental and clinical situations [95]. Osteoblasts contact the implant surface in vivo, are thus are the crucial cells in determining the tissue response at the biomaterial surface. The cell interaction process is dynamic and dependent on several parameters which modulate the cellular response and function (Fig. 13.3) [96,97]. The first event that takes place is protein adsorption, which occurs on contact with body fluids and is influenced by the physico-chemical characteristics of the material and its fabricated form. This is followed by the cell adhesion phase involving various biological molecules such as ECM, cell membrane and cytosketetal protein components [98,99]. These interactions influence cellular responses in terms of migration, cell shape and differentiation. The osteoblast cells will synthesize and deposit bone-like mineral at the implant interface. With biodegradable scaffolds, osteoblasts will proliferate, deposit and maintain mineralization within the degrading scaffold. The new bone tissue will enable controlled functional loading until full recovery is achieved. During this regenerative process, new bone tissue will continuously be formed and remodeled simultaneously to eventually exhibit native bone-like hierarchical structure. The integration or regeneration process will be further influenced by biophysical (mechanical) stimuli experienced under functional or loading conditions.

Bone tissue as discussed earlier is a highly organized hierarchical structure composed of nano-, micro-, and macro-sized building block which includes nanostructures such as non-collageneous proteins, fibrillar collagen and HA crystals, microstructures including lamellae, osteons and Haversian systems, as well as macrostructures such as cancellous and cortical bones [44]. A biomimetic approach will be a scaffold comprising of micro- and nanoscale components providing a surface topography that better mimic the natural bone ECM. In one study, biomimicry was introduced on titanium surfaces by acid etching producing micropits and followed by anodization to form a nanotubular layer (Fig. 13.4) [100]. The microtopography formed by acid etching induced higher initial cell adhesion and osteogenesis-related gene expressions; however, cell response, including proliferation, intracellular total protein synthesis and alkaline phosphatase (ALP) activity, ECM deposition, and mineralization, was significantly reduced. After addition of nanotubes to the micropitted surface, even though cell adhesion and gene expressions decreased slightly, other cell functions such as proliferation, intracellular total protein synthesis, and ALP activity, ECM deposition, and mineralization was maintained or enhanced. It is important to strike a balance between cell proliferation and differentiation behavior. Higher cell proliferation results in more cell coverage on the implant surface leading to a larger mass of bone tissue around the implant. In contrast, faster cell differentiation may result in faster bone maturation around the implant and offer more promise in bone implant integration. The surface topography modulates the cell–cell and cell–scaffold interactions, which subsequently regulate cell function, development, and differentiation [101–103].

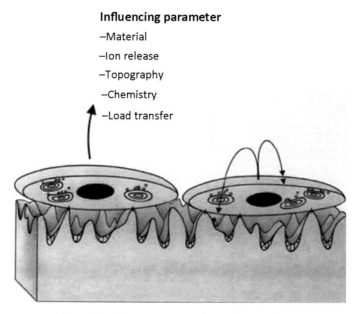

Figure 13.3 Material surface parameters that influence osteoblast behavior [97]. Reprinted from *European Cells and Materials*, 9, Meyer et al., Basic reactions of osteoblasts on structured material surfaces, 39–49, 2005, with kind permission from eCM journal (www.ecmjournal.org).

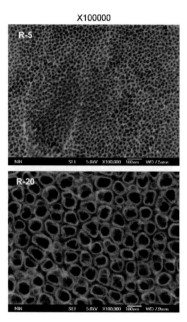

Figure 13.4 SEM pictures of the hierarchical micro/nano-textured and micro titania surfaces (Magnification = 100,000×) [100]. R-5: acid-etched/anodized at 5 V; R-20: acid-etched/anodized at 20 V. Reprinted from *Biomaterials*, **31**(19), Zhao et al., The influence of hierarchical hybrid micro/nano-textured titanium surface with titania nanotubes on osteoblast functions, 5072–5082, 2010, with permission from Elsevier.

With degradable polymers, one of the primary advantages is that it eliminates the need for eventual surgical removal. Early studies were based on biodegradable and biocompatible polymers and co-polymers of poly[esters], poly[anhydrides], and poly[phosphazenes], which were fabricated as 2D matrices and supported the attachment, proliferation, and osteoblast phenotype by the osteoblast-like cell line, MC3T3-E1 cells [104,105]. The micro and nano-hierarchical structure of bone tissue comprising of woven and lamellar bone, interstitial networks and gap-junctions is very difficult to exactly mimic when developing bone substitutes to modulate repair/regeneration. By using porous bone substitutes one could partially mimic the canal systems and interconnected networks present in native bone, and in that direction, 3D macroporous scaffolds were fabricated using salt leaching technique. NaCl crystals of 150–250 μm size were suspended in a dissolved polymer solution and the resulting emulsion was cast to a mold. The NaCl crystals were leached out into deionized water providing a porous, biodegradable, 3D scaffold for tissue regeneration [106,107]. The porosity of these 3D scaffolds was similar to trabecular bone. The increased surface area and the novel surface contours due to entrapped salt supported greater cell adhesion and increased proliferation over a period of 3 weeks. However, salt crystals entrapped within the bulk of the scaffold are not connected to the surface and thus may remain trapped within and not leached out. Efforts to overcome this challenge, led to the development of the sintered microsphere matrix. Using polymeric microspheres made of poly(lactide-*co*-glycolide) (PLAGA), 3D heat sintered scaffold having an interconnected pore structure that resembled the structure of trabecular bone was developed (Fig. 13.5a) [108,109]. The pore structure is a negative template of trabecular bone in structure and volume, and the newly forming bone would occupy the pore structure while the microsphere matrix slowly degraded leaving voids that will form the pore structure of new trabecular bone. These sintered microsphere scaffolds can be tailor made with pore diameter, pore volume, and mechanical properties within a given range. Microspheres of diameter 600–710 μm were sintered yielding an optimal, biomimetic structure with pore diameter in the range of 83–300 μm onto which human osteoblasts seeded were cultured in vitro. On this particular matrix, the cells adhered and proliferated throughout the pore system (Fig. 13.5b). The cells maintained bone phenotype expression on the above-mentioned scaffold as evidenced by osteocalcin staining suggesting its osteoconductive potency (Fig. 13.5c).

In other studies, materials such as synthetic HA, similar to the inorganic component of bone has been combined with other biomaterials such as collagen and PLAGA to introduce osteoinductivity into the bone regenerative scaffold [107,110]. Improved bone cell function has been correlated with reduced grain size of the HA constituent [36,85]. Compared to micro grain sized HA components, the particles of nano-dimensions further improved osteointegration with the host bone tissue. The nano-HA (nHA)/collagen composites more closely mimic native bone composition and structure, and significantly enhance bone cell function and host-integration leading to faster recovery. Composites having nHA exhibited higher mechanical properties compared to those fabricated from micro or bulk-sized HA constituents due to strong interfacial-bonding between the organic and inorganic phases [111]. These nanocomposites are successful in inducing better cellular responses as compared to standard composites due to their similarity with the natural bone structure, and additionally can be processed to have mechanical properties more closely to native bone. Integrating nanotopographical cues is important in engineering complex tissues that have multiple cell types and require precisely defined cell–cell and cell–matrix interactions in a 3D environment. Thus, in a regenerative engineering approach, nanoscale materials/structures play a paramount role in controlling cell fate and the consequent regenerative capacity.

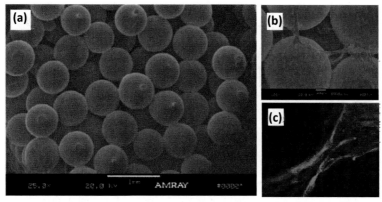

Figure 13.5 (a) Scanning electron micrographs demonstrating the shape and size of sintered microsphere scaffold composed of diameter 600–710 μm diameter microspheres. (Magnification = 25×) [106]. Reprinted from *Clinical Orthopaedics & Related Research*, 447, Cooper et al., The ABJS Nicolas Andry Award: Tissue engineering of bone and ligament: a 15-year perspective, 221–236, 2006, with permission from Lippincott Williams & Wilkins. (b) Scanning electron micrographs showing the morphology of human osteoblasts at 16 days on the microsphere matrix. Micrograph demonstrates cellular adhesion within the matrix and the promotion of several cellular attachment sites between adjacent sintered microspheres [109]. (c) Immunofluorescence staining for osteocalcin to assess the osteoblast phenotypic behavior while cultured on the sintered matrix at 16 days. Micrograph demonstrates osteoblast cells with positive osteocalcin staining at various locations along the matrix [109]. Reprinted from *Biomaterials*, **24**(4), Borden et al., Structural and human cellular assessment of a novel microsphere-based tissue engineered scaffold for bone repair, 597–609, 2003, with permission from Elsevier.

Nanofibers are ECM-mimicking scaffolds characterized by high porosity and surface area, unusual surface properties, and morphological similarity to native bone ECM [112–114]. Nanofiber scaffolds with interconnecting porous structures provide high surface area for cell attachment, growth, and differentiation as well as nutrient transport. Techniques to fabricate nanofiber scaffolds with unique properties include phase separation [115,116], self-assembly [115,117], and electrospinning [115]. Laurencin et al. demonstrated the electrospun nanofiber matrices of poly[bis(p-methylphenoxy)phosphazene] (PNmPh) supported the adhesion and proliferation of osteoblast like MC3T3-E1 cells (Fig. 13.6). These polyphosphazene nanofiber structures closely mimic the ECM architecture and have shown excellent osteoconductivity and osteointegration [118–121].

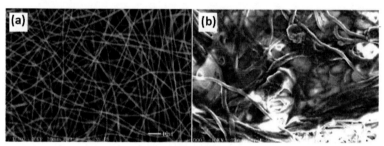

Figure 13.6 Electrospun nanofibers of poly[bis(p-methylphenoxy)phosphazene]. (a) SEM of electrospun PNmPh fibers from chloroform at a concentration of 8% (wt/v) of the polymer at 33 kV using 18 gauge showing the formation of distinct uniform fibers [120]. (b) SEM micrograph presenting MC3T3-E1 cells covering the nanofiber matrix after 7 days of culture. Reprinted with permission from *Biomacromolecules*, 5(6), Nair, et al., Fabrication and optimization of methylphenoxy substituted polyphosphazene nanofibers for biomedical applications, 2212–2220. Copyright 2004 American Chemical Society.

Inspired by the hierarchical structures that enable bone function, a mechanically competent 3D scaffold mimicking the bone marrow cavity, as well as, the lamellar structure of bone by orienting electrospun polyphosphazene-polyester blend nanofibers in a concentric manner with an open central cavity was fabricated (Fig. 13.7) [122]. The 3D biomimetic scaffold exhibited mechanical behavior characteristic to that of native bone. In vitro studies using primary cell culture demonstrated the ability of the biomimetic scaffold to support the osteoblast proliferation and accelerated differentiation throughout the scaffold architecture, which resulted in a similar cell-matrix organization to that of native bone and maintenance of structure integrity. It was thus suggested that the concentric open macrostructures of nanofibers that structurally and mechanically mimic the native bone can be a potential scaffold design for accelerated bone healing.

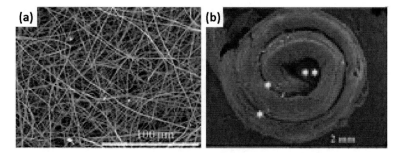

Figure 13.7 SEM image illustrating (a) Polymeric nanofibers fabricated via electrospinning. In electrospinning, a non-woven mat of polymeric nanofibers is created from an electrostatically driven jet of polymer solution. A high electric potential of a few kV is applied to the pendent polymer droplet/melts and a polymer jet is ejected from the charged polymer solution. The polymer jet undergoes a series of bending and stretching instabilities that cause large amounts of plastic stretching resulting in ultrathin fibers. By altering the electrospinning and process parameters, the resultant fiber morphology and structure can be fine-tuned yielding bead-free continuous nanofibers having a mean diameter of ~343 nm. (b) The nanofiber mat rolled into a concentric circle and seeded with cells. ECM deposition is evident throughout 3D scaffold architecture during cell culture after 28 days of culture [122]. Reprinted from *Advanced Functional Materials*, **21**(14), Meng et al., Biomimetic structures: biological implications of dipeptide-substituted polyphosphazene–polyester blend nanofiber matrices for load-bearing bone regeneration, 2641–2651, 2011, with permission from John Wiley & Sons.

In addition to electrospinning, self-assembly [115,117,123,124] or phase separation [115,116] technique is used to fabricate nanofiber scaffolds that emulate natural ECM both structurally and functionally. A novel scaffold that combines robust mechanical aspects of sintered microsphere scaffold with a highly bioactive nanofiber structure was designed [125]. Exploiting the chemistry of two biodegradable polymers, a 3D poly-L-lactide acid (PLLA) nanofiber mesh was successful incorporated within the void spaces between sintered PNEPhA microspheres (Fig. 13.8 a and b). The non-load-bearing fiber portion of these scaffolds is sufficiently porous

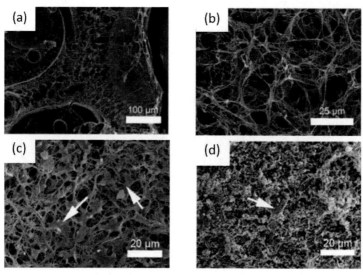

Figure 13.8 Composite nanofiber/microsphere scaffolds bridging nanoscale and microscale architectures to improve bioactivity of mechanically competent constructs for bone regeneration [125]. (a, b) SEM micrographs of the cross-sections of the composite nanofiber/microsphere scaffold demonstrating incorporation of nanofibers of less than 1 μm within the void space generated by sintering microspheres where (a) low magnification image and (b) high magnification image; (c, d) SEM micrographs of preosteoblasts in the interior of composite scaffolds after 3 days (c) and 14 days (d) of culture demonstrating the presence of preosteoblasts and the accumulation of matrix proteins in the interior of the composite scaffold during cell culture. The arrows point to representative cells. Notably, the fibrous portion of the scaffold has been extensively modified through the accumulation of ECM proteins after 14 days, to the extent that identifying the cells is difficult. Reprinted from *Journal of Biomedical Materials Research Part A*, **95A**(4), Brown et al., Composite scaffolds: bridging nanofiber and microsphere architectures to improve bioactivity of mechanically competent constructs, 1150–1158, 2010, with permission from John Wiley & Sons.

to allow cell migration and ECM matrix production throughout the fibrous portion of the scaffold (Fig. 13.8 c and d). These composite nanofiber/microsphere scaffolds promote osteoinduction through focal adhesion kinase activity. The phenotype progression of osteoblast progenitor cells on the composite nanofiber/microsphere scaffolds illustrated a stronger and more rapid progression leading to fully matured osteoblasts by 21 days. This composite scaffold demonstrates an ability to mimic the mechanical environment of trabecular bone while also promoting the osteoinduction of osteoblast progenitor cells [125].

13.6   Stem Cells

Stem cells (SCs) are broadly classified by their developmental potential into pluripotent stem cells and adult stem cells. Pluripotent cells (PSCs) having the broadest differentiation capability and is able to form all the cell lineages [126,127]. Adult stem cells such as mesenchymal stem cells (MSCs) (bone or adipose) are multipotent and is described as having a more limited differentiation potential that can form multiple cell types in one lineage. Since realizing the potential of mesenchymal cells to differentiate and form organs and tissues, self-renew and their regenerative role in healing injury, there has been an explosive growth in novel regenerative strategies to develop therapeutic solutions [128]. Given the right cues, harvested stem cells can be guided from its undifferentiated state into various musculoskeletal tissues, blood vessels, cardiac muscle, skin and various other tissues [129]. For instance, MSCs isolated from the bone marrow can differentiate into bone (osteoblasts) [130], muscle (myoblasts), fat (adipocytes) [131] and cartilage (chrondocytes) [132] cells, while neural stem cells (NSCs) can differentiate into neurons [133]. However, various studies have reported major limitations in reconstituting dead tissue in degenerated organs [134]. It is of extreme importance to reliably control stem cell proliferation and their fate, both prior and subsequent to transplantation. This has been the major challenge in successful application of stem cells for regenerative engineering. For instance, incompletely or incorrectly differentiated cells may become tumorigenic or form undesired tissue negating the therapeutic purpose.

In vivo, the differentiation and self-renewability of stem cells is dominated by signals from their surrounding microenvironment (Fig. 13.9) [134–136]. This microenvironment is composed of other cell types, and in addition numerous chemical, mechanical and topographical cues at the micro- and nanoscale are present and they all serve as signaling factors that modulate the cell behavior [137]. Reliable control of stem cell fate is challenging due to an incomplete understanding of the complex signaling pathways that drive stem cell behavior from early embryogenesis to late adulthood.

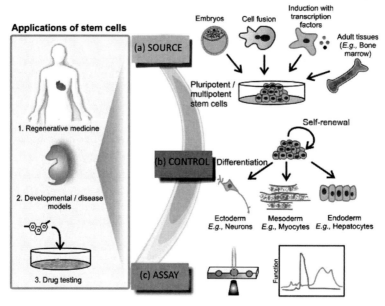

Figure 13.9 Applications of stem cells range from regenerative medicine to developmental and disease models for basic biological studies or drug testing [135]. Most applications involve three basic steps: (a) derivation of a stem cell source either from embryos, from fusing somatic cells with stem cells, via transfecting somatic cells with transcription factors, or from adult tissues, such as bone marrow; (b) controlling the stem cells to induce self-renewal or differentiation into a desired lineage; (c) assaying the resulting (stem) cells to determine their state or function. Reprinted from *Integrative Biology*, **7–8**(2), Toh et al., Advancing stem cell research with microtechnologies: opportunities and challenges, 305–325, 2010, with permission from RSC Publishing.

It is desirable to use increasingly more biomimetic in vitro culture conditions to regulate stem cell differentiation and self-renewal [138]. The success of regenerative strategies will largely be based on their ability to provide a favorable microenvironment that will guide cell differentiation and tissue regeneration. Surface features or topography such as macro-, micro- and nano-sized features can modulate behavioral changes such as cell growth, movement, orientation, and function [85,139–141]. The development of micro- and nano-topography can create stem cell niches providing the critical microenvironment for the maintenance and regulation of the stem cells. Furthermore, these discoveries have been leveraged to control stem cell proliferation, differentiation, and maturation giving rise to the desired regenerative tissue [130,142–144].

A classical presentation of this phenomenon is the basement membrane (BM) which provides the basic substrata for all cellular structures in vertebrates. The BM has a topography composed of grooves, ridges, pits, pores, and an ECM fibrillar meshwork, composed predominantly of collagen and elastin fibers having diameters ranging from 10–300 nm [145]. The ECM fibers exhibit varying degrees of structural organization with which cells interact and give rise to tissues that have unique structure and specific function. For example, parallel-aligned collagen fibers are found in tendon, ligaments, and muscles. In contrast, concentric whorls are noted in bone, and mesh-like lattices are present in the skin.

Micro- and nanoscale techniques enable patterning biomaterial substrate at very high precision, and have been applied to investigate stem cell interaction with their microenvironment to determine the regulatory mechanisms that control cell fate. The early studies in investigating cellular behavior and responses on surfaces was performed by immobilizing cells on micropatterned substrates that were coated with regions of adhesive and non-adhesive molecules. It was determined that primary endothelial cells on smaller surfaces underwent apoptosis while those that were patterned on larger substrates tend to proliferate [27]. In another instance, human mesenchymal stem cells (hMSCs) that were allowed to adhere and flatten on large protein patterns differentiated into osteogenic cells, whereas on smaller patterns they differentiated into adipogenic cells [146]. The change in cell shape alone was sufficient to mediate the switch in hMSC commitment between adipogenic and osteogenic fates. Furthermore, the authors report that the effects of cell shape on proliferation or survival are distinct from those on cell fate determination. Micropatterned microenvironments have been reported to control the differentiation of stem cells exposed to a mixture of pro-differentiative signals. Human mesenchymal stem cells sheets were cultured on micropatterns of controlled shape and exposed them to a cell culture media that was composed of a mixture of pro-osteogenic and pro-adipogenic factors (Fig. 13.10)

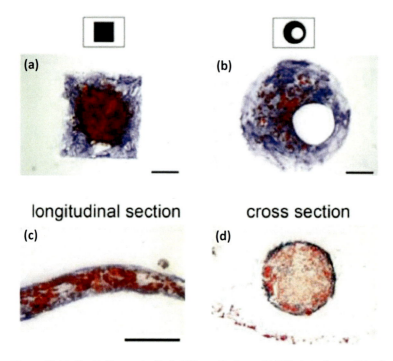

Figure 13.10 Spatially controlled differentiation of MSCs into bony (blue) and fatty tissue (red) [147]. Planar cell adhesive micropatterns, such as a square (a) or an offset annulus (b) provide controlled regions of high and low cytoskeletal stress, thereby influencing differentiation. Scale bar = 250 μm. (c, d) Multicellular 3D constructs differentiate into a fatty core surrounded by bony tissue, similar to natural long bones. Reprinted from *Stem Cells*, **26**(11), Ruiz et al., Emergence of patterned stem cell differentiation within multicellular structures, 2921–2927, 2008, with permission from John Wiley & Sons.

[147]. hMSCs at the edge of multicellular islands differentiate into the osteogenic lineage, while those in the center became adipocytes. Furthermore, by changing the shape of the multicellular sheet the authors were able to modulate the locations of osteogenic versus adipogenic differentiation. The stem cells clearly depicted differentiation dictated by their spatial arrangement and corresponding cytoskeletal stress. The authors used this mechanism to created multicellular stem cell constructs, which mimicked the architecture of normal long bone: a bony tube filled with a fatty core.

Recent studies have reported that subnano, nano, and micro surface features can selectively activate integrin receptors and induce osteoblast differentiation of bone marrow derived MSCs [131]. Titanium surface with controlled topography ranging from subnano (virtually flat) to micron size was fabricated and seeded with hMSCs. Both the nano (150 nm) and nano-micro hybrid (450 nm) surfaces significantly activated integrin–ligand protein interactions through the a-integrin subunits. However, the most influential dimension in promoting osteoblast differentiation was those on the nano-submicron hybrid (450 nm) titanium surfaces. Furthermore, a feature height of 2–4 nm induced significant re-organization of the cellular cytoskeleton, which modulated subsequent osteoblast differentiation as determined by the increased expression of the phenotypic genes.

Vertical TiO_2 nanotubes fabricated by metal anodization have been used to study interactions with MSCs (Fig. 13.11) [144,148,149]. Rat MSCs exhibited pronounced cell adhesion, spreading, mineralization and bone phenotype expression on tubes of diameters ranging from 15 to 30 nm as compared to flat TiO_2. Increased focal adhesion contacts were measured on the smallest nanotubes, which modulated increased upregulation of stem cell differentiation. Similar observations have been reported by others where hMSCs were cultured on TiO_2 tubes of diameters ranging from 70–100 nm [130,150]. Generation of nanotubes by metal anodization onto the surface of titanium based orthopedic implants could enhance their osseous integration. This improvement may be due to mechanical stresses transmitted from the nanostructures to the cell or indirectly by activation of cell adhesive domains or a combination of both [151].

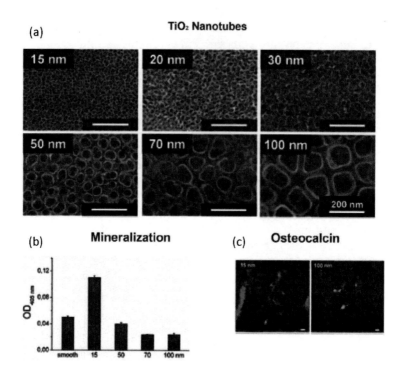

Figure 13.11 (a) Scanning electron micrographs of the TiO_2 nanotubes (15, 20, 30, 50, 70, 100 nm); (b) Plot of ALP versus nanotube diameter; (c) Osteocalcin (red) and F-actin (green) staining of cells seeded on 15 nm and 100 nm TiO_2 nanotubes. The scale bar is 20 μm [144]. Reprinted from *Nano Letters*, **7**(6), Park et al., Nanosize and vitality: TiO_2 nanotube diameter directs cell fate, 1686–1691, 2007, with permission from ACS Publishing.

In another study, hMSCs were seeded onto polyethylene terephthalate (PET) surfaces having controlled nano-topography (Fig. 13.12a) [152]. The depth of the micropatterned surface features was altered to modulate the behavioral responses of hMSCs. Large depths of 100 nm enabled better cell adhesion and spreading, and elicited a collective cell organization forming multilayer networks as compared to other depths of 10 and 50 nm. Increased maturation of focal adhesion contact points was observed in hMSCs cultured on the 100 nm depth substrate and is believed to be responsible for induction of differentiation toward an osteoblastic lineage (Fig. 13.12b). The increased stress induced reorganization of the actin filaments within the cell. Small (10 nm) depth patterns promoted cell adhesion without noticeable differentiation.

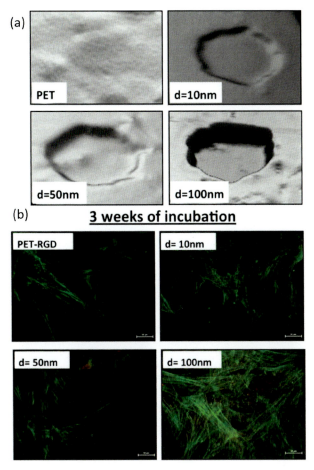

Figure 13.12 (a) Surface of PET topographies with nanoscale depths measured using an Optical 3D Profiler System. Nanoindentation images showing three different nanodepths: d = 10, 50, and 100 nm. (b) Human mesenchymal stem cell at 3 weeks in culture differentiate into osteoblast-like cells on surfaces with 100 nm depth as seen by Runx2 blotting and osteopontin (OPN) staining, respectively. Actin, green; OPN, red. Scale bars: 50 µm [152]. Reprinted from *Journal of Cell Science*, **125** (Pt 5), Zouani et al., Altered nanofeature size dictates stem cell differentiation, 1217–1224, 2012, with permission from The Company of Biologists.

13.7 Conclusions

The regenerative strategies discussed in this chapter provide an insight into the development of ideal bone graft substitutes. Surface topography and the fabricated form of the scaffold mediate cell adhesion, cell migration, proliferation, and differentiation into specific cell lineage. Cells are observed to align, elongate, and migrate parallel to the grooves. The depth of the grooves is found to influence the alignment of the cells. Expression of an osteoblastic phenotype is most prominent on patterned surfaces deposited with calcium phosphate, highlighting the synergy between topography and surface chemistry. The many fabrication technologies allow for precise control of topographical features and structures such as pores, ridges, groves, fibers, nodes and their combinations significantly. These technological advances have been instrumental in understanding the molecular mechanisms governing cells and cell-material interaction to generate better scaffold and implant performance.

With the advent of composite polymers, and micro and nanofabrication techniques, biomaterials can be fabricated into structures that mimic the native bone hierarchical organization. In particular, polymeric nanofiber matrices have been successfully developed to strongly influence bone regeneration. Composite scaffolds with nano-features have been created for load-bearing applications. The regeneration of tissues, organs, or organ systems remains a significant challenge, and requires an integration of physical, chemical, and mechanical cues to regenerate complex biological tissues possessing tissue-type heterogeneity, anisotropic mechanical properties, and well-defined tissue–implant interactions. The next step involves the development of integrated-graft systems for regeneration of multiple tissue components simultaneously. The emergence of induced pluripotent stem cell technology will drive the convergence of advanced topography, developmental biology and regenerative engineering for translational tissue repair. One will sculpt a 3D environment that will specify a unique set of instructions to overcome the regenerative challenges in forming multi-scale tissues and complex organs.

References

1. Vacanti, J. P., Tissue engineering: the design and fabrication of living replacement devices for surgical reconstruction and transplantation. *Lancet*, 1999. **354**: S32.
2. Braddock, M., et al., Born again bone: tissue engineering for bone repair. *News Physiol Sci*, 2001. **16**(5): 208–213.
3. Shors, E. C., Coralline bone graft substitutes. *Orthop Clin North Am*, 1999. **30**(4): 599–613.
4. Joyce, M. J., et al., Musculoskeletal allograft tissue safety. Prepared by: Committee on Biologics Implants Work Group, American Academy of Orthopedics Surgeons, 2008.
5. Webster, T. J., Nanophase ceramics as improved bone tissue engineering materials. *Am Ceram Soc Bull*, 2003. **82**: 23–28.
6. Bauer, T. W., and G. F. Muschler, Bone graft materials: an overview of the basic science. *Clin Orthop Relat Res*, 2000. **371**: 10.
7. Langer, R., and J. Vacanti, Tissue engineering. *Science*, 1993. **260**(5110): 920–926.
8. Laurencin, C. T., et al., Tissue engineering: orthopedic applications. *Annu Rev Biomed Eng*, 1999. **1**(1): 19–46.
9. Deng, M., et al., Biomimetic, bioactive etheric polyphosphazene-poly(lactide-co-glycolide) blends for bone tissue engineering. *J Biomed Mater Res A*, 2010. **92A**(1): 114–125.
10. Deng, M., et al., Polyphosphazene polymers for tissue engineering: an analysis of material synthesis, characterization and applications. *Soft Matter*, 2010. **6**: 3119–3132.
11. Deng, M., et al., Dipeptide-based polyphosphazene and polyester blends for bone tissue engineering. *Biomaterials*, 2010. **31**(18): 4898–4908.
12. Jabbarzadeh, E., et al., Induction of angiogenesis in tissue-engineered scaffolds designed for bone repair: a combined gene therapy-cell transplantation approach. *Proc Natl Acad Sci USA*, 2008. **105**(32): 11099–11104.
13. Jiang, T., et al., Chitosan-poly(lactide-*co*-glycolide) microsphere-based scaffolds for bone tissue engineering: In vitro degradation and in vivo bone regeneration studies. *Acta Biomater*, 2010. **6**(9): 3457–3470.
14. Jarcho, M., Calcium phosphate ceramics as hard tissue prosthetics. *Clin Orthop Relat Res*, 1981. **157**: 259–278.

15. Urist, M. R., et al., Bone regeneration under the influence of a bone morphogenetic protein (BMP) beta tricalcium phosphate (TCP) composite in skull trephine defects in dogs. *Clin Orthop Relat Res*, 1987. (214): 295–304.

16. Tiedeman, J. J., et al., Treatment of nonunion by percutaneous injection of bone marrow and demineralized bone matrix. An experimental study in dogs. *Clin Orthop Relat Res*, 1991. (268): 294–302.

17. Langer, R., Tissue Engineering. *Mol Ther*, 2000. **1**(1): 12–15.

18. Deng, M., et al., In situ porous structures: a unique polymer erosion mechanism in biodegradable dipeptide-based polyphosphazene and polyester blends producing matrices for regenerative engineering. *Adv Funct Mater*, 2010. **20**(17): 2794–2806.

19. Nair, L. S., and C. T. Laurencin, Biodegradable polymers as biomaterials. *Progr Polymer Sci* 2007. **32**(8–9): 762–798.

20. Laurencin, C. T., 6th International Key Symposium NANOMEDICINE, 9-11 September 2009, Stockholm, Sweden.

21. Meng, D., et al., Nanostructured polymeric scaffolds for orthopaedic regenerative engineering. *IEEE Trans NanoBioscience* 2012. **11**(1): 3–14.

22. Kumbar, S. G., et al., Cell behavior toward nanostructured surfaces, in *Biomedical Nanostructures*, (K. Gonsalves, et al., eds.) 2008, John Wiley & Sons: New York. 261–295.

23. Stevens, M. M., and J. H. George, Exploring and engineering the cell surface interface. *Science*, 2005. **310**(5751): 1135–1138.

24. Vitte, J., et al., Is there a predictable relationship between surface physical-chemical properties and cell behaviour at the interface? *Eur Cell Mater*, 2004. **7**: 52–63.

25. Karuri, N. W., et al., Biological length scale topography enhances cell-substratum adhesion of human corneal epithelial cells. *J Cell Sci*, 2004. **117**(15): 3153–3164.

26. Glass-Brudzinski, J., D. Perizzolo, and D. M. Brunette, Effects of substratum surface topography on the organization of cells and collagen fibers in collagen gel cultures. *J Biomed Mater Res*, 2002. **61**(4): 608–618.

27. Chen, C. S., et al., Geometric control of cell life and death. *Science*, 1997. **276**(5317): 1425–1428.

28. Dalby, M. J., et al., Increasing fibroblast response to materials using nanotopography: morphological and genetic measurements of cell response to 13-nm-high polymer demixed islands. *Exp Cell Res*, 2002. **276**(1): 1-9.

29. Dalby, M. J., et al., Attempted endocytosis of nano-environment produced by colloidal lithography by human fibroblasts. *Exp Cell Res*, 2004. **295**(2): 387-394.

30. Chou, L., et al., Effects of titanium substratum and grooved surface topography on metalloproteinase-2 expression in human fibroblasts. *J Biomed Mater Res*, 1998. **39**(3): 437-445.

31. Dalby, M. J., et al., Polymer-demixed nanotopography: control of fibroblast spreading and proliferation. *Tissue Eng*, 2004. **8**(6): 1099-1108.

32. Vance, R. J., et al., Decreased fibroblast cell density on chemically degraded poly-lactic-co-glycolic acid, polyurethane, and polycaprolactone. *Biomaterials*, 2004. **25**(11): 2095-2103.

33. Dalby, M. J., et al., Fibroblast reaction to island topography: changes in cytoskeleton and morphology with time. *Biomaterials*, 2003. **24**(6): 927-935.

34. Dalby, M. J., et al., Osteoprogenitor response to defined topographies with nanoscale depths. *Biomaterials*, 2006. **27**(8): 1306-1315.

35. Price, R., K. Haberstroh, and T. Webster, Enhanced functions of osteoblasts on nanostructured surfaces of carbon and alumina. *Med Biol Eng Comput*, 2003. **41**(3): 372-375.

36. Webster, T. J., et al., Enhanced osteoclast-like cell functions on nanophase ceramics. *Biomaterials*, 2001. **22**(11): 1327-1333.

37. Dalby, M. J., et al., In vitro reaction of endothelial cells to polymer demixed nanotopography. *Biomaterials*, 2002. **23**(14): 2945-2954.

38. Thapa, A., T. J. Webster, and K. M. Haberstroh, Polymers with nano-dimensional surface features enhance bladder smooth muscle cell adhesion. *J Biomed Mater Res A*, 2003. **67A**(4): 1374-1383.

39. Andersson, A.-S., et al., Nanoscale features influence epithelial cell morphology and cytokine production. *Biomaterials*, 2003. **24**(20): 3427-3436.

40. Gallagher, J. O., et al., Interaction of animal cells with ordered nanotopography. *IEEE Trans Nanobiosci*, 2002. **1**(1): 24-28.

41. Bilezikian, J. P., L. G. Raisz, and G. A. Rodan, *Principles of Bone Biology*. 1996, San Diego, CA: Academic Press.

42. Jee, W. S. S., and S. C. Cowin, Integrated bone tissue physiology: anatomy and physiology, in *Bone Mechanics Handbook*. 2001, CRC Press LLC.
43. Kierszenbaum, A. L., Connective tissue, in *Histology and Cell Biology. An Introduction to Pathology.*2002, Mosby Inc.: St. Louis. pp. 118–129.
44. Rho, J.-Y., L. Kuhn-Spearing, and P. Zioupos, Mechanical properties and the hierarchical structure of bone. *Med Eng Phys*, 1998. **20**(2): 92–102.
45. Murugan, R., and S. Ramakrishna, Development of nanocomposites for bone grafting. *Compos Sci Technol*, 2005. **65**(15–16): 2385–2406.
46. Weiner, S., and H. D. Wagner, The material bone: structure-mechanical function relations. *Annu Rev Mater Sci*, 2003. **28**(1): 271–298.
47. Marotti, G., A new theory of bone lamellation. *Calcif Tissue Int*, 1993. **53**(0): S47–S56.
48. Wiesmann, H. P., et al., Aspects of collagen mineralization in hard tissue formation. *Int Rev Cytol*, 2004. **242**: 121–156.
49. van der Rest, M., and R. Garrone, Collagen family of proteins. *FASEB J*, 1991. **5**(13): 2814–2823.
50. Sommerfeldt, D. W., and C. T. Rubin, Biology of bone and how it orchestrates the form and function of the skeleton. *Eur Spine J*, 2001. **10**(0): S86–S95.
51. Weiner, S., and W. Traub, Bone structure: from angstroms to microns. *FASEB J*, 1992. **6**(3): 879–885.
52. Landis, W. J., The strength of a calcified tissue depends in part on the molecular structure and organization of its constituent mineral crystals in their organic matrix. *Bone*, 1995. **16**(5): 533–544.
53. Ziv, V., and S. Weiner, Bone crystal sizes: a comparison of transmission electron microscopic and X-ray diffraction line width broadening techniques. *Connect Tissue Res*, 2009. **30**(3): 165–175.
54. Rey, C., et al., Hydroxyl groups in bone mineral. *Bone*, 1995. **16**(5): 583–586.
55. Beddington, R. S., and E. J. Robertson, Axis development and early asymmetry in mammals. *Cell*, 1999. **96**(2): 195–209.
56. Aubin, J. E., Bone stem cells. *J Cell Biochem Suppl*, 1998. **30–31**: 73–82.
57. Ferrari, S. L., et al., A role for N-cadherin in the development of the differentiated osteoblastic phenotype. *J Bone Miner Res*, 2000. **15**(2): 198–208.
58. Lecanda, F., et al., Gap junctional communication modulates gene expression in osteoblastic cells. *Mol Biol Cell*, 1998. **9**(8): 2249–2258.

59. Liu, X., and P. X. Ma, Polymeric scaffolds for bone tissue engineering. *Ann Biomed Eng*, 2004. **32**(3): 477–486.
60. Li, Z., K. Kong, and W. Qi, Osteoclast and its roles in calcium metabolism and bone development and remodeling. *Biochem Biophys Res Commun*, 2006. **343**(2): 345–350.
61. Blair, H. C., et al., Osteoclastic bone resorption by a polarized vacuolar proton pump. *Science*, 1989. **245**(4920): 855–857.
62. Khan, Y., and C. T. Laurencin, Fracture repair with ultrasound: clinical and cell-based evaluation. *J Bone Joint Surg Am*, 2008. **90**(Suppl 1): 138–144.
63. Laurencin, C., Y. Khan, and S. F. El-Amin, Bone graft substitutes. *Expert Rev Med Devices*, 2005. **3**(1): 49–57.
64. Baroli, B., From natural bone grafts to tissue engineering therapeutics: Brainstorming on pharmaceutical formulative requirements and challenges. *J Pharm Sci*, 2009. **98**(4): 1317–1375.
65. Ilan, D. I., and A. L. Ladd, Bone graft substitutes. *Oper Tech Plast Reconstr Surg*, 2003. **9**(4): 151–160.
66. Laurencin, C. T. and Y. Khan, *Bone Graft Substitute Materials.* http://emedicine.medscape.com/article/1230616-overview.
67. Goulet, J. A., et al., Autogenous iliac crest bone graft. Complications and functional assessment. *Clin Orthop Relat Res*, 1997. **339**: 76–81.
68. Berrey, B., et al., Fractures of allografts. Frequency, treatment, and end-results. *J Bone Joint Surg Am*, 1990. **72**(6): 825–833.
69. Ito, H., et al., Remodeling of cortical bone allografts mediated by adherent rAAV-RANKL and VEGF gene therapy. *Nat Med*, 2005. **11**(3): 291–297.
70. Medtech Insight Report 2006, U.S. *Markets for Orthopedic Biomaterials for Bone Repair and Regeneration*.
71. American Academy of Orthopaedic Surgeons, *The Evolving Role of Bone-Graft Substitutes*, 77th Annual Meeting, New Orleans, Louisiana (http://www.aatb.org/aatb/files/ccLibraryFiles/Filename/000000000322/BoneGraftSubstitutes2010.pdf).
72. Veerman, E. C., et al., SDS-PAGE analysis of the protein layers adsorbing in vivo and in vitro to bone substituting materials. *Biomaterials*, 1987. **8**(6): 442–448.
73. Nojiri, C., et al., In vivo protein adsorption on polymers: visualization of adsorbed proteins on vascular implants in dogs. *J Biomater Sci Polym Ed*, 1992. **4**(2): 75–88.

74. Davies, J. E., Mechanisms of endosseous integration. *Int J Prosthodont*, 1998. **11**(5): 391–401.
75. Soultanis, K., et al., Instrumentation loosening and material of implants as predisposal factors for late postoperative infections in operated idiopathic scoliosis. *Stud Health Technol Inform*, 2006. **123**: 559–564.
76. Kirkpatrick, J. S., et al., Corrosion on spinal implants. *J Spinal Disord Tech*, 2005. **18**(3): 247–251.
77. Laurencin, C. T., et al., The ABJS Nicolas Andry Award: Tissue engineering of bone and ligament: a 15-year perspective. *Clin Orthop Relat Res*, 2006. **447**: 221–236.
78. Einhorn, T. A., The cell and molecular biology of fracture healing. *Clin Orthop Relat Res*, 1998. **355**: S7–21.
79. Schindeler, A., et al., Bone remodeling during fracture repair: the cellular picture. *Semin Cell Dev Biol*, 2008. **19**(5): 459–466.
80. Sung, H. J., et al., The effect of scaffold degradation rate on three-dimensional cell growth and angiogenesis. *Biomaterials*, 2004. **25**(26): 5735–5742.
81. Kuboki, Y., et al., BMP-induced osteogenesis on the surface of hydroxyapatite with geometrically feasible and nonfeasible structures: topology of osteogenesis. *J Biomed Mater Res*, 1998. **39**(2): 190–199.
82. D'Lima, D. D., et al., Bone response to implant surface morphology. *J Arthroplasty*, 1998. **13**(8): 928–934.
83. Sul, Y. T., et al., Characteristics of the surface oxides on turned and electrochemically oxidized pure titanium implants up to dielectric breakdown: the oxide thickness, micropore configurations, surface roughness, crystal structure and chemical composition. *Biomaterials*, 2002. **23**(2): 491–501.
84. Ducheyne, P., and K. de Groot, In vivo surface activity of a hydroxyapatite alveolar bone substitute. *J Biomed Mater Res*, 1981. **15**(3): 441–445.
85. Webster, T. J., et al., Enhanced functions of osteoblasts on nanophase ceramics. *Biomaterials*, 2000. **21**(17): 1803–1810.
86. Lee, C. H., A. Singla, and Y. Lee, Biomedical applications of collagen. *Int J Pharm*, 2001. **221**(1–2): 1–22.
87. Miyata, T., T. Taira, and Y. Noishiki, Collagen engineering for biomaterial use. *Clin Mater*, 1992. **9**(3–4): p. 139–148.
88. Rao, K. P., Recent developments of collagen-based materials for medical applications and drug delivery systems. *J Biomater Sci Polym Ed*, 1995. **7**(7): 623–645.

89. Urist, M. R., Bone: formation by autoinduction. 1965. *Clin Orthop Relat Res*, 2002. (395): 4–10.
90. Sandhu, H. S., and S. D. Boden, Biologic enhancement of spinal fusion. *Orthop Clin North Am*, 1998. **29**(4): 621–631.
91. Wang, E. A., et al., Recombinant human bone morphogenetic protein induces bone formation. *Proc Natl Acad Sci USA*, 1990. **87**(6): 2220–2224.
92. Bianco, P., et al., Bone marrow stromal stem cells: nature, biology, and potential applications. *Stem Cells*, 2001. **19**(3): 180–192.
93. Deng, M., et al., Novel polymer-ceramics for bone repair and regeneration. *Recent Pat Biomed Eng*, 2011. **4**(3): 168–184.
94. Deng, M., et al., Miscibility and in vitro osteocompatibility of biodegradable blends of poly[(ethyl alanato) (*p*-phenyl phenoxy) phosphazene] and poly(lactic acid-glycolic acid). *Biomaterials*, 2008. **29**(3): 337–349.
95. Oreffo, R., and J. Triffitt, Future potentials for using osteogenic stem cells and biomaterials in orthopedics. *Bone*, 1999. **25**(2): 5S–9S.
96. Anselme, K., Osteoblast adhesion on biomaterials. *Biomaterials*, 2000. **21**(7): 667–681.
97. Meyer, U., et al., Basic reactions of osteoblasts on structured material surfaces. *Eur Cell Mater*, 2005. **9**: 39–49.
98. Meyer, U., T. Meyer, and D. Jones, No mechanical role for vinculin in strain transduction in primary bovine osteoblasts. *Biochem Cell Biol*, 1997. **75**(1): 81–87.
99. Boyan, B. D., et al., Role of material surfaces in regulating bone and cartilage cell response. *Biomaterials*, 1996. **17**(2): 137–146.
100. Zhao, L., et al., The influence of hierarchical hybrid micro/nano-textured titanium surface with titania nanotubes on osteoblast functions. *Biomaterials*, 2010. **31**(19): 5072–5082.
101. Civitelli, R., Cell–cell communication in the osteoblast/osteocyte lineage. *Archiv Biochem Biophys*, 2008. **473**(2): 188–192.
102. Marie, P. J., Role of N-cadherin in bone formation. *J Cellular Physiol*, 2002. **190**(3): 297–305.
103. Schiller, P., et al., Gap-junctional communication mediates parathyroid hormone stimulation of mineralization in osteoblastic cultures. *Bone*, 2001. **28**(1): 38–44.
104. Devin, J. E., M. A. Attawia, and C. T. Laurencin, Three-dimensional degradable porous polymer-ceramic matrices for use in bone repair. *J Biomater Sci Polymer Ed*, 1996. **7**(8): 661–669.

105. El-Amin, S., et al., Extracellular matrix production by human osteoblasts cultured on biodegradable polymers applicable for tissue engineering. *Biomaterials*, 2003. **24**(7): 1213–1221.
106. Laurencin, C. T., et al., The ABJS Nicolas Andry Award: Tissue engineering of bone and ligament: A 15-year perspective. *Clin Orthop Relat Res*, 2006. **447**: 221.
107. Laurencin, C., et al., Poly (lactide-co-glycolide)/hydroxyapatite delivery of BMP-2-producing cells: a regional gene therapy approach to bone regeneration. *Biomaterials*, 2001. **22**(11): 1271–1277.
108. Borden, M., et al., Tissue engineered microsphere-based matrices for bone repair: design and evaluation. *Biomaterials*, 2002. **23**(2): 551–559.
109. Borden, M., et al., Structural and human cellular assessment of a novel microsphere-based tissue engineered scaffold for bone repair. *Biomaterials*, 2003. **24**(4): 597–609.
110. Roveri, N., et al., Biologically inspired growth of hydroxyapatite nanocrystals inside self-assembled collagen fibers. *Mater Sci Eng: C*, 2003. **23**(3): 441–446.
111. Webster, T. J., R. W. Siegel, and R. Bizios, Osteoblast adhesion on nanophase ceramics. *Biomaterials*, 1999. **20**(13): 1221–1227.
112. Li, W. J., et al., Electrospun nanofibrous structure: a novel scaffold for tissue engineering. *J Biomed Mater Res*, 2002. **60**(4): 613–621.
113. Nair, L. S., and C. T. Laurencin, Nanofibers and nanoparticles for orthopaedic surgery applications. *J Bone Joint Surg Am*, 2008. **90** (Suppl 1): 128–131.
114. Nair, L. S., S. Bhattacharyya, and C. T. Laurencin, Development of novel tissue engineering scaffolds via electrospinning. *Expert Opin Biol Ther*, 2004. **4**(5): 659–668.
115. Huang, Z. M., et al., A review on polymer nanofibers by electrospinning and their applications in nanocomposites. *Composites Sci Technol*, 2003. **63**: 2223–2253.
116. Ma, P. X., and R. Zhang, Synthetic nano-scale fibrous extracellular matrix. *J Biomed Mater Res*, 1999. **46**(1): 60–72.
117. Whitesides, G. M., and B. Grzybowski, Self-assembly at all scales. *Science*, 2002. **295**(5564): 2418–2421.
118. Bhattacharyya, S., et al., Biodegradable polyphosphazene-nanohydroxyapatite composite nanofibers: scaffolds for bone tissue engineering. *J Biomed Nanotechnol*, 2009. **5**(1): 69–75.

119. Bhattacharyya, S., et al., Electrospinning of poly[bis(ethyl alanato) phosphazene] nanofibers. *J Biomed Nanotechnol*, 2006. **2**(1): 36–45.
120. Nair, L. S., et al., Fabrication and optimization of methylphenoxy substituted polyphosphazene nanofibers for biomedical applications. *Biomacromolecules*, 2004. **5**(6): 2212–20.
121. Conconi, M. T., et al., In vitro evaluation of poly[bis(ethyl alanato)phosphazene] as a scaffold for bone tissue engineering. *Tissue Eng*, 2006. **12**(4): 811–9.
122. Deng, M., et al., Biomimetic structures: biological implications of dipeptide-substituted polyphosphazene-polyester blend nanofiber matrices for load-bearing bone regeneration *Adv Funct Mater*, 2011. **21**(14): 2641–2651.
123. Hartgerink, J. D., E. Beniash, and S.I. Stupp, Self-assembly and mineralization of peptide-amphiphile nanofibers. *Science*, 2001. **294**(5547): 1684–1688.
124. Hartgerink, J. D., E. Beniash, and S. I. Stupp, Peptide-amphiphile nanofibers: a versatile scaffold for the preparation of self-assembling materials. *Proc Natl Acad Sci*, 2002. **99**(8): 5133–5138.
125. Brown, J. L., et al., Composite scaffolds: bridging nanofiber and microsphere architectures to improve bioactivity of mechanically competent constructs. *J Biomed Mater Res A*, 2010. DOI: 10.1002/jbm.a.32934.
126. Yamanaka, S., A fresh look at iPS cells. *Cell*, 2009. **137**(1): 13–17.
127. Jaenisch, R., and R. Young, Stem cells, the molecular circuitry of pluripotency and nuclear reprogramming. *Cell*, 2008. **132**(4): 567–582.
128. Kaur, S. and C. Kartha, Stem Cells: Concepts and Prospects. *Current Trends in Science, Platinum Jubilee Special, Indian Academy of Sciences*, 2009. 438–452.
129. Dolatshahi-Pirouz, A., et al., Micro-and nanoengineering approaches to control stem cell–biomaterial interactions. *J Funct Biomater*, 2011. **2**(3): 88–106.
130. Oh, S., et al., Stem cell fate dictated solely by altered nanotube dimension. *Proc Nat Acad Sci*, 2009. **106**(7): 2130.
131. Kilian, K. A., et al., Geometric cues for directing the differentiation of mesenchymal stem cells. *Proc Natl Acad Sci*, 2010. **107**(11): 4872.
132. Zandstra, P. W. and A. Nagy, Stem cell bioengineering. *Ann Rev Biomed Eng*, 2001. **3**(1): 275–305.

133. Solanki, A., et al., Controlling differentiation of neural stem cells using extracellular matrix protein patterns. *Small*, 2010. **6**(22): 2509–2513.

134. Fukuda, K., Development of regenerative cardiomyocytes from mesenchymal stem cells for cardiovascular tissue engineering. *Artif organs*, 2001. **25**(3): 187–193.

135. Toh, Y. C., K. Blagović, and J. Voldman, Advancing stem cell research with microtechnologies: opportunities and challenges. *Integr. Biol.*, 2010. **2**(7–8): 305–325.

136. Spradling, A., D. Drummond-Barbosa, and T. Kai, Stem cells find their niche. *Nature* (London), 2001: 98–104.

137. Evans, N. D., and M. M. Stevens, Complexity in biomaterials for tissue engineering. *Nat Mater*, 2009. **8**(6): 457–470.

138. Fisher, O. Z., et al., Bioinspired materials for controlling stem cell fate. *Acc Chem Res*, 2009. **43**(3): 419–428.

139. Curtis, A., and C. Wilkinson. New depths in cell behaviour: reactions of cells to nanotopography. *Biochem Soc Symp*, 1999. **65**: 15–26.

140. Nayak, T. R., et al., Thin films of functionalized multiwalled carbon nanotubes as suitable scaffold materials for stem cells proliferation and bone formation. *ACS nano*, 2010. **4**: 7717–7725.

141. Curtis, A. and M. Varde, Control of cell behavior: topological factors. *J Natl Cancer Inst*, 1964. **33**: 15.

142. Dalby, M. J., et al., The control of human mesenchymal cell differentiation using nanoscale symmetry and disorder. *Nat Mater*, 2007. **6**(12): 997–1003.

143. Dalby, M. J., et al., Osteoprogenitor response to semi-ordered and random nanotopographies. *Biomaterials*, 2006. **27**(15): 2980–2987.

144. Park, J., et al., Nanosize and vitality: TiO_2 nanotube diameter directs cell fate. *Nano Lett*, 2007. **7**(6): 1686–1691.

145. Chai, C., and K. W. Leong, Biomaterials approach to expand and direct differentiation of stem cells. *Mol Ther*, 2007. **15**(3): 467–480.

146. McBeath, R., et al., Cell shape, cytoskeletal tension, and RhoA regulate stem cell lineage commitment. *Dev Cell*, 2004. **6**(4): 483–495.

147. Ruiz, S. A. and C. S. Chen, Emergence of patterned stem cell differentiation within multicellular structures. *Stem Cells*, 2008. **26**(11): 2921–2927.

148. Park, J., et al., TiO_2 nanotube surfaces: 15 nm—An optimal length scale of surface topography for cell adhesion and differentiation. *Small*, 2009. **5**(6): 666–671.

149. Park, J., et al., Narrow window in nanoscale dependent activation of endothelial cell growth and differentiation on TiO$_2$ nanotube surfaces. *Nano Lett*, 2009. **9**(9): 3157–3164.
150. Popat, K. C., et al., Influence of engineered titania nanotubular surfaces on bone cells. *Biomaterials*, 2007. **28**(21): 3188–3197.
151. Roach, P., D. Farrar, and C. C. Perry, Surface tailoring for controlled protein adsorption: effect of topography at the nanometer scale and chemistry. *J Am Chem Soc*, 2006. **128**(12): 3939–3945.
152. Zouani, O. F., et al., Altered nanofeature size dictates stem cell differentiation. *J Cell Sci*, 2012. **125**: 1–8.

Chapter 14

Stem Cells and Bone Regeneration

Martin L. Decaris, Kaitlin C. Murphy, and J. Kent Leach

Department of Biomedical Engineering, University of California, Davis, Genome and Biomedical Sciences Facility 2303, 451 Health Sciences Drive, Davis, CA 95616, USA

jkleach@ucdavis.edu

14.1 Introduction

Bone tissue regeneration is characterized by a multistage process that results in vascularization, matrix deposition, mineralization, and structural remodeling at the site of repair. While the self-healing capacity of bone is typically robust, bone loss and non-healing bone defects associated with a variety of clinical conditions often require substitute bone-like materials to induce new bone formation or proper tissue repair. These conditions, which include but are not limited to nonunion fractures, severe skeletal trauma, tumor resections, and spinal fusions, are increasing in number every year and place an enormous financial burden on the world-wide health care system.

Autologous bone grafts represent the current gold standard of treatment for bone defect repair, with over 1.6 million performed annually in the United States alone [99]. Upon transfer to a bone defect site, these grafts deliver osteogenic cell populations and signaling factors set within an osteoconductive scaffold, and are therefore highly efficient at repairing bone defects and bridging fracture gaps. However, there are also several drawbacks associated with autologous grafts including donor site morbidity, costs associated with a secondary surgical site, limited tissue availability, and lack of efficacy in patients suffering from systemic bone disorders [3,16,28]. Allogeneic bone-based materials collected from surgical procedures or harvested from cadavers are also utilized as bone tissue substitutes. However, these materials suffer from numerous drawbacks including potential immunogenic responses, limited availability, and diminished capacity to integrate with host tissue and remodel in response to external mechanical force [67,90].

Tissue-engineered bone constructs offer a potential solution to the limitations associated with bone grafts. This approach to tissue regeneration typically combines biological and synthetic components to create implantable constructs that recapitulate native tissue function and/or stimulate tissue repair [79]. Constructs combining osteogenic cell populations, osteoinductive signaling factors, and osteoconductive scaffolding materials hold the potential to harness each of the positive qualities associated with autologous bone grafts. In fact, bone tissue substitutes combining various osteoconductive materials (e.g., polymers, ceramics, allogeneic bone matrix) with osteoinductive recombinant growth factors (e.g., bone morphogenetic protein-2 (BMP-2), transforming growth factor-ß (TGF-ß)) have demonstrated utility as bone defect fillers and comprise a vast array of commercially available therapeutic products [80]. While growth factor-based approaches to bone regeneration have demonstrated some clinical promise, limitations to this method include the high cost of recombinant protein production, lack of control over protein release kinetics, and the potentially harmful supraphysiological quantities of proteins required to induce a host tissue response [81,85,116]. In addition, the success of growth factor-based constructs is dependent upon the availability of endogenous cell populations, creating a potential challenge for patients lacking sufficient numbers of responsive cells.

Bone tissue substitutes incorporating osteogenic cell populations have the potential to directly participate in bone tissue formation immediately following implantation. In addition, implanted cell populations secrete biological factors in a more physiologically relevant manner through their interaction with the surrounding microenvironment. Stem cells, commonly characterized by the capacity for self-renewal and the potential to differentiate into multiple cell types, provide an exciting source of implantable osteogenic cells that can be isolated from autologous or allogeneic sources, as well as expanded to clinically relevant numbers ex vivo. The purpose of this chapter is to introduce the reader to current research utilizing stem cells for the purposes of bone regeneration. The potential for a number of different stem cell populations to be utilized in therapies directed at bone formation will be discussed. As stem cell differentiation is modulated by both biochemical and physical microenvironmental cues, we will also describe several current approaches to direct stem cells toward a bone-forming phenotype. More specifically, the spatiotemporal presentation of micro- and nanoscale stimuli to stem cells via soluble factors and cell-surface interactions will be addressed in detail. Finally, the ability of cell-based bone tissue constructs to generate new bone tissue, both in vitro and in vivo, will be discussed, along with some of the hurdles remaining to develop synthetically engineered bone tissue substitutes that rival their autologous counterparts.

14.2 Sources of Stem Cells for Bone Regeneration

Stem cells, defined as undeveloped cells capable of self-renewal and differentiation into multiple phenotypes, play a vital role in the development and regeneration of human tissues [134]. These cells can generally be categorized into two groups: pluripotent stem cells (PSCs) and adult stem cells. Pluripotent stem cells, representative of an early stage of embryonic development, have the capacity to differentiate into virtually all mature cell populations. Adult stem cells, on the other hand, possess limited differentiation potential and are present in a wide variety of adult tissues, carrying out day-to-day tissue repair. Here we give a brief introduction to each type of stem cell, discuss their advantages and disadvantages for cell-based therapies, and analyze how they can be utilized in regenerative medicine approaches toward bone repair.

14.2.1 Pluripotent Stem Cells

Embryonic stem cells (ESCs), first established in mice by Evans and Kaufman in 1981 and then with human cells by Thomson et al. in 1998, are the most commonly utilized pluripotent cell population in bone tissue engineering research [32,126]. They are isolated from the inner cell mass of the blastocyst, have unlimited self-renewal properties in culture, and are capable of giving rise to all cell types present in adult tissue [114]. They have therefore been studied in a wide range of cell-based therapies, particularly those where relevant adult stem cell populations cannot be easily isolated or exist in exceedingly small quantities. Embryonic stem cells are typically expanded in an undifferentiated state using fibroblastic feeder cells and defined medium. Upon removal from these conditions, ESCs are capable of forming embryoid bodies, aggregates of cells representative of all three germ layers. Embryonic stem cells collected from undifferentiated colonies or isolated from dissociated embryoid bodies undergo osteogenic differentiation when treated with osteogenic media supplements (e.g., ß-glycerophosphate, ascorbic acid, dexamethasone, vitamin-D3, etc.) [10,63,65]. Several additional techniques have also been developed to increase the osteogenic potential of ESC populations. For example, the culture of ESCs in hepatocyte-conditioned medium enhances mesoderm formation, ESC-derived adult stem cell-like populations have been established that respond to defined methods of osteogenic differentiation associated with those cell types [2,51,52].

The advantages of ESC-derived cell-based therapies for tissue regeneration are plentiful. In addition to their pluripotency and limitless capacity for self-renewal, ESCs provide the potential for an "off-the-shelf" cell-based product as a result of their harvest from allogeneic sources. Embryonic stem cells are also amenable to transfection, allowing for the creation of genetically modified cell-populations that facilitate in-depth analysis of the signaling pathways related to cell differentiation and tissue development [58]. One of the major disadvantages associated with ESCs is their potential to induce an immunogenic response [39]. Since ESCs originate from allogeneic donors, HLA-type matching would be necessary to limit rejection following implantation, barring the development of non-immunogenic ESC-derived cell populations. As the ethical discussion surrounding ESC collection has limited research utilizing this cell population to cells representative of a finite number of donors, the use of ESC populations matched to specific patients is currently unfeasible. The potential for undifferentiated ESCs remaining within the therapeutic cell population to form teratomas, tumors possessing cells representative of each germ layer, also presents a current challenge. Negative selection of undifferentiated cells is necessary to mitigate tumor formation, as well as to remove heterogeneously differentiated cells that could disrupt homogenous tissue formation.

The recent development of a novel pluripotent stem cell population, induced pluripotent stem cells (iPSCs), may address the immunogenic and ethical concerns related to the use of ESCs in cell-based therapies. iPSCs, first established by Yamanaka et al. and then Thomson et al. were originally derived from fibroblast cell populations subjected to heightened expression of several pluripotency genes (e.g., Sox2, Oct4, Klf4, c-Myc, Nanog, Lin 28) through lentiviral-based gene transfer techniques [124,141]. This allows for the establishment of patient specific PSC populations, simultaneously eliminating the immunogenic concerns associated with allogeneic donors and the ethical concerns associated with harvesting ESCs from embryonic tissue. iPSCs behave similarly to ESCs in culture and have the potential to adopt an osteoblastic phenotype [53,84]. One obvious drawback to the original method of obtaining iPSC populations was the use of genetically modified cells. However, novel techniques utilizing alternative methods of inducing pluripotent protein expression have begun to bypass these concerns [120,133]. Additional drawbacks associated with iPSCs include the high cost associated with deriving patient specific cell populations, as well as recent evidence suggesting that iPSCs may still evoke an immune response following implantation in vivo [143]. Further analysis of the epigenetic differences present between ESC-derived and iPSC-derived osteogenic cells may shed light on the potential for iPSCs to be utilized in cell-based bone repair [7].

14.2.2 Adult Stem Cells

Adult stem cells are responsible for the day-to-day regeneration of tissues and organs throughout the body. As terminally differentiated cells die from injury or apoptotic processes, their numbers are replenished by adult stem cells, which are capable of asymmetric division into a phenotypically distinct daughter cell and identical undifferentiated stem cell. This uneven division, made possible by the surrounding microenvironment termed the "stem cell niche," allows stem cells to produce progenitor cell populations that ultimately differentiate into a mature phenotype while simultaneously replenishing the undifferentiated stem cell pool [95]. Although certain adult stem cell populations have been well characterized for stage-specific markers reflective of the distinct cell phenotypes present during differentiation into mature cells (e.g., hematopoietic stem cells), stem cells responsible for bone regeneration have been more difficult to describe.

Bone formation and regeneration occurs through two distinct pathways. Endochondral ossification involves the formation of a transitory cartilage phase prior to mineralized bone deposition, while intramembranous ossification is characterized by the direct formation of mineralized bone tissue. Although much is known regarding both pathways, such as the fact that each process involves the recruitment and condensation of a mesenchymal progenitor cell population, the identity of a specific well-defined stem cell population within bone tissue remains elusive [19,101]. What has been well described in the literature is a heterogeneous stromal cell population present within bone tissue that decreases in number with age and has been linked to several physiological functions including the maintenance of hematopoietic cell activity and the regeneration of mineralized bone tissue [55,121,125,135]. This population, dubbed with monikers including "mesenchymal stem cells" and "multipotent mesenchymal stromal cells," here referred to as MSCs, has been studied in depth for roughly 40 years and shows great promise in cell-based therapeutic approaches to bone repair.

MSCs were first identified by Freidenstein et al. in 1968 as an adherent fibroblastic cell population present in the bone marrow, capable of forming colonies in culture [36]. In the decades since, the isolation and identification of specific subpopulations of these cells has been carried out multiple times, although a distinct clonogenic population has yet to be derived. Bone marrow-derived MSCs are generally defined as a tissue culture plastic adherent cell population isolated from the bone marrow that are CD73+, CD90+, CD105+, CD34-, CD45-, CD14- or CD11b-, CD79alpha- or CD19-, HLA-DR-, and are capable of trilineage differentiation toward the osteogenic, chondrogenic, and adipogenic lineages when cultured under defined media conditions [30]. While additional markers have been utilized to identify and positively or negatively select subpopulations of MSCs with heightened proliferative or differentiation potential, no specific set of markers is maintained by the cells during expansion in culture, and MSCs typically display reduced proliferative and differentiation potential upon extended passaging [82,101,111]. As cells within the heterogeneous population have distinctive proliferative and differentiation capacities, the term "stem cell" is highly dubious when referring to MSCs.

MSCs are the most studied cell population for bone tissue engineering due to their ease of availability and robust osteogenic potential. MSCs exposed to osteogenic media supplements in vitro or osteoinductive growth factors quickly upregulate the expression of the osteogenic transcription factors cbfa-1 (Runx2) and osterix, followed by the expression of several functional proteins including alkaline phosphatase, type 1 collagen, and bone sialoprotein [97,103]. MSC density in culture has also been linked to changes in their capacity for differentiation through cell–cell interactions and the secretion of autocrine factors that modulate downstream signaling pathways [56]. Although MSCs possess a fibroblastic morphology when in an undifferentiated state, they adopt a cuboidal morphology similar to that of mature osteoblasts upon osteogenic induction followed by the deposition of mineralized nodules on their culture surface. Unlike mature osteoblast cell populations, however, MSCs can be isolated from patients through minimally invasive procedures and undergo prolific expansion in culture, potentially providing a clinically relevant number of autologous bone-forming cells for delivery to defective bone tissue. The additional capacity for MSCs to differentiate toward the chondrogenic phenotype also gives them the potential to mimic both the endochondral and intramembranous routes of natural bone formation [34].

Aside from their multilineage differentiation potential, MSCs also demonstrate a number of additional properties that lend themselves to strategies aimed at tissue repair. For instance, MSCs possess the ability to home to injured tissues in vivo, as well as to secrete a wide array of cytokines and growth factors capable of modulating inflammation, apoptosis, and angiogenesis [12,14,107]. MSCs have therefore been studied in numerous therapeutic models unrelated to bone repair including the treatment of ischemic myocardial tissue, graft *vs.* host disease, and spinal cord injury [1,11,33,113]. As inflammation and angiogenesis also play important roles in bone regeneration, and the therapeutic efficacy of MSCs appears to only weakly correlate to long term engraftment following implantation, the secretion of paracrine factors has also been credited with playing an important role in MSC-mediated bone repair [106]. MSC secretion of paracrine factors such as vascular endothelial growth factor (VEGF) correlate with the stage of osteogenic differentiation, with undifferentiated MSCs secreting higher concentrations than osteogenically differentiated cells [47]. Vascular endothelial growth factor is a potent stimulator of endothelial cell migration and proliferation during the early stages of angiogenesis. Utilizing a combination of MSC populations at different stages of differentiation may therefore offer a method of harnessing both the direct osteogenic properties and trophic factor delivery characteristics of MSCs (Fig 14.1) [20,74]. Endothelial cells delivered in combination with MSC populations frequently enhance both vascular formation and mineral deposition in orthotopic models of bone formation [60,72]. Stem cell–based therapies that successfully initiate bone repair may therefore benefit from transplanting multiple cell populations that potentiate the varied processes required for bone regeneration.

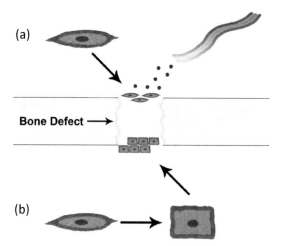

Figure 14.1 Primary approaches to MSC-based bone repair. (a) Trophic factor secretion from undifferentiated MSCs targeting wound healing responses such as angiogenesis and inflammation. (b) Osteogenic pre-conditioning of MSCs targeting direct cell engraftment and mineralized tissue deposition.

In addition to the expression of soluble factors, MSCs also possess extraordinary immunomodulatory properties. Due to their lack of expression of class II major histocompatibility proteins on the cell surface, MSCs may not require immunosuppression when delivered in an allogeneic manner [125]. This could prove extremely advantageous in the treatment of elderly patients, whose own MSC population may be drastically diminished in number and bone-forming potential.

One of the main disadvantages of bone marrow-derived MSCs as a primary cell source for bone tissue repair is the exceedingly small number of cells present in adult tissue. MSCs make up approximately 0.000001% to 0.001% of mononuclear cells in the bone marrow, a fraction that correlates negatively with age [121,142]. However, MSC populations are also present in a wide variety of alternate tissues including adipose, muscle, and the umbilical cord tissue, potentially providing an abundant source of cells for skeletal therapies [21,54,146]. The use of MSCs isolated from fetal tissues such as bone marrow is also being explored, as these cells possess impressive proliferative and differentiation properties along with the potential for allogeneic use as previously discussed [142]. Direct comparison of the MSC populations isolated from different tissues has revealed that MSC concentration, as well as their capacity for proliferation and differentiation, can be highly variable based on tissue source [101]. While bone marrow-derived MSCs represent the most studied population for bone repair applications, more direct comparisons between the various PSC and MSC populations are necessary to determine which population best combines properties related to collection, expansion, and bone tissue formation.

14.3 Osteogenic Induction of Stem Cells

The potential for stem cell–based therapies to enhance skeletal defect repair requires a solid understanding of the mechanisms of stem cell differentiation. Following the collection and expansion of stem cell populations, cells must be directed toward the osteogenic lineage in order to exhibit a robust osteogenic phenotype in vivo, or at the very least, some alternative phenotype that aids in an ancillary pathway to bone repair. Soluble biochemical factors were originally credited as the primary determinant of cell differentiation in vivo.

However, a burgeoning field of study has uncovered that this process is much more complex, involving the spatiotemporal integration of physical, as well as biochemical cues. Cell-extracellular matrix (ECM) and cell–cell interactions play important roles along with local concentrations of autocrine, paracrine, and endocrine factors in modulating cell behavior such as attachment, proliferation, migration, differentiation, and viability. The ECM in particular, once thought of as merely providing structural support to tissues and cells, is now credited with modulating cell behavior in numerous ways including the spatial presentation of instructive peptide sequences, binding and sequestering of growth factors, and mechanotransductive signaling. These interactions activate intracellular signaling pathways that lead to downstream changes in gene expression and ultimately result in an alteration of cell phenotype. Researchers have therefore developed a variety of tools and materials that interact with cells at the micro- and nanometer scale in order to better understand how cells interpret the physical cues that surround them. The following section presents a brief overview of several current techniques to instruct the osteogenic differentiation of stem cell populations. Along with the use of soluble biological factors, we will discuss the use of ECM-mimicking biomaterial substrates, the co-culture of cell populations, and the genetic manipulation of stem cells to enhance their expression of bone related genes.

14.3.1 Soluble Osteogenic Factors

The in situ development and differentiation of endogenous pluripotent and mesenchymal progenitor cells toward specific phenotypes, including that of functional osteoblasts, is tightly regulated by the spatial and temporal presentation of numerous growth factors. Bone morphogenetic proteins (BMPs) are a major contributor to the osteogenic differentiation pathway, activating downstream phosphorylation of Smad proteins and subsequent expression of the major osteogenic transcription factor Runx2 [61]. Members of both the fibroblast growth factor (FGF) and Wnt families of proteins have also been implicated in signaling cascades which regulate both MSC proliferation and osteogenic fate [4]. Microfluidic cell culture systems present a valuable tool to study the effect of growth factor concentration gradients on the differentiation of stem cell populations [88]. Lack of convective mixing in very small volumes allows for establishment of predictable soluble factor gradients. Cells cultured within such gradients can be monitored over time for phenotypic changes.

The use of recombinant proteins mimicking those soluble factors present during natural tissue development presents one approach toward inducing the osteogenic differentiation of stem cells in vitro. Although effective at modulating stem cell fate, recombinant signaling proteins display functional variability and are extremely costly, limiting their extended use in culture. In addition, there is evidence that these factors may not induce the same effects in adult-derived stem cells isolated from alternate tissue sources [145]. While the presentation of recombinant factors in vivo has demonstrated some success for inducing the osteogenic differentiation of stem cells post-implantation, recombinant growth factor-based therapies can also present toxicity issues, as they typically require supraphysiological quantities of proteins to maintain effective concentrations at the implant site [105].

In comparison to recombinant protein-based strategies, more cost effective strategies exist for directing the osteogenic differentiation of stem cells in vitro (Fig. 14.2). For example, both MSC and PSC populations demonstrate enhanced osteogenic differentiation in response to simple media cocktails containing ß-glycerophosphate, ascorbic acid, and dexamethasone [58,66]. ß-glycerophosphate provides a source of extracellular phosphates, which induce osteogenic gene expression and boost cellular capacity for mineralization. In addition, ascorbic acid has demonstrated the capacity to increase Type 1 collagen expression in MSCs, while the corticosteroid dexamethasone further enhances osteogenic gene expression, potentially through the activation of FGF-related signaling pathways [18,40]. Osteogenic differentiation of human MSCs in culture utilizing these factors is commonly performed for approximately 3–4 weeks and is characterized by the early expression of osteogenic transcription factors (e.g., Runx2, osterix) followed by the increased expression of osteogenic proteins (e.g., alkaline phosphatase (ALP), osteocalcin, bone sialoprotein) and ultimately deposition of mineralized nodules.

The osteogenic induction of MSCs prior to delivery to a bone defect site is another common strategy to utilize soluble factors in stem cell-mediated bone repair (Fig. 14.1). The state of MSC differentiation upon implantation significantly affects subsequent bone formation [13,137]. Although MSCs appear to retain their nonimmunogenic state during differentiation, they also markedly reduce the secretion of trophic factors, potentially mitigating their anti-inflammatory and pro-angiogenic properties [47]. MSCs have also been observed to reassume a multipotent phenotype following the removal of soluble osteogenic media factors in culture [118]. These factors must be considered carefully when establishing bone repair strategies that utilize osteogenically induced cells, as cell phenotype present in defined culture conditions may be altered following delivery in vivo. While the use of soluble factors will likely play a major role in cell-based therapies, additional cues that direct stem cell fate may be necessary to guide and maintain the proper phenotype of therapeutic cells throughout the process of bone repair.

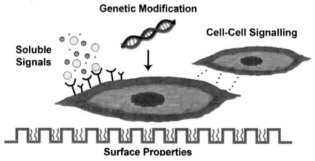

Figure 14.2 Strategies to induce the osteogenic differentiation of stem cells. Soluble factors, cell–cell interactions, genetic modification, surface chemistry, surface topography, bulk material properties, and mechanotransduction each play a role in determining stem cell fate.

14.3.2 Bulk Material Properties

The interaction between stem cells and their physical microenvironment appears to play as much a role in determining phenotypic fate as their exposure to soluble factors. While the ECM was once thought to contribute in a passive, structural manner in many tissues, it is now known to actively modulate cell behavior through structural and biological interactions with the cell surface that regulate gene expression. Biomaterial constructs that harness the cell-instructive properties of the ECM from native tissues will likely be more successful in fostering stem cell-mediated bone repair. Current research in stem cell–based bone repair utilizes a vast array of biomaterial scaffolds to carry out cell delivery and allow for cell-driven tissue regeneration. As the ECM of native bone tissue contains an inorganic component (primarily hydroxyapatite mineral deposits) and an organic component (Type 1 collagen fibers), it should be no surprise that these materials are commonly used to engineer bone tissue replacements. In addition, several other natural and synthetic polymers have also been studied for their potential to support cell delivery and boost bone formation (e.g., fibrin, alginate, chitosan, polyesters, polyanhydrides), possessing tremendous variability in factors such as cost, immunogenicity, reproducibility, deliverability, mechanical properties, and degradation rate. While the sheer number of materials available for bone tissue engineering applications can make the selection of any particular one seem dizzying, this wide variety of materials has enabled the development of many structurally distinct scaffolding types, providing researchers with the tools to uncover how the physical properties of cell substrates direct stem cell fate.

The physical geometry of bone ECM plays an important role in determining cell fate. As bone-forming osteoblasts (approximately 25 µm in diameter) typically interact with collagen fibrils (about 500 nm in diameter) or fibers composed of multiple fibrils, the development of nanofiber scaffolds for bone repair represents an exciting area of research [42]. Several approaches to nanofiber scaffold fabrication have been developed including self-assembly, phase separation, and electrospinning [98]. Electrospinning techniques may hold the most promise for engineering nanofiber scaffolds capable of modulating stem cell behavior, as they can produce long continuous fibers of precise diameter (50–1000 nm) that blend synthetic polymers with additional osteoconductive materials including hydroxyapatite and collagen. Dissolved composite material blends are passed through a needle under high voltage and collected upon a grounded plate, resulting in highly porous nanofiber scaffolds capable of efficient gas and nutrient exchange. These scaffolds also possess a high surface area to volume ratio, thereby facilitating enhanced deposition of proteins that act as sites for cell attachment (Fig. 14.3). Nanofiber scaffolds can modulate the attachment, proliferation, and osteogenic differentiation of MSC and PSC populations in culture [71,93,117]. In addition to fiber diameter, the overall porosity and rate of degradation of biomaterial scaffolds merit consideration. These properties determine the kinetics of host cell infiltration, revascularization, and remodeling at the site of repair, while also demonstrating the capacity to modulate stem cell phenotype [29,64].

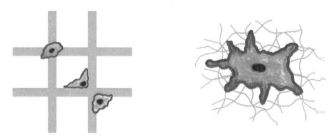

Microscale Adhesion   **Nanoscale Adhesion**

Figure 14.3 Cell-substrate interactions at the micrometer and nanometer scale. Nanoporous scaffolds allow for cell-substrate interactions that more closely mimic the cell's interaction with the native extracellular matrix.

Substrate stiffness is another critical biophysical material property that regulates stem cell phenotype. A seminal study analyzed this relationship by culturing MSCs on collagen coated polyacrylamide gels with adjustable mechanical properties, demonstrating that matrix elasticity can direct cell fate [31]. Markers characteristic of MSC differentiation toward neural, myogenic, or osteogenic lineages were observed simply by adjusting substrate rigidity. In this study, the most rigid substrates (>25 kPa) directed MSCs toward an osteogenic phenotype, as evidenced by increased Runx2 and ALP expression. Subsequent studies utilizing fibrin and polyethylene glycol hydrogels of differing stiffness have also demonstrated a link between substrate compliance and osteogenic differentiation, with the MAP kinase signaling pathway appearing to play an important role [24,68]. The rigid structural properties of native bone ECM may therefore play an important role in the differentiation of osteoprogenitor cells into functional bone-forming cells. MSC migration in vivo may also be influenced by gradients in tissue rigidity, as studies in vitro have demonstrated that MSCs accumulate on stiffer substrates [29]. More recent studies have demonstrated that substrate rigidity can also confer osteogenic signals to MSCs in 3-D culture [50]. Alginate hydrogels modified with cell-adhesive peptides and fabricated with different moduli revealed that matrix stiffness regulates integrin binding and adhesive ligand reorganization in a traction dependent manner, resulting in increased osteogenic differentiation of MSCs at particular rigidities (11–30 kPa).

14.3.3 Material Surface Properties

The physical relationship between cells and their microenvironment is determined via substrate attachment. Integrins, a class of transmembrane cell surface proteins, are responsible for facilitating adhesion of cells to peptide motifs in the ECM. Integrins cluster together to form focal adhesions, which allow cells to apply tension to their substrate, activate intracellular signaling pathways, and/or alter cellular cytoskeletal architecture in a manner that leads to altered gene expression. The important relationship between substrate adhesion and stem cell fate was clearly demonstrated by McBeath et al. [92]. MSC fate was correlated to cell shape by altering the presentation of available surface ligands using fibronectin-coated polydimethylsiloxane. Cells that bound to the substrate over a large area adopted a flattened morphology and underwent osteogenic differentiation, while those forced to maintain a more rounded morphology on a smaller adhesive area became adipocytes. In fact, cell attachment, differentiation, proliferation, migration, cytoskeletal organization, and apoptotic pathways have all been shown to respond to changes in substrate ligand patterning at the nanometer scale [132]. As the osteogenic differentiation of stem cells is highly sought after in bone regenerative therapies, researchers have developed of number of tools to better control how stem cells interact with substrate surfaces, which in turn allow for better control over cell fate.

The direct attachment of stem cells to the bioactive ECM proteins present in bone tissue offers one obvious approach toward the induction of osteogenesis. Type I collagen, for example, activates osteogenic gene expression in MSCs simply through binding mediated by the integrin $\alpha_2\beta_1$ [46]. The attachment of MSCs to fibronectin ($\alpha_5\beta_1$) and vitronectin ($\alpha_v\beta_3$) through distinct integrin-based pathways have also demonstrated the capacity to modulate osteogenesis [75]. The incorporation of ECM proteins into biomaterial substrate design is therefore a popular approach.

Type 1 collagen gels and sponges offer purely natural 3-D substrates, while synthetic substrates are commonly coated with collagen or fibronectin to boost the attachment, proliferation, and/or osteogenic differentiation of stem cell populations. Proteoglycans also constitute an important biological component in bone ECM, having been linked to osteoinductive growth factor binding as well as proper collagen fibrillogenesis [78]. Biglycan and decorin, two small leucine-rich proteoglycans found in bone ECM, modulate osteoblast proliferation and collagen synthesis. Incorporation of glycosaminoglycans into biomaterial design also presents a promising strategy for binding osteogenic growth factors to biomaterial constructs in a manner that mimics that of native tissue, potentially reducing the required quantity and extending duration of efficacy.

As the full span of an ECM protein may not be necessary to mimic their bioactive properties, the addition of short peptide sequences to biomaterial substrates is also a popular field of study. Arginine–glycine–aspartic acid (RGD) tripeptide mediates integrin binding to fibronectin and continues to be a primary area of interest in the field. Biochemical modification of bioinert substrates such as alginate with cyclic RGD peptides confers cell-binding properties to the hydrophilic material, while peptide density is capable of modulating cell proliferation and osteogenic differentiation [132]. A large number of additional peptide sequences (e.g., YIGSR, GFOGER) are currently under investigation for their potential bioactive properties [119].

The use of biomimetic platforms engineered from the ECM present in native bone tissue represents an exciting advance over the presentation of individual protein and peptide-based approaches. Bone ECM contains a complex collection of physical and biochemical cues that direct stem cell fate in situ. Native bone ECM has been utilized as a substrate for MSC populations through the preparation of decellularized and/or demineralized bone tissue scaffolds [37,76,123]. Mechanical agitation combined with chemical treatments are used to drastically reduce the cellularity and mineral content of whole tissues, leaving behind an osteoconductive (and potentially osteoinductive) matrix which can be directly recellularized, or processed into sheets, powders, gels, etc. [22]. While decellularized bone tissue provides a scaffold that closely mimics the structure and composition of native bone ECM, it suffers from several drawbacks similar to that of allogeneic bone grafts including potential for immunogenicity, especially when harvested from xenogeneic sources.

The matrix deposited by cells in culture offers an alternative and potentially autologous means of capturing the cell-instructive properties associated with bone ECM. Cells cultured on biomaterial substrates deposit their own complex matrix that remains intact following decellularization. MSC-derived matrix coatings boost the osteogenic differentiation of freshly deposited undifferentiated MSCs, resulting in accelerated mineral deposition [23,102]. Matrices representative of different stages of MSC differentiation possess distinct osteogenic properties, indicating that the type of matrix present during bone regeneration may induce osteogenesis more effectively than ECM representative of mature healthy bone tissue [25,49]. Recent studies utilizing cell-derived matrix coatings have also explored their potential for binding osteoinductive growth factors, extending MSC multipotency in culture, and restoring the phenotype of MSCs from older donors to that representative of a younger state [5,17,62,77,122]. In addition, methods enabling the solubilization and transfer of matrix coatings from 2-D culture surfaces to more complex 3-D substrates have been established, potentially allowing for their deposition on an array of different stem cell scaffolding materials [26,27].

In addition to modulation of substrate composition, stiffness, and the addition of ECM components, the design of specific surface topographies represents another strategy for controlling stem cell fate. Microtextured implants possessing surface roughness profiles similar to that of fractured bone enhance bone formation in vivo when compared to smooth surfaces [42]. Advances in lithography techniques have enabled the design of pits, grooves, islands, etc., precisely positioned at the nanometer scale (Fig 14.2). These structures have modulated cell shape, focal adhesion formation, motility, gene expression, and differentiation [132]. For example, Oh et al. reported that the diameter of TiO_2 surface-coating nanotubes was a key regulator of MSC phenotype [100]. Cells cultured on 30 nm tubes demonstrated adhesion without differentiation, while cells grown on 70–100 nm tubes exhibited increased cytoskeletal stress and osteogenic differentiation. Nanoscale islands manufactured at specific heights (10–20 nm) also increased ALP activity and mineral deposition from MSCs compared to alternate island sizes and flat surfaces. Although the pathway responsible for the topographical induction of MSC osteogenesis is not fully understood, it likely relates to increased cytoskeletal stress at cellular attachment sites that activate integrin-related signaling cascades [86]. Cell-adhesive proteins such as fibronectin bind with greater efficiency to some nanoscale surface indentations, potentially resulting in higher ligand concentration, focal adhesion formation, and downstream activity of the extracellular signal-regulated kinase (ERK) pathway. Size and scale of nanotopographical structures also likely determine the architecture of focal adhesions at the site of cell binding, thereby modulating cell shape and downstream signaling.

14.3.4 Cell–Cell Interactions

Homotypic and heterotypic interactions play important roles in determining stem cell phenotype in vivo. In addition to soluble biological factors and extracellular matrix, adjacently positioned cells commonly contribute to the maintenance of cell stemness or the differentiation of daughter cells within the stem cell niche. The co-culture of distinct cell populations is therefore under study as a strategy to enhance the osteogenic differentiation of stem cells utilized for bone repair. These techniques can generally be divided into two approaches (Fig. 14.2): (1) direct cell–cell physical interaction; or (2) indirect interactions where phenotypic changes result from paracrine factor signaling. As cell–cell interactions play a vital role in embryonic and fetal development, developmental biology provides an important roadmap in analyzing cell–cell interactions. For example, mesodermal differentiation of PSCs can be enhanced by co-culture with hepatic cells or cell-conditioned media representative of the visceral endoderm to enhance natural mesodermal development [114]. This approach may potentially increase the yield of PSC-derived mesenchymal progenitors that can then be directed toward an osteogenic fate.

MSC culture depends heavily on cell–cell interactions, as the successful maintenance of MSC multipotency relies upon their timely passage prior to confluency. MSC co-culture with different cell populations can also contribute to changes in phenotype. The co-culture of MSCs with osteoblasts and osteocytes, two mature cell populations present in bone tissue, induces osteogenic differentiation [8]. The interaction between MSCs and various populations of endothelial cells (ECs) is also critical, as EC-MSC interactions are capable of both boosting MSC osteogenic differentiation and promoting the formation and stabilization of new vasculature [59,70]. Co-culture experiments demonstrated that ECs induce MSC proliferation and osteogenic differentiation as a function of the cell ratio [6]. Further analysis of the interaction between MSCs and ECs in 3-D spheroid culture uncovered BMP and Wnt–related pathways are involved in EC-induced MSC osteogenesis [112]. Micro- and nanoscale approaches toward the positioning and analysis of both the direct and indirect interactions between cell populations may provide a valuable tool in unlocking new pathways related to stem cell osteogenesis.

Since MSCs also secrete trophic factors that stimulate ECs, there is likely a complex symbiotic signaling relationship between these cell populations. In fact, MSCs can stabilize EC-derived vascular formations through assuming a perivascular phenotype (Fig. 14.1). This has led to a number of studies attempting to utilize EC-MSC co-cultures to accelerate the vascularization of implantable constructs designed for bone regeneration [20,43,128]. As hypoxia-induced cell death represents a major roadblock in the design of large bone constructs, the development of pre-vascularized implants that are quickly perfused following anastamosis with host vasculature presents a possible solution. Vascular infiltration in regenerating bone tissue is also tightly linked with osteoid deposition and new bone formation. MSCs and ECs co-cultured on materials ranging from bioceramic substrates to fibrin gels form longer lasting, more functionally robust vessels [70,130]. These results demonstrate the utility of MSCs as a therapeutic cell source, potentially able to function in multiple tissue forming capacities relevant to bone healing.

14.3.5 Genetic Modification of Stem Cells

The biological and physical cues associated with cells, growth factors, and matrix proteins offer biomimetic approaches toward manipulating stem cell fate. The genetic modification of stem cells, on the other hand, bypasses the signaling cascades associated with natural cell development by directly activating the expression of specific phenotype-determining genes. As MSCs have the potential to enhance bone regeneration through the secretion of trophic factors, as well as through direct differentiation into bone-depositing osteoblasts, strategies utilizing genetically modified MSCs have focused on both enhanced paracrine factor production and the expression of genes responsible for osteogenic differentiation (Fig. 14.2). BMP-2 modified MSCs, for example, have been extensively examined with regard to their bone forming potential. These cells display increased ALP activity and mineral deposition in culture, while also enhancing new bone formation in both ectopic and orthotopic sites following implantation in vivo [48]. Enhanced expression of osteogenic transcription factors such as Runx2 and osterix in MSCs also increases bone forming capacity, with dual expression of BMP-2 and Runx2 potentially having synergistic effects [129,136,144]. The delivery of angiogenic factors from genetically modified MSCs is also being explored as a method for enhancing vascular formation in vivo. Vascular endothelial growth factor-overexpressing MSCs accelerate neovascularization in animal models of tissue ischemia [35]. MSCs modified to upregulate additional proteins such as α_4 integrin and green fluorescent protein have also been studied as methods of enhancing MSC engraftment in bone tissue and for tracking MSC location following implantation, respectively [73,139]. The association of molecular imaging target gene expression with that of osteogenic genes activated through an identical promoter also offers an exciting approach for noninvasive real-time monitoring of changes in stem cell phenotype during osteogenic differentiation.

While each of the techniques discussed within this section offers the potential to direct cell stem fate, it is likely that a combination of these approaches will ultimately be necessary to design stem cell–based therapies that enhance bone regeneration. Osteoinductive soluble factor regimens applied to MSCs or PSCs in culture may be necessary to accumulate physiologically relevant quantities of bone forming cells. Substrate-mediated strategies such as nanotextured ECM-coated biodegradable scaffolding materials may be required to direct cell phenotype in vivo as new bone tissue forms. The engineering of cell-based approaches to bone tissue regeneration will therefore likely combine the spatial and temporal presentation of both biological and physical cues that determine cell fate.

14.4 Stem Cell–Based Approaches to Bone Formation

The regeneration of bone tissue with stem cells requires a multidisciplinary approach. While cell and developmental biologists provide expertise in cell behavior and describing pathways that regulate stem cell differentiation, additional contributions are necessary to engineer delivery systems that sustain cell viability and instruct cell phenotype at the defect site. Material scientists, biomedical engineers, and clinicians have teamed together in the development of various scaffolding materials, culture techniques, and in vivo models of bone formation to assess the efficacy of stem cell–based strategies for bone repair. The following section provides a brief review of these strategies to date.

14.4.1 Ex vivo Bone Formation

The initial analysis of a cell-based skeletal construct's capacity to regenerate bone tissue typically takes place in vitro. Stem cells cultured within biomaterial platforms are monitored for osteogenic gene expression, protein secretion, and calcium deposition in the presence or absence of soluble osteogenic cues. Analysis of cell viability, proliferation, and secretion of trophic factors are also important to consider as they may dramatically affect construct efficacy upon implantation in vivo. While native bone tissue possesses a highly pervasive vascular system to carry out oxygen and nutrient delivery, cell-seeded bone constructs must rely on high scaffold porosities and diffusion of soluble factors from the surrounding media. Under static culture conditions, cell viability is therefore limited to areas 100–200 μm from the scaffold surface, as the cells within that region consume oxygen and nutrients more rapidly than they can diffuse further into the scaffold [131]. This leads to cell death within the scaffold interior, limiting cell-based bone constructs to physiologically irrelevant sizes.

Bioreactor culture systems provide an effective approach to mitigate mass transport issues within cell-based bone constructs through the convective transport of factors within the culture environment. Bioreactors also allow for fine-tuned control over additional culture conditions such as oxygen tension, soluble factor concentration, and the mechanical stimulation of cell populations, thus facilitating ex vivo cultivation of bone tissue constructs in a more physiologically relevant environment [38]. Spinner flasks and rotating wall chambers represent two early model bioreactors studied for their capacity to improve convective flow. These designs rely on the use of magnetic stir bars and the rotation of the culture vessel exterior to keep the culture medium surrounding bone constructs in motion, respectively. While they have both demonstrated the capacity to improve MSC proliferation and osteogenic differentiation within a variety of biomaterial scaffolds, both strategies fail to eliminate transport issues within the scaffold interior [109]. In fact, these approaches may be detrimental to increasing nutrient transport in the construct core by enhancing cell survival and matrix deposition at the outer layer of the construct.

Direct perfusion bioreactors are garnering a great deal of attention in ex vivo bone tissue engineering. Culture medium is physically pumped through the porous scaffold structure at slow but steady velocities, delivering nutrients to and removing waste products from the cells attached within. Direct perfusion systems include those in which the cell-seeded construct is fixated to the reactor walls in such a manner that the culture medium must permeate the scaffold. Frohlich et al. demonstrated that perfusion culture improved the homogeneous distribution of MSCs within a decellularized bone matrix scaffold, while also enhancing osteogenic differentiation and mineralized ECM deposition [37]. Microcomputed tomography analysis of MSC-seeded scaffolds composed of polycaprolactone and Type I collagen revealed a dramatic increase in the mineralization rate of scaffolds under perfusion flow [104].

The mechanical forces applied to cells within bioreactor culture systems, along with improved transport conditions, also play a major role in enhancing construct maturity. Several studies have demonstrated that shear forces ranging from 0.1 to 1.6 dynes/cm^2 can enhance both matrix protein and mineral deposition from MSCs in culture [138]. The relative contributions of shear and enhanced transport on stem cell phenotype were isolated in an elegant set of experiments utilizing dextran to increase media viscosity, allowing for increases in shear while maintaining chemotransport conditions [83]. It was determined that increased shear stress (up to 15 Pa) accelerated MSC osteogenic differentiation and mineralized ECM deposition, while higher rates of mass transport (>3 mL/min) were detrimental to construct mineralization. Although bioreactors are highly effective tools in the study and preparation of cell-seeded tissue engineered bone constructs, the scaffolds cultured therein are generally subject to the same transport concerns present in static culture conditions following delivery in vivo. Novel strategies targeting prevascularization of engineered bone tissue prior to implantation are needed to ensure cell viability throughout constructs of physiologically relevant size.

14.4.2 Bone Formation in vivo

The success or failure of a stem cell–based skeletal regenerative therapy ultimately lies in its capacity to induce bone formation and/or integrate with host tissue in vivo. Experimentation within an in vitro setting typically provides cells with user-defined levels of oxygen, nutrients, and osteoinductive cues within a closed culture environment. However, cells implanted into bone defects in vivo are subjected to highly complex interactions with endogenous host cells, soluble factors, and ECM components under potentially hypoxic and nutrient-deficient conditions, which are virtually impossible to mimic in the laboratory. A number of animal models have been developed to analyze the ability of cell-based therapies to repair bone defects representative of many bone-related pathologies. Although researchers have used such models to perform numerous studies over the past decade to examine the ability of stem cells to generate bone in vivo, little consensus has been reached regarding optimal cell source, biomaterial substrate, or the benefit of ex vivo osteogenic preconditioning prior to implantation. In addition, debate remains as to how best to utilize stem cell populations to induce bone repair. While some researchers target osteoblastic differentiation and direct contribution to tissue mineralization, others point to the anti-inflammatory and proangiogenic nature of stem cells as being more effective in stimulating endogenous bone repair and regeneration.

Preliminary in vivo screening of cell-based regenerative bone therapies is commonly performed in ectopic tissue sites. For example, the murine subcutaneous model offers a minimally invasive approach to monitor construct mineralization and vascularization under a thin layer of skin tissue. The use of immunodeficient animals facilitates the study of human cells within a xenogeneic environment without immunorejection. Human PSCs induced down the osteogenic lineage have demonstrated the capacity to mineralize decellularized bone constructs ex vivo, with further bone maturation occurring over an 8 week period following subcutaneous implantation in immunodeficient mice [91]. Studies performed with murine PSCs have also revealed that subcutaneous bone formation can occur via the endochondral pathway, with the duration of PSC chondrogenic differentiation prior to implantation influencing the subsequent level of mineralization [57]. Bone marrow-derived and adipose-derived MSCs have also demonstrated the ability to mineralize constructs following subcutaneous implantation on polymer/ceramic scaffolds [9,137]. Osteogenic induction of cells prior to implantation, together with simultaneous delivery of osteogenic growth factors, further enhances this process. Tortelli et al. reported that while the subcutaneous implantation of osteoblastic cells results in donor cell bone formation, delivery of undifferentiated MSCs favored induction of angiogenesis followed by bone formation initiated by host cell populations [127]. In order to determine how different cell populations functionally direct tissue regeneration, several techniques have been utilized to track cells following implantation in vivo. These include the implantation of cells previously modified with genes overexpressing marker proteins (e.g., eGFP or luciferase), immunohistochemical staining for species-specific cell markers, and fluorescent in situ hybridization to discern differences in gender between transplanted and host cells [69,139].

Orthotopic models of bone repair offer a more physiologically relevant in vivo environment for testing stem cell–based therapies. Bone defects are created, filled in with the cells/materials of interest, and then monitored for tissue regeneration. For pathologies associated with larger defects, the resected bone tissue should be of a critical size, a defect that does not heal within the normal lifetime of the animal [110]. This ensures that natural healing processes do not compete with the implanted construct. Calvarial, mandibular, and rib defects in rodents and small mammals are a popular choice, as they provide non-weight bearing sites associated with simple fixation techniques. Osteogenically induced MSCs have enhanced bone formation in rodent calvarial defect models on a variety of scaffolding materials [94,140]. This process has been further accelerated using genetically modified MSCs that overexpress osteogenic signaling proteins such as BMPs [15,87]. Segmental defects of the femur and tibia are also commonly utilized as weight-bearing sites of bone repair. Unlike calvarial defects, long bone defects commonly require construct fixation to the surrounding bone tissue. MSCs seeded onto a composite scaffold of poly(lactide-co-glycolide) and ß-tricalcium phosphate repaired 15 mm critically sized radial defects in rabbits [41]. Canine, swine, and ovine models of segmental defect bone repair are also utilized, as their weight and skeletal properties match more closely with those of human bone [110].

Although PSCs have yet to be utilized in any human clinical trials associated with bone regeneration, autologous MSC populations have successful enhanced bone healing in numerous clinical studies. Quarto et al. implanted hydroxyapatite scaffolds seeded with culture-expanded autologous MSCs into 3 human patients with long bone segmental defects [108]. These constructs began integrating with host bone within 2 months, and a follow up study at 6 years reported no apparent complications with the new bone tissue [89]. MSCs seeded on ceramic scaffolding have since also been studied for their capacity to enhance bone repair in maxillary sinus augmentation and tumor resections [96,115]. Concentrated bone marrow aspirate has been used to aid bone regeneration associated with fracture nonunions and osteonecrosis [44,45]. While these studies demonstrate the potential for autologous MSC populations to enhance bone regeneration in various skeletal pathologies, future studies assessing allogeneic MSC-based therapies are necessary to determine the broad efficacy of MSCs in patients with impaired bone healing and reduced progenitor cell concentrations, as well as to determine the precise contribution to tissue repair.

There are several examples of successful bone formation initiated by stem cell populations in vitro and in vivo, yet the best strategy to utilize stem cells in bone regeneration remains unknown. Stem cell engraftment in vivo occurs at very low levels, with hypoxia and lack of speedy construct vascularization resulting in cell death. Recent co-culture studies using MSCs and endothelial cells implanted in vivo have demonstrated that subpopulations of MSCs can be utilized to both carry out mineralization and enhance vascularization within tissue engineered bone constructs [20,128]. These multicellular approaches, along with the use of the spatiotemporal physical and biological cues discussed in the previous section, will undoubtedly lead to more effective stem cell–based approaches to bone tissue repair.

14.5 Conclusions

Stem cell–based therapies targeting bone regeneration offer an exciting therapeutic approach to promote the repair and regeneration of bone defects, bypassing the need to harvest autologous or cadaver tissue. Strategies utilizing stem cells may also offer superior results to those patients with diminished bone healing capacity as a result of age or disease. Although stem cells have already demonstrated the capacity to enhance bone tissue formation in a variety of applications, additional research is necessary to determine the optimal cell source and delivery strategy for different skeletal pathologies. Novel approaches to inducing neovascularization and stem cell differentiation utilizing both biological (e.g., proteins and peptides) and physical (e.g., substrate rigidity and nanotopography) cues may ultimately allow for the design of stem cell microenvironments which mimic those found in vivo, directing and maintaining therapeutic stem cell phenotype post-implantation. In summary, future research combining expertise in developmental and stem cell biology, material science, physiology, biomedical engineering, and orthopedics will be necessary to maximize the utility of stem cells as a therapeutic tool in bone tissue repair.

References

1. Abrams M. B., Dominguez C., Pernold K., Reger R., Wiesenfeld-Hallin Z., Olson L., Prockop D. (2009). Multipotent mesenchymal stromal cells attenuate chronic inflammation and injury-induced sensitivity to mechanical stimuli in experimental spinal cord injury, *Restor. Neurol. Neurosci.*, **27**, 307–321.
2. Arpornmaeklong P., Brown S. E., Wang Z., Krebsbach P. H. (2009). Phenotypic characterization, osteoblastic differentiation, and bone regeneration capacity of human embryonic stem cell-derived mesenchymal stem cells, *Stem. Cells Dev.*, **18**, 955–968.
3. Arrington E. D., Smith W. J., Chambers H. G., Bucknell A. L., Davino N. A. (1996). Complications of iliac crest bone graft harvesting, *Clin. Orthop. Relat. Res.*, **329**, 300–309.

4. Augello A., De Bari C. (2010). The regulation of differentiation in mesenchymal stem cells, *Hum. Gene Ther.*, **21**, 1226–1238.
5. Bhat A., Boyadjiev S. A., Senders C. W., Leach J. K. (2011). Differential growth factor adsorption to calvarial osteoblast-secreted extracellular matrices instructs osteoblastic behavior, *PLoS One*, **6**, e25990.
6. Bidarra S. J., Barrias C. C., Barbosa M. A., Soares R., Amedee J., Granja P. L. (2011). Phenotypic and proliferative modulation of human mesenchymal stem cells via crosstalk with endothelial cells, *Stem Cell Res.*, **7**, 186–197.
7. Bilic J., Izpisua Belmonte J. C. (2012). Concise review: induced pluripotent stem cells versus embryonic stem cells: close enough or yet too far apart?, *Stem Cells* **30**, 33–41.
8. Birmingham E., Niebur G. L., McHugh P. E., Shaw G., Barry F. P., McNamara L. M. (2012). Osteogenic differentiation of mesenchymal stem cells is regulated by osteocyte and osteoblast cells in a simplified bone niche, *Eur. Cell Mater.*, **23**, 13–27.
9. Bodle J. C., Hanson A. D., Loboa E. G. (2011). Adipose-derived stem cells in functional bone tissue engineering: lessons from bone mechanobiology, *Tissue Eng. Part B Rev.*, **17**, 195–211.
10. Buttery L. D., Bourne S., Xynos J. D., Wood H., Hughes F. J., Hughes S. P., Episkopou V., Polak J. M. (2001). Differentiation of osteoblasts and in vitro bone formation from murine embryonic stem cells, *Tissue Eng.*, **7**, 89–99.
11. Caplan A. I. (2007). Adult mesenchymal stem cells for tissue engineering versus regenerative medicine, *J. Cell. Physiol.*, **213**, 341–347.
12. Caplan A. I., Dennis J. E. (2006). Mesenchymal stem cells as trophic mediators, *J. Cell. Biochem.*, **98**, 1076–1084.
13. Castano-Izquierdo H., Alvarez-Barreto J., van den Dolder J., Jansen J. A., Mikos A. G., Sikavitsas V. I. (2007). Pre-culture period of mesenchymal stem cells in osteogenic media influences their in vivo bone forming potential. *J. Biomed. Mater. Res. A*, **82**, 129–138.
14. Chamberlain G., Fox J., Ashton B., Middleton J. (2007). Concise review: mesenchymal stem cells: their phenotype, differentiation capacity, immunological features, and potential for homing, *Stem Cells*, **25**, 2739–2749.
15. Chang S. C., Chung H. Y., Tai C. L., Chen P. K., Lin T. M., Jeng L. B. (2010). Repair of large cranial defects by hBMP-2 expressing bone marrow stromal cells: comparison between alginate and collagen type I systems, *J. Biomed. Mater. Res. A*, **94**, 433–441.

16. Chatterjea A., Meijer G., van Blitterswijk C., de Boer J. (2010). Clinical application of human mesenchymal stromal cells for bone tissue engineering, *Stem Cells Int.*, 2010, 215625.
17. Chen X. D., Dusevich V., Feng J. Q., Manolagas S. C., Jilka R. L. (2007). Extracellular matrix made by bone marrow cells facilitates expansion of marrow-derived mesenchymal progenitor cells and prevents their differentiation into osteoblasts, *J. Bone Miner. Res.*, **22**, 1943–1956.
18. Choi K. M., Seo Y. K., Yoon H. H., Song K. Y., Kwon S. Y., Lee H. S., Park J. K. (2008). Effect of ascorbic acid on bone marrow-derived mesenchymal stem cell proliferation and differentiation, *J. Biosci. Bioeng.*, **105**, 586–594.
19. Colnot C. (2005). Cellular and molecular interactions regulating skeletogenesis, *J. Cell. Biochem.*, **95**, 688–697.
20. Correia C., Grayson W. L., Park M., Hutton D., Zhou B., Guo X. E., Niklason L., Sousa R. A., Reis R. L., Vunjak-Novakovic G. (2011). In vitro model of vascularized bone: synergizing vascular development and osteogenesis, *PLoS One*, **6**, e28352.
21. Covas D. T., Siufi J. L., Silva A. R., Orellana M. D. (2003). Isolation and culture of umbilical vein mesenchymal stem cells, *Braz. J. Med. Biol. Res.*, **36**, 1179–1183.
22. Crapo P. M., Gilbert T. W., Badylak S. F. (2011). An overview of tissue and whole organ decellularization processes, *Biomaterials*, **32**, 3233–3243.
23. Datta N., Holtorf H. L., Sikavitsas V. I., Jansen J. A., Mikos A. G. (2005). Effect of bone extracellular matrix synthesized in vitro on the osteoblastic differentiation of marrow stromal cells, *Biomaterials*, **26**, 971–977.
24. Davis H. E., Miller S. L., Case E. M., Leach J. K. (2011). Supplementation of fibrin gels with sodium chloride enhances physical properties and ensuing osteogenic response. *Acta Biomater.*, **7**, 691–699.
25. Decaris M. L., Leach J. K. (2011). Design of experiments approach to engineer cell-secreted matrices for directing osteogenic differentiation, *Ann. Biomed. Eng.*, **39**, 1174–1785.
26. Decaris M. L., Mojadedi A., Bhat A., Leach J. K. (2012). Transferable cell-secreted extracellular matrices enhance osteogenic differentiation, *Acta Biomater.*, **8**, 744–752.
27. Decaris M. L., Binder B. Y., Soicher M. A., Bhat A., Leach J. K. (2012). Cell-derived matrix coatings for polymeric scaffolds, *Tissue Eng. Part A*, 18(19–20): 2148–2157

28. Dimitriou R., Mataliotakis G. I., Angoules A. G., Kanakaris N. K., Giannoudis P. V. (2011). Complications following autologous bone graft harvesting from the iliac crest and using the RIA: a systematic review, *Injury*, **42**, S3–S15.
29. Discher D. E., Mooney D. J., Zandstra P. W. (2009). Growth factors, matrices, and forces combine and control stem cells, *Science*, **324**, 1673–1637.
30. Dominici M., Le Blanc K., Mueller I., Slaper-Cortenbach I., Marini F., Krause D., Deans R., Keating A., Prockop D., Horwitz E. (2006). Minimal criteria for defining multipotent mesenchymal stromal cells. The International Society for Cellular Therapy position statement, *Cytotherapy*, **8**, 315–317.
31. Engler A. J., Sen S., Sweeney H. L., Discher D. E. (2006). Matrix elasticity directs stem cell lineage specification, *Cell*, **126**, 677–689.
32. Evans M. J., Kaufman M. H. (1981). Establishment in culture of pluripotential cells from mouse embryos, *Nature*, **292**, 154–156.
33. Fan M., Chen W., Liu W., Du G. Q., Jiang S. L., Tian W. C., Sun L., Li R. K., Tian H. (2010). The effect of age on the efficacy of human mesenchymal stem cell transplantation after a myocardial infarction, *Rejuvenation Res.*, **13**, 429–438.
34. Farrell E., Both S. K., Odorfer K. I., Koevoet W., Kops N., O'Brien F. J., Baatenburg de Jong R. J., Verhaar J. A., Cuijpers V., Jansen J., Erben R. G., van Osch G. J. (2011). In vivo generation of bone via endochondral ossification by in vitro chondrogenic priming of adult human and rat mesenchymal stem cells, *BMC Musculoskelet. Disord.*, **12**, 31–39.
35. Fierro F. A., Kalomoiris S., Sondergaard C. S., Nolta J. A. (2011). Effects on proliferation and differentiation of multipotent bone marrow stromal cells engineered to express growth factors for combined cell and gene therapy, *Stem Cells*, **29**, 1727–1737.
36. Friedenstein A. J., Petrakova K. V., Kurolesova A. I., Frolova G. P. (1968). Heterotopic of bone marrow. Analysis of precursor cells for osteogenic and hematopoietic tissues., *Transplantation*, **6**, 230–247.
37. Frohlich M., Grayson W. L., Marolt D., Gimble J. M., Kregar-Velikonja N., Vunjak-Novakovic G. (2010). Bone grafts engineered from human adipose-derived stem cells in perfusion bioreactor culture, *Tissue Eng. Part A*, **16**, 179–189.
38. Grayson W. L., Bhumiratana S., Cannizzaro C., Vunjak-Novakovic G. (2011). Bioreactor cultivation of functional bone grafts, *Methods Mol. Biol.*, **698**, 231–241.

39. Grinnemo K. H., Sylven C., Hovatta O., Dellgren G., Corbascio M. (2008). Immunogenicity of human embryonic stem cells, *Cell Tissue Res.*, **331**, 67–78.

40. Hamidouche Z., Fromigue O., Nuber U., Vaudin P., Pages J. C., Ebert R., Jakob F., Miraoui H., Marie P. J. (2010). Autocrine fibroblast growth factor 18 mediates dexamethasone-induced osteogenic differentiation of murine mesenchymal stem cells, *J. Cell. Physiol.*, **224**, 509–515.

41. Hao W., Pang L., Jiang M., Lv R., Xiong Z., Hu Y. Y. (2010). Skeletal repair in rabbits using a novel biomimetic composite based on adipose-derived stem cells encapsulated in collagen I gel with PLGA-beta-TCP scaffold, *J. Orthop. Res.*, **28**, 252–257.

42. Harvey E. J., Henderson J. E., Vengallatore S. T. (2010). Nanotechnology and bone healing, *J. Orthop. Trauma*, **24**, S25–S30.

43. He J., Decaris M., Leach J. K. (2012) Bioceramic-mediated trophic factor secretion by mesenchymal stem cells enhances in vitro endothelial cell persistence and in vivo angiogenesis, *Tissue Eng. Part A*, 18(13–14): 1520–1528.

44. Hernigou P., Poignard A., Manicom O., Mathieu G., Rouard H. (2005). The use of percutaneous autologous bone marrow transplantation in nonunion and avascular necrosis of bone, *J. Bone Joint Surg. Br.*, **87**, 896–902.

45. Hernigou P., Poignard A., Zilber S., Rouard H. (2009). Cell therapy of hip osteonecrosis with autologous bone marrow grafting, *Indian J. Orthop.*, **43**, 40–45.

46. Hidalgo-Bastida L. A., Cartmell S. H. (2010). Mesenchymal stem cells, osteoblasts and extracellular matrix proteins: enhancing cell adhesion and differentiation for bone tissue engineering, *Tissue Eng. Part B Rev.*, **16**, 405–412.

47. Hoch A. I., Binder B. Y., Genetos D. C., Leach J. K. (2012). Differentiation-dependent secretion of proangiogenic factors by mesenchymal stem cells, *PLoS One*, **7**, e35579.

48. Hong D., Chen H. X., Ge R., Li J. C. (2010). Genetically engineered mesenchymal stem cells: The ongoing research for bone tissue engineering, *Anat. Rec.* (Hoboken), **293**, 531–537.

49. Hoshiba T., Kawazoe N., Tateishi T., Chen G. (2009). Development of stepwise osteogenesis-mimicking matrices for the regulation of mesenchymal stem cell functions, *J. Biol. Chem.*, **284**, 31164–31173.

50. Huebsch N., Arany P. R., Mao A. S., Shvartsman D., Ali O. A., Bencherif S. A., Rivera-Feliciano J., Mooney D. J. (2010). Harnessing traction-mediated manipulation of the cell/matrix interface to control stem-cell fate, *Nat. Mater.*, **9**, 518–526.

51. Hwang N. S., Varghese S., Lee H. J., Zhang Z., Ye Z., Bae J., Cheng L., Elisseeff J. (2008). In vivo commitment and functional tissue regeneration using human embryonic stem cell-derived mesenchymal cells, *Proc. Natl. Acad. Sci. USA*, **105**, 20641–20646.
52. Hwang Y. S., Randle W. L., Bielby R. C., Polak J. M., Mantalaris A. (2006). Enhanced derivation of osteogenic cells from murine embryonic stem cells after treatment with HepG2-conditioned medium and modulation of the embryoid body formation period: application to skeletal tissue engineering, *Tissue Eng.*, **12**, 1381–1392.
53. Illich D. J., Demir N., Stojkovic M., Scheer M., Rothamel D., Neugebauer J., Hescheler J., Zoller J. E. (2011). Concise review: induced pluripotent stem cells and lineage reprogramming: prospects for bone regeneration, *Stem Cells*, **29**, 555–563.
54. Jankowski R. J., Deasy B. M., Huard J. (2002). Muscle-derived stem cells, *Gene Ther.*, **9**, 642–667.
55. Jones E., Yang X. (2011). Mesenchymal stem cells and bone regeneration: current status, *Injury*, **42**, 562–568.
56. Jorgensen C., Gordeladze J., Noel D. (2004). Tissue engineering through autologous mesenchymal stem cells, *Curr. Opin. Biotechnol.*, **15**, 406–410.
57. Jukes J. M., Both S. K., Leusink A., Sterk L. M., van Blitterswijk C. A., de Boer J. (2008). Endochondral bone tissue engineering using embryonic stem cells, *Proc. Natl. Acad. Sci. USA*, **105**, 6840–6845.
58. Jukes J. M., van Blitterswijk C. A., de Boer J. (2010). Skeletal tissue engineering using embryonic stem cells, *J. Tissue Eng. Regen. Med.*, **4**, 165–180.
59. Kaigler D., Krebsbach P. H., West E. R., Horger K., Huang Y. C., Mooney D. J. (2005). Endothelial cell modulation of bone marrow stromal cell osteogenic potential, *FASEB J.*, **19**, 665–667.
60. Kaigler D., Krebsbach P. H., Wang Z., West E. R., Horger K., Mooney D. J. (2006). Transplanted endothelial cells enhance orthotopic bone regeneration, *J. Dent. Res.*, **85**, 633–637.
61. Kang Q., Song W. X., Luo Q., Tang N., Luo J., Luo X., Chen J., Bi Y., He B. C., Park J. K., Jiang W., Tang Y., Huang J., Su Y., Zhu G. H., He Y., Yin H., Hu Z., Wang Y., Chen L., Zuo G. W., Pan X., Shen J., Vokes T., Reid R. R., Haydon R. C., Luu H. H., He T. C. (2009). A comprehensive analysis of the dual roles of BMPs in regulating adipogenic and osteogenic differentiation of mesenchymal progenitor cells, *Stem Cells Dev.*, **18**, 545–559.

62. Kang Y., Kim S., Khademhosseini A., Yang Y. (2011). Creation of bony microenvironment with CaP and cell-derived ECM to enhance human bone-marrow MSC behavior and delivery of BMP-2, *Biomaterials*, **32**, 6119–6130.

63. Karp J. M., Ferreira L. S., Khademhosseini A., Kwon A. H., Yeh J., Langer R. S. (2006). Cultivation of human embryonic stem cells without the embryoid body step enhances osteogenesis in vitro, *Stem Cells*, **24**, 835–843.

64. Kasten P., Beyen I., Niemeyer P., Luginbuhl R., Bohner M., Richter W. (2008). Porosity and pore size of beta-tricalcium phosphate scaffold can influence protein production and osteogenic differentiation of human mesenchymal stem cells: an in vitro and in vivo study, *Acta Biomater.*, **4**, 1904–1915.

65. Kawaguchi J., Mee P. J., Smith A. G. (2005). Osteogenic and chondrogenic differentiation of embryonic stem cells in response to specific growth factors, *Bone*, **36**, 758–769.

66. Khaled E. G., Saleh M., Hindocha S., Griffin M., Khan W. S. (2011). Tissue engineering for bone production- stem cells, gene therapy and scaffolds, *Open Orthop. J.*, **5**, 289–295.

67. Khan Y., Yaszemski M. J., Mikos A. G., Laurencin C. T. (2008). Tissue engineering of bone: material and matrix considerations, *J. Bone Joint Surg. Am.*, **90**, 36–42.

68. Khatiwala C. B., Kim P. D., Peyton S. R., Putnam A. J. (2009). ECM compliance regulates osteogenesis by influencing MAPK signaling downstream of RhoA and ROCK, *J. Bone Miner. Res.*, **24**, 886–898.

69. Kim S., Kim S. S., Lee S. H., Eun Ahn S., Gwak S. J., Song J. H., Kim B. S., Chung H. M. (2008). In vivo bone formation from human embryonic stem cell-derived osteogenic cells in poly(D,L-lactic-*co*-glycolic acid)/hydroxyapatite composite scaffolds, *Biomaterials*, **29**, 1043–1053.

70. Kniazeva E., Kachgal S., Putnam A. J. (2011). Effects of extracellular matrix density and mesenchymal stem cells on neovascularization in vivo, *Tissue Eng. Part A*, **17**, 905–914.

71. Kolambkar Y. M., Peister A., Ekaputra A. K., Hutmacher D. W., Guldberg R. E. (2010). Colonization and osteogenic differentiation of different stem cell sources on electrospun nanofiber meshes, *Tissue Eng. Part A*, **16**, 3219–3230.

72. Koob S., Torio-Padron N., Stark G. B., Hannig C., Stankovic Z., Finkenzeller G. (2011). Bone formation and neovascularization mediated by mesenchymal stem cells and endothelial cells in critical-sized calvarial defects, *Tissue Eng. Part A*, **17**, 311–321.

73. Kumar S., Ponnazhagan S. (2007). Bone homing of mesenchymal stem cells by ectopic alpha 4 integrin expression, *FASEB J.*, **21**, 3917–3927.
74. Kumar S., Wan C., Ramaswamy G., Clemens T. L., Ponnazhagan S. (2010). Mesenchymal stem cells expressing osteogenic and angiogenic factors synergistically enhance bone formation in a mouse model of segmental bone defect, *Mol. Ther.*, **18**, 1026–1034.
75. Kundu A. K., Khatiwala C. B., Putnam A. J. (2009). Extracellular matrix remodeling, integrin expression, and downstream signaling pathways influence the osteogenic differentiation of mesenchymal stem cells on poly(lactide-*co*-glycolide) substrates, *Tissue Eng. Part A*, **15**, 273–283.
76. Kurkalli B. G., Gurevitch O., Sosnik A., Cohn D., Slavin S. (2010). Repair of bone defect using bone marrow cells and demineralized bone matrix supplemented with polymeric materials, *Curr. Stem Cell Res. Ther.*, **5**, 49–56.
77. Lai Y., Sun Y., Skinner C. M., Son E. L., Lu Z., Tuan R. S., Jilka R. L., Ling J., Chen X. D. (2010). Reconstitution of marrow-derived extracellular matrix ex vivo: a robust culture system for expanding large-scale highly functional human mesenchymal stem cells, *Stem Cells Dev.*, **19**, 1095–1107.
78. Lamoureux F., Baud'huin M., Duplomb L., Heymann D., Redini F. (2007). Proteoglycans: key partners in bone cell biology, *Bioessays*, **29**, 758–771.
79. Langer R., Vacanti J. P. (1993). Tissue engineering, *Science*, **260**, 920–926.
80. Laurencin C. T., Magge A., Khan Y., (2012). Bone graft substitute materials. Medscape Reference, Article 1230616.
81. Leach J. K., Mooney D. J. (2004). Bone engineering by controlled delivery of osteoinductive molecules and cells, *Expert Opin. Biol. Ther.*, **4**, 1015–1027.
82. Lee C. C., Christensen J. E., Yoder M. C., Tarantal A. F. (2010). Clonal analysis and hierarchy of human bone marrow mesenchymal stem and progenitor cells, *Exp. Hematol.*, **38**, 46–54.
83. Li D., Tang T., Lu J., Dai K. (2009). Effects of flow shear stress and mass transport on the construction of a large-scale tissue-engineered bone in a perfusion bioreactor, *Tissue Eng. Part A*, **15**, 2773–2783.
84. Li F., Bronson S., Niyibizi C. (2010). Derivation of murine induced pluripotent stem cells (iPS) and assessment of their differentiation toward osteogenic lineage, *J. Cell. Biochem.*, **109**, 643–652.

85. Lieberman J. R., Daluiski A., Einhorn T. A. (2002). The role of growth factors in the repair of bone. Biology and clinical applications, *J. Bone Joint Surg. Am.*, **84-A**, 1032–1044.
86. Lim J. Y., Loiselle A. E., Lee J. S., Zhang Y., Salvi J. D., Donahue H. J. (2011). Optimizing the osteogenic potential of adult stem cells for skeletal regeneration, *J. Orthop. Res.*, **29**, 1627–1633.
87. Lin L., Shen Q., Wei X., Hou Y., Xue T., Fu X., Duan X., Yu C. (2009). Comparison of osteogenic potentials of BMP4 transduced stem cells from autologous bone marrow and fat tissue in a rabbit model of calvarial defects, *Calcif. Tissue Int.*, **85**, 55–65.
88. Lutolf M. P., Gilbert P. M., Blau H. M. (2009). Designing materials to direct stem-cell fate, *Nature*, **462**, 433–441.
89. Marcacci M., Kon E., Moukhachev V., Lavroukov A., Kutepov S., Quarto R., Mastrogiacomo M., Cancedda R. (2007). Stem cells associated with macroporous bioceramics for long bone repair: 6- to 7-year outcome of a pilot clinical study, *Tissue Eng.*, **13**, 947–955.
90. Marolt D., Knezevic M., Novakovic G. V. (2010). Bone tissue engineering with human stem cells, *Stem Cell Res. Ther.*, **1**, 10–19.
91. Marolt D., Campos I. M., Bhumiratana S., Koren A., Petridis P., Zhang G., Spitalnik P. F., Grayson W. L., Vunjak-Novakovic G. (2012). Engineering bone tissue from human embryonic stem cells, *Proc. Natl. Acad. Sci. USA*, **109**, 8705–8709.
92. McBeath R., Pirone D. M., Nelson C. M., Bhadriraju K., Chen C. S. (2004). Cell shape, cytoskeletal tension, and RhoA regulate stem cell lineage commitment, *Dev. Cell.*, **6**, 483–495.
93. McCullen S. D., Zhu Y., Bernacki S. H., Narayan R. J., Pourdeyhimi B., Gorga R. E., Loboa E. G. (2009). Electrospun composite poly (L-lactic acid)/tricalcium phosphate scaffolds induce proliferation and osteogenic differentiation of human adipose-derived stem cells, *Biomed. Mater.*, **4**, 035002.
94. Meinel L., Fajardo R., Hofmann S., Langer R., Chen J., Snyder B., Vunjak-Novakovic G., Kaplan D. (2005). Silk implants for the healing of critical size bone defects, *Bone*, **37**, 688–698.
95. Moore K. A., Lemischka I. R. (2006). Stem cells and their niches, *Science*, **311**, 1880–1885.
96. Morishita T., Honoki K., Ohgushi H., Kotobuki N., Matsushima A., Takakura Y. (2006). Tissue engineering approach to the treatment of bone tumors: three cases of cultured bone grafts derived from patients' mesenchymal stem cells, *Artif Organs*, **30**, 115–118.

97. Nakashima K., Zhou X., Kunkel G., Zhang Z., Deng J. M., Behringer R. R., de Crombrugghe B. (2002). The novel zinc finger-containing transcription factor osterix is required for osteoblast differentiation and bone formation, *Cell*, **108**, 17–29.

98. Ngiam M., Nguyen L. T., Liao S., Chan C. K., Ramakrishna S. (2011). Biomimetic nanostructured materials: potential regulators for osteogenesis?, *Ann. Acad. Med. Singapore*, **40**, 213–210.

99. O'Keefe R. J., Mao J. (2011). Bone tissue engineering and regeneration: from discovery to the clinic—an overview, *Tissue Eng. Part B Rev.*, **17**, 389–392.

100. Oh S., Brammer K. S., Li Y. S., Teng D., Engler A. J., Chien S., Jin S. (2009). Stem cell fate dictated solely by altered nanotube dimension. *Proc. Natl. Acad. Sci. USA*, **106**, 2130–2135.

101. Mafi P., Hindocha S., Mafi R., Griffin M., Khan W. S. (2011). Adult mesenchymal stem cells and cell surface characterization: a systematic review of the literature, *Open Orthop. J.*, **5**, 253–260.

102. Pham Q. P., Kasper F. K., Scott Baggett L., Raphael R. M., Jansen J. A., Mikos A. G. (2008). The influence of an in vitro generated bone-like extracellular matrix on osteoblastic gene expression of marrow stromal cells, *Biomaterials*, **29**, 2729–2739.

103. Pittenger M. F., Mackay A. M., Beck S. C., Jaiswal R. K., Douglas R., Mosca J. D., Moorman M. A., Simonetti D. W., Craig S., Marshak D. R. (1999). Multilineage potential of adult human mesenchymal stem cells, *Science*, **284**, 143–147.

104. Porter B. D., Lin A. S., Peister A., Hutmacher D., Guldberg R. E. (2007). Noninvasive image analysis of 3D construct mineralization in a perfusion bioreactor, *Biomaterials*, **28**, 2525–2533.

105. Porter J. R., Ruckh T. T., Popat K. C. (2009). Bone tissue engineering: a review in bone biomimetics and drug delivery strategies, *Biotechnol. Prog.*, **25**, 1539–1560.

106. Prockop D. J., Kota D. J., Bazhanov N., Reger R. L. Evolving paradigms for repair of tissues by adult stem/progenitor cells (MSCs), *J. Cell. Mol. Med.*, **14**, 2190–2199.

107. Prockop D. J., Oh J. Y. (2012). Mesenchymal stem/stromal cells (MSCs): role as guardians of inflammation, *Mol. Ther.*, **20**, 14–20.

108. Quarto R., Mastrogiacomo M., Cancedda R., Kutepov S. M., Mukhachev V., Lavroukov A., Kon E., Marcacci M. (2001). Repair of large bone defects with the use of autologous bone marrow stromal cells, *N. Engl. J. Med.*, **344**, 385–386.

109. Rauh J., Milan F., Gunther K. P., Stiehler M. (2011). Bioreactor systems for bone tissue engineering, *Tissue Eng. Part B Rev.*, **17**, 263–280.
110. Reichert J. C., Saifzadeh S., Wullschleger M. E., Epari D. R., Schutz M. A., Duda G. N., Schell H., van Griensven M., Redl H., Hutmacher D. W. (2009). The challenge of establishing preclinical models for segmental bone defect research, *Biomaterials*, **30**, 2149–2163.
111. Russell K. C., Lacey M. R., Gilliam J. K., Tucker H. A., Phinney D. G., O'Connor K. C. (2011). Clonal analysis of the proliferation potential of human bone marrow mesenchymal stem cells as a function of potency. *Biotechnol. Bioeng.*, **108**, 2716–2726.
112. Saleh F. A., Whyte M., Genever P. G. (2011). Effects of endothelial cells on human mesenchymal stem cell activity in a three-dimensional in vitro model, *Eur. Cell. Mater.*, **22**, 242–257.
113. Sato K., Ozaki K., Mori M., Muroi K., Ozawa K. (2010). Mesenchymal stromal cells for graft-versus-host disease: basic aspects and clinical outcomes, *J. Clin. Exp. Hematop.*, **50**, 79–89.
114. Seong J. M., Kim B. C., Park J. H., Kwon I. K., Mantalaris A., Hwang Y. S. (2010). Stem cells in bone tissue engineering, *Biomed. Mater.*, **5**, 062001.
115. Shayesteh Y. S., Khojasteh A., Soleimani M., Alikhasi M., Khoshzaban A., Ahmadbeigi N. (2008). Sinus augmentation using human mesenchymal stem cells loaded into a beta-tricalcium phosphate/hydroxyapatite scaffold, *Oral Surg. Oral Med. Oral Pathol. Oral Radiol. Endod.*, **106**, 203–209.
116. Simmons C. A., Alsberg E., Hsiong S., Kim W. J., Mooney D. J. (2004). Dual growth factor delivery and controlled scaffold degradation enhance in vivo bone formation by transplanted bone marrow stromal cells, *Bone*, **35**, 562–569.
117. Smith L. A., Liu X., Hu J., Ma P. X. (2009). The influence of three-dimensional nanofibrous scaffolds on the osteogenic differentiation of embryonic stem cells, *Biomaterials*, **30**, 2516–2522.
118. Song L., Tuan R. S. (2004). Transdifferentiation potential of human mesenchymal stem cells derived from bone marrow. *FASEB J.*, **18**, 980–982.
119. Sreejalekshmi K. G., Nair P. D. (2011). Biomimeticity in tissue engineering scaffolds through synthetic peptide modifications-altering chemistry for enhanced biological response, *J. Biomed. Mater. Res. A*, **96**, 477–491.

120. Stadtfeld M., Nagaya M., Utikal J., Weir G., Hochedlinger K. (2008). Induced pluripotent stem cells generated without viral integration, *Science*, **322**, 945–949.
121. Stolzing A., Jones E., McGonagle D., Scutt A. (2008). Age-related changes in human bone marrow-derived mesenchymal stem cells: consequences for cell therapies, *Mech. Ageing Dev.*, **129**, 163–173.
122. Sun Y., Li W., Lu Z., Chen R., Ling J., Ran Q., Jilka R. L., Chen X. D. (2011). Rescuing replication and osteogenesis of aged mesenchymal stem cells by exposure to a young extracellular matrix, *FASEB J.*, **25**, 1474–1485.
123. Supronowicz P., Gill E., Trujillo A., Thula T., Zhukauskas R., Ramos T., Cobb R. R. (2011). Human adipose-derived side population stem cells cultured on demineralized bone matrix for bone tissue engineering, *Tissue Eng. Part A*, **17**, 789–798.
124. Takahashi K., Yamanaka S. (2006). Induction of pluripotent stem cells from mouse embryonic and adult fibroblast cultures by defined factors, *Cell*, **126**, 663–676.
125. Tare R. S., Kanczler J., Aarvold A., Jones A. M., Dunlop D. G., Oreffo R. O. (2010). Skeletal stem cells and bone regeneration: translational strategies from bench to clinic, *Proc. Inst. Mech. Eng. H.*, **224**, 1455–1470.
126. Thomson J. A., Itskovitz-Eldor J., Shapiro S. S., Waknitz M. A., Swiergiel J. J., Marshall V. S., Jones J. M. (1998). Embryonic stem cell lines derived from human blastocysts, *Science*, **282**, 1145–1147.
127. Tortelli F., Tasso R., Loiacono F., Cancedda R. (2010). The development of tissue-engineered bone of different origin through endochondral and intramembranous ossification following the implantation of mesenchymal stem cells and osteoblasts in a murine model, *Biomaterials*, **31**, 242–29.
128. Tsigkou O., Pomerantseva I., Spencer J. A., Redondo P. A., Hart A. R., O'Doherty E., Lin Y., Friedrich C. C., Daheron L., Lin C. P., Sundback C. A., Vacanti J. P., Neville C. (2010). Engineered vascularized bone grafts, *Proc. Natl. Acad. Sci. USA*, **107**, 3311–3316.
129. Tu Q., Valverde P., Li S., Zhang J., Yang P., Chen J. (2007). Osterix overexpression in mesenchymal stem cells stimulates healing of critical-sized defects in murine calvarial bone, *Tissue Eng.*, **13**, 2431–2440.

130. Unger R. E., Sartoris A., Peters K., Motta A., Migliaresi C., Kunkel M., Bulnheim U., Rychly J., Kirkpatrick C. J. (2007). Tissue-like self-assembly in cocultures of endothelial cells and osteoblasts and the formation of microcapillary-like structures on three-dimensional porous biomaterials, *Biomaterials*, **28**, 3965–3976.

131. Volkmer E., Drosse I., Otto S., Stangelmayer A., Stengele M., Kallukalam B. C., Mutschler W., Schieker M. (2008). Hypoxia in static and dynamic 3D culture systems for tissue engineering of bone, *Tissue Eng. Part A*, **14**, 1331–1340.

132. von der Mark K., Park J., Bauer S., Schmuki P. (2010). Nanoscale engineering of biomimetic surfaces: cues from the extracellular matrix, *Cell Tissue Res.*, **339**, 131–153.

133. Warren L., Manos P. D., Ahfeldt T., Loh Y. H., Li H., Lau F., Ebina W., Mandal P. K., Smith Z. D., Meissner A., Daley G. Q., Brack A. S., Collins J. J., Cowan C., Schlaeger T. M., Rossi D. J. (2010). Highly efficient reprogramming to pluripotency and directed differentiation of human cells with synthetic modified mRNA, *Cell Stem Cell*, **7**, 618–630.

134. Weissman I. L. (2000). Stem cells: units of development, units of regeneration, and units in evolution, *Cell*, **100**, 157–168.

135. Xin Y., Wang Y. M., Zhang H., Li J., Wang W., Wei Y. J., Hu S. S. (2010). Aging adversely impacts biological properties of human bone marrow-derived mesenchymal stem cells: implications for tissue engineering heart valve construction, *Artif. Organs*, **34**, 215–222.

136. Yang S., Wei D., Wang D., Phimphilai M., Krebsbach P. H., Franceschi R. T. (2003). In vitro and in vivo synergistic interactions between the Runx2/Cbfa1 transcription factor and bone morphogenetic protein-2 in stimulating osteoblast differentiation, *J. Bone Miner. Res.*, **18**, 705–715.

137. Ye X., Yin X., Yang D., Tan J., Liu G. (2012). Ectopic bone regeneration by human bone marrow mononucleated cells, undifferentiated and osteogenically differentiated bone marrow mesenchymal stem cells in beta-tricalcium phosphate scaffolds, *Tissue Eng. Part C Methods*, **18**(7): 545–556.

138. Yeatts A. B., Fisher J. P. (2011). Bone tissue engineering bioreactors: dynamic culture and the influence of shear stress, *Bone*, **48**, 171–181.

139. Yin D., Wang Z., Gao Q., Sundaresan R., Parrish C., Yang Q., Krebsbach P. H., Lichtler A. C., Rowe D. W., Hock J., Liu P. (2009). Determination of the fate and contribution of ex vivo expanded human bone marrow stem and progenitor cells for bone formation by 2.3ColGFP, *Mol. Ther.*, **17**, 1967–1978.

140. Yoon E., Dhar S., Chun D. E., Gharibjanian N. A., Evans G. R. (2007). In vivo osteogenic potential of human adipose-derived stem cells/poly(lactide-*co*-glycolic) acid constructs for bone regeneration in a rat critical-sized calvarial defect model, *Tissue Eng.*, **13**, 619–627.

141. Yu J., Vodyanik M. A., Smuga-Otto K., Antosiewicz-Bourget J., Frane J. L., Tian S., Nie J., Jonsdottir G. A., Ruotti V., Stewart R., Slukvin, I. I., Thomson J. A. (2007). Induced pluripotent stem cell lines derived from human somatic cells, *Science*, **318**, 1917–1920.

142. Zhang Z. Y., Teoh S. H., Hui J. H., Fisk N. M., Choolani M., Chan J. K. (2012). The potential of human fetal mesenchymal stem cells for off-the-shelf bone tissue engineering application, *Biomaterials*, **33**, 2656–2672.

143. Zhao T., Zhang Z. N., Rong Z., Xu Y. (2011). Immunogenicity of induced pluripotent stem cells, *Nature*, **474**, 212–215.

144. Zhao Z., Zhao M., Xiao G., Franceschi R. T. (2005). Gene transfer of the Runx2 transcription factor enhances osteogenic activity of bone marrow stromal cells in vitro and in vivo, *Mol. Ther.*, **12**, 247–253.

145. Zuk P., Chou Y. F., Mussano F., Benhaim P., Wu B. M. (2011). Adipose-derived stem cells and BMP2: part 2. BMP2 may not influence the osteogenic fate of human adipose-derived stem cells, *Connect. Tissue Res.*, **52**, 119–132.

146. Zuk P. A., Zhu M., Mizuno H., Huang J., Futrell J. W., Katz A. J., Benhaim P., Lorenz H. P., Hedrick M. H. (2001). Multilineage cells from human adipose tissue: implications for cell-based therapies, *Tissue Eng.*, **7**, 211–228.

Chapter 15

Notch Signaling Biomaterials and Tissue Regeneration

Thanaphum Osathanon,[a] Prasit Pavasant,[a] and Cecilia Giachelli[b]

[a]*Department of Anatomy, Faculty of Dentistry,*
Chulalongkorn University, Bangkok 10330, Thailand
[b]*Department of Bioengineering, School of Medicine,*
University of Washington, Foege N330L, 3720 15th Ave NE,
Seattle, WA 98195, USA

ceci@u.washington.edu

Notch signaling is involved in different functions of both embryonic and mesenchymal stem cells, including cell fate determination and differentiation. The utilization of bioactive materials mimicking Notch signaling could lead to the development of a novel approach for regenerative treatment. The aim of this chapter is to review the role of Notch signaling in stem cell behaviors and bioengineering approaches to induce Notch signaling from biomaterial surfaces. Finally, the promising utilization of Notch ligand–modified surfaces in regenerative medicine is reviewed.

15.1 Introduction

Currently, stem cell research is of great interest to the scientific community due to potential therapeutic applications for a wide array of clinical entities, including dental disease and craniofacial

---

Tissue and Organ Regeneration: Advances in Micro- and Nanotechnology
Edited by Lijie Grace Zhang, Ali Khademhosseini, and Thomas J. Webster
Copyright © 2014 Pan Stanford Publishing Pte. Ltd.
ISBN 978-981-4411-67-7 (Hardcover), 978-981-4411-68-4 (eBook)
www.panstanford.com

regeneration. Stem cells are primitive cells found in a wide variety of tissues and organs that can proliferate and give rise to more stem cells and/or more specialized cells [1]. Stem cells are known to play an important role in the healing and regeneration of tissues [2]. Thus, understanding the mechanisms that control stem cell fate and differentiation is certainly critical in utilizing these cells in regenerative medicine.

The Notch signaling pathway plays critical roles in regulating cell fate determination and differentiation in various cell types. In stem cells, Notch signaling participates in several processes, including maintenance of stemness, cell fate determination, cell proliferation, apoptosis and differentiation [3]. Functions of Notch have been extensively studied in the developmental biology and regeneration of various types of tissues and organs, i.e., nerve [4–6], muscle [7], skeleton [3], and tooth [8]. Hence, modified biomaterials mimicking Notch signaling could be a powerful tool to control stem cells fate in tissue regenerative application.

15.2 The Notch Signaling Pathway

Notch signaling is a conserved pathway in various organisms. The Notch gene was first identified in Drosophila [9]. Notch is a transmembrane receptor that is activated through cell–cell interaction after binding of the extracellular domain with membrane bound Notch ligands on another cell [10]. Notch signaling impairment results in failure in the development of murine embryos, including lack of somitogenesis, vascular defects, delayed closure of the neuropore, and inadequacy of cardiac formation [11–14]. Mutations of Notch signaling components are involved in several diseases in humans. Mutation of Notch-3 is linked to cerebral autosomal dominant ateriopathy with subcortical infarcts and leukoencephalopathy (CADASIL) [15]. Mutation of the Notch ligand, Jagged-1, is one of the causes of Alagille syndrome [16]. In addition, autosomal-recessive spondylocostal dysostosis is caused by mutation of another Notch ligand, Delta-like-3 [16]. Together, these findings strongly indicate a critical role of Notch signaling in development and diseases.

15.2.1 Notch Family of Receptors and Their Ligands

Four Notch receptors (Notch-1, -2, -3, and -4) and five Notch ligands (Delta-like-1, -3, -4, Jagged-1, and -2) have been identified in mammals [3,10,17]. The Notch receptor is synthesized as a full-length precursor protein of 300–350 kDa [27]. After synthesis, Notch is transferred to the trans-Golgi network for maturation and further cleaved by furin-like convertase [18]. This process is called the first cleavage (S1), and results in two subunits: extracellular and transmembrane Notch subunits. These subunits are then organized to form heterodimeric mature Notch receptors that are subsequently translocated to the cell membrane [19,20].

The mature Notch receptor is a type I transmembrane protein, containing three subunits; the large extracellular portion, the transmembrane domain and the small intracellular portion (Fig. 15.1) [21]. The extracellular portion, that interacts with the Notch ligands, comprises a large epidermal growth factor (EGF)-like repeated unit and a Notch negative regulatory region [NRR] [21,22]. The number of EGF-like repeats differs depending on of the specific Notch receptor. Notch-1 and Notch-2 have 36 EGF-like repeats while Notch-3 and Notch-4 have 34 and 29 EGF-like repeats, respectively. While the EGF-like repeated units act as the Notch ligand binding site, the NRR unit regulates receptor activation, acting as an inhibitor to prevent ligand-independent cleavage of the Notch receptor by metalloproteinases [23]. Between the extracellular and intracellular domain of Notch receptors, there are two cysteine residues. The intracellular domain consists of RBP-J associated molecule (RAM) domain, six ankyrin repeats [ANKRs], two nuclear localization sequences (NLS), a transactivation domain [TAD], and a proline-glutamate-serine-threonine-rich (PEST) region [24–26]. The RAM domain is responsible for transcription factor binding and the PEST region is involved in receptor degradation and turnover [24,25,27,28]. When Notch interacts with its ligand, the signaling cascade is initiated and further regulates cell fate decisions to differentiate, proliferation or apoptosis [29–31].

Notch ligands are also single-pass transmembrane proteins containing a Delta, Serrate, LAG (DSL), a Delta-OSM-11 like (DOS) and EGF-like repeat domain (Fig. 15.1) [27,28]. A cysteine-rich DSL domain is crucial for binding to EGF-like domain on Notch receptors

[27,28,32]. Two groups of Notch ligands have been reported in mammals; Delta-like and Jagged. Delta-like and Jagged ligands have a high affinity for the Notch receptors and are involved in the canonical signaling pathway [33]. These canonical ligands contain extracellular N-terminal DSL domain while the non-canonical ligands lack this portion [33]. Jagged ligands have an additional cysteine rich repeat domain near the transmembrane domain.

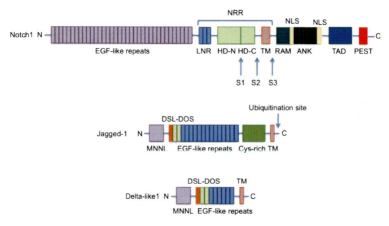

Figure 15.1 Structure of Notch receptor and ligands. NNR, Notch negative regulatory region; LNR, Lin12-Notch repeats; HD, heterodimer domain; TM, transmembrane domain; RAM, RBP-J associated molecule; ANK, ankyrin repeats; NLS, nuclear localization sequences; TAD, transactivation domain; PEST, proline, glutamate, serine and threonine; MNNL, module at N-terminus of Notch ligands; DSL, delta/serrate/LAG; DOS, delta and OSM- Modified from Kovall and Blacklow, 2010 [27].

15.2.2 Notch Signaling

The binding of Notch to its ligand initiates a conformational change that leads to cleavage of Notch by a disintegrin and metalloproteinase (ADAM)/tumor necrosis factor-α converting enzyme (TACE) at an extracellular site about 12 amino acids proximal to the transmembrane domain (Fig. 15.2) [10,21]. This event is termed the second cleavage (S2). Subsequently, a third cleavage (S3) occurs via the action of a Presenilin 1/2, Nicastin, PEN-2, and APH-1 enzyme complex named γ-secretase. Notch extracellular truncation (NEXT), a membrane-tethered intermediate, is cleaved by γ-secretase resulting in release of soluble Notch intracellular domain (NICD) into the cytoplasm [27,28]. NICD initiates intracellular signaling to regulate gene expression. Signaling is terminated upon ubiquitination of NICD and degradation in the proteosome [34].

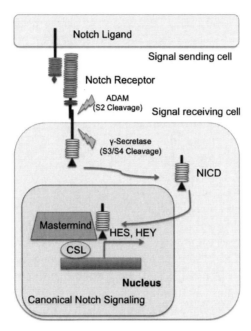

Figure 15.2 Canonical Notch signaling pathway. In the canonical pathway, Notch ligand on signal sending cell binds to Notch receptor on another cell, resulting in the cleavage of Notch by ADAM (S2 cleavage) at an extracellular site. Further, the soluble NICD is released γ-secretase mediated cleavage (S3 cleavage). NICD is then translocated into the nucleus and binds to CSL complex and Mastermind co-activator, turning CSL complex from a transcriptional repressor to a transcriptional activator. Subsequently, Notch target gene expression, i.e., Hes and Hey gene family transcription is induced.

15.2.2.1 Canonical Notch signaling pathway

In the canonical Notch signaling, NICD translocates into the nucleus and activates transcription factors of downstream target genes (Fig. 15.2) [10,21]. NICD binds to the DNA binding protein Epstein-Barr virus latency C promoter binding factor 1 (CBF1), Suppressor of Hairless and Lag1, known as CSL [35].

C promoter binding factor 1, also known as recombinant signal binding protein for immunoglobulin kappa J region (RBP-jk), is a DNA binding transcription factor mediating canonical Notch signaling. Normally, CBF1 binds to specific sequences in the promoter of Notch target gene and regulates their transcription. In the absence of NICD, CBF1 binds to specific transcriptional repressors to inhibit transcription of target genes. In the canonical pathway, the CBF1-NICD complex is activated by Mastermind family co-activators and turns CSL complex from a transcriptional repressor to a transcriptional activator, resulting in the induction of gene transcription, i.e., Hes and Hey family [28].

Hes and Hey gene families are the mammalian counterparts for the primary target genes of the Hairy and Enhancer-of-split genes in *Drosophila* [35]. Both Hes and Hey are basic helix-loop-helix transcription factors, and the major target genes of the canonical Notch signaling pathway [35]. Seven Hes proteins have been identified (Hes1-7). Hes proteins bind to N- and E-box DNA sequences (CACNAG and CANNTG, respectively) [36]. Hes proteins are induced by the Notch signaling pathway (except Hes2, 3, and 6). It has been shown that Hes1, 3, and 5 maintain stem cells in the undifferentiated state [35]. Other major target genes for Notch signaling are members of the Hey family. Three Hey proteins have been identified: Hey1, 2, and L. Minimal differences are noted between Hes and Hey proteins. Hey proteins cannot bind to N-box DNA sequences due to the replacement of glycine in their basic domain [36]. Thus, Hey proteins preferentially bind to E-box DNA sequences [36]. Hey1 and 2 double knockout mice exhibited similar phenotype as those observed in Notch-1 knockout mice [35].

15.2.2.2 Non-canonical Notch signaling pathway

The non-canonical Notch signaling pathway is still poorly understood in mammalian cells. Type I and II non-canonical Notch signaling are defined as NICD dependent-CBF1 independent and NICD independent-CBF1 independent, respectively [37]. In type I non-canonical Notch signaling, the NICD interacts with target proteins other than CBF1 resulting in the activation of different downstream target genes [35,37]. For example, binding of NICD to Deltex or NF-κB, resulting in CSL-NICD-Deltex or NF-κB-NICD complex. The NF-κB-NICD complex enhances NF-κB signaling, resulting in the transcriptional activation of NF-κB inducible genes, i.e., IFNγ [33]. On the other hand, the type II non-canonical Notch signaling pathway does not involve the cleavage of Notch or translocation of NICD to the nucleus to activate notch target genes [37]. For example, FGF-2 is able to activate Hes-1 expression through the direct binding of ATF2 on Hes-1 promoter [38].

15.3 Role of Notch Signaling in Stem Cells

15.3.1 Notch Signaling in Hematopoietic Stem Cells

Hematopoietic stem cells (HSCs) are crucial for maintenance and regeneration of all types of blood cells and their derivatives, including T lymphocytes, B lymphocytes, erythrocytes, neutrophils, basophils, eosinophils, platelets, mast cells, monocytes, macrophages, dendritic cells and osteoclasts [39]. Notch signaling plays important roles in HSC differentiation and self-renewal [40]. HSC self-renewal is increased by activation of the Notch signaling pathway [40]. Correspondingly, Notch-1 activation can inhibit HSC differentiation both in vitro and in vivo [41]. Further, the inhibition of Notch signaling using dominant negative RBP-jk/CSL stimulated differentiation of HSCs in vitro and reduced HSC activity in vivo [42]. These data suggest that Notch signaling preferentially promotes HSC self-renewal.

In regard to progenitor cell differentiation, abnormal expression of NICD increases the number of bone marrow repopulating cells in secondary transplants and promotes their lymphoid differentiation [41]. On the contrary, the activation of Notch signaling inhibited myeloid differentiation [43,44]. Regarding lymphoid lineage differentiation, Notch activation promoted T cells and inhibited B cell fate from a common progenitor [45]. In this respect, the deletion of RBPj/CSL results in increased B cell differentiation and blockage of T-cell development [45]. Distinct roles of Notch ligands in controlling cell fate have previously been reported in HSC. Delta-1, but not Jagged-1, inhibited B cell differentiation from human hematopoietic progenitor cells [46]. Together, these results suggest that Notch signaling is required for maintenance of self-renewal and lymphoid lineage differentiation in HSCs depending on the stage of cell development and type of ligands [41].

15.3.2 Notch Signaling in Adipose-Derived Mesenchymal Stem Cells

Adipose tissues consist of various cell types, i.e., mature adipocytes, preadipocytes, resident monocytes, macrophage, lymphocytes, and fibroblast [47,48]. In addition, adipose tissues also contain a group of cells called the stromal vascular fraction [48]. This fraction is mainly composed of mesenchymal stem cells [47] and several publications suggest that the mesenchymal stem cell niche is located at near blood vessels in adipose tissues [49,50]. Adipose-derived mesenchymal stem cells (ADSCs) have special characteristics that could benefit regenerative medicine such as the ability to perpetually proliferative after transplantation, multipotential differentiation capacity and the ability to release angiogenic growth factors [51,52–54].

Notch signaling has a functional role in proliferation and multi-lineage differentiation in ADSCs [55]. Several Notch ligands and receptors have been identified in ADSCs, i.e., Notch-1, Notch-2, Delta-1, and Delta-4 [56,57]. The proliferation rate of ADSCs decreased when Notch signaling was blocked by γ-secretase inhibitor [55]. The inhibition of Notch signaling in ADSCs in osteogenic culture conditions enhanced the up-regulation of osteogenic markers, including runt-related transcription factor 2 (Runx2), osterix (OSX), and osteocalcin (OCN) [55]. Further, it has also been reported that inhibition of Notch signaling in ADSCs prior to differentiation induced adipogenic differentiation via the enhancement of PPAR-gamma expression and the suppression of DLK-1/Pref-1 expression [58]. Interestingly, ADSCs modulated T lymphocytes activities via cell–cell interaction through Jagged-1, suggesting the involvement of Notch signaling in immunomodulatory mechanism in ADSCs [59].

15.3.3 Notch Signaling in Dental Tissue-Derived Mesenchymal Stem Cells

Stem cells can be isolated from dental pulp tissues of both primary and permanent teeth [60,61] as well as periodontal ligament tissues [62]. The isolated cells were confirmed to be stem cells by their clonogenic, proliferation, expression of stem cell markers and differentiation abilities [60–64]. Dental tissue-derived mesenchymal stem cells were able to differentiate into adipogenic, neurogenic, osteo/odontogenic, chondrogenic, myogenic, cardiomyogenic, and endothelial lineages [61–63,65–73]. These cells also showed immunomodulatory properties as they could significantly reduce the percentage of IL17$^+$IFNg T cell population in CD4$^+$ T cells in vitro [74]. The application of these stem cells in bone regeneration application has been extensively investigated [75,76]. Recently, a potential therapeutic application of dental pulp stem cells in humans was analyzed. The results indicated that dental pulp stem cells could promote better bone formation in extraction sockets [77].

In dental organs, Notch and Notch ligands are expressed [78,79] and have different expression patterns and regulatory mechanisms during normal tooth development and regeneration [80]. Notch-1 and -2 were expressed in human periodontal ligament cells but neither Notch-3 nor Notch-4 was observed [81]. On the contrary, normal rat dental pulp cells expressed Notch-1, -2, and -3, but not Notch-4 [82]. Jagged-2 knockout mice exhibited malformation of molars and defective incisor enamel formation [83]. Sun et al. revealed that Notch-1, -2, -3, Hey1, and Hes1 were expressed in normal rat dental pulp [82]. Moreover, Notch-1, -2, and -3 as well as Delta-like-1 and Jagged-1 were expressed in response to pulp capping (treatment of vital pulp tissues to promote dentin regeneration) [30]. Notch-1 expression was noted in the subodontoblastic zone close to the capping area [30]. Delta-like-1 was also observed around the capping area and dentin walls, whereas Jagged-1 was found in the stromal area of dental pulp [30]. Moreover, up-regulation of Delta-like-1 was also observed in odontoblasts as well as vascular structures [84], a potential niche of dental pulp stem cells [85], suggesting a role of Delta-like-1 in the regenerative process. Expression of Hes1, a downstream target, was also found in adjacent dentin walls [30]. These results suggest a potential role of Notch signaling, especially via the Delta-like-1 ligand, in healing of dental tissues. However, Hey1 was decreased during odontoblast differentiation of rat dental pulp cells [82], suggesting that Hey1 may be negative regulator of odontoblast differentiation.

Recently, it has been reported that co-culture of normal dental pulp stem cells with dental pulp stem cells overexpressing Delta-like-1 resulted in increased cell proliferation and odontoblast differentiation [29], while the over-expression of Jagged-1 in dental pulp stem cells resulted in the inhibition of odontoblast differentiation in vitro and mineralization in vivo [86]. Although, the mechanism for this is unclear, He et al. proposed that these two ligands may be involved in regulating different downstream target genes of Notch, since it has been reported that Hes1 and Deltex regulate CSL dependent and CSL-independent Notch signaling, respectively [29].

While several studies have described expression of Notch ligands in periodontal ligament cells, the role of Notch in periodontal cell function is still very limited. Upon culture, human periodontal ligament cells in osteogenic medium upregulated Delta-like-1 ligands [87]. On the contrary, Nakao et al. suggested a potential role of Jagged-1 in osteoclastogenesis via receptor activator of nuclear factor kappa B ligand (RANKL) in periodontal tissues [81].

15.3.4 Notch Signaling in Epithelial Stem Cells

Notch signaling plays crucial roles in the promotion of epithelial cell differentiation and epidermal stratification [88]. Notch signaling is not required for epithelial stem cell self-renewal but must be suppressed to maintain epithelial stem cells in the basal layer [88]. Notch signaling is essential to induce basal stem cell differentiation [89]. Notch-1 and Notch-2 expression were noted in the epidermal layer while Delta-like-1 expression was restricted at the basal layer [90,91]. The strongest Delta-like-1 expression was observed in the stem cell niche [91]. High expression of Delta-like-1 enhanced epithelial stem cell clustering and averted interactions with neighboring cells, thus protecting epithelial stem cells in their niche, possibly due to Delta-1/Delta-1 homotypic interactions [91,92] as well as *cis*-inhibition mechanism of Notch ligands [28]. However, an optimal level of Delta-like-1 expression stimulated movement of stem cells out of their compartment and initiated differentiation [91]. In addition, Notch/Jagged expression in epithelium appears to act as a positive feedback mechanism enhancing differentiation as epithelial cells migrate out from the basal layer [90]. The expression of early epithelial cell differentiation markers was increased by the induction of Notch-1 and Notch-2 [90]. In contrast, late epithelial cell differentiation markers were downregulated by Notch signaling [90]. From this information, it is likely that Notch signaling is involved in cell fate decisions, including early versus late stage differentiation in epithelial stem cells [90]. However, it was shown that terminal differentiation and cornification were also dependent on Jagged-1/Notch activation [92]. Specific Notch receptor/ligand interactions were identified at each differentiation stage. Delta-like-1 interacts with Notch-1 and Notch-2 in early differentiation, while Jagged-1 interacts with Notch-1, -2, -3, -4 during terminal differentiation and cornification stages [92].

15.4 Notch Signaling Biomaterials

Notch ligands are unlike other signaling ligands such as bone morphogenetic protein, basic fibroblast growth factor, or Wnt in that they require immobilization for proper interaction and activation of Notch. Soluble Notch ligands normally demonstrate no activity or even antagonistic properties unless clustered by antibody [93,94]. This is due to the lack of endocytosis of extracellular domain of Notch ligands by the signal-sending cell, which generates physical force to dissociate the Notch receptor heterodimers [28,95]. Thus, one way to activate Notch signaling in vitro is to immobilize Notch ligands on surface mimicking the signal-sending cells [96,97]. This approach can bypass the requirement of endocytosis pulling process of Notch extracellular domain and ligand complex, although, the exact mechanism is yet unclear [28]. The development of Notch signaling biomaterials could be employed in various applications ranging from in vitro biological study of Notch signaling function to prospective smart biomaterials in clinical regenerative medicine.

15.4.1 Notch Signaling Surfaces

15.4.1.1 Indirect affinity immobilization of Notch ligands

In typical direct immobilization techniques, proteins are non-specifically linked to a surface leading to random orientation and rendering some receptor binding sites inaccessible. Indeed, it has been shown that the concentration of immobilized Notch ligands is not directly correlated with the activation of Notch signaling, however, the correct orientation and availability of active domain of Notch ligands are more crucial [98]. Therefore, we have used an indirect affinity immobilization strategy to enhance the orientation and clustering of Notch ligands.

15.4.1.2 Site-specific binding via Fc domain

Site-specific binding of Notch ligands was achieved using an indirect immobilization technique. In this approach, a Notch ligand fused to the Immunoglobulin Fc domain (Notch ligand/Fc) is selectively bound to either protein G, protein A or antibody directed against Fc (anti-Fc) immobilized to a solid substrate (Fig. 15.3) [96,97,99]. Protein G and anti-Fc contain two immunoglobulin binding domains, while, Protein A contains five immunoglobulin binding domains [96,97,100]. Thus, these binding domains potentially bind several Notch ligand/Fc proteins. This results in an inherent clustering of the ligands, which the direct immobilization scheme lacks [96,97]. Although, both Protein A and G bind to Fc fragment, some differential binding activities are noted. Protein A binds to the high molecular weight Fc fragments but Protein G reacts with both Fab and the low molecular weight Fc fragments [101].

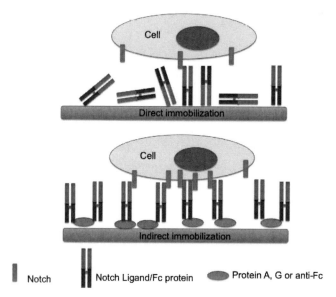

Figure 15.3 Schematic of Notch ligand immobilization using site-specific binding via Fc domain. Direct immobilization approach (upper panel), Notch ligands bind to the surface nonspecifically with random orientation. Indirect affinity immobilization (lower panel), Protein A, Protein G or anti-Fc are coated/immobilized on biomaterial surface, followed by Notch ligand/Fc specific binding, providing correct orientation and availability of ligand binding sites to interact with Notch receptors.

Using Protein G-based indirectly immobilized Jagged-1/Fc, the activity of CBF1 luciferase reporter was significantly increased (3-fold) while directly immobilized Jagged-1/Fc resulted in less activity (1.5-fold) [97]. In addition, soluble Jagged-1/Fc could not activate Notch/CBF1 signaling [96], consistent with the increased potency of indirectly affinity-immobilized Notch ligands on cellular function.

To improve Notch signaling activity, self-assembled monolayers (SAMs) can be employed to modify biomaterials surfaces before indirect immobilization protocols. SAMs are nanoscaled, highly-ordered alkanethiols surfaces. These surfaces can be patterned to expose a variety of functional groups on the surface [98]. Using SAM-modified surfaces, the density of Notch ligands was correctly controlled via indirect immobilization and able to modulate activation levels of Notch signaling in target cells [98].

15.4.1.3 An antigen–antibody reaction combined with biotin-streptavidin chemistry

In this approach, biotinylated antibodies specific for a histidine tag (His) are bound on a streptavidin-coated surface (Fig. 15.4). Subsequently, His-tagged Notch ligands can be immobilized and

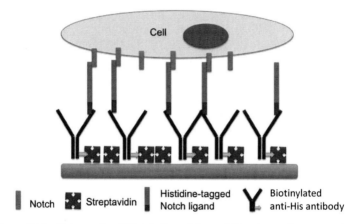

Figure 15.4 Schematic of Notch ligand immobilization using an antigen–antibody reaction combined with biotin-streptavidin chemistry. Streptavidin coated surface is coated with a biotinylated anti-His antibody. Subsequently, His-tagged Notch ligands are immobilized on the surface, resulting in orientated ligands exposed to the cells.

oriented on a biomaterial surface [102]. Using this technique to immobilize His tagged Delta-like-4 on polystyrene microbeads, the functionalization efficiency of microbeads is approximately 65% [102]. Further, Delta-like-4 immobilized microbeads potently inhibited myotube formation by C2C12 myoblast cells, confirming the activity of immobilized protein [102].

15.4.2 Potential Use of Notch Signaling Biomaterials in Regenerative Medicine

15.4.2.1 Notch signaling biomaterials and HSC expansion and differentiation

Notch signaling systems have been previously developed to control proliferation and direct differentiation of HSCs. Jagged-1-immobilized surfaces enhanced proliferation of specific subpopulations of HSCs [99,103], suggesting a potential use of Notch ligand–modified biomaterials in expanding HSC/precursor cell populations. In addition, ex vivo co-culture of HSCs with stromal cell expressing Notch ligands could induce HSC differentiation toward T cells or B cells. For example, co-culture of HSCs with OP9 overexpressing Delta-like-1 promoted T cell differentiation [104,105]. However, this co-culture technique has several limitations, including invariable contamination with the co-cultured cell and high variability. To overcome these problems, Notch ligand–modified biomaterials have been assessed for their ability to direct HSC differentiation. In this regard, Delta-like-4 immobilized polystyrene microbeads and layer-by-layer Delta-like-1 coated polyacrylamide hydrogel have been studied. These Notch ligand–modified biomaterials were successfully used to direct T cell differentiation from HSCs [102,106]. Thus, Notch ligand–modified biomaterials may be useful in controlling HSC proliferation and lineage specific differentiation.

15.4.2.2 Notch signaling biomaterials and bone regeneration

Notch signaling participates in the control of osteoblast differentiation and bone regeneration [107–109]. Up-regulation of Jagged-1 and Notch-2 were observed in mesenchymal cells during tibia and calvarial bone regeneration in mouse [109]. Intrinsic or extrinsic overexpression of Jagged-1 in bone marrow stromal cells led to higher osteogenic differentiation potency, i.e., higher alkaline phosphatase enzymatic activity and mineralization [110–112]. Moreover, Delta-like-1 and Jagged-1 coated poly-D,L-lactic-co-glycolic acid/gelatin sponges seeded with pre-osteoblastic cells could significantly enhance ectopic bone formation in the presence of bone morphogenetic protein 2 in a murine subcutaneous implantation model [113]. The amount of bone trabeculae were markedly increased in Delta-like-1 or Jagged-1 coated biomaterial groups compared to the control [113]. Together, these data indicate that Notch ligand immobilized biomaterials positively regulate osteoblast differentiation and are thus are logical candidates to promote bone tissue regeneration. However, it should be noted that several publications have shown that Notch signaling might also impair osteogenic differentiation [114–116]. Therefore, further investigation is needed to carefully investigate the prospective use of Notch ligand–modified biomaterials in bone regeneration.

15.4.2.3 Notch signaling biomaterials and periodontal tissue regeneration

Periodontal tissue healing is divided into three phases: (1) inflammation, (2) granulation tissue formation and matrix formation, and (3) maturation and remodeling [117]. Uninterrupted, stable fibrin clots positioned between the gingival flap and periodontal compromised root are crucial for periodontal regeneration [118]. The fibrin clot supports cell migration, proliferation, and formation of newly regenerated tissues. However, periodontal healing differs from wound and bone healing during the maturation and remodeling phase since it requires the attachment of collagen fibers to cementum or root dentin and alveolar bone [117]. Four tissues are involved in periodontal regeneration: epithelium, connective tissue, alveolar bone and periodontal ligament [119]. Among these four tissues, epithelium has the highest rate of repair, resulting in a long junctional epithelial attachment and failure of true periodontal tissue regeneration [119]. In addition, the process of periodontal ligament formation is slower than bone. This could lead to ankylosis of the treated tooth in some cases. Together, these data indicate that periodontal tissue regeneration is unique. Therefore, biomaterials that promote periodontal regeneration are likely to require specific design and development strategies.

According to the nature of periodontal healing described above, a guided tissue regeneration technique has been introduced. In this approach, a membrane is placed between the epithelial/connective tissues and the tooth surface before the mucoperiostium flap is placed back and sutured. The membrane prevents soft tissue, especially epithelium, downgrowth and migration into periodontal defect and avoids long junctional epithelium and connective tissue attachment [119]. The membrane also supports fibrin clot development in the defect, which is crucial in the periodontal healing process [119]. In addition, it creates a space in the defect, allowing the concentration of growth factors, progenitor cell migration and periodontal tissue formation in the defect [119].

Notch signaling biomaterials have been investigated as a potential therapeutic approach for periodontal tissue regeneration. Surface modification with indirect affinity immobilization of the Notch ligand, Jagged-1, activated CBF1 luciferase reporter in epithelial cells [97] and increased Notch target gene, Hes-1, expression in human periodontal ligament stem cells [127], indicating that Jagged-1-modified surface were able to activate of Notch signaling in these cell types.

Surface-bound Jagged-1 promoted osteogenic differentiation of HPDLs. In this regard, alkaline phosphatase enzymatic activity and mineralization as well as mRNA expression of ALP, Col 1, and OPN were significantly increased compared to those of control surfaces [127]. In addition, this Notch ligand–modified surface was able to direct the differentiation of epithelial cells [97]. Cells plated on Jagged-1-modified surface rapidly stratified forming multilayers of cells in tight clusters compared to control surface [97]. Jagged-1-modified biomaterials decreased proliferation and increased differentiation of epithelial cells and inhibited epithelial migration along the dermis in a rafted organ culture model [97]. In light of the effects of Jagged-1-modified surfaces on epithelial cells and periodontal ligament stem cells discussed above, Jagged-1-modified surfaces may be particularly useful in developing biomaterials that guide periodontal tissue regeneration.

15.4.2.4 Notch signaling biomaterials and cardiac regeneration

In development, the Notch signaling pathway is crucial for heart formation [120]. Interestingly, Notch signaling has also been identified as one of the key systems involved in myocardial repair and regeneration [121,122]. Notch signaling has a protective role post-infarction as highlighted by studies showing that injection of adenoviral vector expressing NICD could improve function of injured myocardium [123]. In addition, Jagged-1 promoted the differentiation of mesenchymal stem cells toward the cardiomyocytes lineage [124]. Furthermore, mesenchymal stem cells are indirectly involved in cardiac regeneration via the interaction of Jagged-1 and Notch-1 [125]. Jagged-1 ligands on mesenchymal stem cells initiated Notch signaling in cardiomyocytes via Notch-1 receptor, resulting in the enhancement of cardiomyocyte proliferation [125]. Consistent with this, immobilized Jagged-1 was able to enhance cardiomyocyte proliferation [126]. Thus, Notch signaling biomaterials to promote cardiomyocyte proliferation or to direct cardiomyocyte differentiation from stem cells may be useful for post-infarction myocardial regeneration.

15.5 Conclusions

While conventional therapeutics have greatly improved human health, there are still numerous disease and injury states where optimal treatments are lacking. Stem cells and bioengineered materials may lead to novel treatments for such diseases. Understanding the mechanisms that control stem cell proliferation and differentiation will allow development of novel biomaterials that may help control these processes in injury and disease. Notch signaling is a particularly intriguing pathway, since it has been shown to regulate stem cell proliferation and differentiation. Previous study by our group showed that immobilized Notch ligands were able to activate Notch signaling to a greater extent than soluble ligands [96]. In addition, oriented, indirect immobilization of Notch ligands significantly increased Notch signaling compared to unoriented, direct immobilization [96]. Immobilized Jagged-1-modified surfaces were able to control the proliferation and direct the differentiation of epithelial cells [96,97] and periodontal ligament derived mesenchymal stem cell [127]. These data suggest the potential application of Notch ligand–modified biomaterials in tissue regeneration. Further studies to elucidate optimal design criterion for Notch ligand immobilization on biomaterials for specific applications are clearly warranted.

Acknowledgment

The authors were funded by "Integrated Innovation Academic Center: IIAC" Chulalongkorn University Centenary Academic Development Project, National Research University Project of CHE and Ratchadaphiseksomphot Endowment Fund (HR1166I).

References

1. Stocum, D. L. (2001). Stem cells in regenerative biology and medicine, *Wound. Repair. Regen.*, **6**, 429–442.
2. Lin, H. (1997). The tao of stem cells in the germline, *Annu. Rev. Genet.*, **31**, 455–491.
3. Tao, J., Chen, S., Lee, B. (2010). Alteration of Notch signaling in skeletal development and disease, *Ann. N. Y. Acad. Sci.*, **1192**, 257–268.
4. Taylor, M. K., Yeager, K., Morrison, S. J. (2007). Physiological Notch signaling promotes gliogenesis in the developing peripheral and central nervous systems, *Development.*, **134**, 2435–2447.
5. Cornell, R. A., Eisen, J. S. (2005). Notch in the pathway: the roles of Notch signaling in neural crest development, *Semin. Cell. Dev. Biol.*, **16**, 663–672.
6. Pierfelice, T., Alberi, L., Gaiano, N. (2011). Notch in the vertebrate nervous system: an old dog with new tricks, *Neuron.*, **69**, 840–855.
7. Wu, X., Xu, K., Zhang, L., Deng, Y., Lee, P., Shapiro, E., Monaco, M., Makarenkova, H. P., Li, J., Lepor, H., Grishina, I. (2011). Differentiation of the ductal epithelium and smooth muscle in the prostate gland are regulated by the Notch/PTEN-dependent mechanism, *Dev. Biol.*, **356**, 337–349.
8. Borkosky, S. S., Nagatsuka, H., Orita, Y., Tsujigiwa, H., Yoshinobu, J., Gunduz, M., Rodriguez, A. P., Missana, L. R., Nishizaki, K., Nagai, N. (2008). Sequential expressions of Notch-1, Jagged-2 and Math-1 in molar tooth germ of mouse, *Biocell.*, **32**, 251–258.
9. Moohr, O. (1919). Character changes caused by mutation of anterior entire region of a chromosome in drosophila, *Genetics.*, **4**, 275–282.
10. Tien, A. C., Rajan, A., Bellen, H. J. (2009). A Notch updated, *J. Cell. Biol.*, **184**, 621–629.
11. Shi, S., Stanley, P. (2003). Protein O-fucosyltransferase 1 is an essential component of Notch signaling pathways, *Proc. Natl. Acad. Sci. USA*, **100**, 5234–5239.

12. Koo, B. K., Lim, H.S., Song, R., Yoon, M. J., Yoon, K. J., Moon, J. S., Kim, Y. W., Kwon, M. C., Yoo, K. W., Kong, M. P., Lee, L., Chitnis, A. B., Kim, C. H., Kong, Y. Y. (2005). Mind bomb 1 is essential for generating functional Notch ligands to activate Notch, *Development.*, **132**, 3459–3470.

13. Chen, H., Ko, G., Zatti, A., Di Giacomo, G., Liu, L., Raiteri, E., Perucco, E., Collesi, C., Min, W., Zeiss, C., De Camilli, P., Cremona, O. (2009). Embryonic arrest at midgestation and disruption of Notch signaling produced by the absence of both epsin 1 and epsin 2 in mice, *Proc. Natl. Acad. Sci. USA*, **106**, 13838–13843.

14. Donoviel, D. B., Hadjantonakis, A. K., Ikeda, M., Zheng, H., Hyslop, P. S., Bernstein, A. (1999). Mice lacking both presenilin genes exhibit early embryonic patterning defects, *Genes. Dev.*, **13**, 2801–2810.

15. Louvi, A., Arboleda-Velasquez, J. F., Artavanis-Tsakonas, S. (2006). CADASIL: a critical look at a Notch disease, *Dev. Neurosci.*, **28**, 5–12.

16. Gridley, T. (2003). Notch signaling and inherited disease syndromes, *Hum. Mol. Genet.*, **12 Spec No 1**, R9–R13.

17. Miyamoto, A., Lau, R., Hein, P. W., Shipley, J. M., Weinmaster, G. (2006). Microfibrillar proteins MAGP-1 and MAGP-2 induce Notch-1 extracellular domain dissociation and receptor activation, *J. Biol. Chem.*, **281**, 10089–10097.

18. Mumm, J. S., Kopan, R. (2000). Notch signaling: from the outside in, *Dev. Biol.*, **228**, 151–165.

19. Blaumueller, C. M., Qi, H., Zagouras, P., Artavanis-Tsakonas, S. (1997). Intracellular cleavage of Notch leads to a heterodimeric receptor on the plasma membrane, *Cell.*, **90**, 281–291.

20. Logeat, F., Bessia, C., Brou, C., LeBail, O., Jarriault, S., Seidah, N. G., Isreael, A. (1998). The Notch-1 receptor is cleaved constitutively by a furin-like convertase, *Proc. Natl. Acad. Sci. USA*, **95**, 8108–8112.

21. Kopan, R., Ilagan, M. X. (2009). The canonical Notch signaling pathway: unfolding the activation mechanism, *Cell*, **137**, 216–233.

22. Rebay, I., Fleming, R. J., Fehon, R. G., Cherbas, L., Cherbas, P., Artavanis-Tsakonas, S. (1991). Specific EGF repeats of Notch mediate interactions with Delta and Serrate: implications for Notch as a multifunctional receptor, *Cell*, **67**, 687–699.

23. Sanchez-Irizarry, C., Carpenter, A. C., Weng, A. P., Pear, W. S., Aster, J. C., Blacklow, S. C. (2004). Notch subunit heterodimerization and prevention of ligand-independent proteolytic activation depend, respectively, on a novel domain and the LNR repeats, *Mol. Cell. Biol.*, **24**, 9265–9273.

24. Weinmaster, G. (1997). The ins and outs of Notch signaling, *Mol. Cell. Neurosci.*, **9**, 91–102.
25. Fleming, R. J. (1998). Structural conservation of Notch receptors and ligands, *Semin. Cell. Dev. Biol.*, **9**, 599–607.
26. Baron, M. (2003). An overview of the Notch signalling pathway, *Semin. Cell. Dev. Biol.*, **14**, 113–119.
27. Kovall, R. A., Blacklow, S. C. (2010). Mechanistic insights into Notch receptor signaling from structural and biochemical studies, *Curr. Top. Dev. Biol.*, **92**, 31–71. Modified from Kovall and Blacklow, 2010 [27]
28. D'Souza, B., Meloty-Kapella, L., Weinmaster, G. (2010). Canonical and non-canonical Notch ligands, *Curr. Top. Dev. Biol.*, **92**, 73–129.
29. He, F., Yang, Z., Tan, Y., Yu, N., Wang, X., Yao, N., Zhao, J. (2009). Effects of Notch ligand Delta-1 on the proliferation and differentiation of human dental pulp stem cells in vitro, *Arch. Oral. Biol.*, **54**, 216–222.
30. Lovschall, H., Tummers, M., Thesleff, I., Fuchtbauer, E. M., Poulsen, K. (2005). Activation of the Notch signaling pathway in response to pulp capping of rat molars, *Eur. J. Oral. Sci.*, **113**, 312–317.
31. Engin, F., Lee, B. (2010). NOTCHing the bone: insights into multi-functionality, *Bone.*, **46**, 274–280.
32. Glittenberg, M., Pitsouli, C., Garvey, C., Delidakis, C., Bray, S. (2006). Role of conserved intracellular motifs in Serrate signalling, cis-inhibition and endocytosis, *EMBO. J.*, **25**, 4697–4706.
33. Katoh, M. (2007). Notch signaling in gastrointestinal tract (review). *Int. J. Oncol.*, **30**, 247–251.
34. Kopan, R. (1999). All good things must come to an end: how is Notch signaling turned off?, *Sci. STKE.*, **1999**, PE1.
35. Zanotti, S., Canalis, E. (2010). Notch and the skeleton, *Mol. Cell. Biol.*, **30**, 886–896.
36. Fischer, A., Gessler, M. (2007). Delta-Notch–and then? Protein interactions and proposed modes of repression by Hes and Hey bHLH factors, *Nucleic. Acids. Res.*, **35**, 4583–4596.
37. Sanalkumar, R., Dhanesh, S. B., James, J. (2010). Non-canonical activation of Notch signaling/target genes in vertebrates, *Cell. Mol. Life. Sci.*, **67**, 2957–2968.
38. Sanalkumar, R., Indulekha, C. L., Divya, T. S., Divya, M. S., Anto, R. J., Vinod, B., Vidyanand, S., Jagatha, B., Venugopal, S., James, J. (2010). ATF2 maintains a subset of neural progenitors through CBF1/Notch independent Hes-1 expression and synergistically activates the expression of Hes-1 in Notch-dependent neural progenitors, *J. Neurochem.*, **113**, 807–818.

39. Dzierzak, E., Speck, N. A. (2008). Of lineage and legacy: the development of mammalian hematopoietic stem cells, *Nat. Immunol.*, **9**, 129–136.
40. Varnum-Finney, B., Xu, L., Brashem-Stein, C., Nourigat, C., Flowers, D., Bakkour, S., Pear, W. S., Bernstein, I. D. (2000). Pluripotent, cytokine-dependent, hematopoietic stem cells are immortalized by constitutive Notch-1 signaling, *Nat. Med.*, **6**, 1278–1281.
41. Stier, S., Cheng, T., Dombkowski, D., Carlesso, N., Scadden, D. T. (2002). Notch-1 activation increases hematopoietic stem cell self-renewal in vivo and favors lymphoid over myeloid lineage outcome, *Blood.*, **99**, 2369–2378.
42. Duncan, A. W., Rattis, F. M., DiMascio, L. N., Congdon, K. L., Pazianos, G., Zhao, C., Yoon, K., Cook, J. M., Willert, K., Gaiano, N., Reya, T. (2005). Integration of Notch and Wnt signaling in hematopoietic stem cell maintenance, *Nat. Immunol.*, **6**, 314–322.
43. Bigas, A., Martin, D. I., Milner, L. A. (1998). Notch-1 and Notch-2 inhibit myeloid differentiation in response to different cytokines, *Mol. Cell. Biol.*, **18**, 2324–2333.
44. Milner, L. A., Bigas, A., Kopan, R., Brashem-Stein, C., Bernstein, I. D., Martin, D. I. (1996). Inhibition of granulocytic differentiation by mNotch-1, *Proc. Natl. Acad. Sci. USA*, **93**, 13014–13019.
45. Han, H., Tanigaki, K., Yamamoto, N., Kuroda, K., Yoshimoto, M., Nakahata, T., Ikuta, K., Honjo, T. (2002). Inducible gene knockout of transcription factor recombination signal binding protein-J reveals its essential role in T versus B lineage decision, *Int. Immunol.*, **14**, 637–645.
46. Jaleco, A. C., Neves, H., Hooijberg, E., Gameiro, P., Clode, N., Haury, M., Henrique, D., Parreira, L. (2001). Differential effects of Notch ligands Delta-1 and Jagged-1 in human lymphoid differentiation, *J. Exp. Med.*, **194**, 991–1002.
47. Brown, S. A., Levi, B., Lequeux, C., Wong, V. W., Mojallal, A., Longaker, M. T. (2010). Basic science review on adipose tissue for clinicians, *Plast. Reconstr. Surg.*, **126**, 1936–1946.
48. Wilson, A., Butler, P. E., Seifalian, A. M. (2010). Adipose-derived stem cells for clinical applications: a review, *Cell. Prolif.*, **44**, 86–98.
49. Crisan, M., Yap, S., Casteilla, L., Chen, C. W., Corselli, M., Park, T. S., Andriolo, G., Sun, B., Zheng, B., Zhang, L., Norotte, C., Teng, P. N., Traas, J., Schugar, R., Deasy, B. M., Badylak, S., Buhring, H. J., Giacobino, J. P., Lazzari, L., Huard, J., Peault, B. (2008). A perivascular origin for mesenchymal stem cells in multiple human organs, *Cell. Stem. Cell.*, **3**, 301–313.

50. da Silva Meirelles, L., Caplan, A. I., Nardi, N. B. (2008). In search of the in vivo identity of mesenchymal stem cells, *Stem. Cells.*, **26**, 2287–2299.

51. Miranville, A., Heeschen, C., Sengenes, C., Curat, C. A., Busse, R., Bouloumie, A. (2004). Improvement of postnatal neovascularization by human adipose tissue-derived stem cells, *Circulation.*, **110**, 349–355.

52. Moon, M. H., Kim, S. Y., Kim, Y. J., Kim, S. J., Lee, J. B., Bae, Y. C., Sung, S. M., Jung, J. S. (2006). Human adipose tissue-derived mesenchymal stem cells improve postnatal neovascularization in a mouse model of hindlimb ischemia, *Cell. Physiol. Biochem.*, **17**, 279–290.

53. Planat-Benard, V., Silvestre, J. S., Cousin, B., Andre, M., Nibbelink, M., Tamarat, R., Clergue, M., Manneville, C., Saillan-Barreau, C., Duriez, M., Tedgui, A., Levy, B., Penicaud, L., Casteilla, L. (2004). Plasticity of human adipose lineage cells toward endothelial cells: physiological and therapeutic perspectives, *Circulation.*, **109**, 656–663.

54. Zuk, P. A., Zhu, M., Mizuno, H., Huang, J., Futrell, J. W., Katz, A. J., Benhaim, P., Lorenz, H. P., Hedrick, M. H. (2001). Multilineage cells from human adipose tissue: implications for cell-based therapies, *Tissue. Eng.*, **7**, 211–228.

55. Jing, W., Xiong, Z., Cai, X., Huang, Y., Li, X., Yang, X., Liu, L., Tang, W., Lin, Y., Tian, W. (2010). Effects of gamma-secretase inhibition on the proliferation and vitamin D(3) induced osteogenesis in adipose derived stem cells, *Biochem. Biophys. Res. Commun.*, **392**, 442–447.

56. Kingham, P. J., Mantovani, C., Terenghi, G. (2009). Notch independent signalling mediates Schwann cell-like differentiation of adipose derived stem cells, *Neurosci. Lett.*, **467**, 164–168.

57. Andersen, D. C., Schroder, H. D., Jensen, C. H. (2008). Non-cultured adipose-derived CD45-side population cells are enriched for progenitors that give rise to myofibres in vivo, *Exp. Cell. Res.*, **314**, 2951–2964.

58. Huang, Y., Yang, X., Wu, Y., Jing, W., Cai, X., Tang, W., Liu, L., Liu, Y., Grottkau, B. E., Lin, Y. (2010). Gamma-secretase inhibitor induces adipogenesis of adipose-derived stem cells by regulation of Notch and PPAR-gamma, *Cell. Prolif.*, **43**, 147–156.

59. Shi, D., Liao, L., Zhang, B., Liu, R., Dou, X., Li, J., Zhu, X., Yu, L., Chen, D., Zhao, R. C. (2011). Human adipose tissue-derived mesenchymal stem cells facilitate the immunosuppressive effect of cyclosporin A on T lymphocytes through Jagged-1-mediated inhibition of NF-kappaB signaling, *Exp. Hematol.*, **39**, 214–224 e211.

60. Gronthos, S., Mankani, M., Brahim, J., Robey, P. G., Shi, S. (2000). Postnatal human dental pulp stem cells (DPSCs) in vitro and in vivo, *Proc. Natl. Acad. Sci. USA*, **97**, 13625–13630.
61. Miura, M., Gronthos, S., Zhao, M., Lu, B., Fisher, L. W., Robey, P. G., Shi, S. (2003). SHED: stem cells from human exfoliated deciduous teeth, *Proc. Natl. Acad. Sci. USA*, **100**, 5807–5812.
62. Seo, B. M., Miura, M., Gronthos, S., Bartold, P. M., Batouli, S., Brahim, J., Young, M., Robey, P. G., Wang, C. Y., Shi, S. (2004). Investigation of multipotent postnatal stem cells from human periodontal ligament, *Lancet*, **364**, 149–155.
63. Huang, C. Y., Pelaez, D., Dominguez-Bendala, J., Garcia-Godoy, F., Cheung, H. S. (2009). Plasticity of stem cells derived from adult periodontal ligament, *Regen. Med.*, **4**, 809–821.
64. Park, J. C., Kim, J. M., Jung, I. H., Kim, J. C., Choi, S. H., Cho, K. S., Kim, C. S. (2011). Isolation and characterization of human periodontal ligament (PDL) stem cells (PDLSCs) from the inflamed PDL tissue: in vitro and in vivo evaluations, *J. Clin. Periodontol.*, **38**, 721–731.
65. Osathanon, T., Nowwarote, N., Pavasant, P. (2011). Basic fibroblast growth factor inhibits mineralization but induces neuronal differentiation by human dental pulp stem cells through a FGFR and PLCgamma signaling pathway, *J. Cell. Biochem.*, **112**, 1807–1816.
66. Gronthos, S., Brahim, J., Li, W., Fisher, L. W., Cherman, N., Boyde, A., DenBesten, P., Robey, P. G., Shi, S. (2002). Stem cell properties of human dental pulp stem cells, *J. Dent. Res.*, **81**, 531–535.
67. Spath, L., Rotilio, V., Alessandrini, M., Gambara, G., De Angelis, L., Mancini, M., Mitsiadis, T. A., Vivarelli, E., Naro, F., Filippini, A., Papaccio, G. (2010). Explant derived human dental pulp stem cells enhance differentiation and proliferation potentials, *J. Cell. Mol. Med.*, **14**, 1635–1644.
68. Huang, G. T., Gronthos, S., Shi, S. (2009). Mesenchymal stem cells derived from dental tissues vs. those from other sources: their biology and role in regenerative medicine, *J. Dent. Res.*, **88**, 792–806.
69. Zhang, W., Walboomers, X. F., Van Kuppevelt, T. H., Daamen, W. F., Van Damme, P. A., Bian, Z., Jansen, J. A. (2008). In vivo evaluation of human dental pulp stem cells differentiated towards multiple lineages, *J. Tissue. Eng. Regen. Med.*, **2**, 117–125.
70. Arthur, A., Rychkov, G., Shi, S., Koblar, S. A., Gronthos, S. (2008). Adult human dental pulp stem cells differentiate toward functionally active neurons under appropriate environmental cues, *Stem. Cells.*, **26**, 1787–1795.

71. Sakai, V. T., Zhang, Z., Dong, Z., Neiva, K. G., Machado, M. A., Shi, S., Santos, C. F., Nor, J. E. (2010). SHED differentiate into functional odontoblasts and endothelium, *J. Dent. Res.*, **89**, 791–796.
72. Chadipiralla, K., Yochim, J. M., Bahuleyan, B., Huang, C. Y., Garcia-Godoy, F., Murray, P. E., Steinicki, E. J. (2010). Osteogenic differentiation of stem cells derived from human periodontal ligaments and pulp of human exfoliated deciduous teeth, *Cell. Tissue. Res.*, **340**, 323–333.
73. Wang, J., Wang, X., Sun, Z., Yang, H., Shi, S., Wang, S. (2010). Stem cells from human-exfoliated deciduous teeth can differentiate into dopaminergic neuron-like cells, *Stem. Cells. Dev.*, **19**, 1375–1383.
74. Yamaza, T., Kentaro, A., Chen, C., Liu, Y., Shi, Y., Gronthos, S., Wang, S., Shi, S. (2010). Immunomodulatory properties of stem cells from human exfoliated deciduous teeth, *Stem. Cell. Res. Ther.*, **1**, 5.
75. Seo, B. M., Sonoyama, W., Yamaza, T., Coppe, C., Kikuiri, T., Akiyama, K., Lee, J. S., Shi, S. (2008). SHED repair critical-size calvarial defects in mice, *Oral. Dis.*, **14**, 428–434.
76. Zheng, Y., Liu, Y., Zhang, C. M., Zhang, H. Y., Li, W. H., Shi, S., Le, A. D., Wang, S. L. (2009). Stem cells from deciduous tooth repair mandibular defect in swine, *J. Dent. Res.*, **88**, 249–254.
77. d'Aquino, R., De Rosa, A., Lanza, V., Tirino, V., Laino, L., Graziano, A., Desiderio, V., Laino, G., Papaccio, G. (2009). Human mandible bone defect repair by the grafting of dental pulp stem/progenitor cells and collagen sponge biocomplexes, *Eur. Cell. Mater.*, **18**, 75–83.
78. Mitsiadis, T. A., Henrique, D., Thesleff, I., Lendahl, U. (1997). Mouse Serrate-1 (Jagged-1): expression in the developing tooth is regulated by epithelial-mesenchymal interactions and fibroblast growth factor-4, *Development.*, **124**, 1473–1483.
79. Mitsiadis, T. A., Lardelli, M., Lendahl, U., Thesleff, I. (1995). Expression of Notch-1, 2 and 3 is regulated by epithelial-mesenchymal interactions and retinoic acid in the developing mouse tooth and associated with determination of ameloblast cell fate, *J. Cell. Biol.*, **130**, 407–418.
80. Mitsiadis, T. A., Hirsinger, E., Lendahl, U., Goridis, C. (1998). Delta-notch signaling in odontogenesis: correlation with cytodifferentiation and evidence for feedback regulation, *Dev. Biol.*, **204**, 420–431.
81. Nakao, A., Kajiya, H., Fukushima, H., Fukushima, A., Anan, H., Ozeki, S., Okabe, K. (2009). PTHrP induces Notch signaling in periodontal ligament cells, *J. Dent. Res.*, **88**, 551–556.
82. Sun, H., Kawashima, N., Xu, J., Takahashi, S., Suda, H. (2010). Expression of Notch signalling-related genes in normal and differentiating rat dental pulp cells, *Aust. Endod. J.*, **36**, 54–58.

83. Mitsiadis, T. A., Graf, D., Luder, H., Gridley, T., Bluteau, G. (2010). BMPs and FGFs target Notch signalling via jagged-2 to regulate tooth morphogenesis and cytodifferentiation, *Development.*, **137**, 3025–3035.

84. Mitsiadis, T. A., Fried, K., Goridis, C. (1999). Reactivation of Delta-Notch signaling after injury: complementary expression patterns of ligand and receptor in dental pulp, *Exp. Cell. Res.*, **246**, 312–318.

85. Shi, S., Gronthos, S. (2003). Perivascular niche of postnatal mesenchymal stem cells in human bone marrow and dental pulp, *J. Bone. Miner. Res.*, **18**, 696–704.

86. Zhang, C., Chang, J., Sonoyama, W., Shi, S., Wang, C. Y. (2008). Inhibition of human dental pulp stem cell differentiation by Notch signaling, *J. Dent. Res.*, **87**, 250–255.

87. Liu, L., Ling, J., Wei, X., Wu, L., Xiao, Y. (2009). Stem cell regulatory gene expression in human adult dental pulp and periodontal ligament cells undergoing odontogenic/osteogenic differentiation, *J. Endod.*, **35**, 1368–1376.

88. Xin, Y., Lu, Q., Li, Q. (2011). IKK1 control of epidermal differentiation is modulated by Notch signaling, *Am. J. Pathol.*, **178**, 1568–1577.

89. Iglesias-Bartolome, R., Gutkind, J. S. (2011). Signaling circuitries controlling stem cell fate: to be or not to be, *Curr. Opin. Cell. Biol.*, **23**, 716–723.

90. Rangarajan, A., Talora, C., Okuyama, R., Nicolas, M., Mammucari, C., Oh, H., Aster, J. C., Krishna, S., Metzger, D., Chambon, P., Miele, L., Aguet, M., Radtke, F., Dotto, G. P. (2001). Notch signaling is a direct determinant of keratinocyte growth arrest and entry into differentiation, *EMBO. J.*, **20**, 3427–3436.

91. Lowell, S., Jones, P., Le Roux, I., Dunne, J., Watt, F. M. (2000). Stimulation of human epidermal differentiation by delta-notch signalling at the boundaries of stem-cell clusters, *Curr. Biol.*, **10**, 491–500.

92. Nickoloff, B. J., Qin, J. Z., Chaturvedi, V., Denning, M. F., Bonish, B., Miele, L. (2002). Jagged-1 mediated activation of notch signaling induces complete maturation of human keratinocytes through NF-kappaB and PPARgamma, *Cell. Death. Differ.*, **9**, 842–855.

93. Small, D., Kovalenko, D., Kacer, D., Liaw, L., Landriscina, M., Di Serio, C., Prudovsky, I., Maciag, T. (2001). Soluble Jagged-1 represses the function of its transmembrane form to induce the formation of the Src-dependent chord-like phenotype, *J. Biol. Chem.*, **276**, 32022–32030.

94. Hicks, C., Ladi, E., Lindsell, C., Hsieh, J. J., Hayward, S. D., Collazo, A., Weinmaster, G. (2002). A secreted Delta-1-Fc fusion protein functions both as an activator and inhibitor of Notch-1 signaling, *J. Neurosci. Res.*, **68**, 655–667.

95. Varnum-Finney, B., Wu, L., Yu, M., Brashem-Stein, C., Staats, S., Flowers, D., Griffin, J. D., Bernstein, I. D. (2000). Immobilization of Notch ligand, Delta-1, is required for induction of notch signaling, *J. Cell. Sci.*, **113**, 4313–4318.

96. Beckstead, B. L., Santosa, D. M., Giachelli, C. M. (2006). Mimicking cell–cell interactions at the biomaterial-cell interface for control of stem cell differentiation, *J. Biomed. Mater. Res. A.*, **79**, 94–103.

97. Beckstead, B. L., Tung, J. C., Liang, K. J., Tavakkol, Z., Usui, M. L., Olerud, J. E., Giachelli, C. M. (2009). Methods to promote Notch signaling at the biomaterial interface and evaluation in a rafted organ culture model, *J. Biomed. Mater. Res. A.*, **91**, 436–446.

98. Goncalves, R. M., Martins, M. C., Almeida-Porada, G., Barbosa, M. A. (2009). Induction of notch signaling by immobilization of jagged-1 on self-assembled monolayers, *Biomaterials.*, **30**, 6879–6887.

99. Toda, H., Yamamoto, M., Kohara, H., Tabata, Y. (2011). Orientation-regulated immobilization of Jagged-1 on glass substrates for ex vivo proliferation of a bone marrow cell population containing hematopoietic stem cells, *Biomaterials.*, **32**, 6920–6928.

100. Moks, T., Abrahmsen, L., Nilsson, B., Hellman, U., Sjoquist, J., Uhlen, M. (1986). Staphylococcal protein A consists of five IgG-binding domains, *Eur. J. Biochem.*, **156**, 637–643.

101. Aybay, C. (2003). Differential binding characteristics of protein G and protein A for Fc fragments of papain-digested mouse IgG, *Immunol. Lett.*, **85**, 231–235.

102. Taqvi, S., Dixit, L., Roy, K. (2006). Biomaterial-based notch signaling for the differentiation of hematopoietic stem cells into T cells, *J. Biomed. Mater. Res. A.*, **79**, 689–697.

103. Varnum-Finney, B., Purton, L. E., Yu, M., Brashem-Stein, C., Flowers, D., Staats, S., Moore, K. A., Le Roux, I., Mann, R., Gray, G., Artavanis-Tsakanas, S., Bernstein, I. D. (1998). The Notch ligand, Jagged-1, influences the development of primitive hematopoietic precursor cells, *Blood.*, **91**, 4084–4091.

104. Awong, G., Herer, E., Surh, C. D., Dick, J. E., La Motte-Mohs, R. N., Zuniga-Pflucker, J. C. (2009). Characterization in vitro and

engraftment potential in vivo of human progenitor T cells generated from hematopoietic stem cells, *Blood.*, **114**, 972–982.

105. Kutlesa, S., Zayas, J., Valle, A., Levy, R. B., Jurecic, R. (2009). T-cell differentiation of multipotent hematopoietic cell line EML in the OP9-DL1 coculture system, *Exp. Hematol.*, **37**, 909–923.

106. Lee, J., Kotov, N. A. (2009). Notch ligand presenting acellular 3D microenvironments for ex vivo human hematopoietic stem-cell culture made by layer-by-layer assembly, *Small.*, **5**, 1008–1013.

107. Lin, G. L, Hankenson, K. D. (2011). Integration of BMP, Wnt, and notch signaling pathways in osteoblast differentiation, *J. Cell. Biochem.*, **112**, 3491–3501.

108. Shimizu, T., Tanaka, T., Iso, T., Matsui, H., Ooyama, Y., Kawai-Kowase, K., Arai, M., Kurabayashi, M. (2011). Notch signaling pathway enhances bone morphogenetic protein 2 (BMP2) responsiveness of Msx2 gene to induce osteogenic differentiation and mineralization of vascular smooth muscle cells, *J. Biol. Chem.*, **286**, 19138–19148.

109. Dishowitz, M. I., Terkhorn, S. P., Bostic, S. A., Hankenson, K. D. (2012). Notch signaling components are upregulated during both endochondral and intramembranous bone regeneration, *J. Orthop. Res.*, **30**, 296–303.

110. Balduino, A., Hurtado, S. P., Frazao, P., Takiya, C. M., Alves, L. M., Nasciutti, L. E., El-Cheikh, M. C., Borojevic, R. (2005). Bone marrow subendosteal microenvironment harbours functionally distinct haemosupportive stromal cell populations, *Cell. Tissue. Res.*, **319**, 255–266.

111. Fujita, S., Toguchida, J., Morita, Y., Iwata, H. (2008). Clonal analysis of hematopoiesis-supporting activity of human mesenchymal stem cells in association with Jagged-1 expression and osteogenic potential, *Cell. Transplant.*, **17**, 1169–1179.

112. Ugarte, F., Ryser, M., Thieme, S., Fierro, F. A., Navratiel, K., Bornhauser, M., Brenner, S. (2009). Notch signaling enhances osteogenic differentiation while inhibiting adipogenesis in primary human bone marrow stromal cells, *Exp. Hematol.*, **37**, 867–875, e861.

113. Nobta, M., Tsukazaki, T., Shibata, Y., Xin, C., Moriishi, T., Sakano, S., Shindo, H., Yamaguchi, A. (2005). Critical regulation of bone morphogenetic protein-induced osteoblastic differentiation by Delta-1/Jagged-1-activated Notch-1 signaling, *J. Biol. Chem.*, **280**, 15842–15848.

114. Xing, Q., Ye, Q., Fan, M., Zhou, Y., Xu, Q., Sandham, A. (2010). Porphyromonas gingivalis lipopolysaccharide inhibits the osteoblastic

differentiation of preosteoblasts by activating Notch-1 signaling, *J. Cell. Physiol.*, **225**, 106–114.

115. Hilton, M. J., Tu, X., Wu, X., Bai, S., Zhao, H., Kobayashi, T., Kronenberg, H. M., Teitelnaum, S. L., Ross, F. P., Kopan, R., Long, F. (2008). Notch signaling maintains bone marrow mesenchymal progenitors by suppressing osteoblast differentiation, *Nat. Med.*, **14**, 306–314.

116. Zanotti, S., Smerdel-Ramoya, A., Canalis, E. (2011). Reciprocal regulation of Notch and nuclear factor of activated T-cells (NFAT) c1 transactivation in osteoblasts, *J. Biol. Chem.*, **286**, 4576–4588.

117. Wikesjo, U. M., Selvig, K. A. (1999). Periodontal wound healing and regeneration, *Periodontol. 2000.*, **19**, 21–39.

118. Baker, D. L., Stanley Pavlow, S. A., Wikesjo, U. M. (2005). Fibrin clot adhesion to dentin conditioned with protein constructs: an in vitro proof-of-principle study, *J. Clin. Periodontol.*, **32**, 561–566.

119. Darby, I. (2011). Periodontal materials, *Aust. Dent. J.*, **56 Suppl 1**, 107–118.

120. Pedrazzini, T. (2007). Control of cardiogenesis by the notch pathway, *Trends. Cardiovasc. Med.*, **17**, 83–90.

121. Sofi, F. A., Ahmed, S. H., Dar, M. A., Nabhi, D. G., Mufti, S., Bhat, M. A., Tabassum, P. N. (2010). Nontraumatic massive right-sided Bochdalek hernia in an adult: an unusual presentation, *Am. J. Emerg. Med.*, **29**, 356 e355–357.

122. Li, Y., Hiroi, Y., Liao, J. K. (2010). Notch signaling as an important mediator of cardiac repair and regeneration after myocardial infarction, *Trends. Cardiovasc. Med.*, **20**, 228–231.

123. Gude, N. A., Emmanuel, G., Wu, W., Cottage, C. T., Fischer, K., Quijada, P., Muraski, J. A., Alvarez, R., Rubio, M., Schaefer, E., Sussman, M. A. (2008). Activation of Notch-mediated protective signaling in the myocardium, *Circ. Res.*, **102**, 1025–1035.

124. Li, H., Yu, B., Zhang, Y., Pan, Z., Xu, W. (2006). Jagged-1 protein enhances the differentiation of mesenchymal stem cells into cardiomyocytes, *Biochem. Biophys. Res. Commun.*, **341**, 320–325.

125. Sassoli, C., Pini, A., Mazzanti, B., Quercioli, F., Nistri, S., Saccardi, R., Zecchi-Oralandini, S., Bani, D., Formigli, L. (2011). Mesenchymal stromal cells affect cardiomyocyte growth through juxtacrine Notch-1/Jagged-1 signaling and paracrine mechanisms: clues for cardiac regeneration, *J. Mol. Cell. Cardiol.*, **51**, 399–408.

126. Collesi, C., Zentilin, L., Sinagra, G., Giacca, M. (2008). Notch-1 signaling stimulates proliferation of immature cardiomyocytes, *J. Cell. Biol.*, **183**, 117–128.

127. Osathanon, T., Ritprajak, P., Nowwarote, N., Manokawinchoke, J., Giachelli, C. M., Pavasant, P. (2013). Surface-bound orientated Jagged-1 enhances osteogenic differentiation of human periodontal ligament derived mesenchymal stem cells, *J. Biomed. Mater. Res. A.*, **101**, 358–167. (Accepted Jun 18, 2012).

Chapter 16

Stem Cell-Based Dental, Oral, and Craniofacial Tissue Engineering

Sahng G. Kim,[a,b] Chang Hun Lee,[a] Jian Zhou,[a] Mo Chen,[a] Ying Zheng,[a] Mildred C. Embree,[a] Kimi Kong,[a] Karen Song,[a] Susan Y. Fu,[a] Shoko Cho,[a] Nan Jiang,[a] and Jeremy J. Mao[a]

[a]*Center for Craniofacial Regeneration, Columbia University, 630 W. 168 St. PH7Stem #128, New York, NY 10032, USA*
[b]*Division of Endodontics, College of Dental Medicine, Columbia University, 630 W. 168 St. PH7E, New York, NY 10032, USA*

jmao@columbia.edu

16.1 Introduction

Orofacial structures not only are of critical importance for esthetics but also serve indispensible functions, including breathing, eating, hearing, sight, and smell. Although substantial progress has been made, much is yet to be learned toward both fundamental understanding of orofacial stem/progenitor cells and clinical translation [47].

16.2 Challenges of Orofacial Tissue Regeneration

Some of the characteristics of orofacial structures are unusual or even unique. For example, a tooth develops by an epithelial-mesenchymal interaction that results in the formation of highly mineralized and hierarchical structures, including the enamel, dentin, and cementum as well as a specialized loose connective tissue, dental pulp [8,24,45]. Encased in highly mineralized dentin, the dental pulp contains mainly interstitial fibroblasts in the center, and odontoblasts lining the dentin surface at the periphery, as well as other cells such as nerve fibers, endothelial cells, and stem/progenitor cells that presumably replenish all pulp cells in tissue turnover and injury. The periodontium includes the cementum on the surface of tooth root, the periodontal ligament, and the alveolar bone. The periodontium withstands the physiological forces and maintains homeostasis. Some of the distinctive features of orofacial structures present challenges for tissue regeneration:

- frequently heterogeneous structures originating from both epithelium and mesenchyme
- Small-scale but highly complex structures that exert multiple functionality
- esthetically demanding in addition to anatomically intricate
- oral cavity presenting a highly contaminated environment but nonetheless heals with little scar tissue

Two approaches have been practiced in experimental studies of orofacial regeneration studies:

(1) cell transplantation entailing isolation of cells, including stem/progenitor cells, and ex vivo cell manipulation, followed by delivery of cells as an in vivo graft to the host
(2) cell homing by delivery of signaling molecules, rather than cells, into the host to induce cell migration, attachment, proliferation, and differentiation of endogenous stem/progenitor cells

16.3 Orofacial Stem/Progenitor Cells

Recently, orofacial stem/progenitor cells have been critically reviewed with regard to their properties, limitations, and benefits toward potential use in tissue regeneration [47]. There are two types of orofacial stem/progenitor cells: (1) epithelium stem cells and (2) connective tissue or mesenchyme stem/progenitor cells. Epithelium stem cells and connective stem/progenitor cells of dental origin are separately discussed below.

16.3.1 Dental Epithelial Stem Cells

Dental epithelium stem cells derive from neural crest cells and differentiate into ameloblasts that form tooth enamel. Dental epithelium stem cells are located in the stellate reticulum of the developing teeth. In humans, ameloblasts are irretrievably lost after tooth eruption, with the perhaps fortunate caveat that some dental epithelium stem cells are left behind in the periodontal ligament in postnatal life, known as the epithelial cell rests of Malassez (ECRM) [23]. Rodent incisors continue to grow and erupt throughout life, displaying continuous enamel matrix formation by ameloblasts on the labial surface only, along with corresponding dentin formation on both the labial and lingual sides [33,48]. During development of rodent incisors, dental epithelium stem cells migrate from the stellate reticulum to the labial surface and replenish a population of proliferating, transit amplifying cells, which continue to differentiate into ameloblasts and deposit enamel matrix [77]. The lack of enamel on the lingual surface of the rodent teeth is attributed to the spatial differences in the expression of activin and follistatin, an activin antagonist [77]. Given the disappearance of dental epithelium stem cells in humans following tooth eruption, there is yet a demonstration of whether postnatal human dental epithelium stem cells are of therapeutic value in the regeneration of tooth structures, regardless of the third molars or the epithelium cell rests of Malassez.

16.3.2 Dental Mesenchyme Stem/Progenitor Cells

16.3.2.1 Periodontal ligament

The majority of cells in the periodontal ligament (PDL) are fibroblasts that engage in matrix synthesis and maintenance of homeostasis [61], in addition to odontoblasts that align dentin surface, macrophages, mast cells, and endothelial cells of blood vessels. Among abundant fibroblasts, there are rare cells with stem/progenitor cell properties [61]. Cells that are positive to STRO-1 and CD146/MUC18 differentiate into cementoblasts, adipocytes, collagen forming cells in vitro. Periodontal ligament stem/progenitor cells incorporated in hydroxyapatite (HA)/tricalcium phosphate (TCP) form cementum-like and PDL-like structures in immunodeficient rats [61]. Cryopreserved PDL stem/progenitor cells apparently maintain some of the properties and continue to form mineralized tissues in vivo [62].

16.3.2.2 Dental pulp

Dental pulp stem/progenitor cells are typically isolated from dental pulp of extracted deciduous or permanent teeth and commonly express CD146, α-smooth muscle actin and pericyte-associated antigen (3G5) among other markers [15,64]. Stem/progenitor cells from dental pulp differentiate into dentinogenic/osteogenic, chondrogenic, adipogenic, myogenic, and neurogenic lineages ex vivo in chemically defined media [4,16,39,85] even after cryopreservation [78,85]. Upon pulpal injury, stem/progenitor cells are activated and migrate toward the site of injury [72]. Serial transplantion of pulp stem/progenitor cells retain some of the original capcity to form dentin/pulp-like structure [4]. In addition to the permanent teeth, dental pulp of deciduous teeth also harbor cells that differentiate into adipocytes and form bone/dentin-like tissues when placed in TCP in the dorsum of immunodeficient mice [4,15,24,51,63]. Apical papilla is the portion of dental papilla prior to full closure and development of the root. Cells with stem/progenitor cell properties have been isolated from apical papilla prior to the completion of root development (http://www.cartilage.org/index.php?pid=22). When transplanted in hydroxyapatite scafolds, cells from apical papilla yield mineralized tissue and a PDL-like structure in tooth extraction sockets [66,67].

16.3.2.3 Dental follicle

Dental follicle develops into the PDL and alveolar bone, and cementum [50]. Certain cells isolated from dental follicle express putative stem/progenitor markers such as Notch-1 and Nestin. Dental follicle cells differntiatite into cementoblast-like cells that are positive to cementum attachment protein (CAP) and cementum protein-23 (CP-23) [34] and form cementum-like matrix in severe combined immunodeficency (SCID) mice [18]. Dental follicle cells immortalized by a retrovirus-expressing human papilloma virus formed PDL-like and bone-like tissues after subcutaneous transplantion into SCID mice [82].

16.4 Tooth Regeneration

The understanding of tooth development reveals important clues for tooth regeneration. Reciprocal interactions between oral epithelium and mesenchyme are indispensible for tooth development. Localized thickening of oral epithelium invaginates into the underlying mesenchyme and signals the initiation of tooth development [73,74]. Signaling molecules released from oral epithelium such as FGF8, BMP4, Shh, and Wnt induce the differentiation of underlying mesenchyme cells toward dental mesenchyme [33]. The patterning of dentition is further regulated by the expression of homeobox genes such as Msx-1 and -2, Dlx-1 and -2, and Barx-1 in the underlying mesenchyme [73]. Epithelial and mesenchymal cells eventually form a bell shaped crown or the tooth germ that loses its connection to oral epithelium. During crown formation, mesenchymally derived dental papilla cells differentiate into odontoblasts. Root formation begins after crown formation and is characterized by odontoblast differentiation upon interactions with the inner epithelial cells of Hertwig's epithelial root sheath. Dental follicle cells give rise to cementoblasts, PDL cells, and alveolar bone cells.

To date, the majority of tooth regeneration strategies have attempted to mimic the developmental process of tooth formation [46,47]. Ohazama et al. [55] showed in a mouse model that recombination between cells from nondental cell derived mesenchyme, including embryonic stem cells, neural stem cells and bone marrow cells, and oral epithelial cells, could trigger odontogenesis in the mesenchyme from different sources. When transplanted into a renal capsule, the recombinant formed the tooth-like structure consisting of enamel, dentin, and dental pulp as well as ameloblasts and odontoblasts, all of which were donor derived. Hu et al. [21] demonstrated that dissociated epithelial cells/tissues and mesenchymal cells/tissues re-organized in vitro and formed the bell shape tooth germ structure with functional differentiation of ameloblasts and odontoblasts. After 2 week transplantation under the skin of adult mice, the development of root and PDL was observed with the developing bone. Furthermore, it was suggested that tooth morphogenesis using dissociated cells/tissues could be modulated by increasing the number of mesenchymal cells re-organized with the epithelial cells/tissues.

Another strategy is to transplant biomaterial scaffolds seeded with the tooth forming cells such as tooth bud cells and mesenchymal stem cells. In a study by Young et al. [83], dissociated tooth bud cells from third molars of 6 month-old pigs were seeded in polyglycolate/poly-L-lactate (PGA/PLLA) and poly-L-lactate-co-glycolate (PLGA) tooth scaffolds, and implanted in the omenta of athymic rats. After 20 to 30 week implantation, tooth crown-like structures consisting of enamel, dentin, pulp chamber with odontoblasts as well as cementum and cementoblasts were regenerated. Kuo et al. [38] obtained dental bud cells (DBCs) in a similar way from 1.5 month-old pigs. Dental bud cells then were seeded onto gelatin–chondroitin–hyaluronan tri-copolymer scaffold and implanted into the original extraction site. Thirty-six weeks after implantation, tooth-like structures containing pulp-dentin complex with odontoblasts and vasculature in the pulp and cellular cementum surrounded by PDL and bone were observed. Although two of six animals showed the tooth regeneration, it was suggested that the morphology of the regenerated tooth could be controlled by the size of the scaffold seeded with DBCs [38]. Sonoyama et al. [66] combined apical papilla cells and PDL cells onto HA/TCP carrier and gelfoam, respectively, and inserted into the extraction socket of a lower incisor in a swine model. After eight weeks post transplantation, tooth root and PDL complex was regenerated. Another experiment by Young et al. [84] showed that a partially regenerated tooth crown using PGA/PLLA scaffolds seeded with swine tooth bud cells as shown in the previous experiment [83] when combined and sutured with PLGA scaffolds seeded with osteoblasts induced from swine bone marrow stem/stromal cells could generate a tooth-bone hybrid construct with PDL-like structure at the interface in the rat omentum.

Cell homing has been recently attempted to form tooth roots by recruitment of tissue forming cells, including stem/progenitor cells, to biomaterial scaffolds by signaling molecules. The fabrication of the bioscaffolds with the same shape and dimension as real sized teeth is attainable with the three-dimensional (3D) bioprinting method through 3D layer-by-layer apposition [36,70,81]. In a study by Kim et al. [36], the anatomically shaped human molar scaffolds and rat incisor scaffolds with 200 μm-diameter microchannels were fabricated by this method with a composite of poly-ε-caprolactone (PCL) and HA. The scaffolds were infused with collagen gels loaded with two signaling molecules, including stromal-derived factor-1 (SDF1) and bone morphogenetic protein-7 (BMP7). The two signaling molecules are considered to be of critical importance in regenerating a tooth. SDF1 is a chemoattractant involved in the mobilization of cells, including hematopoietic stem cells [79], mesenchymal stromal cells [9], and immune cells [79] by binding to the chemokine receptor CXCR4 [49]. BMP7 is known to induce osteogenic and dentinogenic differentiation in mesenchymal cells [29,59,65,76]. The scaffolds with bioactive cues were implanted orthotopically and ectopically into rats [36]. Nine weeks post surgery, the incisor scaffolds harvested from the socket of rat lower incisors revealed PDL and new bone formation between the scaffolds and native alveolar bone. Although this study was not designed to regenerate enamel, cell homing strategy could be useful in the regeneration of tooth roots that are designed to support clinical, prosthetic crowns.

16.5 Dental Pulp and Dentin Regeneration

Dental pulp and dentin regeneration is likely a low-hanging fruit in orofacial tissue engineering. Clinical acceptance for dentin-pulp regeneration is quite high, per the American Dental Association (ADA) and the American Association of Endodontists [2]. Dentin-pulp regeneration is to restore the functionality of the pulp-dentin complex. Complete dentin-pulp regeneration includes pulp vasculature, nociceptive and sympathetic/parasympathetic nerve fibers, functional odontoblasts lining the dentin surface, and interstitial fibroblasts as well as stem/progenitor cells that serve to replenish all pulp cells lost from normal turnover or injury.

Dental pulp revascularization is a separate process and has been pursued by anecdotal observations involving successful clinical case series/reports with the use of antibiotics and/or induced bleeding into the root canal space or a platelet rich plasma delivery system [3,28,30,54,58,75]. Dental pulp regeneration inevitably includes pulp revascularization but pulp revascularization arguably is only a component of all pulp tissues that are to be regenerated [37].

A small number of experimental studies have shown regeneration of pulp-like tissues using two separate strategies: cell transplantation and cell homing. In several studies, the ectopic in vivo transplantation of dental pulp stem cells or other stem/progenitor cells could generate pulp-like tissues. In a study by Cordeiro et al. [7], the formation of vascular pulp-like tissue was observed when SHED, seeded onto gels in a tooth slice, were transplanted subcutaneously into immunodeficient mice. Huang et al. [24] also demonstrated the formation of pulp-like tissue with odontoblastic layers in root fragments when synthetic scaffolds seeded with stem/progenitor cells from the apical papilla and dental pulp were implanted into the dorsum of mice. In addition to the ability to control the number of cells to be transplanted, the cell transplantation approach has other major benefits, including the selection of the best subpopulation of transplanted cells. Iohara et al. [25,26] showed that side population (SP) cells from the dental pulp had higher self-renewal and multipotentiality compared to the heterogeneous non-SP cells, while maintaining differentiation potential such as high angiogenic ability that could promote neovascularization in the pulp. These fractionated cells may have a greater utility to induce the formation of pulp-like tissues consisting of nerves, vasculature, and dentin [27].

Cell homing has recently been attempted in dental pulp regeneration. Kim et al. [35] used several growth factors, including basic fibroblast growth factors (bFGFs), vascular endothelial growth factors (VEGFs), platelet-derived growth factors (PDGFs), nerve growth factors (NGFs), and bone morphogenetic protein-7 (BMP7) in an ectopic tooth implantation model in mice. Human extracted teeth were endodontically treated without root canal filling so that the root canal space could allow for tissue regeneration. The emptied root canal space without any biological or organic substances was filled with collagen scaffolds that were impregnated with the growth factors. After 3- to 6 week in vivo subcutaneous tooth implantation in mice, vascular pulp-like tissues with nerves and odontoblast-like cells were observed in the entire length of root canals. This was the first demonstration that the pulp-like tissues in a root canal space could be regenerated by the homing of endogenous cells from the host, guided by growth factors, without cell transplantation. A cocktail of growth factors in this study served a multitude of functions that induce the formation of the pulp-dentin complex. bFGF, VEGF, and PDGF played a role in chemotaxis; PDGF and VEGF in angiogenesis; NGF in neuronal growth and survival; and BMP-7 in mineralization. Cell homing strategy by recruitment of host endogenous cells circumvents some of barriers in association with cell transplantation such as cell isolation, ex vivo cell manipulation with the potential of altering cell phenotype, as well as safety issues, including immunorejection, pathogen transmission, and tumorigenesis [46].

16.6 Periodontal Regeneration

Periodontal regeneration aims to restore the functionality of the periodontium, consisting of cementum, PDL, and alveolar bone. Clinically, certain periodontal defects fail to heal and lead to tooth loss. Defective area after surgical debridement is prone to be filled with long junctional oral epithelial cells rather than PDL fibroblasts and bone cells that contribute to the restoration of the original architecture and function of the periodontium. In order to induce periodontal healing, various types of periodontal regenerative surgery have been attempted. These include guided tissue regeneration (GTR) [31] with/without bone grafts and delivery of biochemical mediators with natural and synthetic polymers [20,60]. The GTR method utilizes the principle of selecting and allowing slowly growing but favorable cells to repopulate the periodontal defects by blocking the fast-growing long junctional epithelial cells with barrier membranes. The biochemical mediators such as growth factors [6,53,69] and enamel matrix derivatives (Emdogain®) [12,17,57] have been shown to stimulate the cell attachment, proliferation, and differentiation as well as cell homing. The clinical usefulness of these approaches, however, has only been established in limited clinical situations because of the constant challenges of contamination and reinfection at the surgical site by oral microflora. Additionally, there is uncertainty as to the predictability of the natural/synthetic materials that have been used in periodontal regenerative procedures.

There have been a limited number of clinical studies with an end goal to regenerate the periodontium with various biological mediators in scaffolds. Lynch et al. [44] showed that alveolar bone and cementum were formed 2 weeks after the application of an aqueous gel of PDGF and insulin-like growth factor-1 (IGF-1) to surgically created periodontal defects in beagle dogs while no new bone or cementum formation was observed in controls. Giannobile et al. [13] further compared the effect of PDGF and IGF-1 in two animal models, including beagle dogs and nonhuman primates.

There were significant increases in new bone and attachment formation in periodontal defects 1 month after the use of PDGF/IGF-1 compared to controls. Although there were some differences in response to the growth factors between the two animal species, in general PDGF/IGF-1 promoted significant periodontal regeneration. Similar results were reported in another study by Giannobile et al. [14] in a nonhuman primate model. In this study, the results showed that IGF-1 alone did not significantly promote periodontal healing but PDGF-bb and PDGF-bb/IGF-1 did significantly increase the periodontal tissue healing. Nevins et al. [52] recently showed that in their multicenter human randomized controlled trials, significant improvements in clinical periodontal healing parameters such as clinical attachment level gain and linear bone growth were observed in local periodontal bony defects three years after local PDGF-bb delivery with a synthetic bioscaffold (β-TCP). Other growth factors such as bFGF [1,51], BMP [5,68], and transforming growth factor β (TGFβ) [40,71] have also been suggested for periodontal regenerative therapy.

Cell-based strategies have shown some promise for periodontal regeneration in animal models. Periodontal or bone marrow stem/progenitor cells have been delivered to periodontal defects to investigate their efficacy in regenerating periodontal tissues. Liu et al. [43] used ex vivo expanded PDL stem/progenitor cells in a minipig model. Local osseous defects were surgically created in the mesial region of upper and lower first molars to generate periodontal lesions [43]. HA/TCP scaffolds with or without autologous cells were transplanted into the local periodontal defects [43]. Twelve weeks post transplantation, improved periodontal tissue regeneration was observed clinically and histologically in cell delivery group than HA/TCP alone. The immunogenetic property of periodontal stem/progenitor cells is low and may be used for allogeneic transplanted, owing to suppression of T-cell proliferation through prostaglandin E2.

Kawaguchi et al. [32] investigated periodontal tissue regeneration in beagle dogs after auto-transplantation of bone marrow stem/stromal cells into class III furcation defects. Bone marrow cells isolated from bone marrow aspirates from iliac crest in beagle dogs were expanded and mixed with atelocollagen (2% type I collagen) before being transplanted into surgically created type III furcation defects of mandibular premolars in each dog.

One month post transplantation, significantly higher amounts of new bone and cementum were observed in the cell-atelocollagen groups compared to the atelocollagen control groups based on histomorphometric analysis. A further study by Hasegawa et al. [19] in the same experimental model revealed that transplanted GFP-labeled bone marrow cells contributed to the regenerated tissues in furcation defects as evidenced by the presence of GFP-positive differentiated cells in the area. Li et al. [42] showed that bone marrow cells were able to retain their regenerative capacity after cryopreservation for 1 month in vitro and in vivo. The cryopreserved bone marrow cells were shown to have in vitro cell behaviors such as cell viability, cell attachment, osteogenic differentiation similar to those of the unfrozen bone marrow cells. When surgically created periodontal bone fenestrations in vivo were filled with cryopreserved and noncryopreserved bone marrow cells seeded onto collagen scaffolds in beagle dogs, respectively, there were no significant differences between the two cell groups in the percentage of alveolar bone, cementum, and PDL regeneration. Periodontal regeneration was significantly higher in both cell delivery groups compared to the control (scaffold alone) group, suggesting the potential use of cryopreserved bone marrow cells for periodontal regeneration.

16.7 Calvarial Bone Regeneration

Craniofacial skeletal defects, resulting from traumatic injuries, tumor resection as well as various craniofacial syndromes can severely affect a patient's quality of life by deforming the esthetic and functional roles of the original skeletal structures. The reconstruction of craniofacial skeletal structures remains a challenge for contemporary surgical approaches [11]. Advances in craniofacial tissue engineering may hold a promise to address this demand, among which calvarial bone regeneration is perhaps most likely to meet the clinical needs in the near future.

A breakthrough study by Cowan et al. [8] demonstrated that adipose stem/progenitor cells (ASCs) healed critical-size calvarial bone defects in mice. Mouse ASCs seeded onto apatite-coated synthetic scaffolds were transplanted into 4 mm critical-size parietal defects in 2 month-old mice. The osteogenic ability of ASCs in the calvarial defects was compared to bone marrow stromal cells, calvarial-derived osteoblasts, and dura mater cells. Significant bone formation was observed in all groups except for the control (no cell) group but mineralization was highest in the calvarial-derived osteoblasts group and lowest in dura mater cell group, which is equivalent to the control. Intramembranous bone formation was shown to be the mechanism of ossification as evidenced by the absence of cartilage. Similar bone formation and mineralization were observed between ASCs and bone marrow stromal cells. The use of ASCs in calvarial defects may have several benefits, including a higher harvest rate, an easier harvesting technique, faster ex vivo cell expansion, and the avoidance of issues related to bone grafting [8]. A similar study was performed with the use of human ASCs, harvested from lipoaspirate, in mouse calvarial defects by Levi et al. [41]. It was shown that human ASCs healed critical-size mouse cranial defects with enhanced regeneration from BMP-2 supplementation.

A recent study by Osugi et al. [56] showed that culture conditioned media from human BMMSCs could be used to augment calvarial bone regeneration without cell transplantation. The cell culture conditioned media were collected after 2 day incubation of cultured human bone marrow stem/stromal cells in serum free media and stored for the subsequent experiments. Cell migration, proliferation, and expression of osteogenic markers such as OCN and Runx2 were increased using the conditioned media in vitro, which is presumed to be due to the presence of growth factors such as IGF-1 and VEGF detected in the media by enzyme-linked immunosorbent assays. Further in vivo experiments revealed that the culture conditioned media in agarose gels regenerated a higher amount of bone in circular calvarial bone defects (5 mm in diameter) than BMMSC/agarose, serum free medium/agarose, PBS/agarose, and control (defect alone) groups. The origin of cells contributing to the regenerated tissues was investigated using the tracing of DiR-labeled cells injected into caudal veins and GFP positive cells in transgenic mice. The cell tracing using in vivo imaging and immunohistochemical staining showed that endogenous host cells were recruited to the calvarial defects for regeneration. In another recent study by Dumas et al. [10], extensive new bone bridging with higher mineralization was observed when injectable lysine-derived polyurethane/allograft biocomposites with BMP-2 were implanted into 15 mm critical size calvarial defects in rabbits.

Significantly enhanced calvarial regeneration was reported when PDGF-BB and BMMSCs with β-TCP scaffolds were transplanted compared with BMMSCs/β-TCP, PDGF-BB/β-TCP, and β-TCP only group in a study by Xu et al. [80] using a rat critical-size calvarial defect model.

16.8 Clinical Engagement and Training for Regenerative Therapies

Practitioners are the final key factor in the delivery of regenerative therapies. It is vital for clinical practitioners to be involved in the innovation of regenerative therapies. Clinical input is indispensable for the creation of regenerative therapies, for without clinical input, the novel regenerative therapies may not be applicable in a clinical setting. The majority of clinicians currently lack the expertise to handle and grow cells in the laboratory. As described above, regenerative therapies may present in two forms: cell transplantation and cell homing. The lack of knowledge and skills in cell handling can be a significant barrier in therapeutic applications of cell therapy. Cell homing offers a more readily approach for practitioners, given that bioactive cues can be prepackaged and made available in a hospital or medical/dental office.

One of the major concerns in cell delivery by inexperienced practitioners is the contamination of donor cells during the transplantation procedure. A practitioner's office is infection controlled but nonetheless is not a sterile environment. Cell handling, however, should be performed in a sterile or at least highly disinfected environment. Cell manipulation, especially when combined with scaffold preparation for cell transplantation cannot be performed in a chair side setting. It perhaps requires laboratory equipment that allows for a disinfected clinical atmosphere even though the stem cell product is most likely resistant to a low-grade infection challenge, due to the antimycotic-antibiotics supplementation. If cells are contaminated during handling, a various degree of clinical failures can be expected to occur, such as the death of viable cells at grafting sites, morbidity by infection and immunorejection at the recipient site, and severe tissue destruction due to inflammation and infections.

Orofacial structures are also prone to infections due to their anatomical and physiological characteristics, thereby making cell engraftment more challenging than other tissue regeneration. For example, oral structures are constantly challenged by exogenous and endogenous microorganisms and are, in most instances, under physiological function as in talking, chewing, swallowing, etc. Practitioners should have surgical training to perfect wound management after the cell delivery. An expanded level of surgical training can be provided to practitioners depending on the type of tissues that need to be regenerated.

Table 16.1 Challenges and strategies for clinical translation of orofacial regeneration

	Challenges	**Strategies**
Cell source	Limited number of stem cells in mature tissues; surgical harvesting technique	Cell homing to recruit endogenous cells; potential use of iPS cells
Scale up	Time and costs required for ex vivo expansion	Identify true stem cells; only need a small number of true stem cells for regeneration
Delivery method	Coordinated release of growth factors and scaffold degradation	Use of tailored scaffolds specifically for tissues of interest
Practitioner training	Ex vivo cell manipulation; wound management to prevent cell contamination	Training for cell handling and growth factor delivery

16.9 Summary

Orofacial tissues are structurally complex; all are of vital importance for esthetics. The majority of orofacial structures are connective tissues rather than vital organs. At least, risks of clinical trials of regenerative therapies for orofacial tissues are not as high as for vital organs. Novel approaches are being developed for the regeneration of teeth, dental pulp, periodontium, and orofacial bones. Much has been learned from cell transplantation, including stem/progenitor cells, in the regeneration of orofacial structures. However, cell transplantation encounters a multitude of barriers toward clinical translation. Cell homing, on the other hand, may circumvent some of the barriers in association with cell transplantation. Clinical practitioners need to be involved in the creation of regenerative therapies and begin to learn the knowledge of stem cells and tissue regeneration.

Acknowledgments

We thank Dr. Charles Solomon for critiques and F. Guo, H. Keyes, and J. Melendez for technical and administrative assistance. The effort for the composition of this article is supported by NIH grants R01DE018248, R01EB009663, and RC2DE020767 to J. J. Mao.

References

1. Akman, A. C., Tiğli, R. S., Gümüşdereliöğlu, M., and Nohutcu, R. M. (2010). bFGF-loaded HA-chitosan: a promising scaffold for periodontal tissue engineering, *J. Biomed. Mater. Res A*, **92**, 953–962.
2. American Dental Association. (2010). Changes to the code 2011–2012. *Curr. Dent. Terminol.*, 89.
3. Banchs, F., and Trope. M. (2004). Revascularization of immature permanent teeth with apical periodontitis: new treatment protocol?, *J. Endod.*, **30**, 196–200.
4. Batouli, S., Miura, M., Brahim, J., Tsutsui, T. W., Fisher, L. W., Gronthos, S., Robey, P. G., and Shi, S. (2003). Comparison of stem-cell-mediated osteogenesis and dentinogenesis, *J. Dent. Res.*, **82**, 976–981.
5. Chen, F. M., Zhao, Y. M., Zhang, R., Jin, T., Sun, H. H., Wu, Z. F., and Jin, Y. (2007). Periodontal regeneration using novel glycidyl methacrylated dextran (Dex-GMA)/gelatin scaffolds containing microspheres loaded with bone morphogenetic proteins. *J. Control. Release*, **121**, 81–90.
6. Chen, F. M., Shelton, R. M., Jin, Y., and Chapple, I. L. (2009). Localized delivery of growth factors for periodontal tissue regeneration: role, strategies, and perspectives, *Med. Res. Rev.*, **29**, 472–513.
7. Cordeiro, M. M., Dong, Z., Kaneko, T., Zhang, Z., Miyazawa, M., Shi, S., Smith, A. J., and Nör, J. E. (2008). Dental pulp tissue engineering with stem cells from exfoliated deciduous teeth, *J. Endod.*, **34**, 962–969.
8. Cowan, C. M., Shi, Y. Y., Aalami, O. O., Chou, Y. F., Mari, C., Thomas, R., Quarto, N., Contag, C. H., Wu B., and Longaker, M. T. (2004). Adipose-derived adult stromal cells heal critical-size mouse calvarial defects, *Nat. Biotechnol.*, **22**, 560–567.

9. Dar, A., Kollet, O., and Lapidot, T. (2006). Mutual, reciprocal SDF-1/CXCR4 interactions between hematopoietic and bone marrow stromal cells regulate human stem cell migration and development in NOD/SCID chimeric mice, *Exp. Hematol.*, **34**, 967–975.
10. Dumas, J. E., Brownbaer, P. B., Prieto, E. M., Guda, T., Hale, R. G., Wenke, J. C., and Guelcher, S. A. (2012). Injectable reactive biocomposites for bone healing in critical-size rabbit calvarial defects. *Biomed. Mater.*, **7**, 024112.
11. Fisher, M., Dorafshar, A., Bojovic, B., Manson, P. N., and Rodriguez, E. D. (2012). The evolution of critical concepts in aesthetic craniofacial microsurgical reconstruction, *Plast. Reconstr. Surg.*, **130**, 389–398 (Epub ahead of print).
12. Gestrelius, S., Andersson, C., Lidström, D., Hammarström, L., and Somerman, M. (1997). In vitro studies on periodontal ligament cells and enamel matrix derivative, *J. Clin. Periodontol.*, **24**, 685–692.
13. Giannobile, W. V., Finkelman, R. D., and Lynch, S. E. (1994). Comparison of canine and non-human primate animal models for periodontal regenerative therapy: results following a single administration of PDGF/IGF-I, *J. Periodontol.*, **65**, 1158–1168.
14. Giannobile, W. V., Hernandez, R. A., Finkelman, R. D., Ryan, S., Kiritsy, C. P., D'Andrea, M., and Lynch, S. E. (1996). Comparative effects of platelet-derived growth factor-BB and insulin-like growth factor-I, individually and in combination, on periodontal regeneration in Macaca fascicularis, *J. Periodontal. Res.*, **31**, 301–312.
15. Gronthos, S., Mankani, M., Brahim, J., Robey, P. G., and Shi, S. (2000). Postnatal human dental pulp stem cells (DPSCs) in vitro and in vivo, *Proc. Natl. Acad. Sci. USA*, **97**, 13625–13630.
16. Gronthos, S., Brahim, J., Li, W., Fisher, L. W., Cherman, N., Boyde, A., DenBesten, P., Robey, P. G., and Shi, S. (2002). Stem cell properties of human dental pulp stem cells, *J. Dent. Res.*, **81**, 531–535.
17. Haase, H. R., and Bartold, P. M. (2001). Enamel matrix derivative induces matrix synthesis by cultured human periodontal fibroblast cells, *J. Periodontol.*, **72**, 341–348.
18. Handa, K., Saito, M., Tsunoda, A., Yamauchi, M., Hattori, S., Sato, S., Toyoda, M., Teranaka, T., and Narayanan, A. S. (2002). Progenitor cells from dental follicle are able to form cementum matrix in vivo, *Connect. Tissue Res.*, **43**, 406–408.
19. Hasegawa, N., Kawaguchi, H., Hirachi, A., Takeda, K., Mizuno, N., Nishimura, M., Koike, C., Tsuji, K., Iba, H., Kato, Y., and Kurihara, H. (2006). Behavior of transplanted bone marrow-derived

mesenchymal stem cells in periodontal defects, *J. Periodontol.*, **77**, 1003–1007.

20. Herberg, S., Siedler, M., Pippig, S., Schuetz, A., Dony, C., Kim, C. K., and Wikesjö, U. M. (2008). Development of an injectable composite as a carrier for growth factor-enhanced periodontal regeneration, *J. Clin. Periodontol.*, **35**, 976–984.

21. Hu, B., Nadiri, A., Kuchler-Bopp, S., Perrin-Schmitt, F., Peters, H., and Lesot, H. (2006). Tissue engineering of tooth crown, root, and periodontium, *Tissue Eng.*, **12**, 2069–2075.

22. Huang, G. T., Sonoyama, W., Liu, Y., Liu, H., Wang, S., and Shi, S. (2008). The hidden treasure in apical papilla: the potential role in pulp/dentin regeneration and bioroot engineering, *J. Endod.*, **34**, 645–651.

23. Rincon, J. C., Young, W. G., and Bartold, P. M. (2006). The epithelial cell rests of Malassez: a role in periodontal regeneration? *J. Periodontol. Res.*, **41**, 245–2527

24. Huang, G. T., Yamaza, T., Shea, L. D., Djouad, F., Kuhn, N. Z., Tuan, R. S., and Shi, S. (2010). Stem/progenitor cell-mediated de novo regeneration of dental pulp with newly deposited continuous layer of dentin in an in vivo model, *Tissue Eng. Part A*, **16**, 605–615.

25. Iohara, K., Zheng, L., Ito, M., Tomokiyo, A., Matsushita, K., and Nakashima, M. (2006). Side population cells isolated from porcine dental pulp tissue with self-renewal and multipotency for dentinogenesis, chondrogenesis, adipogenesis, and neurogenesis, *Stem Cells*, **24**, 2493–2503.

26. Iohara, K., Zheng, L., Ito, M., Ishizaka, R., Nakamura, H., Into, T., Matsushita, K., and Nakashima, M. (2009). Regeneration of dental pulp after pulpotomy by transplantation of CD31(-)/CD146(-) side population cells from a canine tooth, *Regen. Med.*, **4**, 377–385.

27. Iohara, K., Imabayashi, K., Ishizaka, R., Watanabe, A., Nabekura, J., Ito, M., Matsushita, K., Nakamura, H., and Nakashima, M. (2011). Complete pulp regeneration after pulpectomy by transplantation of CD105+ stem cells with stromal cell-derived factor-1, *Tissue Eng. Part A*, **17**, 1911–1920.

28. Iwaya, S. I., Ikawa, M., and Kubota, M. (2001). Revascularization of an immature permanent tooth with apical periodontitis and sinus tract, *Dent. Traumatol.*, **17**, 185–187.

29. Jepsen, S., Albers, H. K., Fleiner, B., Tucker, M., and Rueger, D. (1997). Recombinant human osteogenic protein-1 induces dentin formation: an experimental study in miniature swine, *J. Endod.*, **23**, 378–382.

30. Jung, I. Y., Lee, S. J., and Hargreaves, K. M. (2008). Biologically based treatment of immature permanent teeth with pulpal necrosis: a case series, *J. Endod.*, **34**, 876–887.
31. Karring, T., Nyman, S., Gottlow, J., and Laurell, L. (1993). Development of the biological concept of guided tissue regeneration—animal and human studies, *Periodontol.*, 2000, **1**, 26–35.
32. Kawaguchi, H., Hirachi, A., Hasegawa, N., Iwata, T., Hamaguchi, H., Shiba, H., Takata, T., Kato, Y., and Kurihara, H. (2004). Enhancement of periodontal tissue regeneration by transplantation of bone marrow mesenchymal stem cells, *J. Periodontol.*, **75**, 1281–1287.
33. Kawano, S., Saito, M., Handa, K., Morotomi, T., Toyono, T., Seta, Y., Nakamura, N., Uchida, T., Toyoshima, K., Ohishi, M., and Harada, H. (2004). Characterization of dental epithelial progenitor cells derived from cervical-loop epithelium in a rat lower incisor, *J. Dent. Res.*, **83**, 129–133.
34. Kémoun, P., Laurencin-Dalicieux, S., Rue, J., Farges, J. C., Gennero, I., Conte-Auriol, F., Briand-Mesange, F., Gadelorge, M., Arzate, H., Narayanan, A. S., Brunel, G., and Salles, J. P. (2007). Human dental follicle cells acquire cementoblast features under stimulation by BMP-2/-7 and enamel matrix derivatives (EMD) in vitro, *Cell Tissue Res.*, **329**, 283–294.
35. Kim, J. Y., Xin, X., Moioli, E. K., Chung, J., Lee, C. H., Chen, M., Fu, S. Y., Koch, P. D., and Mao, J. J. (2010). Regeneration of dental-pulp-like tissue by chemotaxis-induced cell homing, *Tissue. Eng. Part A*, **16**, 3023–3031.
36. Kim, K., Lee, C. H., Kim, B. K., and Mao, J. J. (2010). Anatomically shaped tooth and periodontal regeneration by cell homing, *J. Dent. Res.*, **89**, 842–847.
37. Kim, S. G., Zhou, J., Solomon, C., Zheng, Y., Suzuki, T., Chen, M., Song, S., Jiang, N., Cho, S., and Mao, J. J. (2012). Effects of growth factors on dental stem/progenitor cells. *Dent. Clin. North. Am.*, **56**, 563–575.
38. Kuo, T. F., Huang, A. T., Chang, H. H., Lin, F. H., Chen, S. T., Chen, R. S., Chou, C. H., Lin, H. C., Chiang, H., and Chen, M. H. (2008). Regeneration of dentin-pulp complex with cementum and periodontal ligament formation using dental bud cells in gelatin–chondroitin–hyaluronan tri-copolymer scaffold in swine, *J. Biomed. Mater. Res A*, **86**, 1062–1068.
39. Laino, G., d'Aquino, R., Graziano, A., Lanza, V., Carinci, F., Naro, F., Pirozzi, G., and Papaccio, G. (2005). A new population of human adult dental pulp stem cells: a useful source of living autologous fibrous bone tissue (LAB), *J. Bone. Miner. Res.*, **20**, 1394–1402.

40. Lee, J. S., Wikesjö, U. M., Jung, U. W., Choi, S. H., Pippig, S., Siedler, M., and Kim, C. K. (2010). Periodontal wound healing/regeneration following implantation of recombinant human growth/differentiation factor-5 in a beta-tricalcium phosphate carrier into one-wall intrabony defects in dogs, *J. Clin. Periodontol.*, **37**, 382–389.

41. Levi, B., James, A. W., Nelson, E. R., Vistnes, D., Wu, B., Lee, M., Gupta, A., and Longaker, M. T. (2010). Human adipose derived stromal cells heal critical size mouse calvarial defects, *PLoS One*, **5**, e11177.

42. Li, H., Yan, F., Lei, L., Li, Y., and Xiao, Y. (2009). Application of autologous cryopreserved bone marrow mesenchymal stem cells for periodontal regeneration in dogs, *Cells Tissues Organs.*, **190**, 94–101.

43. Liu, Y., Zheng, Y., Ding, G., Fang, D., Zhang, C., Bartold, P. M., Gronthos, S., Shi, S., and Wang, S. (2008). Periodontal ligament stem cell-mediated treatment for periodontitis in miniature swine, *Stem Cells*, **26**, 1065–1073.

44. Lynch, S. E., Williams, R. C., Polson, A. M., Howell, T. H., Reddy, M. S., Zappa, U. E., and Antoniades, H. N. (1989). A combination of platelet-derived and insulin-like growth factors enhances periodontal regeneration, *J. Clin. Periodontol.*, **16**, 545–548.

45. Lynch, S. E., de Castilla, G. R., Williams, R. C., Kiritsy, C. P., Howell, T. H., Reddy, M. S., and Antoniades, H. N. (1991). The effects of short-term application of a combination of platelet-derived and insulin-like growth factors on periodontal wound healing, *J. Periodontol.*, **62**, 458–467.

46. Mao, J. J., Kim, S. G., Zhou, J., Ye, L., Cho, S., Suzuki, T., Fu, S. Y., Yang, R., and Zhou, X. (2012). Regenerative endodontics: barriers and strategies for clinical translation, *Dent. Clin. North. Am.,* **56**, 639–649.

47. Mao, J. J., Robey, P. G., and Prockop, D. J. (2012). Stem cells in the face: tooth regeneration and beyond, *Cell Stem Cell*, **11**, 291–301.

48. Mitsiadis, T. A., Barrandon, O., Rochat, A., Barrandon, Y., and De Bari, C. (2007). Stem cell niches in mammals, *Exp. Cell. Res.*, **313**, 3377–3385.

49. Mizoguchi, T., Verkade, H., Heath, J. K., Kuroiwa, A., and Kikuchi, Y. (2008). Sdf1/Cxcr4 signaling controls the dorsal migration of endodermal cells during zebrafish gastrulation, *Development.*, **135**, 2521–2529.

50. Morsczeck, C., Götz, W., Schierholz, J., Zeilhofer, F., Kühn, U., Möhl, C., Sippel, C., and Hoffmann, K. H. (2005). Isolation of precursor cells (PCs) from human dental follicle of wisdom teeth, *Matrix. Biol.*, **24**, 155–165.

51. Nakahara, T., Nakamura, T., Kobayashi, E., Inoue, M., Shigeno, K., Tabata, Y., Eto, K., and Shimizu, Y. (2003). Novel approach to regeneration of periodontal tissues based on in situ tissue engineering: effects of controlled release of basic fibroblast growth factor from a sandwich membrane, *Tissue Eng.*, **9**, 153–162.

52. Nevins, M., Kao, R. T., McGuire, M. K., McClain, P. K., Hinrichs, J. E., McAllister, B. S., Reddy, M. S., Nevins, M. L., Genco, R. J., Lynch, S. E., and Giannobile, W. V. (2012). PDGF promotes periodontal regeneration in localized osseous defects: 36 month extension results from a randomized, controlled, double-masked clinical trial, *J. Periodontol.*, **84**, 456–464 (Epub ahead of print).

53. Nikolidakis, D., and Jansen, J. A. (2008). The biology of platelet-rich plasma and its application in oral surgery: literature review, *Tissue. Eng. Part B. Rev.*, **14**, 249–258.

54. Nosrat, A., Seifi, A., and Asgary, S. (2011). Regenerative endodontic treatment (revascularization) for necrotic immature permanent molars: a review and report of two cases with a new biomaterial, *J. Endod.*, **37**, 562–567.

55. Ohazama, A., Modino, S. A., Miletich, I., and Sharpe P. T. (2004). Stem-cell-based tissue engineering of murine teeth, *J. Dent. Res.*, **83**, 518–522.

56. Osugi, M., Katagiri, W., Yoshimi, R., Inukai, T., Hibi, H., and Ueda, M. (2012). Conditioned media from mesenchymal stem cells enhanced bone regeneration in rat calvarial bone defects, *Tissue Eng. Part A,* **18**, 1479–1489 (Epub ahead of print).

57. Ramis, J. M., Rubert, M., Vondrasek, J., Gayà, A., Lyngstadaas, S. P., and Monjo, M. (2012). Effect of enamel matrix derivative and of proline-rich synthetic peptides on the differentiation of human mesenchymal stem cells toward the osteogenic lineage, *Tissue Eng. Part A,* **18**, 1253–1263 (Epub ahead of print).

58. Reynolds, K., Johnson, J. D., and Cohenca, N. (2009). Pulp revascularization of necrotic bilateral bicuspids using a modified novel technique to eliminate potential coronal discolouration: a case report, *Int. Endod. J.*, **42**, 84–92.

59. Rutherford, R. B., and Gu, K. (2000). Treatment of inflamed ferret dental pulps with recombinant bone morphogenetic protein-7, *Eur. J. Oral. Sci.*, **108**, 202–206.

60. Saito, A., Saito, E., Handa, R., Honma, Y., and Kawanami, M. (2009). Influence of residual bone on recombinant human bone morphogenetic protein-2-induced periodontal regeneration in experimental periodontitis in dogs, *J. Periodontol.*, **80**, 961–968.

61. Seo, B. M., Miura, M., Gronthos, S., Bartold, P. M., Batouli, S., Brahim, J., Young, M., Robey, P. G., Wang, C. Y., and Shi, S. (2004). Investigation of multipotent postnatal stem cells from human periodontal ligament, *Lancet*, **364**, 149–155.
62. Seo, B. M., Miura, M., Sonoyama, W., Coppe, C., Stanyon, R., and Shi, S. (2005). Recovery of stem cells from cryopreserved periodontal ligament, *J. Dent. Res.*, **84**, 907–912.
63. Seo, B. M., Sonoyama, W., Yamaza, T., Coppe, C., Kikuiri, T., Akiyama, K., Lee, J. S., and Shi, S. (2008). SHED repair critical-size calvarial defects in mice, *Oral. Dis.* **14**, 428–434.
64. Shi, S., and Gronthos, S. (2003). Perivascular niche of postnatal mesenchymal stem cells in human bone marrow and dental pulp, *J. Bone. Miner. Res.*, **18**, 696–704.
65. Six, N., Lasfargues, J. J., and Goldberg, M. (2002). Differential repair responses in the coronal and radicular areas of the exposed rat molar pulp induced by recombinant human bone morphogenetic protein 7 (osteogenic protein 1), *Arch. Oral. Biol.*, **47**, 177–187.
66. Sonoyama, W., Liu, Y., Fang, D., Yamaza, T., Seo, B. M., Zhang, C., Liu, H., Gronthos, S., Wang, C. Y., Wang, S., and Shi, S. (2006). Mesenchymal stem cell-mediated functional tooth regeneration in swine, *PLoS One*, **1**, e79.
67. Sonoyama, W., Liu, Y., Yamaza, T., Tuan, R. S., Wang, S., Shi, S., and Huang, G. T. (2008). Characterization of the apical papilla and its residing stem cells from human immature permanent teeth: a pilot study, *J. Endod.*, **34**, 166–171.
68. Sorensen, R. G., Wikesjö, U. M., Kinoshita, A., and Wozney, J. M. (2004). Periodontal repair in dogs: evaluation of a bioresorbable calcium phosphate cement (Ceredex) as a carrier for rhBMP-2, *J. Clin. Periodontol.*, **31**, 796–804.
69. Stavropoulos, A., and Wikesjö, U. M. (2012). Growth and differentiation factors for periodontal regeneration: a review on factors with clinical testing, *J. Periodontal. Res.*, **47,** 545–553 (Epub ahead of print).
70. Stosich, M. S., Moioli, E. K., Wu, J. K., Lee, C. H., Rohde, C., Yousref, A. M., Ascherman, J., Diraddo, R., Marion, N. W., and Mao, J. J. (2009). Bioengineering strategies to generate vascularized soft tissue grafts with sustained shape, *Methods*, **47**, 116–121.
71. Tatakis, D. N., Wikesjö, U. M., Razi, S. S., Sigurdsson, T. J., Lee, M. B., Nguyen, T., Ongpipattanakul, B., and Hardwick, R. (2000). Periodontal repair in dogs: effect of transforming growth factor-beta 1 on alveolar bone and cementum regeneration, *J. Clin. Periodontol.*, **27**, 698–704.

72. Téclès, O., Laurent, P., Zygouritsas, S., Burger, A. S., Camps, J., Dejou, J., and About, I. (2005). Activation of human dental pulp progenitor/stem cells in response to odontoblast injury, *Arch. Oral. Biol.*, **50**, 103–108.
73. Thesleff, I., and Sharpe, P. (1997). Signalling networks regulating dental development, *Mech. Dev.*, **67**, 111–123.
74. Thesleff, I., Keränen, S., and Jernvall, J. (2001). Enamel knots as signaling centers linking tooth morphogenesis and odontoblast differentiation, *Adv. Dent. Res.*, **15**, 14–18.
75. Torabinejad, M., and Turman, M. (2011). Revitalization of tooth with necrotic pulp and open apex by using platelet-rich plasma: a case report, *J. Endod.*, **37**, 265–268.
76. Tsiridis, E., Bhalla, A., Ali, Z., Gurav, N., Heliotis, M., Deb, S., and DiSilvio, L. (2006). Enhancing the osteoinductive properties of hydroxyapatite by the addition of human mesenchymal stem cells, and recombinant human osteogenic protein-1 (BMP-7) in vitro, *Injury*, **37** Suppl 3, S25–S32.
77. Wang, X. P., Suomalainen, M., Felszeghy, S., Zelarayan, L. C., Alonso, M. T., Plikus, M. V., Maas, R. L., Chuong, C. M., Schimmang, T., and Thesleff, I. (2007). An integrated gene regulatory network controls stem cell proliferation in teeth, *PLoS Biol.*, **5**, e159.
78. Woods, E. J., Perry, B. C., Hockema, J. J., Larson, L., Zhou, D., and Goebel, W. S. (2009). Optimized cryopreservation method for human dental pulp-derived stem cells and their tissues of origin for banking and clinical use, *Cryobiology*, **59**, 150–157.
79. Wright, N., Hidalgo, A., Rodríguez-Frade, J. M., Soriano, S. F., Mellado, M., Parmo-Cabañas, M., Briskin, M. J., and Teixidó, J. (2002). The chemokine stromal cell-derived factor-1 alpha modulates alpha 4 beta 7 integrin-mediated lymphocyte adhesion to mucosal addressin cell adhesion molecule-1 and fibronectin, *J. Immunol.*, **168**, 5268–5277.
80. Xu, L., Lv, K., Zhang, W., Zhang, X., Jiang, X., and Zhang, F. (2012). The healing of critical-size calvarial bone defects in rat with rhPDGF-BB, BMSCs, and β-TCP scaffolds, *J. Mater. Sci. Mater. Med.*, **23**, 1073–1084.
81. Yildirim, S., Fu, S. Y., Kim, K., Zhou, H., Lee, C. H., Li, A., Kim, S. G., Wang, S., and Mao, J. J. (2011). Tooth regeneration: a revolution in stomatology and evolution in regenerative medicine, *Int. J. Oral. Sci.*, **3**, 107–116.
82. Yokoi, T., Saito, M., Kiyono, T., Iseki, S., Kosaka, K., Nishida, E., Tsubakimoto, T., Harada, H., Eto, K., Noguchi, T., and Teranaka, T. (2007). Establishment of immortalized dental follicle cells for generating periodontal ligament in vivo, *Cell Tissue Res.*, **327**, 301–311.

83. Young, C. S., Terada, S., Vacanti, J. P., Honda, M., Bartlett, J. D., and Yelick, P. C. (2002). Tissue engineering of complex tooth structures on biodegradable polymer scaffolds, *J. Dent. Res.*, **81**, 695–700.
84. Young, C. S., Abukawa, H., Asrican, R., Ravens, M., Troulis, M. J., Kaban, L. B., Vacanti, J. P., and Yelick, P. C. (2005). Tissue-engineered hybrid tooth and bone, *Tissue. Eng.*, **11**, 1599–1610.
85. Zhang, W., Walboomers, X. F., Shi, S., Fan, M., and Jansen, J. A. (2006). Multilineage differentiation potential of stem cells derived from human dental pulp after cryopreservation, *Tissue Eng.*, **12**, 2813–2823.

Chapter 17

Engineering Functional Bone Grafts for Craniofacial Regeneration

Pinar Yilgor Huri and Warren L. Grayson

*Johns Hopkins University, Department of Biomedical Engineering,
Translational Tissue Engineering Center,
400 N. Broadway, Smith 5023, Baltimore, MD 21231, USA*

wgrayson@jhmi.edu

17.1 Introduction

The craniofacial unit is among the most complex tissue regions in the body, providing a delicate juxtaposition of bone, cartilage, cranial nerves, soft tissues, and blood vessels. The remediation of craniofacial bone deformities is uniquely challenging since one must manage the close interactions of bone and surrounding tissues within this most aesthetically demanding part of the body. Craniofacial bone loss arising from congenital defects, surgical treatments (e.g., mandibulectomy or bone tumor resection) or trauma requires special consideration since the bone provides the structural basis underlying a patient's physical appearance (and sense of identity), protects vital organs such as the brain and the eyes, and facilitates necessary functions such as mastication and speech. Regeneration of craniofacial bone defects should effectively

---

Tissue and Organ Regeneration: Advances in Micro- and Nanotechnology
Edited by Lijie Grace Zhang, Ali Khademhosseini, and Thomas J. Webster
Copyright © 2014 Pan Stanford Publishing Pte. Ltd.
ISBN 978-981-4411-67-7 (Hardcover), 978-981-4411-68-4 (eBook)
www.panstanford.com

address these functional outcomes preferably with the use of personalized grafts designed to match the defect site.

Current clinical applications in the reconstruction of cranial bone defects include autogenic, allogenic, and xenogenic grafts. The use of autografts remains the most preferred procedure. However, problems associated with the limited supply of autologous bone for transplantation, donor site morbidity, increased hospitalization times, and significantly increased operation durations and blood loss limit their use. Although the development of tissue engineering strategies and their craniofacial application has impacted the production of implantable bone substitutes, several key issues should be addressed before they can be considered viable alternatives. These include: Selection of an ideal cell source, development of isolation and expansion procedures capable of yielding clinically relevant cell counts, a better understanding of biomaterial properties, and improved graft vascularization are all necessary to provide postimplant survival.

17.1.1 Overview of Bone Tissue Engineering for Craniofacial Applications

Bone has important functions as an endocrine organ, regulating global levels of calcium, insulin, seratonin, and other hormones [1–3]. However, bone treatments primarily emphasize restoring structural function. As a result, anatomically shaped inorganic materials have sufficed to treat cranial defects or to recapitulate maxillofacial structures. Alternatively, bone tissue engineering (BTE) uses biological components. The major difference is the new tissue's ability to integrate with host tissues and remodel in response to environmental cues. The traditional BTE approach combines osteoprogenitor cells with scaffolds and growth factors. Potential cell sources include mesenchymal stem cells derived from various sites within the body including bone marrow and adipose tissues. These cells are readily available with limited morbidity, and can be easily differentiated into bone-forming cells through exposure to growth factors or other biophysical stimuli. Several objective parameters are assessed to determine the choice of scaffold biomaterial including its mechanical properties, osteoconductivity, and osteoinductivity. While the classical BTE approach employs a combination of cells with biomaterials to induce tissue regeneration, the economic and regulatory hurdles associated with cell-based therapies have also led to the proliferation of cell-free biomaterial approaches, which stimulate the activity of endogenous stem cells. For large craniomaxillofacial defects, the damage to physical appearance has negative psychosocial effects on the patients and the cosmetic outcome has become a primary consideration.

In this chapter we describe in detail the application of BTE principles to the facial skeleton with special emphasis on cells, scaffolds, growth factors, and bioreactor technologies used to obtain bone substitutes. We focus on the relative success of these approaches in animal studies and human trials. Additionally, we report on the impact of recent advances in the fields of micro- and nanotechnology on scaffold properties, modulation of cell-scaffold interactions, and growth factor delivery. The clinical impact and limitations of these approaches are also discussed.

17.2 Principles of Craniofacial Graft Design

The traditional strategy for BTE-mediated repair of nonhealing defects is to isolate cells (most commonly mesenchymal stem cells or progenitor cells), expand them in vitro, and seed them onto biocompatible and biodegradable scaffolds that meet the structural and mechanical requirements of the defect site. Appropriate growth factors are added to accelerate healing, initiate proliferation, and differentiation of local osteoprogenitor cells and improve bone formation. After in vitro maturation and mineralization of this cell-seeded construct, preferably in bioreactors, it is implanted at the target site. In time, the biodegradable scaffold is resorbed while the cells produce their own ECM and replace the implant. In this section, these components—cells, biomaterials, growth-factors, and bioreactors—are described in detail in the particular context of craniofacial graft design.

17.2.1 Cell Sources for Craniofacial Bone Tissue Engineering

It is widely assumed that exogenous cells are required to stimulate functional bone regeneration. Implantation of viable cells within appropriate scaffolds is indeed beneficial for BTE, since soft callus formation after surgery often depends on bone formation by the transplanted osteoblasts. Possible sources of cells for tissue engineering include autogenic, allogenic and xenogenic cells. The use of allogenic cells is restricted due to possible immunogenic responses of the host [4], while the use of xenogenic cells is limited to research purposes and application in humans is rare [5]. In tissue engineering, an appropriate source is autologous cells taken from a healthy region of the patient's damaged tissue. However, due to limited availability of the healthy tissue as well as difficulty in tissue harvesting for mature cell isolation (especially in the case of bone), other cell sources have been considered.

Stem cells are widely used in the engineering of bone substitutes. The use of pluripotent embryonic stem cells (ESCs) in BTE is promising [6] as they are capable of indefinite undifferentiated proliferation in vitro and can provide an unlimited supply of cells [7]. However, there are technical and ethical issues that have to be addressed before they can be used in clinical applications. Ethical issues may be circumvented by the use of induced pluripotent stem (iPS) cells, which have similar characteristics to ESCs [8,9]. Although this technique has remarkable potential in tissue engineering and stem cell therapy, current limitations such as low efficiency and risks associated with tumor formation and viral transgenes should be eliminated before use in a clinical setting [10].

Multipotent mesenchymal stem cells (MSCs) are of great interest to tissue engineers. In the current clinical practice, MSCs can be differentiated into the osteogenic lineage by culturing in the presence of osteogenic supplements [11]. MSCs and bone repair cells [12] from bone marrow have been shown to enhance craniofacial bone regeneration in both orthotopic and ectopic models (Table 17.1). Bone marrow MSCs isolated from beagle dogs were labeled with green fluorescent protein (GFP) and were implanted into periodontal defects within collagen matrices [13]. At 4 weeks, histological evaluation revealed that the defect was fully regenerated by GFP-positive cementoblasts, osteoblasts, osteocytes, and fibroblasts indicating the extent of differentiation of MSCs in orthotopic defect sites. In another recent orthotopic implantation study, bone marrow MSCs were again harvested from beagle dogs, encapsulated within HAp particles, and this time implanted within jaw cleft defects [14]. At 6 months' follow-up, complete regeneration of the defect was reported by histological and radiological analysis. The potential of bone marrow-derived MSCs was also verified in ectopic models.

Table 17.1 Representative examples of cell types and applications in craniofacial bone tissue engineering

Cell type	Cell source	Carrier	Application site	Harvest*	Outcome	Ref.
Periodontal cells	Tissue block of periodontal ligament and alveolar bone	Collagen gel	0.6 mm defect created in mesial root of the first molar	2	Stimulate alveolar bone formation in rat model	[24]
Cementoblasts	Immortalized cell line	PLGA sponge	3 mm × 2 mm rat mandibular defect	3	Complete bone bridging and periodontal ligament formation	[25]
Bone repair cells	Bone marrow	Gelatin sponge	2 mm × 7 mm jawbone defect	6	Formation of highly vascular bone within the defect	[12]
Mesenchymal stem cells	Bone marrow	Carbonated HAp particles	5 mm × 10 mm jaw cleft defect in dogs	24	Complete bone regeneration	[14]
Mesenchymal stem cells	Adipose tissue	PLGA scaffold by solvent casting/particulate leaching	5 mm parietal bone defect in mice	12	Complete bone regeneration	[18]
Periodontal ligament stem cells	Periodontal ligament	HAp/TCP particles	2 mm² buccal cortex of the mandibular molar in rats	8	Cementum/periodontal regeneration	[21]
Dental pulp stem cells	Human exfoliated deciduous teeth	PLLA scaffold by salt leaching	Subcutaneous implantation in mice	4	Dentin and dental pulp regeneration	[19]
Apical papilla stem cells	Root apical papilla of swine teeth	Root-shaped HAp/TCP block	Place of lower incisor after extraction in minipig	8	Regeneration of root/periodontal ligament tissues	[22]
Dental follicle stem cells	Human third molar	N/A	8 mm parietal defect in rat	4	Enhanced bone regeneration	[23]
BMP-7 gene induced dermal fibroblasts	Skin biopsy	Gelatin sponge	3 mm × 2 mm periodontal alveolar bone defect	7	Osteogenesis and cementogenesis followed by bridging of the bone defect	[26]

*Weeks post surgery

Human iliac crest-derived cells were seeded into HAp/TCP cylinders (D: 3.2 mm, L: 5 mm) and were subcutaneously implanted into SCID mice [15]. At 6 months, production of bone-specific markers at the defect site such as bone sialoprotein and osteocalcin implied the potential of MSCs to produce osteogenic factors.

Stem cells can be more readily isolated from adipose tissue [16] than from bone marrow and the potential of these cells for the regeneration of craniofacial bone defects has been shown [17]. Cowan et al. (2004) seeded mice adipose stromal cells into apatite coated PLGA sponges and implanted them within parietal bone defects [18]. Twelve weeks after implantation, new bone formation was assessed within the defect even without the application of growth factors or genetic modification.

Stem cells from other tissues have been used successfully for craniofacial regeneration. These include dental pulp stem cells [19,20], periodontal ligament stem cells [21], stem cells from apical papilla [22] and dental follicle cells [23]. These have been shown to express osteogenic and odontogenic markers and have been used successfully to regenerate bone, dentin and periodontal ligament in the craniofacial region (Table 17.1). Periodontal ligament stem cells were isolated from extracted human third molars, encapsulated within HAp/TCP particles, and implanted into the defects created in the buccal cortex of the mandibular molar of rats [21]. After 8 weeks, histological analysis revealed the regeneration of cementum and periodontal tissues. In another study using stem cells from the apical papilla, swine-derived cells were seeded into root-shaped HAp/TCP blocks and the scaffolds were implanted into the place of the extracted lower incisors [22]. Three months after implantation, it was radiologically and histologically revealed that the root and the periodontal tissue were successfully regenerated.

Primary cells have also been used for the regeneration of craniofacial bone defects. For example, primary periodontal cells were labeled either by fluorescent beads or modified to express β-galactosidase to track their contribution in the periodontal regeneration. These cells were then implanted within the periodontal defects in rats within collagen carriers [24]. It was observed that labeled cells participated in the regeneration of the periodontal ligament and alveolar bone 2 weeks after implantation. In another study, primary cementoblasts were implanted within the bony defects created on the first mandibular molar of rats within PLGA sponges [25]. At the end of 6 weeks, mineralization and bridging of the bone defect as well as cementum formation was verified by histological analysis.

As another strategy, genetically modified cells (such as BMP-7 transduced skin fibroblasts) have been used in BTE for periodontal regeneration [26]. In this study, transduced cells were seeded onto gelatin scaffolds and were implanted into alveolar bone defects in rats. Results showed that implantation of BMP-7 transduced cells improved chondrogenesis followed by osteogenesis and bony union to a significant degree compared to control groups. Similarly, BMP-2-transfected autologous bone marrow MSCs were used within alginate/collagen scaffolds and implanted into the cranial defects in miniature swine. Three months after implantation, complete regeneration of the defects was shown with alginate/collagen scaffolds where no bone regeneration was observed when β-gal-transected MSCs were used as a control [27].

It has been shown that the progenitor cells isolated from the maxillofacial region have distinct characteristics that differentiate them from their other skeletal counterparts [28,29]. For example, stromal cells isolated from the maxilla and mandible showed higher proliferation rates, delayed senescence, and increased levels of alkaline phosphatase expression and mineral deposition compared to stromal cells of the iliac crest isolated from the same individual [29]. Mandibular MSCs exhibited higher mineralized matrix formation when compared with bone marrow MSCs in a mouse calvarial defect model [30]. These site-specific differences in cellular characteristics were thought to emanate from the different developmental origins of mandibular cells (neural crest) compared to bone marrow cells obtained from the appendicular skeleton (mesoderm). Therefore, specific considerations to be addressed in cells used for the engineering of craniofacial bone grafts include the developmental origin of the cells, culture conditions, growth factors, and dosage forms to maximize osteogenesis and mineralization, mechanical properties and infrastructure of the scaffold to host the cells.

17.2.2 Scaffold Biomaterials

Bones in the craniofacial region are subject to stresses and strains mainly due to mastication. For mandibular bones, these stresses range 120–450 MPa and 11000–30000 MPa in the absence and presence of dentition, respectively [31]. It is therefore highly beneficial to use mechanically competent scaffolds to deliver cells to defect sites. Scaffold biomaterials capable of withstanding these loads have developed continuously over the last several decades. Besides mechanical integrity, the main design parameters for craniofacial bone scaffolds are osteoconductivity, osteoinductivity, and degradability. First-generation scaffolds were mainly structural templates. Subsequent scaffolds were capable of delivering cells and/or growth factors. The development of cells into functional tissues is dictated by the properties of the scaffold materials such as intrinsic biocompatibility, surface architecture, and chemistry. Hence, more recent scaffold systems deliver cells and growth factors as well as induce the formation of vascular networks within the graft and are capable of regulating cell-graft interactions through topographical cues such as surface nano- and microtopography [32].

A wide range of materials have been employed for the engineering of craniofacial bone. Natural polymers were used as extracellular matrix (ECM)-based scaffold materials because of their osteoconductivity and biochemical similarity to native tissues. Collagen [33], fibroin [34], chitosan [35], calcium alginate either in injectable [36] or 3D hydrogel forms [27], hyaluronic acid [37], and composites [38] have been shown to be osteoconductive bone fillers mainly in cranial defect models in rodents (Table 17.2). These studies indicate the importance of scaffold materials with biomimetic properties. For example, in the study of Chang et al. (2010), BMP-2 gene transfected bone marrow MSCs were used to repair 5 cm^2 cranial defects in miniature swine [27]. Cells were encapsulated either in alginate or collagen hydrogels to compare the effects of the two biomaterials. Histological, mechanical and CT examinations 3 months after implantation verified that almost no bone regeneration occurred within the defects when alginate was used as the scaffold material, while collagen scaffolds induced improved bone regeneration. The need to provide a more bioactive environment to enhance bone regeneration was similarly demonstrated in another study where alginate was used in combination with nano-hydroxyapatite/collagen particles [36]. Two months post implantation, bone regeneration within the 5 mm-diameter rat cranial defects could only be achieved in the presence of mineralized material.

Table 17.2 Scaffolds in craniofacial bone tissue engineering

	Material	Production technique	Application	Harvest*	Outcome	Reference
Natural polymeric	Silk fibroin	Solvent casting-Particulate leaching	5 mm × 8 mm parietal defect	4	Mature bone formation and defect correction	[34]
	Collagen	Lyophilization	8 mm rat calvarial defect	4	Complete bone fill when used in combination with Activin	[33]
		Cross-linking COL fibers with HA	5 mm × 3 mm rat cranial defect	3	Adequate osteoconductive potential in case of COL/HA application	[38]
	Chitosan	Fiber bonding	5 mm × 1 mm defect in nude mice	8	Good integration with the surrounding tissue and significant bone formation	[35]
	Alginate	Injectable hydrogel	5 mm diameter rat cranial defect	8	Bone healing only when used in combination with nano HAp/COL particles	[36]
		Hydrogel	5 cm² cranial bone defect in swine	6	No bone regeneration	[27]
	HA	Hydrogel	5 mm diameter rat calvarial defect	6	Mineralization in case of BMP-2 delivery	[37]

(Continued)

Table 17.2 (Continued)

	Material	Production technique	Application	Harvest*	Outcome	Reference
Synthetic polymeric	PLGA	Solvent casting—particulate leaching	4 mm mouse calvarial defect	8	Succesful healing of defects	[39]
	PLLA	Electrospining	5 mm rat parietal defect	12	Better ossification when used in combination with BMP-2	[52]
		Gas foaming	8 mm rat calvarial defect	18	Complete bone ingrowth	[44]
	PEG	Photopolymerization in mold	Mandibular condyle scaffold preparation in mice dorsum	12	Succesful preparation of osteochondral construct	[43]
	PCL	3D printing	Mandibular condyle subcutaneous implantation	6	Production of vascularized and mineralized tissue within construct	[41]
Ceramic-based	TCP	Impregnation/Incubation	5 mm rat calvarial bone defect	8	β-TCP combined with rhPDGF or BMSCs promote new bone formation	[47]
	HAp/TCP	Sintering	Sinus elevation clinical application	36	Osseointegration	[48]
	HAp/PA	SLS	Mandibular condyle clinical application	96	Successful facial reconstruction	[50]

*Weeks post surgery.
Note: COL, collagen; HA, hyaluronic acid; HAp, hydroxyapatite; PA, polyamide; SLS, selective laser sintering.

Synthetic biocompatible polymers can also be used to provide the necessary structural integrity for bone reconstruction. These materials are more readily available, processable, and nonantigenic. Synthetic polymers such as polylactic acid (PLA), polyglycolic acid PGA, and their copolymers in various ratios (PLGA) [39], polymethyl methacrylate (PMMA) [40], polycaprolactone (PCL) [41], polypropylene fumarate (PPF) [42], and polyethylene glycol (PEG) [43] have been prepared as custom osteoconductive matrices and used in the regeneration of craniofacial components such as the calvarium and the mandibular condyle (Table 17.2). In one example, disc-shaped PLA scaffolds prepared by foaming supercritical gas (D: 8 mm, H: 3 mm) were implanted into rat calvarial defects. After 18 weeks, complete bone bridging was verified by histological and radiographic analysis [44]. Osteochondral grafts have also been engineered. Bone marrow MSCs were differentiated into chondrocytes and osteoblasts in monolayer, detached and resuspended in PEG hydrogels. First the chondrogenic, then the osteogenic layers were photopolymerized in a mold shaped as a human mandibular condyle [43]. These scaffolds were implanted ectopically in mice and histopathological assessment 3 months after implantation demonstrated the successful maintenance of spatially distinct osseous and chondrogenic regions. Alternatively, biphasic scaffolds composed of decellularized bone and agarose have been used to induce a single population of MSCs into bone and cartilage tissues. The chemical and mechanical cues provided by the substrates were combined with biological factors and perfusion of culture medium to form osteochondral constructs in vitro [45].

The osteoconductivity of scaffolds is often enhanced by using HAp and tricalcium phosphate (TCP) either alone or in combination with natural and synthetic polymers as they mimic the mineralized component of the native tissue [46]. Due to their brittle nature, their application alone is mostly limited to nonstress craniofacial areas such as the calvarium and maxillary sinus [47,48]. When used in combination with other polymeric materials such as polyamide (PA), the HAp/PA composite seeded with bone marrow MSCs showed enhanced bone regeneration in the marrow-poor rabbit mandibular angle defects 3 months after implantation [49]. HAp/PA has also been used in the preparation of custom-made human mandibular condyle scaffolds, and was successfully used in the clinical treatment of a 27-year-old woman. At 24 months after the surgery, the patient regained proper jaw appearance and joint function [50].

17.2.3 Engineering Anatomically Shaped Craniofacial Grafts

The functionality of bone grafts used for craniofacial reconstruction relies heavily on both the internal architecture and the gross geometry. The internal structure or porosity impacts nutrient and oxygen diffusion into the scaffold, cellular in-growth and vascular invasion. Several techniques have been employed to produce porous 3D structures to fill cranial defects that have pore interconnectivity and controlled pore size such as solvent casting-particulate leaching [39], phase separation [51], fiber bonding [35], electrospinning [52], melt molding [53] and gas foaming [44] (Table 17.2). HAp/PA composite scaffolds prepared by phase separation/particle leaching were punch-shaped (D: 8 mm, H: 2 mm) and implanted into 8 mm rat cranial defects to completely regenerate bone after 16 weeks [51]. A similar production technique was used to produce porous tyrosine-derived polycarbonate scaffolds with 15 mm diameter that were subsequently implanted into rabbit calvarial defects [54]. Although the successful regeneration of large bone defects was reported in these and similar studies, such scaffold production techniques are not well suited to the production of anatomically shaped scaffolds.

In contrast, computer-aided design (CAD) technologies such as rapid prototyping (RP) using biodegradable polymers, facilitate the production of patient-specific, anatomically shaped tissue engineering scaffolds. Multiple studies have focused on the mandibular condyle, which is challenging to repair due to its irregular shape and the nature of the loads imparted to it (compression and shear). Furthermore, damage to the condyle leads to debilitating diseases and significant reduction in the quality of life. Anatomically shaped mandibular condyle grafts have been successfully produced by 3D printing [41] (Figs. 17.1a,b) and selective laser sintering (SLS) [55] (Figs. 17.1c,d) as well as CNC milling of decellularized trabecular bone [56] (Figs. 17.1e,f). In pioneering studies, CT scans of the animal were used to obtain the anatomical shape and the mandibular condyle and ramus of a minipig were fabricated as a single unit through SLS of PCL powder [57,58]. A later study used 3D printing of PCL/HAp to obtain scaffolds in the shape of a human condyle. This scaffold was seeded with human MSCs encapsulated in PEG to produce vascularized osteochondral grafts in a rat model [41]. More recently, human mandibular condylar grafts were reconstructed from clinical CT scans using a CNC machine to shape decellularized trabecular bone [56]. Cultivation of completely viable functional anatomically shaped bone grafts was reported within perfusion bioreactors. Besides polymeric materials, CaP ceramics and polymer/ceramic composites can be used for the production of personalized craniofacial implants by RP techniques [59,50] (Figs. 17.1g,h). It was shown that CaP implants could be successfully custom-made by 3D printing to provide a perfect fit with the defects on the calvarium, zygoma, orbital rim, and mandibula [59] in a human cadaveric study. Mechanical and physical characterization of the RP scaffolds revealed promising results for use in craniofacial BTE.

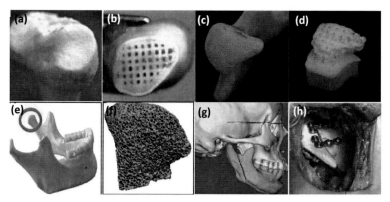

Figure 17.1 Production of anatomically shaped scaffolds by rapid prototyping technology. The anatomical model (a, c, e, g) and produced mandibular condyl scaffolds in accordance with these models by (b) 3D printing [41], (d) SLS [55], (f) CNC manufacturing [56], (h) Laser prototyping [50].

17.2.4 Growth Factors and Delivery Strategies

During bone regeneration, multiple growth factors such as transforming growth factor-beta (TGF-β) superfamily proteins (including bone morphogenetic proteins (BMPs), inhibins, and activin), insulin-like growth factor (IGF), fibroblast growth factor (FGF), platelet derived growth factor (PDGF), and vascular endothelial growth factor (VEGF) function in unison in a time- and concentration-dependent manner to regulate different aspects of the repair process. TGF-βs have multiple functions and couple the migration of osteoprogenitor cells with the inhibition and subsequent activation of osteoclasts. This coupling enables ossification during the early phases of bone repair and regulates the production of collagen and other ECM proteins [60]. Bone morphogenetic proteins induce osteoblastic and chondroblastic differentiation of MSCs. IGF-1 is an important agent during early fracture healing and stimulates osteoprogenitor cell mitosis and differentiation, thereby increasing the number of functionally mature osteoblasts [61]. FGFs act together with heparin sulfate-containing proteoglycans to modulate cell migration, angiogenesis, bone development, and repair [62]. EGF has been shown to promote bone remodeling while PDGF and VEGF have significant roles in angiogenesis and vasculogenesis, both of which are crucial for successful healing [63].

Since growth factors have such important regulatory functions, their incorporation into tissue engineering strategies is central to achieving functional constructs. The conventional strategy for growth factor administration during in vitro and in vivo studies is to apply the agent in the form of large doses by either single or repeated applications. However, in such cases a considerable proportion of the agent is lost through leakage from the site by biodistribution and/or by denaturation. Encapsulation of growth factors in protective carrier structures is of utmost importance for the protection of their bioactivity and sustained local concentration over an extended time-period at the target site. Micro- or nano-encapsulation prolongs growth factor availability and enhances their penetration through natural barriers. These capsules may also be adsorbed onto scaffolds to increase osteoinductivity and enhance the effectiveness of the construct.

Various growth factors have been used within 3D or injectable carrier structures to achieve enhanced bone regeneration in the craniofacial region (Table 17.3). In particular, BMP-2, PDGF, and FGF-2 have been effective in inducing craniofacial bone regeneration in multicentric, highly randomized clinical trials [64–66]. In the study of Triplett et al. (2009), 160 patients, who were followed up for 5 years in a total of 21 US centers, received 1.50 mg/mL BMP-2 within collagen sponges for the maxillary sinus floor augmentation and the results were compared with autograft application. Patients revealed proper tissue integration and functional recovery starting from 6 months after application.

Table 17.3 Studies including growth factor mediated tissue engineered craniofacial constructs

Study model	Growth factor	Carrier	Application site	Harvest*	Outcome	Ref.
Clinical Trial (Human)	BMP-2	Collagen sponge	Maxillary sinus floor	24	Comparable results with autograft	[65]
	BMP-7	HAp blocks within titanium mesh	Mandibular replacement after maturation of the construct within latissimus dorsi	38	Successful bone regeneration	[69]
	PDGF	TCP matrix	Periodontal osseous defect	24	Increased bone regeneration compared to carrier alone	[64]
	FGF-2	Hydroxypropyl cellulose gel	Periodontal vertical bone defect	36	Increased bone fill	[66]
Primate	TGF-β3	Matrigel® gelatinous protein mixture	Mandibular molar defect	4	Enhanced periodontal regeneration	[67]
Sheep	BMP-7	Collagen matrix	35 mm mandibular osteoperiosteal continuity defect	12	Modest bone regeneration	[68]
Canine	IGF-1/ PDGF	Methylcellulose gel	Implantation into extraction sockets	12	Better bone/implant contact compared to carrier alone	[74]

*Weeks post surgery

Other growth factors such as TGF-β3 [67] and BMP-7 [68] were used in preclinical animal models, while TGF-β3 (1.5 µg/application) was especially reported to be a strong mediator of mandibular defect regeneration in primates. The use of 1.0 mg/cm^3 of BMP-7 alone within a collagen matrix revealed only modest (no effect/positive effect) regeneration of ovine mandibular defects [68]; however, its use within HAp blocks with a total dose of 7 mg led to successful bone healing in a clinical study of mandibular replacement [69].

One of the most recent advancements in growth factor delivery for BTE is the combined delivery of multiple growth factors in a time-dependent manner. The use of BMP-7 in combination with BMP-2 in a nanoparticulate sequential controlled delivery system (providing early BMP-2/late BMP-7 release) to mimic the natural bone regeneration cascade was shown to provide enhanced bone regeneration both in in vitro and in vivo studies. These included free nanoparticulate form as well as nanoparticles incorporated within porous scaffolds [70–72]. Encapsulation of doses as low as 40 ng BMP/mL was shown to be effective in inducing osteogenesis in vitro. The combination of BMP-2/BMP-7 with a total BMP amount of 50 ng/mL induced cementoblastic differentiation of dental follicle cells in vitro [73]. The co-administration of these two growth factors is promising for use in the craniofacial region. However, further studies are needed to validate their effectiveness. Other growth factor cocktails have also been shown to be effective: the cocktail of IGF-1/PDGF (total: 5 µg/mL) within methylcellulose gel carriers showed that bone/implant contact and ossification could be enhanced when implanted into extraction sockets in a canine model [74].

The effectiveness of platelet rich plasma (PRP) was investigated as an easily accessible source of growth factors in periodontal defects [75,76]. Results of these studies revealed conflicting results, suggesting that the effects of composition and dose of PRP should be better understood prior to routine clinical uses. Besides growth factors, strategies incorporating the controlled release of antimicrobial agents within osteoinductive scaffolds could have a functional therapeutic outcome during bone regeneration particularly in infectious environments such as the oral cavity.

17.2.5 Bone Bioreactor

BTE bioreactors are used to regulate the presentation of biological, mechanical, and physiological cues within the cellular microenvironment. The spatial and temporal specificity with which these cues arise during development directs the cell and matrix organization within the tissue. Using bioreactors to recapitulate these spatiotemporal profiles in vitro, it is possible to provide cell-based constructs with physiologically relevant stimuli to guide their conversion into functional tissue types. The earliest iterations of bioreactors—spinner-flasks and rotating wall vessels (RWV)— were used to improve mass transfer in engineered bone grafts. Currently, perfusion bioreactors are most commonly employed for engineered bone applications as they enable predictable flow patterns through the interstitial pore spaces and uniform tissue development.

In addition to improving the transport of nutrients and oxygen, medium perfusion induces shear stresses, which enhances the osteogenic differentiation and mineral deposition of cells seeded within tissue constructs [77]. Consequently, constructs cultured within perfusion bioreactor systems exhibited superior tissue formation properties relative to those cultured under static conditions. Matrix and mineral depositions exhibit dose-dependent relationships with flow-rates: Bancroft et al. reported increases in matrix and mineral content with increased flow-rate [78]. Cartmell and coworkers reported the opposite trend i.e. there was decreased matrix and increased cell death at higher flow-rates [79], while the study done by Grayson et al. demonstrated an optimal flow rate for matrix assembly and deposition of bone specific proteins II (BSP II), osteocalcin, and osteopontin [80]. Differences in cell types, biomaterial composition and structure, and bioreactor designs make it challenging to compare these various findings or understand the discrepancies in results. An attempt was made to decouple the effects of enhanced nutrient transfer from the effects of flow-induced shear forces. To investigate the roles of increased shear stress specifically, Sikavitsas and coworkers [81] added dextran to increase the viscosity of the osteoinductive culture medium used to culture rat marrow stromal cells. In this way, the flow-rate (and hence, nutrient transfer rates) could be maintained constant while varying shear stresses in the various culture conditions. The authors demonstrated that cells within the 3D constructs did exhibit higher mineral and matrix deposition when higher viscosity media (i.e. increased shear stress) was used for perfusion.

The complex patterns of flow through these porous constructs render it unfeasible to experimentally determine the actual values of shear stress imparted to cells in the constructs and extensive use is made of computational modeling. Grayson et al. (2011) [80] used simplified models that neglected the tortuosity of the flow through the pore spaces to evaluate the relative levels of shear and reported that it was significantly lower than the 1–3 Pa reported for cells in native bone [82]. In spite of its simplicity, this was consistent with earlier reports that used more extensive finite element analysis (FEA) for modeling 3D flow through porous architecture [83]. However, these studies only provide approximations as changes in cell density and matrix deposition in the scaffold throughout culture would affect flow patterns and shear distribution over time. When analyzed together with computational models of oxygen distribution, it was concluded that the effects of shear had a greater impact on tissue development within these scaffolds than the improved oxygen delivery to cells [80].

Knowledge gleaned from aforementioned studies, which have all employed cylindrical grafts, has been applied to develop more complex bioreactors capable of housing and perfusing human bone grafts having the geometry of the temporomandibular joint condyle (TMJ) [56]. In this study, a computerized tomography (CT) scan of a patient was obtained and the region of interest segmented to obtain the geometry of the TMJ. The computerized image was used to design a perfusion bioreactor based on FEA models of the flow patterns through the grafts. As a result of the highly irregular shapes, constructs were placed into tightly fit molds to force medium to flow through the interstitial pore spaces. Medium perfusion dramatically enhanced cell number, matrix formation and organization, and mineral deposition throughout the centimeter-sized grafts during the in vitro culture period. The ability to engineer cellularized, anatomically shaped bone grafts has specific significance for craniofacial regeneration given the complex geometry of many of the bones in that region and the importance of aesthetics on the well-being of the individual.

17.3 Impact of Micro- and Nano-Technologies in Craniofacial Bone Tissue Engineering

The natural ECM of bone tissue is a complex array of proteins and glycosaminoglycans, which exhibit hierarchical organization from the nano- to micro- and milliscale. By imitating the intrinsic architecture of ECM for scaffold production, it is possible to influence cellular behavior and enhance bone regeneration. Two approaches have been adopted to incorporate advances in micro- and nanotechnologies into BTE. These include the formation of nanofibrous scaffolds, which directly mimic the ECM structure and the modification of scaffold surfaces with nano-topographical cues to regulate cellular behavior.

17.3.1 Biomimetic Nanofibrous Scaffolds

Among the scaffold production techniques previously discussed, only a few lead to the formation of structures with nanoscale features to mimic the natural ECM structure. These include production of nanofibers by various techniques including electrospinning, self-assembly, and thermally induced phase separation. Electrospinning is based on production of fibers on a grounded collector from a polymer solution by the application of an electric field. This recently established technique is widely used with both natural (e.g., collagen [84]) and synthetic (e.g., PCL, [85]) polymers or blends of both (e.g., PGA/Chitin, [86] as well as inorganic materials such as bioactive glass [87] to produce scaffolds with fibers within the nanometer or micron size range. Thin fiber layers (mats) obtained through electrospinning are generally used as multilamellar 3D structures [88]. Alternatively, nanofibers can be electrospun onto a preformed microfibrous scaffold [89,90] or micro- and nanofibers could be co-electrospun [91] to better mimic the hierarchical features of the natural tissue. Electrospun mats have been combined with macroporous material layers in a sandwich like design to increase the functionality of the scaffold [92]. An alternative approach to producing 3D structures with electrospinning has been to add leachable porogens to the system in the form of either co-electrospun fibers [93] or salt particles [94] to increase cellular infiltration and attachment throughout the inner regions of the scaffold.

Self-assembled nanofibers mimic the collagenous nanofibrillar structure of bone. They form by molecular interactions such as van der Waals forces and are produced through bottom-up formation from small building blocks like nucleic acids and peptides. Chemically synthesized peptide amphiphiles [95] and oligopeptides [96] have also been used to produce self-assembled nonwoven nanofibrous structures. Although these techniques offer simple and spontaneous fabrication methods, insufficient mechanical properties and limited material choices have restricted the use of this technique in scaffold production [97]. As another method to produce macroporous scaffolds with nanofiber features, thermally induced phase separation together with porogen leaching has been used. Various studies have shown that this technique can produce nanofibrous 3D scaffolds having macro and micropores suitable for BTE with a variety of cell types and composite materials [98]. Nanofibers can also be incorporated into anatomically shaped mandibular scaffolds produced within RP molds [99].

17.3.2 Topographical Cues

Cells within natural ECM are subject to distinct topographical features. In vitro studies have demonstrated that cells recognize and react accordingly to surface properties by reorganizing their cytoskeleton, leading to morphological as well as functional alterations. This phenomenon is called contact guidance and is defined as the effect of surface properties, such as topography and roughness, on cell behavior. Bone is essentially a nanocomposite material composed of collagen fibers, HAp minerals, and proteoglycans, having a high degree of structural hierarchy. Mimicking the intrinsic structure of the bone microenvironment at the nanometer scale has been shown to provide enhanced ossification results.

Various techniques have been described in the literature to produce nanostructured scaffolds with ridges, grooves, channels, fibers, and nodes on their surfaces [100]. The most common example of these techniques is photolithography, in which the wafer to be patterned is coated with a photoresist and exposed to high-energy radiation through a mask, creating a pattern on the photoresist. The gaps in the photoresist allow the surface to be subsequently chemically or physically etched. The resultant patterned wafer can then be used as a template from which an inverse pattern is obtained with a polymer solution by solvent casting [101].

Several studies have investigated the influence of nano- and micro-topographic features on cellular responses, bone regeneration, and mineral deposition. In the study of Dalby et al. (2007), nanostructured PMMA substrates with nanopits (D: 120 nm, H: 100 nm) on the surface in an organization ranging from highly ordered to random, were produced by e-beam lithography [102]. It was reported that human MSCs exhibited higher osteoblastic differentiation activity (as measured by osteocalcin and osteopontin expression) when provided with a nanoscale ordered topography. The effect of the nanotopography on the cellular differentiation response was comparable to the osteogenic effects obtained via dexamethasone induction. It was also reported that microgrooves and micropits on poly(3-hydroxybutyrate-co-3-hydroxyvalerate) (PHBV) surface enhanced MSC derived osteoblast adhesion and alignment leading to increased osseointegration [103]. Oriented electrospun nanofibers were also used to align seeded primary osteoblasts in a biomimetic scaffold structure and elevated phenotype expression was reported compared to nonwoven scaffolds [104].

17.4 Summary

Recent studies have demonstrated the considerable potential for engineering functional bone grafts for craniofacial regeneration. Advances in biomaterial design, drug delivery, and bioreactor technologies along with improved understanding of stem cell biology are quickly transforming tissue engineering into a viable therapeutic alternative. However, tissue engineering approaches have only been used to regenerate craniofacial defects in a handful of clinical studies. Achieving widespread clinical application in the future requires the successful hurdling of regulatory, practical, commercial, and biological challenges. As such, advancements in automated bioreactor technologies to perform cell culture tasks may be useful in addressing quality control and manufacturing concerns, which have restricted the implementation of cell-based therapies. The properties of clinically relevant bioreactors for engineering bone grafts have been recently described [105]. Similarly, improved understanding of cell–biomaterial interactions is leading to better designs in the structure and composition of biomaterials that can induce vascular invasion as well as promote tissue development and integration. In essence, technological advances continue to yield improved functional outcomes, driving engineered bone grafts closer to becoming a clinical reality for the repair and regeneration of massive bone defects.

Acknowledgements

We gratefully acknowledge the support of the Johns Hopkins University Biomedical Engineering Department, the Maryland Stem Cell Research Fund (2010-MSCRFE-0150-00 and 2012-MSCRFF-165), and the US Department of Defense (DM090323) for the work described in this chapter.

References

1. Clemens, T. L., and Karsenty, G. (2011). The osteoblast: an insulin target cell controlling glucose homeostasis, *J Bone Miner Res*, **4**, 677–680.
2. Karsenty, G., and Ferron, M. (2012). The contribution of bone to whole-organism physiology, *Nature*, **7381**, 314–320.
3. Karsenty, G., and Oury, F. (2012). Biology without walls: the novel endocrinology of bone, *Annu Rev Physiol*, 87–105.
4. Niemeyer, P., Seckinger, A., Simank, H. G., Kasten, P., Sudkamp, N., and Krause, U. (2004). Allogenic transplantation of human mesenchymal stem cells for tissue engineering purposes: an in vitro study, *Orthopade*, **12**, 1346–1353.
5. Leyh, R. G., Wilhelmi, M., Rebe, P., Fischer, S., Kofidis, T., Haverich, A., and Mertsching, H. (2003). In vivo repopulation of xenogeneic and allogeneic acellular valve matrix conduits in the pulmonary circulation, *Ann Thorac Surg*, **5**, 1457–1463.
6. Marolt, D., Campos, I. M., Bhumiratana, S., Koren, A., Petridis, P., Zhang, G., Spitalnik, P. F., Grayson, W. L., and Vunjak-Novakovic, G. (2012). Engineering bone tissue from human embryonic stem cells, *Proc Natl Acad Sci USA*, **22**, 8705–8709.
7. Jukes, J. M., Both, S. K., Leusink, A., Sterk, L. M., van Blitterswijk, C. A., and de Boer, J. (2008). Endochondral bone tissue engineering using embryonic stem cells, *Proc Natl Acad Sci USA*, **19**, 6840–6845.

8. Takahashi, K., Tanabe, K., Ohnuki, M., Narita, M., Ichisaka, T., Tomoda, K., and Yamanaka, S. (2007). Induction of pluripotent stem cells from adult human fibroblasts by defined factors, *Cell*, **5**, 861–872.
9. Yu, J., Vodyanik, M. A., Smuga-Otto, K., Antosiewicz-Bourget, J., Frane, J. L., Tian, S., Nie, J., Jonsdottir, G. A., Ruotti, V., Stewart, R., Slukvin, II, and Thomson, J. A. (2007). Induced pluripotent stem cell lines derived from human somatic cells, *Science*, **5858**, 1917–1920.
10. Yamanaka, S. (2009). A fresh look at iPS cells, *Cell*, **1**, 13–17.
11. Friedenstein, A. J., Chailakhyan, R. K., and Gerasimov, U. V. (1987). Bone marrow osteogenic stem cells: in vitro cultivation and transplantation in diffusion chambers, *Cell Tissue Kinet*, **3**, 263–272.
12. Kaigler, D., Pagni, G., Park, C. H., Tarle, S. A., Bartel, R. L., and Giannobile, W. V. (2010). Angiogenic and osteogenic potential of bone repair cells for craniofacial regeneration, *Tissue Eng Part A*, **9**, 2809–2820.
13. Hasegawa, N., Kawaguchi, H., Hirachi, A., Takeda, K., Mizuno, N., Nishimura, M., Koike, C., Tsuji, K., Iba, H., Kato, Y., and Kurihara, H. (2006). Behavior of transplanted bone marrow-derived mesenchymal stem cells in periodontal defects, *J Periodontol*, **6**, 1003–1007.
14. Yoshioka, M., Tanimoto, K., Tanne, Y., Sumi, K., Awada, T., Oki, N., Sugiyama, M., Kato, Y., and Tanne, K. (2012). Bone regeneration in artificial jaw cleft by use of carbonated hydroxyapatite particles and mesenchymal stem cells derived from iliac bone, *Int J Dent*, 352510.
15. Cooper, L. F., Harris, C. T., Bruder, S. P., Kowalski, R., and Kadiyala, S. (2001). Incipient analysis of mesenchymal stem-cell-derived osteogenesis, *J Dent Res*, **1**, 314–320.
16. Zuk, P. A., Zhu, M., Ashjian, P., De Ugarte, D. A., Huang, J. I., Mizuno, H., Alfonso, Z. C., Fraser, J. K., Benhaim, P., and Hedrick, M. H. (2002). Human adipose tissue is a source of multipotent stem cells, *Mol Biol Cell*, **12**, 4279–4295.
17. Nacamuli, R. P., and Longaker, M. T. (2005). Bone induction in craniofacial defects, *Orthod Craniofac Res*, **4**, 259–266.
18. Cowan, C. M., Shi, Y. Y., Aalami, O. O., Chou, Y. F., Mari, C., Thomas, R., Quarto, N., Contag, C. H., Wu, B., and Longaker, M. T. (2004). Adipose-derived adult stromal cells heal critical-size mouse calvarial defects, *Nat Biotechnol*, **5**, 560–567.
19. Cordeiro, M. M., Dong, Z., Kaneko, T., Zhang, Z., Miyazawa, M., Shi, S., Smith, A. J., and Nor, J. E. (2008). Dental pulp tissue engineering with stem cells from exfoliated deciduous teeth, *J Endod*, **8**, 962–969.

20. Rios, H. F., Lin, Z., Oh, B., Park, C. H., and Giannobile, W. V. (2011). Cell- and gene-based therapeutic strategies for periodontal regenerative medicine, *J Periodontol*, **9**, 1223–1237.

21. Seo, B. M., Miura, M., Gronthos, S., Bartold, P. M., Batouli, S., Brahim, J., Young, M., Robey, P. G., Wang, C. Y., and Shi, S. (2004). Investigation of multipotent postnatal stem cells from human periodontal ligament, *Lancet*, **9429**, 149–155.

22. Sonoyama, W., Liu, Y., Fang, D., Yamaza, T., Seo, B. M., Zhang, C., Liu, H., Gronthos, S., Wang, C. Y., Wang, S., and Shi, S. (2006). Mesenchymal stem cell-mediated functional tooth regeneration in swine, *PLoS One*, e79.

23. Honda, M. J., Imaizumi, M., Suzuki, H., Ohshima, S., Tsuchiya, S., and Satomura, K. (2011). Stem cells isolated from human dental follicles have osteogenic potential, *Oral Surg Oral Med Oral Pathol Oral Radiol Endod*, **6**, 700–708.

24. Lekic, P. C., Rajshankar, D., Chen, H., Tenenbaum, H., and McCulloch, C. A. (2001). Transplantation of labeled periodontal ligament cells promotes regeneration of alveolar bone, *Anat Rec*, **2**, 193–202.

25. Zhao, M., Jin, Q., Berry, J. E., Nociti, F. H., Jr., Giannobile, W. V., and Somerman, M. J. (2004). Cementoblast delivery for periodontal tissue engineering, *J Periodontol*, **1**, 154–161.

26. Jin, Q. M., Anusaksathien, O., Webb, S. A., Rutherford, R. B., and Giannobile, W. V. (2003). Gene therapy of bone morphogenetic protein for periodontal tissue engineering, *J Periodontol*, **2**, 202–213.

27. Chang, S. C., Chung, H. Y., Tai, C. L., Chen, P. K., Lin, T. M., and Jeng, L. B. (2010). Repair of large cranial defects by hBMP-2 expressing bone marrow stromal cells: comparison between alginate and collagen type I systems, *J Biomed Mater Res A*, **2**, 433–441.

28. Mao, J. J., Giannobile, W. V., Helms, J. A., Hollister, S. J., Krebsbach, P. H., Longaker, M. T., and Shi, S. (2006). Craniofacial tissue engineering by stem cells, *J Dent Res*, **11**, 966–979.

29. Akintoye, S. O., Lam, T., Shi, S., Brahim, J., Collins, M. T., and Robey, P. G. (2006). Skeletal site-specific characterization of orofacial and iliac crest human bone marrow stromal cells in same individuals, *Bone*, **6**, 758–768.

30. Chung, I. H., Yamaza, T., Zhao, H., Choung, P. H., Shi, S., and Chai, Y. (2009). Stem cell property of postmigratory cranial neural crest cells and their utility in alveolar bone regeneration and tooth development, *Stem Cells*, **4**, 866–877.

31. Zaky, S. H., and Cancedda, R. (2009). Engineering craniofacial structures: facing the challenge, *J Dent Res*, **12**, 1077–1091.
32. Ward, B. B., Brown, S. E., and Krebsbach, P. H. (2010). Bioengineering strategies for regeneration of craniofacial bone: a review of emerging technologies, *Oral Dis*, **8**, 709–716.
33. Bateman, J. P., Safadi, F. F., Susin, C., and Wikesjo, U. M. (2012). Exploratory study on the effect of osteoactivin on bone formation in the rat critical-size calvarial defect model, *J Periodontal Res*, **2**, 243–247.
34. Riccio, M., Maraldi, T., Pisciotta, A., La Sala, G. B., Ferrari, A., Bruzzesi, G., Motta, A., Migliaresi, C., and De Pol, A. (2012). Fibroin scaffold repairs critical-size bone defects in vivo supported by human amniotic fluid and dental pulp stem cells, *Tissue Eng Part A*, **9–10**, 1006–1013.
35. Costa-Pinto, A. R., Correlo, V. M., Sol, P. C., Bhattacharya, M., Srouji, S., Livne, E., Reis, R. L., and Neves, N. M. (2012). Chitosan-poly(butylene succinate) scaffolds and human bone marrow stromal cells induce bone repair in a mouse calvaria model, *J Tissue Eng Regen Med*, **1**, 21–28.
36. Tan, R., Feng, Q., Jin, H., Li, J., Yu, X., She, Z., Wang, M., and Liu, H. (2011). Structure and biocompatibility of an injectable bone regeneration composite, *J Biomater Sci Polym Ed*, **14**, 1861–1879.
37. Patterson, J., Siew, R., Herring, S. W., Lin, A. S., Guldberg, R., and Stayton, P. S. (2010). Hyaluronic acid hydrogels with controlled degradation properties for oriented bone regeneration, *Biomaterials*, **26**, 6772–6781.
38. Liu, L. S., Thompson, A. Y., Heidaran, M. A., Poser, J. W., and Spiro, R. C. (1999). An osteoconductive collagen/hyaluronate matrix for bone regeneration, *Biomaterials*, **12**, 1097–1108.
39. Levi, B., James, A. W., Nelson, E. R., Vistnes, D., Wu, B., Lee, M., Gupta, A., and Longaker, M. T. (2010). Human adipose derived stromal cells heal critical size mouse calvarial defects, *PLoS One*, **6**, e11177.
40. Shi, M., Kretlow, J. D., Spicer, P. P., Tabata, Y., Demian, N., Wong, M. E., Kasper, F. K., and Mikos, A. G. (2011). Antibiotic-releasing porous polymethylmethacrylate/gelatin/antibiotic constructs for craniofacial tissue engineering, *J Control Release*, **1**, 196–205.
41. Lee, C. H., Marion, N. W., Hollister, S., and Mao, J. J. (2009). Tissue formation and vascularization in anatomically shaped human joint condyle ectopically in vivo, *Tissue Eng Part A*, **12**, 3923–3930.

42. Henslee, A. M., Gwak, D. H., Mikos, A. G., and Kasper, F. K. (2012). Development of a biodegradable bone cement for craniofacial applications, *J Biomed Mater Res A*, **100**, 2252–1159.

43. Alhadlaq, A., and Mao, J. J. (2005). Tissue-engineered osteochondral constructs in the shape of an articular condyle, *J Bone Joint Surg Am*, **5**, 936–944.

44. Montjovent, M. O., Mathieu, L., Schmoekel, H., Mark, S., Bourban, P. E., Zambelli, P. Y., Laurent-Applegate, L. A., and Pioletti, D. P. (2007). Repair of critical size defects in the rat cranium using ceramic-reinforced PLA scaffolds obtained by supercritical gas foaming, *J Biomed Mater Res. Part A*, **1**, 41–51.

45. Grayson, W. L., Bhumiratana, S., Grace Chao, P. H., Hung, C. T., and Vunjak-Novakovic, G. (2010). Spatial regulation of human mesenchymal stem cell differentiation in engineered osteochondral constructs: effects of pre-differentiation, soluble factors and medium perfusion, *Osteoarthritis Cartilage*, **5**, 714–723.

46. Cancedda, R., Giannoni, P., and Mastrogiacomo, M. (2007). A tissue engineering approach to bone repair in large animal models and in clinical practice, *Biomaterials*, **29**, 4240–4250.

47. Xu, L., Lv, K., Zhang, W., Zhang, X., Jiang, X., and Zhang, F. (2012). The healing of critical-size calvarial bone defects in rat with rhPDGF-BB, BMSCs, and beta-TCP scaffolds, *J Mater Sci Mater Med*, **4**, 1073–1084.

48. Shayesteh, Y. S., Khojasteh, A., Soleimani, M., Alikhasi, M., Khoshzaban, A., and Ahmadbeigi, N. (2008). Sinus augmentation using human mesenchymal stem cells loaded into a beta-tricalcium phosphate/hydroxyapatite scaffold, *Oral Surg Oral Med Oral Pathol Oral Radiol Endod*, **2**, 203–209.

49. Guo, J., Meng, Z., Chen, G., Xie, D., Chen, Y., Wang, H., Tang, W., Liu, L., Jing, W., Long, J., Guo, W., and Tian, W. (2012). Restoration of critical-size defects in the rabbit mandible using porous nanohydroxyapatite-polyamide scaffolds, *Tissue Eng Part A*, **11–12**, 1239–1252.

50. Li, J., Hsu, Y., Luo, E., Khadka, A., and Hu, J. (2011). Computer-aided design and manufacturing and rapid prototyped nanoscale hydroxyapatite/polyamide (n-HA/PA) construction for condylar defect caused by mandibular angle ostectomy, *Aesthetic Plast Surg*, **4**, 636–640.

51. Khadka, A., Li, J., Li, Y., Gao, Y., Zuo, Y., and Ma, Y. (2011). Evaluation of hybrid porous biomimetic nano-hydroxyapatite/polyamide 6 and bone marrow-derived stem cell construct in repair of calvarial critical size defect, *J Craniofac Surg*, **5**, 1852–1858.

52. Schofer, M. D., Roessler, P. P., Schaefer, J., Theisen, C., Schlimme, S., Heverhagen, J. T., Voelker, M., Dersch, R., Agarwal, S., Fuchs-Winkelmann, S., and Paletta, J. R. (2011). Electrospun PLLA nanofiber scaffolds and their use in combination with BMP-2 for reconstruction of bone defects, *PLoS One*, **9**, e25462.

53. Oh, S. H., Kang, S. G., Kim, E. S., Cho, S. H., and Lee, J. H. (2003). Fabrication and characterization of hydrophilic poly(lactic-*co*-glycolic acid)/poly(vinyl alcohol) blend cell scaffolds by melt-molding particulate-leaching method, *Biomaterials*, **22**, 4011–4021.

54. Kim, J., Magno, M. H., Waters, H., Doll, B. A., McBride, S., Alvarez, P., Darr, A., Vasanji, A., Kohn, J., and Hollinger, J. O. (2012). Bone regeneration in a rabbit critical-sized calvarial model using tyrosine-derived polycarbonate scaffolds, *Tissue Eng Part A*, **11–12**, 1132–1139.

55. Williams, J. M., Adewunmi, A., Schek, R. M., Flanagan, C. L., Krebsbach, P. H., Feinberg, S. E., Hollister, S. J., and Das, S. (2005). Bone tissue engineering using polycaprolactone scaffolds fabricated via selective laser sintering, *Biomaterials*, **23**, 4817–4827.

56. Grayson, W. L., Frohlich, M., Yeager, K., Bhumiratana, S., Chan, M. E., Cannizzaro, C., Wan, L. Q., Liu, X. S., Guo, X. E., and Vunjak-Novakovic, G. (2010). Engineering anatomically shaped human bone grafts, *Proc Natl Acad Sci USA*, **8**, 3299–3304.

57. Hollister, S. J., Lin, C. Y., Saito, E., Schek, R. D., Taboas, J. M., Williams, J. M., Partee, B., Flanagan, C. L., Diggs, A., Wilke, E. N., Van Lenthe, G. H., Muller, R., Wirtz, T., Das, S., Feinberg, S. E., and Krebsbach, P. H. (2005). Engineering craniofacial scaffolds, *Orthod Craniofac Res*, **3**, 162–173.

58. Smith, M. H., Flanagan, C. L., Kemppainen, J. M., Sack, J. A., Chung, H., Das, S., Hollister, S. J., and Feinberg, S. E. (2007). Computed tomography-based tissue-engineered scaffolds in craniomaxillofacial surgery, *Int J Med Robot*, **3**, 207–216.

59. Klammert, U., Gbureck, U., Vorndran, E., Rodiger, J., Meyer-Marcotty, P., and Kubler, A. C. (2010). 3D powder printed calcium phosphate implants for reconstruction of cranial and maxillofacial defects, *J Craniomaxillofac Surg*, **8**, 565–570.

60. Centrella, M., Casinghino, S., Ignotz, R., and McCarthy, T. L. (1992). Multiple regulatory effects by transforming growth factor-beta on type I collagen levels in osteoblast-enriched cultures from fetal rat bone, *Endocrinology*, **6**, 2863–2872.

61. Spencer, E. M., Liu, C. C., Si, E. C., and Howard, G. A. (1991). In vivo actions of insulin-like growth factor-I (IGF-I) on bone formation and resorption in rats, *Bone*, **1**, 21–26.

62. Nishimura, T., Utsunomiya, Y., Hoshikawa, M., Ohuchi, H., and Itoh, N. (1999). Structure and expression of a novel human FGF, FGF-19, expressed in the fetal brain, *Biochim Biophys Acta*, **1**, 148–151.

63. Allori, A. C., Sailon, A. M., and Warren, S. M. (2008). Biological basis of bone formation, remodeling, and repair-part I: biochemical signaling molecules, *Tissue Eng Part B Rev*, **3**, 259–273.

64. Nevins, M., Giannobile, W. V., McGuire, M. K., Kao, R. T., Mellonig, J. T., Hinrichs, J. E., McAllister, B. S., Murphy, K. S., McClain, P. K., Nevins, M. L., Paquette, D. W., Han, T. J., Reddy, M. S., Lavin, P. T., Genco, R. J., and Lynch, S. E. (2005). Platelet-derived growth factor stimulates bone fill and rate of attachment level gain: results of a large multicenter randomized controlled trial, *J Periodontol*, **12**, 2205–2215.

65. Triplett, R. G., Nevins, M., Marx, R. E., Spagnoli, D. B., Oates, T. W., Moy, P. K., and Boyne, P. J. (2009). Pivotal, randomized, parallel evaluation of recombinant human bone morphogenetic protein-2/absorbable collagen sponge and autogenous bone graft for maxillary sinus floor augmentation, *J Oral Maxillofac Surg*, **9**, 1947–1960.

66. Kitamura, M., Akamatsu, M., Machigashira, M., Hara, Y., Sakagami, R., Hirofuji, T., Hamachi, T., Maeda, K., Yokota, M., Kido, J., Nagata, T., Kurihara, H., Takashiba, S., Sibutani, T., Fukuda, M., Noguchi, T., Yamazaki, K., Yoshie, H., Ioroi, K., Arai, T., Nakagawa, T., Ito, K., Oda, S., Izumi, Y., Ogata, Y., Yamada, S., Shimauchi, H., Kunimatsu, K., Kawanami, M., Fujii, T., Furuichi, Y., Furuuchi, T., Sasano, T., Imai, E., Omae, M., Watanuki, M., and Murakami, S. (2011). FGF-2 stimulates periodontal regeneration: results of a multi-center randomized clinical trial, *J Dent Res*, **1**, 35–40.

67. Ripamonti, U., Ferretti, C., Teare, J., and Blann, L. (2009). Transforming growth factor-beta isoforms and the induction of bone formation: implications for reconstructive craniofacial surgery, *J Craniofac Surg*, **5**, 1544–1555.

68. Abu-Serriah, M., Ayoub, A., Wray, D., Milne, N., Carmichael, S., and Boyd, J. (2006). Contour and volume assessment of repairing mandibular osteoperiosteal continuity defects in sheep using recombinant human osteogenic protein-1, *J Craniomaxillofac Surg*, **3**, 162–167.

69. Warnke, P. H., Wiltfang, J., Springer, I., Acil, Y., Bolte, H., Kosmahl, M., Russo, P. A., Sherry, E., Lutzen, U., Wolfart, S., and Terheyden, H. (2006). Man as living bioreactor: fate of an exogenously prepared customized tissue-engineered mandible, *Biomaterials*, **17**, 3163–3167.

70. Yilgor, P., Hasirci, N., and Hasirci, V. (2010). Sequential BMP-2/BMP-7 delivery from polyester nanocapsules, *J Biomed Mater Res A*, **2**, 528–536.

71. Yilgor, P., Sousa, R. A., Reis, R. L., Hasirci, N., and Hasirci, V. (2010). Effect of scaffold architecture and BMP-2/BMP-7 delivery on in vitro bone regeneration, *J Mater Sci Mater Med*, **11**, 2999–3008.

72. Yilgor, P., Yilmaz, G., Onal, M. B., Solmaz, I., Gundogdu, S., Keskil, S., Sousa, R. A., Reis, R. L., Hasirci, N., and Hasirci, V. (2012). An in vivo study on the effect of scaffold geometry and growth factor release on the healing of bone defects, *J Tissue Eng Regen Med*, **7**, 687–696.

73. Kemoun, P., Laurencin-Dalicieux, S., Rue, J., Farges, J. C., Gennero, I., Conte-Auriol, F., Briand-Mesange, F., Gadelorge, M., Arzate, H., Narayanan, A. S., Brunel, G., and Salles, J. P. (2007). Human dental follicle cells acquire cementoblast features under stimulation by BMP-2/-7 and enamel matrix derivatives (EMD) in vitro, *Cell Tissue Res*, **2**, 283–294.

74. Stefani, C. M., Machado, M. A., Sallum, E. A., Sallum, A. W., Toledo, S., and Nociti, F. H., Jr. (2000). Platelet-derived growth factor/insulin-like growth factor-1 combination and bone regeneration around implants placed into extraction sockets: a histometric study in dogs, *Implant Dent*, **2**, 126–131.

75. Kotsovilis, S., Markou, N., Pepelassi, E., and Nikolidakis, D. (2010). The adjunctive use of platelet-rich plasma in the therapy of periodontal intraosseous defects: a systematic review, *J Periodontal Res*, **3**, 428–443.

76. Del Fabbro, M., Bortolin, M., Taschieri, S., and Weinstein, R. (2011). Is platelet concentrate advantageous for the surgical treatment of periodontal diseases? A systematic review and meta-analysis, *J Periodontol*, **8**, 1100–1111.

77. Owan, I., Burr, D. B., Turner, C. H., Qiu, J., Tu, Y., Onyia, J. E., and Duncan, R. L. (1997). Mechanotransduction in bone: osteoblasts are more responsive to fluid forces than mechanical strain, *Am J Physiol*, 3 Pt 1, C810–C815.

78. Bancroft, G. N., Sikavitsas, V. I., van den Dolder, J., Sheffield, T. L., Ambrose, C. G., Jansen, J. A., and Mikos, A. G. (2002). Fluid flow increases mineralized matrix deposition in 3D perfusion culture of marrow stromal osteoblasts in a dose-dependent manner, *Proc Natl Acad Sci USA*, **20**, 12600–12605.

79. Cartmell, S. H., Porter, B. D., Garcia, A. J., and Guldberg, R. E. (2003). Effects of medium perfusion rate on cell-seeded three-dimensional bone constructs in vitro, *Tissue Eng*, **6**, 1197–1203.
80. Grayson, W. L., Marolt, D., Bhumiratana, S., Frohlich, M., Guo, X. E., and Vunjak-Novakovic, G. (2011). Optimizing the medium perfusion rate in bone tissue engineering bioreactors, *Biotechnol Bioeng*, **5**, 1159–1170.
81. Sikavitsas, V. I., Bancroft, G. N., Holtorf, H. L., Jansen, J. A., and Mikos, A. G. (2003). Mineralized matrix deposition by marrow stromal osteoblasts in 3D perfusion culture increases with increasing fluid shear forces, *Proc Natl Acad Sci USA*, **25**, 14683–14688.
82. Zeng, Y., Cowin, S. C., and Weinbaum, S. (1994). A fiber matrix model for fluid flow and streaming potentials in the canaliculi of an osteon, *Ann Biomed Eng*, **3**, 280–292.
83. Porter, B., Zauel, R., Stockman, H., Guldberg, R., and Fyhrie, D. (2005). 3-D computational modeling of media flow through scaffolds in a perfusion bioreactor, *J Biomech*, **3**, 543–549.
84. Matthews, J. A., Wnek, G. E., Simpson, D. G., and Bowlin, G. L. (2002). Electrospinning of collagen nanofibers, *Biomacromolecules*, **2**, 232–238.
85. Yu, H. S., Jang, J. H., Kim, T. I., Lee, H. H., and Kim, H. W. (2009). Apatite-mineralized polycaprolactone nanofibrous web as a bone tissue regeneration substrate, *J Biomed Mater Res A*, **3**, 747–754.
86. Park, K. E., Kang, H. K., Lee, S. J., Min, B. M., and Park, W. H. (2006). Biomimetic nanofibrous scaffolds: preparation and characterization of PGA/chitin blend nanofibers, *Biomacromolecules*, **2**, 635–643.
87. Kim, H.W., Kim, H.E., Knowles, J.C. (2006). Production and potential of bioactive glass nanofibers as a next generation biomaterial. *Adv Funct Mater*, **16**, 1529-1535..
88. Chen, L., Zhu, C., Fan, D., Liu, B., Ma, X., Duan, Z., and Zhou, Y. (2011). A human-like collagen/chitosan electrospun nanofibrous scaffold from aqueous solution: electrospun mechanism and biocompatibility, *J Biomed Mater Res A*, **3**, 395–409.
89. Tuzlakoglu, K., Santos, M. I., Neves, N., and Reis, R. L. (2011). Design of nano- and microfiber combined scaffolds by electrospinning of collagen onto starch-based fiber meshes: a man-made equivalent of natural extracellular matrix, *Tissue Eng Part A*, **3–4**, 463–473.

90. Santos, M. I., Tuzlakoglu, K., Fuchs, S., Gomes, M. E., Peters, K., Unger, R. E., Piskin, E., Reis, R. L., and Kirkpatrick, C. J. (2008). Endothelial cell colonization and angiogenic potential of combined nano- and micro-fibrous scaffolds for bone tissue engineering, *Biomaterials*, **32**, 4306–4313.

91. Kim, S. J., Jang, D. H., Park, W. H., and Min, B. M. (2010). Fabrication and characterization of 3-dimensional PLGA nanofiber/microfiber composite scaffolds, *Polymer*, **6**, 1320–1327.

92. Park, S. H., Kim, T. G., Kim, H. C., Yang, D. Y., and Park, T. G. (2008). Development of dual scale scaffolds via direct polymer melt deposition and electrospinning for applications in tissue regeneration, *Acta Biomater*, **5**, 1198–1207.

93. Baker, B. M., Gee, A. O., Metter, R. B., Nathan, A. S., Marklein, R. A., Burdick, J. A., and Mauck, R. L. (2008). The potential to improve cell infiltration in composite fiber-aligned electrospun scaffolds by the selective removal of sacrificial fibers, *Biomaterials*, **15**, 2348–2358.

94. Nam, J., Huang, Y., Agarwal, S., and Lannutti, J. (2007). Improved cellular infiltration in electrospun fiber via engineered porosity, *Tissue Eng*, **9**, 2249–2257.

95. Beniash, E., Hartgerink, J. D., Storrie, H., Stendahl, J. C., and Stupp, S. I. (2005). Self-assembling peptide amphiphile nanofiber matrices for cell entrapment, *Acta Biomater*, **4**, 387–397.

96. Zhang, S., Holmes, T. C., DiPersio, C. M., Hynes, R. O., Su, X., and Rich, A. (1995). Self-complementary oligopeptide matrices support mammalian cell attachment, *Biomaterials*, **18**, 1385–1393.

97. Zhang, Z., Hu, J., and Ma, P. X. (2012). Nanofiber-based delivery of bioactive agents and stem cells to bone sites, *Adv Drug Deliv Rev*, **64**, 1129–1141.

98. Gupte, M. J., and Ma, P. X. (2012). Nanofibrous scaffolds for dental and craniofacial applications, *J Dent Res*, **3**, 227–234.

99. Chen, V. J., Smith, L. A., and Ma, P. X. (2006). Bone regeneration on computer-designed nano-fibrous scaffolds, *Biomaterials*, **21**, 3973–3979.

100. Zorlutuna, P., Annabi, N., Camci-Unal, G., Nikkhah, M., Cha, J. M., Nichol, J. W., Manbachi, A., Bae, H., Chen, S., and Khademhosseini, A. (2012). Microfabricated biomaterials for engineering 3D tissues, *Adv Mater*, **14**, 1782–1804.

101. Falconnet, D., Csucs, G., Grandin, H. M., and Textor, M. (2006). Surface engineering approaches to micropattern surfaces for cell-based assays, *Biomaterials*, **16**, 3044–3063.

102. Dalby, M. J., Gadegaard, N., Tare, R., Andar, A., Riehle, M. O., Herzyk, P., Wilkinson, C. D. W., and Oreffo, R. O. C. (2007). The control of human mesenchymal cell differentiation using nanoscale symmetry and disorder, *Nat Mater*, **12**, 997–1003.

103. Kenar, H., Kocabas, A., Aydinli, A., and Hasirci, V. (2008). Chemical and topographical modification of PHBV surface to promote osteoblast alignment and confinement, *J Biomed Mater Res A*, **4**, 1001–1010.

104. Deng, M., Kumbar, S. G., Nair, L. S., Weikel, A. L., Allcock, H. R., and Laurencin, C. T. (2011). Biomimetic structures: biological implications of dipeptide-substituted polyphosphazene-polyester blend nanofiber matrices for load-bearing bone regeneration, *Adv Funct Mater*, **14**, 2641–2651.

105. Salter, E., Goh, B., Hung, B., Hutton, D., Ghone, N., and Grayson, W. L. (2012). Bone tissue engineering bioreactors: a role in the clinic?, *Tissue Eng Part B Rev*, **1**, 62–75.

Chapter 18

Nanotechnology in Osteochondral Regeneration

Nathan J. Castro,[a] Joseph R. O'Brien,[b] and Lijie Grace Zhang[a]

[a]*Department of Mechanical and Aerospace Engineering and Department of Medicine, The George Washington University, 801 22nd Street, NW, 726 Phillips Hall, Washington, DC 20052, USA*
[b]*Department of Orthopedic Surgery, The George Washington University, 2150 Pennsylvania Avenue, NW, Washington, DC 20037, USA*

lgzhang@gwu.edu

With the development of nanotechnology, a better understanding of the role of feature size (nano, micro, and macro) on cell and tissue behavior, and a focused effort of regenerative medicine and tissue engineering (TE) research on mimicking native tissue dimension and composition, staunch advancements have been made in the areas of tissue and organ regeneration. Through the course of this chapter, we will discuss and explore technological advancements at the nanoscale with emphasis in osteochondral (bone–cartilage) tissue regeneration. We will begin with a brief overview of the anatomy and physiology of osteochondral tissue then explore regenerative approaches for the disparate tissues (bone and cartilage) which comprise the osteochondral tissue unit. Next we will delve in to current strategies and techniques for the manufacture of gradient and stratified scaffolds for regeneration

---

Tissue and Organ Regeneration: Advances in Micro- and Nanotechnology
Edited by Lijie Grace Zhang, Ali Khademhosseini, and Thomas J. Webster
Copyright © 2014 Pan Stanford Publishing Pte. Ltd.
ISBN 978-981-4411-67-7 (Hardcover), 978-981-4411-68-4 (eBook)
www.panstanford.com

of the entire tissue unit with emphasis on synthetic and natural nanocomposite materials.

18.1 Introduction

Acute and chronic osteochondral defects caused by degenerative joint disease (such as osteoarthritis (OA)) and trauma present a common and serious clinical problem. Currently, 48 million Americans are afflicted with this condition and 67 million Americans are projected to suffer from OA by 2030 [8,42] leading to a pressing need for new treatment options to address these defects. Clinically, OA is defined as the progressive degeneration of hyaline cartilage leading to structural and functional failure at the bone–cartilage interface [5]. In severe cases, the cartilage may be missing completely and the subchondral bone is exposed. Not surprisingly, bone-on-bone contact leads to inhibited joint motion and increased pain. Currently, there is no cure for OA and the course of treatment is determined by the severity, type, size, and location of the defect.

Several traditional surgical treatment options are available for focal defects, (>5mm) which include autografts, autologous chondrocyte implantation, allografts, debridement [1], microfracture [11], and mosaicplasty [51]. Even though they are clinically viable options, they are still not perfect. The "gold standard" for osteochondral repair (autograft) largely involves the harvest and transplantation of autologous tissue. In this procedure, cylindrical osteochondral "plugs," which include cartilage and subchondral bone tissue, are harvested from sites within the patient's body that do not experience much mechanical stress and transplanted to defect site(s) wherein greater mechanical stress is experienced [51]. This procedure is considerably limited due to insufficient donor tissue and donor site morbidity. For patients with severe and advanced OA, total joint arthroplasty (TJA) is a common treatment option [57]. Total joint arthroplasty is an invasive procedure wherein the articulating surfaces of the joint are replaced by complex systems comprised of metallic, ceramic, and polymeric components. While generally minor in prevalence, complications such as infection, particulate induced bone loss (osteolysis), and reaction to metal ions can affect the longevity of TJA. Since all mechanical and implanted devices have the potential for failure, treatment of a diseased or damaged joint with an implantable biodegradable single-unit scaffold is appealing. In particular, TE approaches may one day offer the possibility of treating and potentially curing the progression of degenerative joint disease in younger patients thus minimizing the need for TJA. With an increasingly active lifestyle, TE approaches to osteochondral repair may also offer a favorable alternative that enables patients to return to high-impact activities like skiing and running or competitive sports, which are not recommended for patients with TJA.

Therefore, the interdisciplinary field of TE holds great promise for the development of novel therapeutic approaches for the treatment of traumatic injuries, diseases and congenital defects that may overcome the body's natural healing capacity [40,52]. In the following, we will provide an overview of the anatomy and physiology of osteochondral tissue within articulating joints with emphasis on the nanostructured composition of this complex tissue.

18.2 Osteochondral Anatomy and Physiology

Within articulating joints, the osteochondral interface is the junction between hyaline cartilage and the underlying bone. Hyaline cartilage is a multiphase tissue composed of four distinct zones (i.e., superficial, middle, deep and calcified zones), the deepest of which is in direct contact with subchondral bone. From the superficial zone to the calcified region (as shown in Table 18.1), each is primarily classified by chondrocyte cell density and morphology; collagen type [48]; collagen fibril size (30–80 nm) and orientation; and extracellular matrix (ECM) composition [64,69].

Various gradients of water, proteins, chondrocytes, and collagen fibers exist throughout articular cartilage and are purported to be essential for load transfer. For example, aggrecan is a supramolecular proteoglycan, which is linked to hyaluronan and can be found sparingly in the superficial zone but is more concentrated in the middle zone. Aggrecan plays a crucial role in the overall function of articular cartilage mediating compressive stresses through osmotic resistance [31]. When examined from the superficial to the deep zone, a gradual decrease in collagen and water content is evident. In addition, the collagen fiber diameter increases (Table 18.1) along with a transition in chondrocyte morphology (round to elliptical). It should be evident through the course of this discussion that natural human osteochondral tissue ECM can be considered a nanocomposite material due to the nanometer scale of the essential components (such as proteoglycans, collagen, other noncollagenous proteins, and nanocrystalline hydroxyapatite (nHA)) [32].

Table 18.1 Chondrocyte morphology, collagen fiber dimension, and composition of the four distinct articular cartilage layers

Component		Superficial zone	Middle zone	Deep zone	Calcified zone
Chondrocytes	morphology	flattened	round	round or ellipsoid	small and inert
Collagen fibrils	% dry weight [50]	86%	between	67%	ND
	Diameter [41,50,65]	30–35 nm	between	40–80 nm	ND
Proteoglycan	% dry weight [30]	15%	25%	20%	ND
Water	% wet weight [22]	84%	between	40–60%	ND
Total thickness	% total tissue [17]	10–20%	40–60%	20–30%	ND

Source: Data obtained from [17,22,30,41,50,58,65]; ND, no data.

At the superficial zone, the nano collagen fibrils are oriented parallel to the articulating surface [41]. The superficial zone is the most hydrated of all the layers with minimal proteoglycan content and mainly consists of type II collagen [18,19]. The middle zone is a transition between the parallel superficial orientation of the collagen fibrils and the orthogonally oriented fibrils of the deep zone. This region contains more spherically shaped chondrocytes distributed amongst randomly oriented collagen fibrils. Within the deep zone, chondrocytes are packed in columns parallel to the organized collagen fibers [69]. Moreover, cells in the deep zone show a 10-fold increase in synthetic activity even though they only have twice as much surface area and volume when compared to cells located in the superficial zone [69]. Collagen fibrils increase in diameter from the superficial to the deep zone while water content decreases. A basophilic staining region, referred to as the tidemark, is visible in thin sections at the juncture between the non-calcified deep zone and the underlying calcified cartilage. The tidemark region is believed to serve as a mechanism for attachment of the collagen fibrils [31], as well as a mode of nutrient diffusion through small gaps located within the structure [49]. The calcified cartilage zone below is void of proteoglycans and contains collagen type X [69]. It is connected to the subchondral bone through a series of interdigitations, which assist in transforming the shear stresses of articulation into tensile and compressive stresses for load bearing [35]. Type I collagen is primarily found in bone and comprises the bulk collagen character of subchondral bone.

18.3 Osteochondral Tissue Regeneration

18.3.1 Introduction

Interfacial tissue engineering (ITE) is an approach that addresses the complex bi- or multiphasic nature of tissue defects where two or more disparate tissues are proximally located. One of the main caveats of ITE is the presence of shared biochemical and physical characteristics of the tissues being connected (bone–cartilage, tendon/ligament-bone, muscle-tendon) as well as retention of regions of distinct composition and biological function [59]. Current osteochondral ITE strategies commonly employ a combination of cells, a biocompatible/biodegradable three-dimensional (3D) support structure, and chemical or biological factor(s) to promote cell adhesion and proliferation during *de novo* tissue formation. The basic premise relies on the introduction or elicitation of cells to the defect site by means of an appropriate scaffold, which results in directed spatial and temporal tissue remodeling. Several key scaffold parameters shown to affect the success of osteochondral regeneration are: (1) biocompatibility and bioactivity to maximize tissue growth, (2) appropriate mechanical properties to enable the patient's rapid return to mobility while protecting developing tissue, (3) controllable biodegradability where degradation rates closely match the rate of new tissue formation, and (4) interconnected porous structure to improve nutrient diffusion and waste transport

[33,69]. In addition, osteochondral ITE can be classified in to two distinct approaches. The first approach addresses the interface as an independent structure bridging two tissues, the second approach addresses the interface as a component of a specific "tissue unit" transitioning from one tissue type to another [59].

Owing to the aforementioned differences in tissue composition and mechanical properties of osteochondral tissue, researchers have engineered cartilage and bone constructs independently, then suture and/or adhere two distinct constructs together. This approach addresses the heterogeneity in composition and mechanical properties found in each tissue, by means of manufacturing a univariate system. Typically, bone and cartilage are categorized as hard and soft tissues, respectively. Therefore, the base materials employed in the fabrication of each bone and cartilage scaffold are chosen from biomaterials that exhibit similar mechanical and physical properties to the native tissue [23]. For example, natural polymers such as collagen and polysaccharides or water soluble low-molecular weight synthetic polymers (<5 kDa) such as poly(ethylene) glycol and poly(ethylene) oxide allow for easy incorporation of tissue-specific morphogenetic factors have been used for cartilage regeneration. Rigid bone scaffolds traditionally are manufactured from high-molecular weight synthetic polymers, ceramics, and metals with the precursor material usually in solid form. Approaches in the extension of multiple commercially available biomaterials have been explored to address osteochondral defects. For example, Scotti et al. [53] developed and evaluated osteochondral composites generated by the combination of three clinically compliant biomaterials: Chondro-Gide (containing human chondrocytes), Tutobone, and Tisseel. The clinically relevant osteochondral graft exhibited good bonding via biological ECM interactions while exhibiting stability and processability thus facilitating a quick implementation within the clinical arena.

Advances in scaffold design have also included biochemical cues that mimic those found within articular cartilage and subchondral bone exhibiting improved cell adhesion, proliferation, directed differentiation, and phenotypic expression [9,25]. Extended culture approaches, where cartilage-like tissue is secreted by mature cells, have also been employed to overcome the inherent complexity of manufacturing functional tissue in combination with scaffold-based strategies, but limitations with these approaches persist. In addition to biomaterial limitations of traditional TE approaches with respect to spatial and temporal control of tissue formation, the mechanical properties of single tissue-specific constructs has also proven challenging. Therefore, applying nanotechnology (i.e., nanobiomaterials and 3D nanofabrication) to manufacture novel biomimetic osteochondral constructs linking two distinct tissues within certain biological and mechanical constraints merits considerable focused attention. In the following sections, we will explore the role of cutting-edge nanotechnology for osteochondral regeneration.

18.3.2 Nanobiomaterials for Osteochondral Regeneration

With the advent of novel nanobiomaterials, the design of biomimetic and bioactive osteochondral tissue scaffolds with improved biocompatibility and functional properties [73,74] has greatly increased. The underlying advantage of nanoscaled structures is the ability to mimic the native tissue ECM environment, as well as favorably modulate cell function. Several proposed mechanisms for the improved nanomaterial–cell interaction have been correlated to structural (surface topography and surface area) and physicochemical (surface chemistry, energy, and wettability) cues that can regulate cellular behavior, but the basic principles have yet to be identified [55]. In the following, we will discuss several promising nanobiomaterials for osteochondral regeneration.

18.3.2.1 Self-assembling nanobiomaterials

Since natural tissues are constructed via a bottom-up self-assembly method, self-assembling supramolecular nanobiomaterials hold great potential to facilitate the construction of complex tissue environments [32]. Advances in nanotechnology are greatly increasing the design of these types of sophisticated nanobiomaterials. For instance, Hartgerink et al. reported that a peptide-amphiphile (PA) with the cell-adherent RGD (Arg-Gly-Asp) peptide can self-assemble into supramolecular nanofibers and align nHA along their long axis similar to the pattern of bone ECM [26]. Hosseinkhani et al. showed significantly enhanced osteogenic differentiation of stem cells in a 3D PA scaffold when compared to 2D static tissue culture [29]. Also, Shah et al. recently designed PA nanofibers that display a high density of transforming growth factor β1 (TGF-β1) binding sites for improved cartilage regeneration [3,54].

In addition to the promising results obtained with PA nanofibers, another promising direction is the development of new self-assembling nanotubes that mimics cellular (such as DNA) and ECM components while displaying signals in a spatiotemporally controlled manner. Our lab has developed these types of highly innovative self-assembling rosette nanotubes (RNTs, Fig. 18.1) with controllable surface chemistry. Specifically, RNTs are a new class of biologically inspired supramolecular nanobiomaterials obtained through the self-assembly of low-molecular-weight DNA base pair motifs (Guanine^Cytosine, G^C) in an aqueous solution. In our previous pioneering work, we designed multiple DNA-based RNTs with varying peptide and amino acid side chains via a bottom-up self-assembly method, which has shown great potential for cartilage and bone regeneration [10,20,56,68,70–72]. Figure 18.1 illustrates the morphology of two types of twin DNA-based RNTs. For the twin DNA-based RNTs, two covalently linked G^C bases can self-assemble into a six member twin rosette maintained by 36 hydrogen bonds. The RNTs have a very stable nanotubular structure with a hydrophobic core and hydrophilic outer surface via electrostatic forces, base stacking interactions, and hydrophobic effects. The outer diameter and the length of all nanotubes are ~3–4 nm and several hundred nm, respectively. Another intriguing feature of RNTs is their flexibility in design, which makes their length, diameter, and surface chemistry tunable. In our lab's recent work, we explored human bone marrow mesenchymal stem cell (MSC) adhesion, proliferation and 4-week chondrogenic differentitiaon in twin-based RNTs conjugated with cell adherent RGDSK (TB-RNT-RGDSK) peptide adsorbed upon poly-L-lactic acid (PLLA) scaffolds [10]. Our results demonstrated that these biomimetic twin-based nanoutbes can significantly enhance MSC ahesion, proliferation and chondrogenic differentiation (such as glycosaminoglycan (GAG), collagen and protein synthesis) when compared to controls. Histological examination (Fig. 18.2) confirmed that TB-RNT-RGDSK can greatly improve tissue formation when compared to controls without nanotubes.

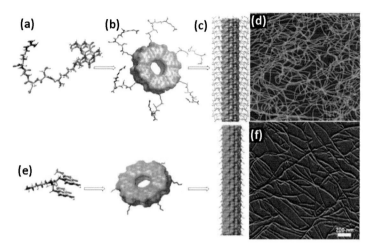

Figure 18.1 Schematic illustration of self-assembly process of RNTs. (a) Twin G^C motifs with a RGDSK peptide; (b) rosette-like supermacrocycle assembled from six motifs; and (c) rosettes stack up into stable helical nanotubes with a 11 Å hollow core, 3–4 nm in diameter and up to several μm long. Atomic force microscopy image of (d) twin DNA-based RNTs with RGDSK peptide. (e) and (f) twin DNA-based RNTs with an aminobutane linker (TBL).

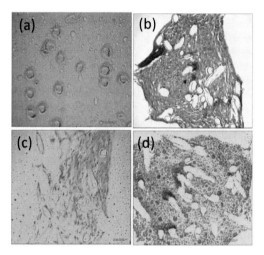

Figure 18.2 Hemotoxylin and eosin staining of (a, c) PLLA controls; and (b, d) TB-RNT-RGDSK PLLA scaffolds for MSC chondrogenic differentiation at weeks 1 and 2.

Self-assembling RNTs have several unique features which renders them ideal for osteochondral tissue regeneration, including: (1) nanostructure and nanotubular architecture creating an environment similar to the dimensions of natural osteochondral ECM; (2) high density of functionalizable surface groups allowing for the incorporation of bioactive peptides with tunable spatial distribution and density via co-assembly; and (3) collagen-like soft nature for improved protein adsorption and cell function. Theoretically, any cell-favorable short peptide can be conjugated onto the G^C motifs to modulate surface chemistry, rendering RNTs as a biomimetic nano-template for tissue regeneration. Based on the current available studies, supramolecular biomimetic self-assembling nanobiomaterials have great potential in regenerating osteochondral tissue.

18.3.2.2 Carbon-based nanobiomaterials

Carbon-based nanobiomaterials such as carbon nanotubes (CNTs) (Fig. 18.3) have also garnered great attention for osteochondral tissue regeneration owing to their excellent mechanical properties, outstanding electrical and surface properties. Although the use of CNTs in tissue regeneration is still in its infancy, they are considered an exciting alternative for osteochondral tissue growth. Morphologically, CNTs exhibit dimensions similar to those of native ECM components (i.e., collagen nanofibers), which cells are accustomed to interacting with. This property renders them an excellent candidate to induce positive cellular responses when combined with traditional biomaterials [67]. In addition, their superior mechanical properties are efficient for use as a nanoscale reinforcing material for high-load-bearing applications [2,15,37,43,45]. Their unique chemical properties they possess permit them to be functionalized with varying chemical groups for the promotion of cell growth [60].

To date, CNTs have primarily been employed in bone tissue engineering where rigid and robust scaffolds must be able to withstand considerable mechanical load. Notwithstanding, CNTs have shown to be beneficial in cartilage regeneration applications as well [27]. For instance, recently Holmes et al. used H_2-purified multi-walled carbon nanotubes (MWCNTs, Fig. 18.3a) coated with poly-L-lysine within a biocompatible PLLA polymer to electrospin CNT-doped microfibers for cartilage regeneration [27]. It was found that scaffolds made from these fibers had mechanical properties quite similar to native articular cartilage. When compared to a pure PLLA control, scaffolds with MWCNTs showed no adverse effects on MSC proliferation, and, more importantly, displayed enhanced MSC chondrogenesis. The purified H_2-treated nanotubes also showed enhanced differentiation over scaffolds containing untreated tubes (Fig. 18.3b).

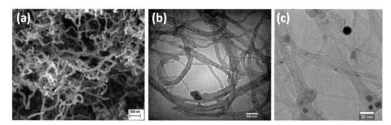

Figure 18.3 Scanning electron microscopy (SEM) image of (a) hydrogen purified multiwalled carbon nanotubes (MWCNTs); Transmission electron microscopy (TEM) images of (b) untreated MWCNTs and (c) magnetically treated single-walled carbon nanotubes (SWCNTs).

Although cytotoxicity concerns have been raised, carbon-based nanobiomaterials have exhibited great potential for a variety of tissue regenerative applications. With the rapid development of highly reproducible synthesis methods, greater controlled production, and experimental analysis, highly purified and novel functionalized carbon nanotubes/fibers with various bioactive molecules have been prepared and have shown better cell or tissue responses. Moving forward, the underlying mechanism of interaction between carbon nanotubes/fibers or composites and cells particularly at the molecular level will be thoroughly clarified in order to design ever more cytocompatible nanotubes/fibers in an effort to advance the clinical application of carbon-based nanobiomaterial.

18.3.2.3 Other therapeutic encapsulated nanobiomaterials

In addition to the increased attention and implementation of the aforementioned nanobiomaterials, extended delivery of tissue-specific growth factors through the manufacture of growth factor encapsulated nanospheres has also shown great promise for improved osteochondral tissue growth. Nanoparticle fabrication for therapeutic encapsulation has long been an area of research with widespread applications [4,21,24,46,47]. As in the case with osteochondral tissue regeneration, availability of candidate nanomaterials for efficient growth factor encapsulation is still sparse. Our lab has begun exploring the use of electrosprayed core–shell nanospheres for highly efficient encapsulation of growth factors and therapeutics.

Electrospraying, as depicted in Fig. 18.4, employs the same basic principle as traditional electrospinning wherein a voltage potential is generated between one electrode (needle) and another electrode (collector plate) to overcome the inherent surface tension of the polymer solution. Unlike electrospinning where the polymer solution is a fairly viscous liquid, polymer solutions employed in electrospraying are quite dilute allowing for the formation of a droplet stream composed of nanospheres. This technique allows for better regulation of particle size with similar or greater encapsulation when compared to traditional emulsion techniques. Although traditional emulsion-based micro/nanosphere fabrication techniques have exhibited positive results, limitations regarding initial burst and uncontrolled release have inhibited their full clinical potential partially due to the disparity in particle size. Coaxial electrospraying can produce nanospheres with good size distribution (Fig. 18.4a). Our recent study has revealed that electrosprayed core–shell polydioxanone nanospheres can steadily release encapsulated therapeutics over 18 days without initial burst release [7]. In addition, the flexibility of this technique allows for a wide range of polymer materials to be used as controlled delivery vesicles.

Another commonly used nanoparticle biomaterial for osteochondral regeneration is nHA. It is the key bioactive and osteoconductive chemical component in subchondral bone and calcified cartilage. Through a hydrothermal treatment method [34, 56,61,62,66,72], nHA can be readily synthesized with excellent control of the crystallinity and surface morphology at the nanoscale (Fig. 18.5a). It has been shown that nHA particles can directly nucleate and align along the long axis of RNTs (Fig. 18.5b) [72] similar to the self-assembled pattern of nHA and collagen in subchondral bone. Owing to the disparate mechanical properties of native osteochondral tissue, osteogenic nHA particles have been used to reinforce various natural and synthetic "soft" materials such as collagen and hydrogels to create a stiffness gradient emanating from the dense, rigid subchondral region to the ceramic-free superficial articular cartilage zone [38].

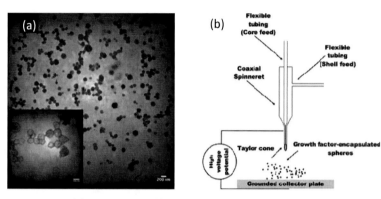

Figure 18.4 (a) TEM image of bone morphogenetic protein-2 encapsulated polydioxanone nanospheres. (b) Graphical representation of a coaxial electrospray technique for the manufacture of growth factor-encapsulated nanospheres.

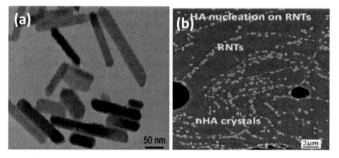

Figure 18.5 (a) TEM image of rod-like nHAs. (b) SEM image of nHA nucleation on RNTs.

In summary, several examples have been provided illustrating the effectiveness of nanobiomaterials for osteochondral tissue regeneration. Although nanobiomaterials have been widely investigated in many other regenerative applications to include bone [74], there are still limited studies for complex osteochondral tissue regeneration. Since cells directly interact with (and create) nanostructured osteochondral ECM, the biomimetic features and excellent physiochemical properties of nanomaterials play a key role in stimulating cell growth as well as guided tissue regeneration, thus holding great potential for clinical applications. The following section will further explore 3D spatiotemporal nanocomposite scaffold manufacturing techniques for osteochondral defect repair.

18.3.3 Three-Dimensional Nanocomposite Scaffolds For Osteochondral Regeneration

Generally, traditional TE efforts have focused on the manufacture of homogenous constructs exhibiting mechanical properties and characteristics similar to those of one particular tissue type. As previously discussed, the osteochondral interface is the juncture between disparate bone and cartilage tissue; therefore it is not only imperative to mimic the composition of one tissue, but of all the tissues present. Consequently, current research has focused on the fabrication of 3D spatiotemporal stratified/graded nanocomposite scaffolds that better mimic native osteochondral tissue.

18.3.3.1 3D stratified/graded nano osteochondral scaffolds

Three-dimensional scaffold architecture and geometric cues play a major role in directing cell behavior and tissue regeneration [39]. For osteochondral studies, conventional 3D scaffold fabrication methods such as electrospinning, particle leaching, and freeze drying have been used to fabricate 3D biphasic and graded osteochondral scaffolds which have shown to influence cell behavior and improve tissue regeneration [6,7,14,28]. Stratified and graded scaffolds aim to collectively induce osteochondral tissue formation through physiochemical and/or mechanical stimulation of cells leading to the growth of mature healthy tissue. Castro et al. developed a novel approach to fabricate a stratified biphasic osteochondral construct (Fig. 18.6) containing tissue-specific nanobiomaterials, including nHA, bone morphogenetic protein-2 (BMP-2), and TGF-β1-loaded core–shell nanospheres. The work illustrated the feasibility of manufacturing a biomimetic osteochondral nanocomposite scaffold with controlled growth factor release leading to increased MSC growth and osteochondral differentiation. Other systems have also focused on the fabrication of stratified scaffolds through novel methods of adhering discrete tissue-specific layers [36,44] to address the mechanical requirements of each tissue type. In addition, Erisken et al. [16] fabricated graded poly(caprolactone)/nHA composite fiber meshes via a hybrid twin-screw extrusion/electrospinning technique with excellent nanoparticle spatial control. Fibrous meshes were subsequently seeded with mouse pre-osteoblast cells and after a four-week culture period, a deposited ECM was observed exhibiting gradations of collagen type I and calcium. Wang et al. [63] developed a silk microsphere/scaffold gradient system wherein recombinant BMP-2 and insulin-like growth factor-1 (IGF-1) were encapsulated within silk microspheres for controlled release and spatially distributed within the silk scaffold for directed human MSC differentiation. This study shows that MSCs exhibited osteogenic and chondrogenic phenotypic expression along the BMP-2 gradient and combination of BMP-2/IGF-1 after culturing the seeded scaffolds in a medium containing osteogenic and chondrogenic factors.

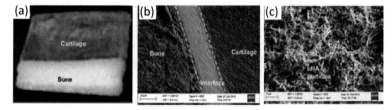

Figure 18.6   Optical (left) and SEM images (middle and right) of biomimetic biphasic 3D osteochondral scaffolds for joint defect repair. High magnification SEM images illustrate a nHA-reinforced polycaprolactone bone layer with a well-integrated poly(ethylene) glycol hydrogel cartilage layer.

18.3.3.2   Emerging 3D printed nanocomposite osteochondral scaffolds

For osteochondral studies, conventional 3D scaffold fabrication methods offer limited control over scaffold geometry, pore size and distribution, pore interconnectivity, as well as internal channel construction. Random, spontaneously generated and disconnected pores significantly decrease nutrient transportation, cell migration, and survival especially in the center of the scaffold limiting their clinical feasibility. As an emerging biotechnology, 3D printing (such as stereolithography, fused deposition modeling, inkjet printing, selective laser sintering) offers great precision and control of the internal architecture and outer shape of a scaffold, allowing for the fabrication of complicated structures that closely mirror the architecture of biological tissue [13]. Based on computer-aided design (CAD) data reconstructed from MRI images of defects, 3D printers can easily fabricate an osteochondral construct with anatomically relevant gross shape for a near-perfect fit within a defect site. Recently Cui et al. successfully inkjet bioprinted a poly (ethylene glycol) dimethacrylate solution containing chondrocytes into a defect formed in an osteochondral plug [12]. They observed greater proteoglycan deposition at the interface of the printed implant and native tissue.

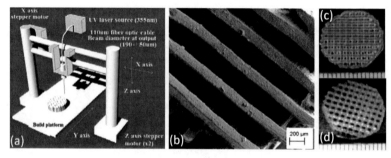

Figure 18.7 (a) Schematic illustration of a new table top stereolithography 3D bioprinter. (b) SEM image of 3D printed poly(ethylene glycol) diacrylate nano osteochondral scaffold with nHA particles. (c, d) 3D printed poly(ethylene glycol) diacrylate hydrogel scaffold without nHA.

3D printing technologies allow for the fabrication of osteochondral scaffolds through a layer-by-layer process in which nanobiomaterials can be readily incorporated within or upon 3D scaffolds for greater spatiotemporal control. The extension of 3D printing technologies in the design and fabrication of spatiotemporal osteochondral scaffolds can further aid in the development of raw and composite nanobiomaterials designed specifically for the technology employed. Manufacturing constraints and available nanobiomaterials with suitable physical and biological properties have limited the clinical applicability of bioprinted constructs for osteochondral applications, but more focused investigations have leveraged nanomaterials such as those previously described in fabricating more biomimetic osteochondral scaffolds. Our lab has developed a table-top stereolithography apparatus for the manufacture of osteochondral scaffolds containing graded nHA particles (Fig. 18.7). Through the integration of nanobiomaterials and 3D printing, we are inching ever more closer to a biomimetic and bioactive remedy for osteochondral defects.

18.4 Conclusions

From traditional homogenous constructs to contemporary functionally graded scaffolds, osteochondral ITE has evolved as novel nanobiomaterials, 3D nano/microfabrication techniques, and a greater understanding of cell–ECM interactions have progressed in a concerted effort to direct multi-tissue regeneration. Despite the challenges that lie ahead, significant evidence now exists elucidating that nanotechnology represents an important and transformative area of research that will most certainly aid in improving osteochondral implant efficacy. By extending the capabilities of current TE strategies and nanotechnology in a concerted effort toward an often overlooked and complex research area, advancements in the development of clinically relevant implantable osteochondral constructs may soon be realized.

References

1. Aaron, R. K., A. H. Skolnick, S. E. Reinert, and D. M. Ciombor, Arthroscopic debridement for osteoarthritis of the knee. *J Bone Joint Surg-Am*, 2006. **88**(5), 936–43.
2. Abarrategi, A., M. C. Gutierrez, C. Moreno-Vicente, M. J. Hortiguela, V. Ramos, J. L. Lopez-Lacomba, M. L. Ferrer, and F. del Monte, Multiwall carbon nanotube scaffolds for tissue engineering purposes. *Biomaterials*, 2008. **29**(1), 94–102.
3. Aida, T., E. W. Meijer, and S. I. Stupp, Functional supramolecular polymers. *Science*, 2012. **335**(6070), 813–817.
4. Anchordoquy, T., and L. Xu, Drug delivery trends in clinical trials and translational medicine: challenges and opportunities in the delivery of nucleic acid-based therapeutics. *J Pharm Sci*, 2011. **100**(1), 38–52.
5. Buckwalter, J. A., J. Martin, and H. J. Mankin, Synovial joint degeneration and the syndrome of osteoarthritis. *Instr Course Lect*, 2000. **49**, 481–489.

6. Castro, N. J., S. A. Hacking, and L. G. Zhang, Recent progress in interfacial tissue engineering approaches for osteochondral defects. *Ann Biomed Eng*, 2012. **40**(8), 1628–1640.
7. Castro, N. J., C. O'Brien, and L. G. Zhang, Biomimetic biphasic 3D nanocomposite scaffold for osteochondral regeneration AICHE Journal 2014. **60**(2), 432-442.
8. CDC,http://www.cdc.gov/arthritis/arthritis/osteoarthritis.htm.2008, National Center for Chronic Disease Prevention and Health Promotion.
9. Chen, J., H. Chen, P. Li, H. Diao, S. Zhu, L. Dong, R. Wang, T. Guo, J. Zhao, and J. Zhang, Simultaneous regeneration of articular cartilage and subchondral bone in vivo using MSCs induced by a spatially controlled gene delivery system in bilayered integrated scaffolds. *Biomaterials*, 2011. **32**(21), 4793–4805.
10. Childs, A., U. D. Hemraz, N. J. Castro, H. Fenniri, and L. G. Zhang, Novel biologically-inspired rosette nanotube PLLA scaffolds for improving human mesenchymal stem cell chondrogenic differentiation. *Biomed Mater*, 2013. **8**(6), 065003.
11. Chuckpaiwong, B., E. M. Berkson, and G. H. Theodore, Microfracture for osteochondral lesions of the ankle: outcome analysis and outcome predictors of 105 cases. *Arthroscopy J Arthroscopic Relat Surg*, 2008. **24**(1), 106–112.
12. Cui, X., K. Breitenkamp, M. G. Finn, M. Lotz, and D. D. D'Lima, Direct human cartilage repair using three-dimensional bioprinting technology. *Tissue Eng Part A*, 2012. **18**(11–12), 1304–1312.
13. Derby, B., Printing and prototyping of tissues and scaffolds. *Science*, 2012. **338**(6109), 921–926.
14. Dormer, N. H., M. Singh, L. Wang, C. J. Berkland, and M. S. Detamore, Osteochondral interface tissue engineering using macroscopic gradients of bioactive signals. *Ann Biomed Eng*, 2010. **38**(6), 2167–2182.
15. Edwards, S. L., J. A. Werkmeister, and J. A. Ramshaw, Carbon nanotubes in scaffolds for tissue engineering. *Expert Rev Med Devices*, 2009. **6**(5), 499–505.
16. Erisken, C., D. M. Kalyon, and H. Wang, Functionally graded electrospun polycaprolactone and beta-tricalcium phosphate nanocomposites for tissue engineering applications. *Biomaterials*, 2008. **29**(30), 4065–4073.

17. Ethier, C. R., and C. A. Simmons, *Introductory Biomechanics—From Cells to Organisms*. 2007: Cambridge University Press 459.
18. Eyre, D., Collagen of articular cartilage. *Arthritis Res*, 2002. **4**(1), 30–35.
19. Eyre, D. R., M. A. Weis, and J. J. Wu, Articular cartilage collagen: an irreplaceable framework? *Eur Cell Mater*, 2006. **12,** 57–63.
20. Fine, E., L. Zhang, H. Fenniri, and T. J. Webster, Enhanced endothelial cell functions on rosette nanotube-coated titanium vascular stents. *Int J Nanomed*, 2009. **4**, 91–97.
21. Foldvari, M., M. Elsabahy, and A. Nazarali, Non-viral nucleic acid delivery: key challenges and future directions. *Curr Drug Deliv*, 2011. **8**(3), 235–244.
22. Freeman, M. A. R., *Adult Articular Cartilage*. 1979, Tunbridge Wells: Pitman Medical. 590.
23. Ge, Z., C. Li, B. C. Heng, G. Cao, and Z. Yang, Functional biomaterials for cartilage regeneration. *J Biomed Mater Res Part A*, 2012. **100**(9), 2526–2536.
24. Grund, S., M. Bauer, and D. Fischer, Polymers in drug delivery-state of the art and future trends. *Adv Eng Mater*, 2011. **13**(3), B61–B87.
25. Guo, X., H. Park, S. Young, J. D. Kretlow, J. J. van den Beucken, L. S. Baggett, Y. Tabata, F. K. Kasper, A. G. Mikos, and J. A. Jansen, Repair of osteochondral defects with biodegradable hydrogel composites encapsulating marrow mesenchymal stem cells in a rabbit model. *Acta Biomater*, 2010. **6**(1), 39–47.
26. Hartgerink, J. D., E. Beniash, and S. I. Stupp, Self-assembly and mineralization of peptide-amphiphile nanofibers. *Science*, 2001. **294**(5547), 1684–1688.
27. Holmes, B., N. J. Castro, J. Li, M. Keidar, and L. G. Zhang, Enhanced human bone marrow mesenchymal stem cell functions in novel 3D cartilage scaffolds with hydrogen treated multi-walled carbon nanotubes. *Nanotechnology*, 2013. **24**(36), 365102.
28. Holmes, B., N. J. Castro, L. G. Zhang, and E. Zussman, Electrospun fibrous scaffolds for bone and cartilage tissue generation: recent progress and future developments. *Tissue Eng Part B Rev*, 2012. **18**(6), 478–486.
29. Hosseinkhani, H., M. Hosseinkhani, F. Tian, H. Kobayashi, and Y. Tabata, Osteogenic differentiation of mesenchymal stem cells in self-assembled peptide-amphiphile nanofibers. *Biomaterials*, 2006. **27**(22), 4079–4086.

30. Hu, J., Chondrocyte self-assembly and culture in bioreactors, in Department of Bioengineeirng 2005, Rice University: Houston. PhD thesis, p. 276.

31. Huber, M., S. Trattnig, and F. Lintner, Anatomy, biochemistry, and physiology of articular cartilage. *Invest Radiol*, 2000. **35**(10), 573–580.

32. Huebsch, N., and D. J. Mooney, Inspiration and application in the evolution of biomaterials. *Nature*, 2009. **462**(7272), 426–432.

33. Hutmacher, D. W., Scaffolds in tissue engineering bone and cartilage. *Biomaterials*, 2000. **21**(24), 2529–2543.

34. Im, O., J. Li, M. Wang, L. G. Zhang, and M. Keidar, Biomimetic three-dimensional nanocrystalline hydroxyapatite and magnetically synthesized single-walled carbon nanotube chitosan nanocomposite for bone regeneration. *Int J Nanomed*, 2012. **7**, 2087–2099.

35. Imhof, H., I. Sulzbacher, S. Grampp, C. Czerny, S. Youssefzadeh, and F. Kainberger, Subchondral bone and cartilage disease— A rediscovered functional unit. *Invest Radiol*, 2000. **35**(10), 581–588.

36. Jiang, C. C., H. Chiang, C. J. Liao, Y. J. Lin, T. F. Kuo, C. S. Shieh, Y. Y. Huang, and R. S. Tuan, Repair of porcine articular cartilage defect with a biphasic osteochondral composite. *J Orthop Res*, 2007. **25**(10), 1277–1290.

37. Kawaguchi, M., T. Fukushima, T. Hayakawa, N. Nakashima, Y. Inoue, S. Takeda, K. Okamura, and K. Taniguchi, Preparation of carbon nanotube-alginate nanocomposite gel for tissue engineering. *Dent Mater J*, 2006. **25**(4), 719–725.

38. Khanarian, N. T., J. Jiang, L. Q. Wan, V. C. Mow, and H. H. Lu, A hydrogel-mineral composite scaffold for osteochondral interface tissue engineering. *Tissue Eng Part A*, 2011. **18**(5–6), 533–545.

39. Kilian, K. A., B. Bugarija, B. T. Lahn, and M. Mrksich, Geometric cues for directing the differentiation of mesenchymal stem cells. *Proc Natl Acad Sci U S A*, 2010. **107**(11), 4872–4877.

40. Langer, R., and J. P. Vacanti, Tissue engineering. *Science*, 1993. **260**(5110), 920–926.

41. Langsjo, T. K., M. Hyttinen, A. Pelttari, K. Kiraly, J. Arokoski, and H. J. Helminen, Electron microscopic stereological study of collagen fibrils in bovine articular cartilage: volume and surface densities are best obtained indirectly (from length densities and diameters) using isotropic uniform random sampling. *J Anat*, 1999. **195** (Pt 2), 281–293.

42. Lawrence, R. C., D. T. Felson, C. G. Helmick, L. M. Arnold, H. Choi, R. A. Deyo, S. Gabriel, R. Hirsch, M. C. Hochberg, G. G. Hunder, J. M. Jordan, J. N. Katz, H. M. Kremers, and F. Wolfe, Estimates of the prevalence of arthritis and other rheumatic conditions in the United States. Part II. *Arthritis Rheum*, 2008. **58**(1), 26–35.

43. MacDonald, R. A., B. F. Laurenzi, G. Viswanathan, P. M. Ajayan, and J. P. Stegemann, Collagen-carbon nanotube composite materials as scaffolds in tissue engineering. *J Biomed Mater Res Part A*, 2005. **74**(3), 489–496.

44. Oliveira, J. M., M. T. Rodrigues, S. S. Silva, P. B. Malafaya, M. E. Gomes, C. A. Viegas, I. R. Dias, J. T. Azevedo, J. F. Mano, and R. L. Reis, Novel hydroxyapatite/chitosan bilayered scaffold for osteochondral tissue-engineering applications: Scaffold design and its performance when seeded with goat bone marrow stromal cells. *Biomaterials*, 2006. **27**(36), 6123–6137.

45. Pan, L., X. Pei, R. He, Q. Wan, and J. Wang, Multiwall carbon nanotubes/polycaprolactone composites for bone tissue engineering application. *Colloids Surf B Biointerfaces*, 2012. **93**, 226–234.

46. Park, K., J. Y. Kim, S. Kim, and R. Pinal, Hydrotropic polymer micelles as versatile vehicles for delivery of poorly water-soluble drugs. *J Control Release*, 2011. **152**(1), 13–20.

47. Parveen, S., R. Misra, and S. K. Sahoo, Nanoparticles: a boon to drug delivery, therapeutics, diagnostics and imaging. *Nanomed-Nanotechnol Biol Med*, 2012. **8**(2), 147–166.

48. Reddi, A. H., R. Gay, S. Gay, and E. J. Miller, Transitions in collagen types during matrix-induced cartilage, bone, and bone-marrow formation. *Proc Natl Acad Sci U S A*, 1977. **74**(12), 5589–5592.

49. Redler, I., V. C. Mow, M. L. Zimny, and J. Mansell, The ultrastructure and biomechanical significance of the tidemark of articular cartilage. *Clin Orthop Relat Res*, 1975. (112), 357–362.

50. Responte, D. J., R. M. Natoli, and K. A. Athanasiou, Collagens of articular cartilage: structure, function, and importance in tissue engineering. *Crit Rev Biomed Eng*, 2007. **35**(5), 363–411.

51. Robert, H., Chondral repair of the knee joint using mosaicplasty. *Orthop Traumatol Surg Res*, 2011. **97**(4), 418–429.

52. Santo, V. E., M. E. Gomes, J. F. Mano, and R. L. Reis, From nano- to macro-scale: nanotechnology approaches for spatially controlled delivery of bioactive factors for bone and cartilage engineering. *Nanomedicine (Lond)*, 2012. **7**(7), 1045–1066.

53. Scotti, C., D. Wirz, F. Wolf, D. J. Schaefer, V. Burgin, A. U. Daniels, V. Valderrabano, C. Candrian, M. Jakob, I. Martin, and A. Barbero, Engineering human cell-based, functionally integrated osteochondral grafts by biological bonding of engineered cartilage tissues to bony scaffolds. *Biomaterials*, 2010. **31**(8), 2252–2259.

54. Shah, R. N., N. A. Shah, M. M. Del Rosario Lim, C. Hsieh, G. Nuber, and S. I. Stupp, Supramolecular design of self-assembling nanofibers for cartilage regeneration. *Proc Natl Acad Sci U S A*, 2010. **107**(8), 3293–3298.

55. Streicher, R. M., M. Schmidt, and S. Fiorito, Nanosurfaces and nanostructures for artificial orthopedic implants. *Nanomedicine (Lond)*, 2007. **2**(6), 861–874.

56. Sun, L., L. Zhang, U. D. Hemraz, H. Fenniri, and T. J. Webster, Bioactive rosette nanotube-hydroxyapatite nanocomposites improve osteoblast functions. *Tissue Eng Part A*, 2012. **18**(17–18), 1741–1750.

57. Tavazoie, S. F., C. Alarcon, T. Oskarsson, D. Padua, Q. Wang, P. D. Bos, W. L. Gerald, and J. Massague, Endogenous human microRNAs that suppress breast cancer metastasis. *Nature*, 2008. **451**(7175), 147–152.

58. Temenoff, J. S., and A. G. Mikos, Review: tissue engineering for regeneration of articular cartilage. *Biomaterials*, 2000. **21**(5), 431–440.

59. Temenoff, J. S., and P. J. Yang, Engineering orthopedic tissue interfaces. *Tissue Eng Part B-Rev*, 2009. **15**(2), 127–141.

60. Tran, P. A., L. Zhang, and T. J. Webster, Carbon nanofibers and carbon nanotubes in regenerative medicine. *Adv Drug Deliv Rev*, 2009. **61**(12), 1097–1114.

61. Wang, M., N. J. Castro, J. Li, M. Keidar, and L. G. Zhang, Greater osteoblast and mesenchymal stem cell adhesion and proliferation on titanium with hydrothermally treated nanocrystalline hydroxyapatite/magnetically treated carbon nanotubes. *J Nanosci Nanotechnol*, 2012. **12**(10), 7692–7702.

62. Wang, M., X. Cheng, W. Zhu, B. Holmes, M. Keidar, and L. G. Zhang, Design of biomimetic and bioactive cold plasma-modified nanostructured scaffolds for enhanced osteogenic differentiation of bone marrow-derived mesenchymal stem cells. *Tissue Eng Part A*, 2013. doi:10.1089/ten.tea.2013.0235.

63. Wang, X., E. Wenk, X. Zhang, L. Meinel, G. Vunjak-Novakovic, and D. L. Kaplan, Growth factor gradients via microsphere delivery in

biopolymer scaffolds for osteochondral tissue engineering. *J Control Release*, 2009. **134**(2), 81–90.

64. Watanabe, H., and K. Kimata, The roles of proteoglycans for cartilage. *Clin Calcium*, 2006. **16**(6), 1029–1033.

65. Weiss, C., L. Rosenberg, and A. J. Helfet, An ultrastructural study of normal young adult human articular cartilage. *J Bone Joint Surg Am*, 1968. **50**(4), 663–674.

66. Zhang, L., Y. Chen, J. Rodriguez, H. Fenniri, and T. J. Webster, Biomimetic helical rosette nanotubes and nanocrystalline hydroxyapatite coatings on titanium for improving orthopedic implants. *Intl J Nanomed*, 2008. **3**(3), 323–333.

67. Zhang, L., B. Ercan, and T. J. Webster, Carbon nanotubes and nanofibers for tissue engineering applications, in *Carbon* (C. Liu, ed.), 2009, Research Signpost.

68. Zhang, L., U. D. Hemraz, H. Fenniri, and T. J. Webster, Tuning cell adhesion on titanium with osteogenic rosette nanotubes. *J Biomed Mater Res A*, 2010. **95**(2), 550–563.

69. Zhang, L., J. Hu, and K. A. Athanasiou, The role of tissue engineering in articular cartilage repair and regeneration. *Crit Rev Biomed Eng*, 2009. **37**(1–2), 1–57.

70. Zhang, L., F. Rakotondradany, A. J. Myles, H. Fenniri, and T. J. Webster, Arginine-glycine-aspartic acid modified rosette nanotube-hydrogel composites for bone tissue engineering. *Biomaterials*, 2009. **30**(7), 1309–1320.

71. Zhang, L., S. Ramsaywack, H. Fenniri, and T. J. Webster, Enhanced osteoblast adhesion on self-assembled nanostructured hydrogel scaffolds. *Tissue Eng Part A*, 2008. **14**(8), 1353–1364.

72. Zhang, L., J. Rodriguez, J. Raez, A. J. Myles, H. Fenniri, and T. J. Webster, Biologically inspired rosette nanotubes and nanocrystalline hydroxyapatite hydrogel nanocomposites as improved bone substitutes. *Nanotechnology*, 2009. **20**(17), 175101.

73. Zhang, L., S. Sirivisoot, G. Balasundaram, and T. J. Webster, Nanoengineering for bone tissue engineering, in *Micro and Nanoengineering of the Cell Microenvironment: Technologies and Applications* (A. Khademhosseini, et al., eds.), 2008, Artech House. pp. 431–460.

74. Zhang, L., and T. J. Webster, Nanotechnology and nanomaterials: promises for improved tissue regeneration. *Nanotoday*, 2009. **4**(1), 66–80.

Chapter 19

Aortic Heart Valve Tissue Regeneration

Bin Duan, Laura A. Hockaday, Kevin H. Kang, and Jonathan T. Butcher

Department of Biomedical Engineering, Cornell University, 304 Weill Hall, Ithaca, NY 14853, USA

jtb47@cornell.edu

Heart valve disease is a serious and growing public health problem for which prosthetic replacement is most commonly indicated. Current prosthetic devices are inadequate for younger adults and growing children. Tissue engineering is an alternative therapeutic strategy with the potential to provide a living valve replacement capable of integration with host tissue and growth. This chapter briefly reviews the functional characteristics of the aortic valve and roles of valve endothelial and interstitial cells. Then it focuses on the principles of tissue-engineered heart valve (TEHV) highlighting scaffold fabrication/process, cell sources, dynamic culture systems, and in vivo animal models. It presents some ongoing challenges in engineering trileaflet semilunar valves. The chapter provides an overview of recent trends in understanding and incorporating multiscale complexity within engineered semilunar heart valves and highlights the future directions of TEHV.

Tissue and Organ Regeneration: Advances in Micro- and Nanotechnology
Edited by Lijie Grace Zhang, Ali Khademhosseini, and Thomas J. Webster
Copyright © 2014 Pan Stanford Publishing Pte. Ltd.
ISBN 978-981-4411-67-7 (Hardcover), 978-981-4411-68-4 (eBook)
www.panstanford.com

19.1 Introduction

Heart valve disease is a serious and growing public health problem in both developed and developing regions of the world. Each year, approximately 100,000 heart valve surgeries were performed in the United States and 300,000 worldwide, the majority of which were performed on the aortic valve [1]. Heart valve disease surgery is the second most common cardiovascular procedure, and the most common heart valve operation is aortic valve replacement to treat aortic stenosis or aortic insufficiency [2]. The incidence of heart valve disease requiring surgery is expected to triple by 2030 [3]. While some diseased valves can be surgically repaired, the majority of patients undergo prosthetic valve replacement using a mechanical or biological substitute. Most MHV contain a hinge, stent, leaflet and sewing ring [4], and the design have moved from the original ball-and-cage valve to tilting disc and bi-leaflet designs [5]. Mechanical valves are durable but require lifelong coagulation management therapy and significant risks of bleeding events due to blood contact with the artificial surfaces [5]. Biologically derived valves, such as porcine and bovine xenografts, do not have the attendant hemocompatibility co-morbidities requiring medication but instead suffer from reduced durability [6]. BHV were found to have a high incidence of calcification and structural deterioration probably due to fixation of the glutaraldehyde [7]. While mature adults, particularly over 65 years old, can expect 20 years or more of prosthetic valve functionality, the effectiveness of these devices drops off considerably for younger patients [2]. These nonliving substitutes cannot repair themselves nor grow, thus requiring multiple resizing operations in children. A third method for valve replacement is the Ross procedure. Instead of using a prosthetic valve to replace the aortic valve, this procedure transplants the patient's pulmonary valve into the aortic position and implant a pulmonary allograft or prosthesis into the less demanding pulmonary position. This procedure has been employed more frequently to decrease morbidity and costs comparable with those of standard mechanical aortic valve replacement, and it has been shown to be superior to homograft aortic valves in adults [8]. However, recent studies suggest that the pulmonary conduit may pathologically dilate and result in severe stenosis, particularly in growing children [9,10].

Tissue engineering is an alternative therapeutic strategy with the potential to provide a living valve replacement capable of integration with host tissue and growth [11]. The classical tissue engineering concept is to fabricate a temporary scaffold that can support cell adhesion and signaling and eventually be remodeled into the patient's own tissue. Heart valves are particularly challenging because the scaffold must function mechanically the moment it is implanted. The aortic valve is situated in one of the most demanding mechanical environments in the body [12]. Tissue-engineered heart valves have required dynamic in vitro conditioning in a bioreactor that simulates in vivo flow conditions prior to implantation [11]. To fulfill strenuous requirements of geometry, mechanical strength, and biological function in aortic valve tissue engineering, successful strategies must thus consider cell source, scaffold parameters, fabrication techniques, and bioreactor design. This chapter reviews recent trends in understanding and incorporating multiscale complexity within engineered semilunar heart valves. First, we briefly review the functional characteristics of the aortic valve and roles of valve endothelial and interstitial cells. Then we discuss the principles of TEHV highlighting scaffold fabrication/process, cell sources, dynamic culture systems, and in vivo animal models. Then we present some ongoing challenges in engineering trileaflet semilunar valves.

19.2 Heart Valve Function, Structure, and Physiology

19.2.1 Heart Valve Function and Structure

Heart valves ensure unidirectional blood flow through the cardiovascular system. Heart valves typically open and close approximately 40 million times a year and over 3 billion times over a lifetime [14]. The four heart valves in the human heart are categorized into the atrioventricular valves (mitral valve [MV] and tricuspid valves [TV]) and semilunar valves (aortic valves [AV] and pulmonary valves [PV]). The coordinated movements, mechanical integrity, and durability of the valves are maintained by the complex, dynamic, and highly responsive tissue macro- and microstructure [15].

The aortic valve is composed of three semilunar cusps (also called "leaflets") and their respective aortic sinus complexes that make up the aortic root (Fig. 19.1). The aortic root is a bulb-shaped fibrous structure to which the aortic leaflets are attached. It is

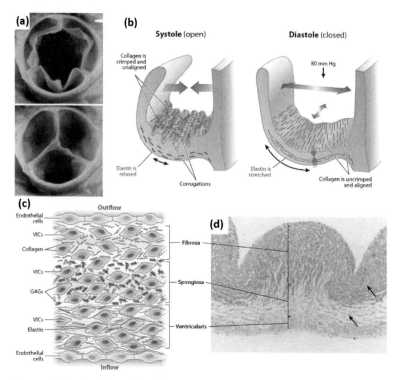

Figure 19.1 Aortic valve functional structure at macroscopic and microscopic levels. (a) Outflow aspect of aortic valve in open (top) and closed (bottom) configurations, corresponding to systole and diastole, respectively. (b) Schematic representation of architecture and configuration of aortic valve cusp in cross section and of collagen and elastin in systole and diastole. (c) Schematic diagram of the detailed cellular and extracellular matrix architecture of a normal aortic valve. (d) Tissue architecture, shown as low-magnification photomicrograph of cross-section cuspal configuration in the nondistended state (corresponding to systole), emphasizing three major layers: ventricularis, spongiosa, and fibrosa. Valvular interstitial cells (VICs) are denoted by arrows. The outflow surface is at the top. Original magnification: 100×. Hematoxylin and eosin stain. [15,17,18].

also populated with blood-vessel like endothelial, medial smooth muscle, and adventitial fibroblasts [3]. Being sufficiently thin to be nourished through hemodynamic convection and diffusion from the blood, aortic valve leaflets exhibit a complex tri-layer striation (Fig. 19.1c,d): (a) The fibrosa, which is located on the aortic side of the leaflet, is composed of numerous circumferentially aligned dense collagen bundles. (b) The spongiosa comprises primarily glycosaminoglycans (GAG) with a few loosely connected fibrous proteins. (c) The ventricularis, which contains a laminate of collagen and elastin. Collagen is the major stress-bearing component of the aortic valve and can transfer the load from the leaflets to the aortic wall when the valve is closed [15]. The elastin within the ventricularis restores the contracted configuration of the cusp during systole and facilitates the rearrangements of collagen during opening. Glycosaminoglycans can absorb shocks during the valve cycle and also facilitate the relative internal rearrangements to reduce valve damage [16].

This complex microstructure creates anisotropic, nonlinear tissue mechanical properties [19]. The leaflets are extremely compliant in the radial direction, but are relatively stiff in the circumferential direction [19]. These properties enable easy opening but strong closure, with increased coaptation area as blood pressure increases. During the majority of their in vivo strain range (<20%), valve leaflets are very extensible and compliant, which permits rapid and efficient opening (modulus ~54 kPa for aortic leaflet and ~40 kPa for pulmonary leaflets in radial direction [20–23]. The sinus root wall, however, is significantly more rigid (aortic root modulus ~140–180 kPa and pulmonary root modulus ~50–85 kPa [3,24,25]).

19.2.2 Aortic Valve Cellular Composition

The aortic valve root wall and leaflets are populated by different subtypes of cells. The root wall microstructure is similar to that of blood vessels, with an endothelial-lined internal elastic lamina, smooth muscle filled medial wall, and fibroblast populated adventitia. Aortic valve leaflets, on the other hand, contain very little smooth muscle and their indigenous cell population is much more heterogeneous. They are populated by interstitial cells and the blood contacting surfaces lined with endothelial cells.

19.2.2.1 Valvular endothelial cells

Similar to arterial endothelial cells, valvular endothelial cells (VEC) maintain a nonthrombogenic surface layer and regulate immune and inflammatory reactions [26,27]. Gene expression and functional studies have established that VEC are a unique endothelial phenotype [12,28–31]. Unlike vascular endothelial cells, VEC aligns perpendicular to the direction of blood flow, which suggests that their mechanosensation is distinct. Valvular endothelial cells may also exhibit different behaviors between the fibrosa and ventricularis layer surfaces. Inflammatory and calcific degeneration for aortic valves are reported to initiate on the fibrosa side of the valve [32,33]. One reason is that aortic endothelial cells showed significantly less expression of multiple inhibitors of cardiovascular calcification [34]. The ventricularis (inflow) surface is exposed to a rapid and pulsatile shear stress with cycle averaged magnitude of 20 dynes/cm^2 (70 dynes/cm^2 peak), while the fibrosa (outflow) surface experiences low oscillatory shear stress [35]. It is not yet clear whether side specific valve endothelial expression differences are the result of intrinsic differences in phenotype or the product of their unique hemodynamic environments.

19.2.2.2 Valve interstitial cells

Aortic valve interstitial cells (VIC) are a heterogeneous population with up to five distinct phenotypes identified: embryonic-like progenitor, quiescent fibroblast, activated myofibroblast, adult progenitor-derived, and osteoblast-like [36]. The predominant VIC phenotype in healthy adult valves is quiescent fibroblasts, with only 2–5% expressing myofibroblast markers [37]. In contrast, 50–80% of VIC isolated from heart valves cultured in vitro express high levels of myofibroblastic markers such as α-smooth muscle actin (αSMA), likely due to high stiffness of plastic culture substrates [38]. The origins and differentiation progression of each sub-phenotype have yet to be clarified, but it has been suggested that there may exist a continuum of phenotype ranging from progenitor to fibroblast to myofibroblast to osteoblast-like cell [3,36,39,40]. Valve interstitial cells are very sensitive to changes in their microenvironment, but also rapidly remodel their local matrix by synthesizing matrix components, growth factors, cytokines, and matrix remodeling enzymes such as matrix metalloproteinases (MMPs) and their tissue inhibitors (TIMPs) [41–43]. Valve interstitial cells, therefore, play a critical role in maintaining homeostasis and driving tissue remodeling within the dynamic environment of the valve, understanding which will be essential for the success of tissue engineering strategies.

19.2.3 Interaction between Valve Interstitial Cells and Microenvironment

In response to a valve injury, VIC can be activated and differentiated from fibroblast-like phenotype into myofibroblast-like phenotype with elevated expression of αSMA, which is a normal process responsible for repairing and replacing damaged ECM [44,45]. Valve interstitial cells were reported to maintain a quiescent VIC fibroblastic phenotype in VIC-VEC 3D collagen co-culture model [46]. The removal of VEC layer promoted the formation of calcific nodules, indicating that VEC may protect VIC from calcification [47].

Growth factors and ECM have been shown to affect VIC phenotype. Transforming growth factor-β1 (TGF-β1) is one of the most efficient mediators of VIC phenotype transition [48]. The effects of TGF-β1 is dose dependent and also mediated by ECM molecules [37,49]. ECM components, such as fibronectin and heparin, with TGF-β1 binding sites were reported to activate VIC. TGF-β prevents excessive heart valve growth under normal physiological conditions while it promotes cell proliferation in the early stages of repair [50]. In addition, fibroblast growth factor-2 promoted in vitro VIC wound repair, at least in part, through the TGF-β/Smad2/3 signaling pathway [51]. Vascular endothelial growth factor (VEGF) significantly inhibited the formation of calcific nodules independent of ECM coating [52]. The migration, proliferation and differentiation of encapsulated VIC within MMP-degradable poly(ethylene glycol) (PEG) hydrogels are controlled by polymer concentration and arginine–glycine–aspartic acid (RGD) peptide density [53]. Similar to 2D culture, addition of TGF-β1 increased expression of αSMA in MMP-PEGDA hydrogels and methacrylated gelatin hydrogels [53,54].

Normally, myofibroblastic VICs are gradually lost by apoptosis when wound healing is relieved. However, if this de-activation is misregulated and the myofibroblastic phenotype persists, fibrosis may occur due to increased matrix modulus and may further induce calcification [55]. Even single ECM component can affect phenotypes and calcification of VIC. Fibronecin and collagen were reported to repress the calcification of VIC, while fibrin enhanced VIC calcification [56,57]. Hyaluronic acid (HA) is another important ECM component that can regulate phenotype and calcification of VIC in both 2D and 3D [58].

Valve interstitial cells cultured on high stiffness substrates have a higher population of myofibroblast-like cells with elevated αSMA expression. Myofibroblastic VIC can be de-activated to fibroblasts in situ by decreasing the tissue modulus of photodegradable hydrogels UV light [59]. Valve interstitial cells cultured on soft polyacrylamide (PA) gels (with storage modulus of 0.3 kPa) exhibited a small rounded morphology, significantly smaller and less spread than those on stiff substrates [60,61]. Following equibiaxial cyclic stretch, VIC cultured on soft PA gel spread to the extent of cells cultured on stiff substrates [60]. Increasing TGF-β1 levels, in the presence of cyclic stretch, resulted in synergistic increases in contractile and biosynthetic proteins in VIC in 2D culture [62]. External forces and internal mechanical rigidity both influence VIC phenotype in a manner somewhat dependent on age and anatomic region [63]. Recently, Gould et al. seeded VIC in 3D collagen hydrogels and implemented cyclic anisotropic strain to the constructs [41]. Increasing anisotropy of biaxial strain resulted in increased cellular orientation and collagen fiber alignment along the principal directions of strain. The cyclic strain also modulated several of the osteogenic markers such as calcium content, Runx2, and alkaline phosphatase enzyme activity for VIC cultured in 3D collagen gels [64]. 3D systems for characterizing VIC function and pathobiology are of increasing importance for understanding valve disease and regenerating function valve tissue. We also observed that strain modulates.

19.3 Tissue-Engineered Aortic Heart Valve

19.3.1 Principles and Criteria

As previously mentioned, the clinical need for a living valve replacement is greatest for pediatric populations, where growth and biological integration is essential. Tissue engineering scaffolds must meet several requirements. The engineered scaffold must be a temporary environment that enables cells to adhere, grow, proliferate, differentiate, and produce a native-like matrix architecture. Scaffolds must accommodate somatic growth of the recipient and last the lifetime of the patient [3,14]. In addition, implanted scaffold materials must be biodegradable, biocompatible, and robust [65]. In addition, TEHV constructs should be nonobstructive, nonthrombogenic, and nonimmunogenic. Several strategies for engineering TEHV have been explored to meet these significant demands. These strategies can be categorized into (1) decellularization of heart valve scaffolds; (2) cell-seeded natural biodegradable scaffolds; (3) cell-seeded synthetic biodegradable polymer scaffolds; and (4) in vivo–engineered valve-shaped tissues via endogenous pathophysiologic processes (Fig. 19.2).

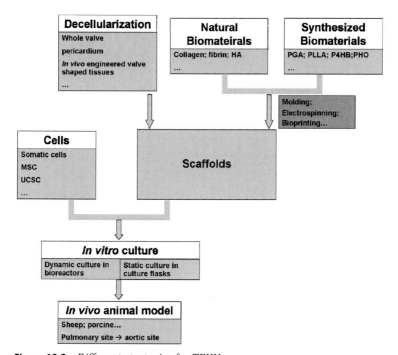

Figure 19.2 Different strategies for TEHV.

19.3.1.1 Decellularized valves

Decellularization strategies are intent on removing all cellular and nuclear material to prevent immune response while preserving the native ultrastructure and composition of ECM. For this strategy, studies have derived native tissues from bovine/porcine pericardium, porcine small intestinal submucosa, and porcine or ovine heart valves as promising matrix for tissue engineering of valve replacements, as shown in Fig. 19.3a [66–69]. The isolated tissues were washed with ionic, nonionic, or zwitterionic detergents (e.g., Triton-X, SDS, and CHAPS), enzymes (e.g., trypsin), and/or nucleases (DNase and RNase) to remove native cells [70]. Different decellularization techniques have shown varying impacts on ECM preservation, valve cell removal efficiency, and biomechanics. For instance, trypsin or a nonionic detergent such as Triton X-100 followed by RNase digestion was reported to have only an incomplete removal of cells [71]. It has also been shown that SDS treatment can preserve the mechanical properties of bovine pericardium [72] and ensure complete removal of cells, but other studies showed that SDS can also destabilize the collagen triple helical domain and swell the elastin network [73]. Total GAG contents and collagen decreased over time, suggesting that ECM-integrity may be compromised with prolonged incubation. The decellularization of ovine, baboon, and human heart valves by Jiao and his colleagues was reported to cause only modest changes in viscoelastic properties [74]. In addition, for the same species, tissues (leaflets, sinus wall, and great vessel wall) from aortic valves were stiffer than the corresponding tissues from pulmonary valves after decellularization. The overall extensibility of decellularized pig aortic valve leaflets increased after treatment with SDS, trypsin, and Triton X-100, but a profound loss of stiffness was observed [75].

Although tissue mechanics are somewhat decreased after decellularization process, decellularized aortic valve allografts largely retain their native geometry, which, therefore, translates to improved hemodynamics. da Costa et al. have demonstrated low rate of calcification in selected patients [76]. Synergraft from Cryolife is a decellularized–cryopreserved cardiac valve allograft that has been used in adult valve replacement with clinical promising results [77,78]. Efficiency of insoluble collagen extraction from xenogeneic valves increased proportionally with decellularization time [79]. In order to avoid any immune response a thorough decellularization of 24 h was reported to be mandatory. Comparing to decellularized xenogenous heart valves, the decellularization of human pulmonary heart valve strongly diminishes the migration of human monocytes toward the valve tissue, which indicated a more completely nonimmunogenic heart valve scaffold [80]. These encouraging results and support from animal studies motivated a clinical trial for decellularized valves in children. Synergraft valves were implanted in four male children (age 2.5 to 11 years) in 2001, and three children died, two suddenly, with severely degenerated Synergraft valves after 6 week and 1 year implantation [81]. The early failure indicates that decellularized scaffold may be not suitable for pediatric application at this point but also raise concerns about the utility of the standard animal model.

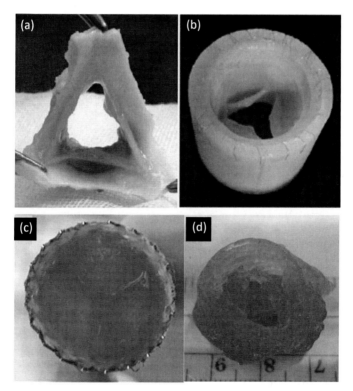

Figure 19.3 Recent TEHV conduits fabricated by different strategies. (a) Decellularized juvenile ovine aortic valves prior to implantation [69]; (b) fibrin-based valves with three leaflets and conduit wall generated by mould [82]; (c) TEHV fabricated from nonwoven PGA meshes coated with P4HB. The construct was then integrated into radially self-expandable nitinol stents and seeded with bone marrow-derived mononuclear cell [83]; (d) Bioprinted aortic valve conduit with alginate/gelatin hydrogel [84].

The limited remodeling to date seen in decellularized valves has motivated studies to recellularize acellular valve scaffolds. Platelet adhesion and aggregate formation were reported to occur on the surface of decellualarized porcine heart valve conduits without seeding with human umbilical vein endothelial cells (HUVEC) [85]. Recellularization of endothelial cells onto detergent decellularized ovine pulmonary valve conduits were achieved under simulated physiological circulation conditions using a dynamic bioreactor system [86]. Alternatively, acellular valve scaffolds conjugated with an antibody against CD90 enabled trapping and adhesion of circulating mesenchymal stem cells to the surface [87]. Further research is needed to determine the extent to which surface seeded cells can invade and remodel acellular valve scaffolds.

19.3.1.2 Natural biomaterials for TEHV

A variety of naturally derived biomaterials have been employed as scaffold materials for heart valve tissue engineering. Type 1 collagen is responsible for most of the nonlinear biomechanics of valve leaflets, and is nontoxic, biocompatible, biodegradable, and easily absorbable [88]. Purified collagen hydrogels have been used to fabricate valve leaflets and whole conduits [46,89], each developing preferential cell and matrix fiber alignment. Alternatively, collagen can be freeze dried into a porous sponge with somewhat tunable mechanical properties without compromising its adhesive and biological activity. Valve interstitial cells and other cells cultured within collagen matrices significantly compact the matrix, necessitating careful design of the mold geometry to ensure appropriate final dimensions [90]. After this compaction phase, VIC cultured within collagen gels express a fibroblast like phenotype, but exhibit limited mechanical strengthening that does not appear to be maintained over culture [91]. While some attempts have been made at developing a humanized collagen source, it is yet unclear what source of collagen would be applicable for clinical use [92].

Fibrin is a natural biopolymer that is a key structural component of initial blood clot and granulation tissue matrix [93,94]. Fibrin hydrogels are formed spontaneously by combining fibrinogen and thrombin. Fibrinogen can be procured from the patient's own blood and, therefore, can be used as an autologous 3D scaffold for the seeded cells without toxic degradation or inflammatory reactions [95]. Cells cultured within fibrin gels exhibit enhanced collagen synthesis and mechanical strengthening over collagen alone [96,97]. Flanagan et al. synthesized a completely autologous fibrin-based heart valve structure by molding the fibrin hydrogels and seeding with ovine carotid artery-derived cells, as shown in Fig. 19.3b [82]. The engineered valve leaflets showed reduced tissue shrinkage when cultured under simulated flow conditions compared to conduits cultured in stirred media. Fibrin-based valves implanted in the lumen of the pulmonary trunk, or interposed between two sectioned ends of the pulmonary trunk using a sheep model, the explanted valve roots remained intact and showed qualitatively similar matrix organization [98]. However, leaflets significantly contracted, leading to pronounced insufficiency.

Unlike collagen and fibrin, hyaluronic acid (HA) is an anionic linear polysaccharide and nonsulfated glycosaminoglycan with no protein backbone. Hyaluronic acid comprises 60% of the total glycosaminoglycan content in the heart valve, and is abundant in the spongiosa layer of the valve leaflet [99,100]. Hyaluronic acid is hypoallergenic and has multiple reactive groups for surface modification. Recent evidence suggests that HA incorporated into valve scaffolds renders them less susceptible to calcification and also promote cell endothelialization [101,102]. Surface modification of bioprosthetic heart valves obtained from with HA derivatives can reduce the calcification [103,104]. Hyaluronic acid, however, exhibits significant swelling in hydrated environments, making control of both TEHV geometry and mechanics difficult.

19.3.1.3 Biodegradable synthetic polymers

Unlike biological polymers, synthetic polymers have a defined and tunable chemical composition, can be produced with high precision, and in large quantities more easily. Frequently used synthetic biomaterials for TEHV include poly(glycolic acid) (PGA), poly(lactic acid) (PLA), poly(ε-caprolactone) (PCL), and polyhydroxyalkanoates (PHA) [16]. Mayer and his colleagues pioneered the use of synthetic polymers for TEHV [105,106]. They implemented fibrous scaffold composing of a PLA woven mesh sandwiched between two nonwoven PGA mesh sheets and seeded autologous myofibroblasts and endothelial cells [107–109]. Some limitations emerged due to the thickness, initial stiffness, and inflexibility of the scaffold material made with aliphatic polyesters that led to stenosis. To increase scaffold flexibility, Mayer et al. also fabricated a bilayer trileaflet heart valve scaffold with a combination of PGA and PHA or polyhydroxyoctanoate (PHO) [107,108,110,111]. The PGA/PHO composite scaffolds showed a much longer degradation profile than PGA or PLA, and they also showed increasing cellular and extracellular matrix contents without thrombus after 24 week implantation in the low-pressure pulmonary position [112]. Poly-4-hydroxybutyrate (P4HB), one member of PHA family which is linear polyesters produced as intracellular granules by bacterial fermentation of sugar or lipids, can be used to dip-coat onto PGA nonwoven scaffolds for creation of tissue-engineered trileaflet pulmonic valve replacements [113]. The PGA-P4HB scaffolds can also be attached to ring shaped supports or self-expanding nitinol stent for in vitro study and minimally invasive implantation (Fig. 19.3c) [83,114,115]. Most recently, autologous amniotic fluid cells were isolated from pregnant sheep and seeded onto stented PGA-P4HB constructs [116]. The TEHV constructs were then implanted orthotopically into the pulmonary position using an in utero closed-heart hybrid approach. Preliminary results after 1 week implantation showed that this conduit maintained valve function in vivo with absence of thrombus formation. It remains to be seen how well this valve design will integrate and function in the long term.

Most, but not all, of these synthetic polymers are not water soluble. This necessitates fabricating the scaffold first, and then seeding the material with cells afterwards. The residual organic solvent and acidic degradation products may be toxic to the seeded cells [117]. In addition, the polymer-based heart valve scaffolds have much higher stiffness compared to native tissue in the physiological strain range (<20%). The seeded valve cells/stem cells may not properly respond to the microenvironment and show pathological phenotypes [118].

19.3.1.4 In vivo–engineered valve-shaped tissues

TEHV strategies involving shaping biomaterials into constructs have disadvantages in long-term in vitro culture, risk of infection and cost-intensive infrastructures [119]. Alternatively, in vivo–engineered tissues rely on the natural foreign body response to synthesize autologous tissue around an implant material [3]. This approach was pioneered by Campbell for blood vessels, who showed that bone marrow derived mesothelial and mesenchymal cells were recruited to and remodeled these neo-matrices [120]. For the case of heart valves, Yamanami et al. implanted a valve-shaped molde of silicone polyurethane into the dorsal subcutaneous space of a rabbit [121]. These valves were able to close and open rapidly in synchrony with the backward and forward pulsatile flow in vitro. The tensile strength of the leaflets was on the same order as native leaflets. However, when implanted orthotopically into dogs, the valve surfaces were much less antithrombogenic than natural controls [122].

19.3.2 Strategies for TEHV Scaffold Fabrication

Because of the limitations of each individual biomaterial strategy and natural complexity of the valve, recent efforts have explored combining multiple materials into valve scaffolds. As previously mentioned, the use of a hydrogel cell carrier can increase the homogeneity and penetration of seeding of a valve scaffold [111,123]. Alternatively, Tedder and colleagues created a layered TEHV by vacuum pressing multiple acellular matrices against a valve-like mold and seeding with mesenchymal stem cells [124]. Preliminary results showed viable cells expressing fibroblast markers, but it is unclear how well the layers bonded.

Electrospinning has also been employed to create TEHV with fiber structure. Electrospinning can generate fibers with diameters ranging from 5 nm to several micrometers under a high voltage electrostatic field operated between a metallic capillary of a syringe and a grounded collector [125,126]. With high surface-to-volume ratio and porosity, studies suggested that nonwoven membranes of electrospun nanofibers can mimic natural ECM and consequently promote cell adhesion, migration and proliferation [127,128]. This technique was also advanced by modifying the jet pathway through controlling the mechanically movement of the collector and electrostatic inducement to generate highly aligned ultrafine fibers [129]. Electrospinning can thus produce fibrous structures and anisotropy that can potentially mimic the microstructure and material behavior of heart valves [130,131].

Engineering heart valve constructs with complex anatomical structure and heterogeneous tissue biomechanics is still challenging. Recently, more and more attention has been given to rapid prototyping techniques that can generate 3D structures with anatomical architecture and heterogeneous tissue biomechanics [132]. Sodian et al. demonstrated that stereolithography can create intricate 3D shapes by photo-cross-linking liquid resin [133]. Conversely, two-photon laser-based photo-cross-linking can create directly encapsulated 3D tissues, but only on the order of a few mm, far smaller than what would be needed clinically [134,135]. More recently, Butcher et al. engineered entire heart valve conduits using an inexpensive open source solid freeform fabrication (SFF), (or 3D printing) platform (Fab@Home) [136]. Using multiple deposition syringes loaded with different hydrogel formulations (i.e., poly(ethylene glycol) diacrylate (PEGDA) with different molecular weight; alginate/gelatin hybrid hydrogel) and cell sources (both VIC from aortic valve leaflets and aortic root sinus SMC), studies have demonstrated that valve and root specific microenvironments can be engineered while maintaining anatomical geometry [84,136]. In addition, the stiffness of PEGDA-based hydrogels is tunable by changing PEGDA molecular weight and comparable to those of aortic leaflets and root in the physiological strain range.

Most recently, the trileaflet heart valve scaffolds fabricated from nonwoven PGA meshes coated with P4HB were seeded with ovine vascular derived cells and cultured in dynamic environment. The TEHV constructs were decellularized and then recellularized with MSC [137]. In vivo/in vitro–engineered valve-shaped conduits can provide largely available "off-the-shelf" heart valve scaffolds with endothelialization and tissue-regeneration potential for heart valve replacement.

19.3.3 Cell Sources

The success of TEHV strategies depend on effective remodeling and maintenance by resident cells. Early studies demonstrated that allogenic cell sources cause an acute inflammatory response even in the presence of immunosuppressant treatment [105]. Subsequent strategies have focused on autologous differentiated cells and stem cells as sources for populating TEHV. Marker expression studies indicate that VIC exhibit phenotypes that are similar between the four valves (aortic, pulmonary, mitral, and tricuspid), but have significantly different expression profiles compared to other sources (arterial smooth muscle, vein, skin, pericardium) [138–141]. Maish et al. proposed tricuspid valve biopsy as a method for obtaining autologous VIC and VEC for and aortic TEHV, and their supporting study in sheep demonstrated that tricuspid valve cells could be isolated, cultured, and the tricuspid valve could remain functional [141]. Unfortunately, the risk of operative morbidity or damage to the tricuspid valve has dampened the acceptance of the procedure. Valve interstitial cells phenotype appears to fall between vascular smooth muscle cells and skin fibroblasts, and both of these cell types have been explored as potential TEHV cell sources [105,142]. In engineered leaflets vascular smooth muscle cells isolated from veins and arteries performed better than dermal fibroblasts [143].

Autologous stem cells are being explored as a source of cells for TEHV, to see if they can be differentiated to duplicate the phenotype and function of native valve cells. Studies using in vitro bioreactors and implantation into an animal model have shown that bone marrow derived and circulating progenitors have the capacity to form both endothelial-like and interstitial-like cells when seeded on valve scaffolds [144–147]. Additionally, preliminary experiments with adipose-derived mesenchymal stem cells (ADSC) indicate they could be suitable for TEHV [148,149]. Adipose-derived mesenchymal stem cells can be isolated in comparatively high numbers, can form endothelial-like cells [149], and have been shown in a partial tissue bioreactor study to have the ability to synthesize and process valve ECM components and are responsive to mechanical stress [148]. Hoerstrup and colleagues have developed protocols and have carried out feasibility studies for several stem cell sources unique for pediatric applications. These cell sources include amniotic fluid, placenta, umbilical cord blood, and chorionic villi [114,115,150–152]. Autologous pediatric stem cells could be procured prenatally or perinatally and used to fabricate a TEHV or stored in a cell bank for future use [116,153]. There is already some existing infrastructure for tissue banking with public and private tissue banks that store amniotic fluid derived cells and umbilical cord blood cells [154]. More research is necessary to determine if stem cell sources can adequately mimic native valve phenotypes and if they maintain that phenotype in the long term. Stem cell multilineage potential and plasticity may require that the biomaterials and the culture conditions be optimized for valve cell differentiation. A recent study highlights this, as stem cells can shift toward cartilage and osteogenic lineages that could predispose TEHV to calcification [155].

19.3.4 Heart Valve Tissue Bioreactors

Native heart valves develop and function under dynamic conditions. Bioreactors designed to mimic the physiological stress and hemodynamics heart valves experience are integral to tissue engineering strategies for heart valve regeneration. Numerous studies have demonstrated that TEHVs cultured in bioreactors have improved ECM content and organization, mechanical properties, and function upon implantation compared to those that are statically cultured [82,98,145,156,157]. The magnitude and distribution of mechanical loading and flow changes during the cardiac cycle, and it changes during the course of heart valve development, as shown in Fig. 19.4 and Table 19.1 [158–160]. Two main classes of bioreactors have been used for these studies: component bioreactors and whole organ bioreactors.

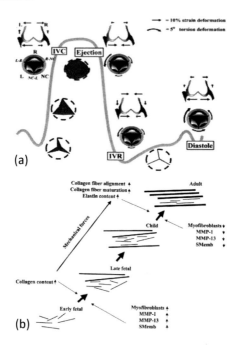

Figure 19.4 Native valve loading and flow conditions change during cardiac cycle and as the valve develops. (a) In addition to the leaflets, the aortic root and sinuses deform during the cardiac cycle [3,158]. (b) Changing mechanical forces during cardiac valve development are tied to matrix organization and cell activity. Modified from [159].

Table 19.1 Native valve loading and flow conditions change as the valve develops [3,158,159,161]

Age/stage	Aorta blood pressure sys/dias	Pulmonary artery blood pressure sys/dias	Heart rate [bpm]
Fetal	50/15 mmHg	50/15 mmHg	140–180
Postnatal	70/40 mmHg	30/15 mmHg	100–160
Toddler (2 years old)	95–105/ 53–66 mm Hg	?	80–140
Adult	120/80 mmHg	20/9 mmHg	60–80

19.3.4.1 Component bioreactors

Component bioreactors are designed to apply a single specific mechanical stimulus to identify how and by what mechanism it effects cell differentiation and/or scaffold remodeling. Biomechanical components of the environment tested with specialized bioreactors include cyclic stretch, cyclic flexure, and oscillating shear stress and flow [162]. Some of the major findings of these three types of partial tissue bioreactor studies are summarized in Table 19.2.

To apply defined fluid shear stress to tissues and cell-seeded scaffolds, different designs of a parallel plate flow chamber combined with a pump have been used. Butcher et al. found that valve endothelial cells align perpendicular to flow while vascular endothelial cells align parallel to flow within 24 h when steady, unidirectional shear stress (20 dynes/cm^2) is applied [26]. They also found that the signaling pathways mediating the alignment response was different between the two cell types [46]. Jockenhoevel et al. included a second nutrient chamber and a multiframe setup to hold multiple seeded scaffolds [163]. An infusion pump removed media from the nutrient chamber and a gravity feed replenished it. It was found that aortic myofibroblasts seeded into a PGA hydrogel scaffold responded to shear stress by producing hydroxyproline, indicating collagen deposition.

The effects of defined tensile strain on native and engineered valve tissues and cells have been studied using a variety of stretch bioreactor designs. These bioreactors deform the tissue or culture using either a pressure/vacuum or a linear actuator and have varying degrees of geometric control. The commercially available Flexcell

Table 19.2 Miniaturized/partial tissue bioreactors

Bioreactor types	Cell/scaffold types	Bioreactor features in specific study	Mechanistic findings	Ref.
Flow	Cell monolayer (VEC)	Steady, laminar, unidirectional shear stress (20 dynes/cm^2)	Valve endothelial cells are distinct from vascular endothelial cells in behavior and signaling pathways; valve endothelial cells align perpendicular to flow	[26]
Flow	VIC + VEC collagen slab construct	Steady, laminar, unidirectional shear stress (20 dynes/cm^2)	Valvular interstitial cells proliferate when not in communication with valvular endothelial cells; VIC ECM secretion is dependent on endothelial cells and on flow	[46]
Flow	PGA fiber scaffold aortic myofibroblasts	Flow rate 250–500 mL/min	Collagen synthesis increases in response to shear	[163]
Stretch (Flexcell)	Confluent VICs and MSC plated on collagen I coated membrane	Flexible membrane culture surface stretched across posts by applied vacuum; 0.6 Hz; radial stretch 7%, 10%, 14%, 20%	VIC and MSC increase collagen synthesis in response to cyclic stretch	[164]
Stretch (Flexcell)	PGA fiber scaffold coated with P4HB seeded with human venousmyofibroblasts with fibrin gel cell carrier	Scaffold ends reinforced and attached to Flexcell well with silicone rubber. Intermittent straining at 4% 1 Hz	Intermittent straining engineered tissues increased collagen production, cross-link density, collagen organization, and mechanical properties faster than constrained controls; stronger tissues in shorter culture time	[97, 165]

Bioreactor types	Cell/scaffold types	Bioreactor features in specific study	Mechanistic findings	Ref.
Uniaxial stretch (linear actuator)	Aortic valve leaflet circumferential direction	10%,15%, and 20% strain at 1.167 Hz (70 beats/min)	10% cyclic stretch "normal" maintains native matrix remodeling activity; cell proliferation and apoptosis increase as cyclic stretch increases from normal to pathologic levels (15%, 20%); increase in matrix remodeling enzyme activity and expression at elevated cyclic stretch (15%, 20%)	[166]
Stretch (linear actuator)	Aortic valve leaflets circumferential direction	Uniaxial tension delivered with actuating arm; tissues threaded with stainless steel springs; 15% stretch, 1 Hz	Cyclic stretch + biochemical factor TGFB1 increase contractile and biosynthetic proteins in VICs	[62]
Stretch (biaxial)	Mitral VIC or chordal cells seed in collagen gels	10% strain, 1.167 Hz. Alternate stretch and relaxation every 24 h; collagen gel anchored by mesh holders	GAG secretion up regulated during cyclic stretch and down regulated during relaxation. VICs adapt to high cyclic strains indicated by proportion of GAG classes changing; for chordal cell constructs GAG classes remain consistent	[167]
Stretch (Biaxial and anisotropy)	Aortic VIC seeded into collagen gels	Equibiaxial and controlled anisotropic strain; collagen gel anchored/formed in a compression spring	Increasing anisotropy of biaxial strain increases cell orientation and collagen fiber alignment along principle directions of	[41]

(Continued)

Table 19.2 (Continued)

Bioreactor types	Cell/scaffold types	Bioreactor features in specific study	Mechanistic findings	Ref.
			strain; cells orient before fibers reorganize. Results suggest strain field anisotropy regulates VIC fibroblast phenotype, proliferation, apoptosis, and matrix organization	
Flex (linear actuator)	PGA vs. PLLA scaffolds each coated with P4HB (No cells)	Three point bending with controlled strain rate; 1 Hz	Decrease in stiffness both materials after 2, 3, and 5 weeks of flexure	[168]
Flex (linear actuator)	Ovine vascular smooth muscle cells seeded into PGA and PLLA scaffolds	Three point bending, flexure angle 62%, 1 Hz; multiple wells to hold rectangular specimens (isolated from each other)	Cyclic flexure increased effective stiffness, collagen, vimentin expression of cell-seeded scaffolds	[169]
Flow + Stretch + Flex (bending and stretch with a linear actuator, shear flow induced by a paddle wheel)	Bone marrow mesenchymal stem cells from juvenile sheep seeded into PGA and PLLA scaffolds	Can study flex, stretch, flow each independently or coupled; 12 rectangular scaffolds at once; spiral metal binders threaded through ends of scaffolds. 0.012–1.875 dynes/cm^2; up to 75% tensile strain	Cyclic flexure and laminar flow synergistically accelerate BMSC mediated tissue formation; collagen content and effective stiffness was higher for flex-flow conditions compared to flex and flow only conditions; comparable collagen and effective stiffness for flex only conditions to SMC seeded scaffolds	[170, 171]

bioreactor deforms flexible membranes that are set into a multiwell plate. A vacuum applied to the underside of the well deforms the membrane across a post. The flexible membrane setup has been used to condition cell monolayers [164] and has been adapted to condition engineered heart valve tissues [165]. A recent bioreactor specifically designed to hold hydrogel-based tissues, deforms a silicone rubber slab that can hold different mold shapes to control strain direction to introduce anisotropy into tissues [41].

During each cardiac cycle, bending stresses are caused by the reversal of the curvature of the leaflets when leaflets open and close in response to pressure gradient changes [3,172]. Dynamic flexure bioreactors have enabled study of cell-seeded scaffolds for valve engineering and valve tissues in bending. The flexure and bending mode of these bioreactors is generally driven by a linear actuator. Engelmayr et al. developed multiple bioreactors for testing scaffolds in flexure [168–171]. The flex bioreactor applies three-point bending to a scaffold inside a well.

19.3.4.2 Whole valve scale bioreactors

Whole valve scale bioreactors, while not able to target mechanisms of a specific stimulus, simulate the entire hemodynamic and mechanical microenvironment on TEHV to understand how cells and scaffold materials would interact and remodel toward clinically useful valve conduits. Aspects of this 3D environment include (1) leaflet stretching and deformation during opening and coaptation; (2) deformation of the valve root and pressure induced vessel stretch; and (3) non-laminar flow in the coronary sinuses [162]. They generally comprise the following basic components: (1) a driving force or pump for fluid movement; (2) a reservoir usually containing culture media; (3) a holder or test section containing the heart valve; (4) a fluid capacitance to store and release energy every pump cycle; (5) a resistance element to help control the overall system pressure; and (6) a means of gas exchange [162]. The culture bioreactor must also maintain physiological temperature and maintain sterility throughout long-term culture. The different designs of bioreactors produce different hemodynamics conditions, degrees of control, and throughput. There are four main bioreactor types: pneumatic diaphragm/balloon, plate-piston, pump, and splash (Fig. 19.5, Table 19.3).

Table 19.3 Whole valve bioreactors

Operation/components	Cell/scaffold types	Hemodynamic/biomechanical conditions	Mechanistic findings/features of study	Ref.
Pneumatic diaphragm				
Diaphragm between an air chamber and media chamber deforms to pulse media through a valve.	Trileaflet valve construct of bioabsorbable polymers seeded with ovine myofibroblasts and endothelial cells	Systole 10–240 mmHg, 0.05 L/min to 2.0 L/min	Constructs cultured for 14 days in gradually increasing pulsatile flow, then implanted into the pulmonary position of lambs, were functional up to 5 months; at 20 weeks ECM and DNA content equal to and greater than native, and the mechanical strength comparable to native valves.	[156, 179]
Air-driven diaphragm deforms to pulse fluid through valve, and system also includes a capacitance chamber to control transvalvular pressure	1st study PGA/PLA scaffold seeded with ovine smooth muscle cells, 2nd study PGA/PLLA trileaflet valve scaffold seeded with bone marrow MSCs	Systole/Diastole 35/20 mmHg-125/85 mmHg, 0–6 L/min. Valves cultured under pulmonary artery conditions although the bioreactor has a wide range of possible conditions	3 week static and then 3 week bioreactor culture; media supplemented with bFGF and AA2P accelerated collagen formation compared to standard media; dynamic conditioning increases collagen production; note: (1) reduction in GAG content with increased culture time; (2) flexibility of scaffold material a limitation for replicating deformation and motion of native leaflets	[145, 173]
Air-driven diaphragm deforms to pulse fluid through valve, and system also includes a capacitance chamber to control transvalvular pressure; universal valve holder mounting design	Decellularized porcine scaffolds seeded with porcine aortic endothelial cells	Systole/diastole 40/15 mmHg-80/70 mmHg, 5–23 mL stroke volume	17 days of bioreactor culture; cells adhere and form cobblestone morphology, but incomplete endothelialization, probably due to low seeding concentration; valve opening and closing monitored with video system	[180]

Operation/ components	Cell/scaffold types	Hemodynamic/ biomechanical conditions	Mechanistic findings/features of study	Ref.
Balloon				
Pressure chamber with bladder on the outflow side of the valve; negative pressure causes back flow on the valve to close it, positive pressure to get flow through open valve	Decellularized porcine valves seeded with ovine carotid artery endothelial cells and myofibroblasts	Systole/Diastole 60/40 mmHg-180/120 mmHg, 25 mL/min-3 L/min	Hydrodynamic reseeding of a scaffold more effective than static reseeding; hydrodynamic seeded scaffolds had more cell mass, collagen and elastin content, and strength than static controls	[188, 189]
Silicone blub compressed by piston – TE valve holder – compliance chamber and resistance – reservoir with aerator – mechanical valve	Checked system for biocompatibility using endothelial cells; bioreactor materials put into media for 2 weeks for leaching, and media then fed to cells	Systole/Diastole 120/80 mmHg-40/25 mmHg, 1.68 L/min-3.44 L/min, Stroke volume: 35–76 mL	The rubber sealing material and rubber used for left ventricle was cytotoxic; ethylene oxide (EtO) vs. glutaraldehyde (2%) (GA) sterilization of all the bioreactor materials: silicone tubing, silicone ventricle, rubber sealing, Teflon sealing, Plexiglass, glue, glued pieces of Plexiglass and/or polyvinyl chloride [PVC]), PVC tubes, and PVC angles	[190]
Plate-piston				
Plate-piston	Tested with commercial bioprosthetic and mechanical valves	Systole/Diastole 120/80 mmHg 180/100 mmHg, ΔP: 0–120 mmHg; vertical movement range associated with stroke volume	Bioreactor evaluated with an aqueous xanthan gum solution to give media blood-like rheological properties and a blood-like salt solution; valves opening and closing monitored with video system	[174, 175]

(Continued)

Table 19.3 (Continued)

Operation/components	Cell/scaffold types	Hemodynamic/biomechanical conditions	Mechanistic findings/features of study	Ref.
Pump				
Pump Deformation + Flow -latex tube -TEHV mount -flow circuit for stretch -flow circuit or nutrient supply -reciprocating syringe pump -peristaltic pump	Fibrin-based valve construct seeded with human dermal fibroblasts	Cyclic loading of valve root. 0–15% Root Strain Low flow rate 10–15 mL/min	3 weeks of cyclic stretching with incrementally increasing strain amplitude; TEHV leaflets after culture had circumferential fiber alignment and had tensile stiffness and anisotropy similar to sheep pulmonary valves	[97]
Pump deformation w/Fluid Minimal flow/shear	Human saphenous vein cells seeded into PGA/P4Hb scaffolds using fibrin cell carrier.	Diastole; applied pressure difference over leaflets; dynamic transvalvular pressure: 0–80 mmHg; dynamic strain 0–25%; low shear stress	Dynamically loaded leaflets have higher UTS, modulus, and tissue formation compared non-loaded tissue strips after 4 weeks of culture; mechanical behavior of loaded leaflets nonlinear and strips was linear; prestrain induced by the stent (3–5%) also affects the mechanical and tissue organization	[183]
Developed a proportional integral-derivative (PID) feedback controller to regulate deformation in their TEHV bioreactor system; results indicated a	Molded valve scaffold of PGA coated with P4HB, then coated with PCL and bonded to a polycarbonate cylinder.	Diastole; applied pressure difference over leaflets. Up to 100 mmHg transvalvular pressure; slow media circulation 4 mL/min.	12 days culture in low speed media circulation then dynamic pressure differences applied for 16 days at 1 Hz; with increased culture time the leaflets became less stiff, more flexible, and less leaky; no significant modulus difference between loading protocols, but anisotropic mechanical properties (circumferential vs. radial) induced by both	[176]

Operation/components	Cell/scaffold types	Hemodynamic/biomechanical conditions	Mechanistic findings/features of study	Ref.
good correspondence between the measured and the prescribed deformation values	which was seeded with human saphenous vein endothelial cells using fibrin cell carrier		Study goal to facilitate development of an optimal conditioning protocol using deformation feedback.	
-Capacitance chamber; -Pulsatile pump; -Cell seeding inlets; -Fits into Incubator; direct control of flow rate using pulsatile pump; roller pump enabled gas exchange in an oxygenation chamber	Decellularized ovine pulmonary valves seeded with jugular vein endothelial cells	Mean system pressure was maintained at 25 ± 4 mmHg, 0.1 L/min to 2.0 L/min	Valves were seeded using the bioreactor and then implanted into lambs for 3 months; valves were completely endothelialzed following bioreactor culture; found that moderate pulsatile flow with bioreactor stimulated EC proliferation, and high flow damaged endothelium and caused loss of cellularity; after explant both reseeded valves and bare decellularized valves had interstitial cells, but a confluent monolayer of EC only present on recellularized valves; more thrombotic formations on bare decellularized valves	[181, 182]
Splash				
As the chamber rotates, the culture medium flows past the tissue surface, imparting normal and shear forces to the surface and causing deformation of the organ culture	Porcine mitral valve segments including strut chordae	3 mL/s	Native mitral valves lose microstructure and ECM expression patterns when cultured under static conditions and were better maintained in dynamic culture; proliferation of cells throughout the leaflet was also effected	[177, 191]

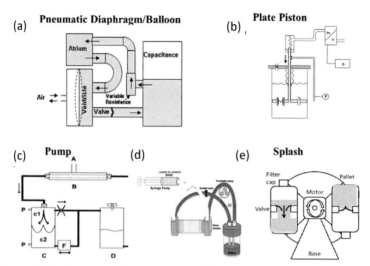

Figure 19.5 Four main bioreactor types. (a) Pneumatic diaphragm/balloon [173]; (b) plate piston [174,175]; (c, d) pump driven [97,176], and (e) splash [177].

Pneumatic diaphragm or balloon bioreactors use a deformable elastic membrane to drive fluid through a flow loop (Fig. 19.5A). With this type of design, it is possible to induce leaflet stretching and coaptation and to create non-laminar flow in the valve sinuses. The most elaborate of this type of design models the left side of the heart [145,173,178]. In this design media is drawn from an "atrium" media reservoir in to a "ventricle" chamber where air deforms a diaphragm in a "ventricle" chamber that pushes media through an aortic valve construct. A pressurized capacitance tank following the valve allows for control of the transvalvular pressure and fluid recycles to the atrium reservoir. Systole and diastole can be mimicked with this type of design, and it enables a high degree of flow and pressure control. One of the major disadvantages of a pneumatic diaphragm/balloon design is that a large number of components are needed to achieve a high level of control. As these bioreactors become increasingly intricate, the bioreactor system gets larger [156,173,179,180]. If the system must fit into a culture incubator to regulate temperature and CO_2, size becomes one of the major limitations to high-throughput culture of multiple valves.

A plate-piston bioreactor physically moves valves through liquid to condition them (Fig. 19.5b) [174]. Multiple valves are mounted in a plate that is submerged in liquid. A steel tube that is driven up and down by a piston is attached to the plate. By moving the valve back and forth through the liquid, it is possible to mimic systole and diastole, leaflet stretching and coaptation, and flow eddies in the sinuses. The vertical range of movement in the system is coupled to the stroke volume for this system. This design has the benefit of being relatively high throughput although the multiple valves are not isolated from one another. The piston-plate bioreactor design enables a wide range of loading conditions and enable loading of multiple valves simultaneously [174]. The major disadvantage of the system is that the valves are not isolated from one another during culture, which means it is difficult to test multiple conditions (for example cell type or media composition) and contamination would affect the entire set of TEHVs. Additionally the plate-piston periodically requires time to reset the position, which can alter the "cardiac" cycle conditions.

Pump bioreactors such as diaphragm bioreactors move fluid through flow loops. For convenient sterile culture, the syringe pumps and peristaltic pumps have been incorporated into these designs. Lichtenberg et al. designed a bioreactor specifically for seeding TEHV with a pulsatile pump, valve reservoir and holder, and oxygenation compliance chamber [181,182]. Cell inlets were incorporated above and below the heart valve. Several pump bioreactor designs mimic both valve leaflet and root deformation with particular emphasis on the diastolic phase of the cardiac cycle (Fig. 19.5c,d) [97,176,183]. Diastolic pressure differences can be applied over the leaflets, with minimal shear flow using a bioreactor consisting of a valve holding container and a medium container. Using a pump a pulse of media of controlled volume and pressure is applied to the outflow side of the leaflets, and the valve deformation can be regulated [176] (Fig. 19.5c). In another bioreactor design there are two separate flow loops-a stretch circuit for applying strain to the valve root wall and leaflets, and a flow circuit for nutrient supply (Fig. 19.5d) [97]. The Syedain design is one of the few that specifically attempts to recreate valve root deformation biomechanics. The advantage of these pump-driven bioreactor designs is that they are very compact compared to other bioreactors and multiple systems can fit into an incubator. Pump-driven systems have been used to replicate specific elements of the cardiac cycle such as blood flow through the leaflets during systole [181], diastolic loading [176] and root deformation

[97] and several compact designs have been demonstrated. However, duplicating the full cardiac cycle with a pump-driven design may involve the same component and complexity increase associated with control that affects the diaphragm/balloon bioreactors.

The final bioreactor type is a splash bioreactor (Fig. 19.5e). A valve segment is mounted between two chambers, one of which is filled with media. As the chamber rotates, the culture medium flows past the tissue surface, imparting normal and shear forces to the surface and causing deformation of the valve leaflet [177]. The splash bioreactor has the advantage of having self-contained sterile conditioning of individual valves, and can be scaled up to have multiple chambers for high-throughput [177]. However, the current splash bioreactor design is more suited to the mitral valve, and may not be suitable for aortic or pulmonary TEHV. It does not allow for control of pressure, flow rate, or stroke volume.

In vitro bioreactor studies have demonstrated that hemodynamic conditioning affects TEHV development and can improve tissue function. However, optimal magnitudes of biomechanical conditioning still need to be identified. In vitro conditioning is critically important for TEHV strategies that begin with cellularized scaffolds unable to immediately function under physiologic levels of cyclic stretch, flexure, and shear stress upon implantation [82,98]. Many of the new materials developed for valve and stem cell culture [184–187], if fabricated into scaffolds may fall into this category. As the field of biomaterials expands, the need for high throughput in vitro evaluation and conditioning of different materials for TEHV is also expanding.

19.3.5 In vivo Animal Models and Approaches for Heart Valve Regeneration

Ultimately, TEHV needs to be evaluated in animal models prior to human trials. While a standard animal model for testing TEHV has not been established, larger animals such as sheep and pig have been used for accommodating tissue-engineered constructs [98,192–194]. The porcine model has similar physiology to humans and can develop aortic valve calcification spontaneously, but grow very rapidly to sizes much larger than humans [195,196]. Invasive surgeries in pig are poorly tolerated and significant cost limits the application. Sheep, on the other hand, are easier to intervene and tolerate surgeries well. They also grow less rapidly, permitting better controlled time course studies. While not developing valve calcification spontaneously, they have been shown to accelerate and enhance mineralization within implanted biomaterials including on valves [195]. The sheep is the only FDA-approved animal model for heart valve replacement evaluation [197,198]. Since large animal models are very expensive and require long-term follow-up, small animal models for valves have been explored. Kallenbach et al. developed a rat model to test the recellularized aortic valvular grafts in the descending aorta [199]. In another case, a rat abdominal aorta model was also developed to test the biocompatibility of composite polymer materials in a physiological pulsatile flow condition and blood-contacting environment [200]. Because the aortic root sizes for rodents are on the order of 1–3 mm in diameter, it is unlikely that engineered complete conduits will be tested in these models. Nevertheless, the rat model can be a more economical means to screen materials for in vivo function and durability.

19.4 Future Direction

Tissue engineering provides a promising solution to the problems encountered by the use of currently available mechanical and biological heart valves. In order to create a fully functional tissue-engineered heart valve, optimal scaffolds with suitable cell source distributed on/within the scaffolds are required and followed by conditioning in bioreactor to ensure dynamic properties in vivo. All of these components, i.e., selection of scaffold materials and fabrication techniques, cell source, and culture condition, will affect the final properties of the constructs and thus should be carefully taken under consideration during the design of a TEHV. However, currently there is no ideal scaffold to satisfy all the requirements and mimic the native tissue. Thus, composite scaffolds with different components or different layers may be the best choice. Another issue is whether it is necessary to generate heart valve conduits with anatomical shape, or whether they can be tailored from a flat tissue sheet formed before implantation [16]. If the native geometry is important, advanced fabrication techniques such as 3D bioprinting are highly recommended, due to the complex architecture and biomechanical heterogeneity of the heart valve. In addition, understanding the interactions between the scaffolds and the conditioned cells is of significance to recognize the remodeling of the scaffolds and cell behaviors. Although there are many potential cell sources, current research on progenitor and stem cells in vitro is highly ineffective, since we lack a sufficient understanding of the biomarker of heart valve cells and have no means of controlling cells differentiation. Advanced bioreactors are able to accommodate cells with a complex hemodynamic environment that can provide various mechanical stimuli, maintain and stimulate desirable cell phenotype, and promote the remodeling of scaffolds [201]. Another major challenge is successful translation of the conduit from preclinical animal models into clinical studies [202]. The TEHV would need to be proved effective in a high-pressure environment comparable with human left-side circulation. In addition, there are requirements for the development of mini-invasive procedures, including catheterization techniques, suitable stents, fine instruments for valve implantation, and advanced imaging systems, e.g., 3D echocardiography and computer tomography (CT) [202].

19.5 Conclusions

The currently used mechanical and biological heart valve prostheses have serious disadvantages and are unsuitable for young patients. TEHV is a promising alternative to fulfill the urgent need for pediatric population. The concept of TEHV requires fabrication of valve conduit–shaped scaffolds, control of cell function, and importantly the need to produce functional leaflets that are strong enough to withstand the hemodynamic forces and implantation. With a good understanding of the valvular cell biology, microenvironment, and intricate multiscale hierarchical arrangements, researchers can mimic the native heart valve structure and generate the living valve with the capacity to maintain and remodel the ECM via mechanical signals. Although the approaches for the development of TEHV still face many hurdles and unresolved questions, tissue engineering is currently the only technology with the potential to generate living tissue analogous to a native human heart valve and have the potential to revolutionize cardiac surgery of the future.

References

1. Friedewald VE, Bonow RO, Borer JS, Carabello BA, Kleine PP, Akins CW, et al. The editor's roundtable: cardiac valve surgery. *American Journal of Cardiology* 2007; **99**: 1269–1278.
2. Kidane AG, Burriesci G, Cornejo P, Dooley A, Sarkar S, Bonhoeffer P, et al. Current developments and future prospects for heart valve replacement therapy. *Journal of Biomedical Materials Research Part B—Applied Biomaterials* 2009; **88B**: 290–303.
3. Butcher JT, Mahler GJ, Hockaday LA. Aortic valve disease and treatment: the need for naturally engineered solutions. *Advanced Drug Delivery Reviews* 2011; **63**: 242–268.
4. Mohammadi H, Mequanint K. Prosthetic aortic heart valves: modeling and design. *Medical Engineering and Physics* 2011; **33**: 131–147.
5. Butany J, Ahluwalia MS, Munroe C, Fayet C, Ahn C, Blit P, et al. Mechanical heart valve prostheses: identification and evaluation. *Cardiovascular Pathology* 2003; **12**: 322–344.
6. Butany J, Leask R. The failure modes of biological prosthetic heart valves. *Journal of Long-Term Effects of Medical Implants* 2001; **11**: 115–135.
7. Senthilnathan V, Treasure T, Grunkemeier G. Heart valves: which is the best choice? *Cardiovascular Surgery* 1999; **7**: 393–397.
8. Jaggers J, Harrison JK, Bashore TM, Davis RD, Glower DD, Ungerleider RM. The Ross procedure: shorter hospital stay, decreased morbidity, and cost effective. *Annals of Thoracic Surgery* 1998; **65**: 1553–1557.
9. Brown JW, Ruzmetov M, Rodefeld MD, Mahomed Y, Turrentine MW. Incidence of and risk factors for pulmonary autograft dilation after ross aortic valve replacement. *Annals of Thoracic Surgery* 2007; **83**: 1781–1789.
10. Xie GY, Bhakta D, Smith MD. Echocardiographic follow-up study of the Ross procedure in older versus younger patients. *American Heart Journal* 2001; **142**: 331–335.
11. Gandaglia A, Bagno A, Naso F, Spina M, Gerosa G. Cells, scaffolds and bioreactors for tissue-engineered heart valves: a journey from basic concepts to contemporary developmental innovations. *European Journal of Cardio-Thoracic Surgery* 2011; **39**: 523–531.
12. Butcher JT, Simmons CA, Warnock JN. Review: Mechanobiology of the aortic heart valve. *Journal of Heart Valve Disease* 2008; **17**: 62–73.

13. Concha M, Aranda PJ, Casares J, Merino C, Alados P, Munoz I, et al. The Ross procedure. *Journal of Cardiac Surgery* 2004; **19**: 401–409.
14. Sacks MS, Schoen FJ, Mayer JEJ. Bioengineering challenges for heart valve tissue engineering. *Annual Review of Biomedical Engineering* 2009; **11**: 289–313.
15. Schoen FJ. Mechanisms of fuction and disease of natural and replacement heart valves. *Annual Review of Pathology—Mechanisms of Disease* 2012; **7**: 161–183.
16. Filova E, Straka F, Mirejovsky T, Masin J, Bacakova L. Tissue-engineered heart valves. *Physiological Research* 2009; **58**: S141–S158.
17. Schoen FJ. Aortic valve structure-function correlations: role of elastic fibers no longer a stretch of the imagination. *Journal of Heart Valve Disease* 1997; **6**: 1–6.
18. Rajamannan NM, Evans FJ, Aikawa E, Grande-Allen KJ, Demer LL, Heistad DD, et al. Calcific aortic valve disease: not simply a degenerative process. A review and agenda for research from the national heart and lung and blood institute aortic stenosis working group. *Circulation* 2011; **124**: 1783–1791.
19. Weinberg EJ, Shahmirzadi D, Mofrad MRK. On the multiscale modeling of heart valve biomechanics in health and disease. *Biomechanics and Modeling in Mechanobiology* 2010; **9**: 373–387.
20. Mavrilas D, Missirlis Y. An approach to the optimization of preparation of bioprosthetic heart valves. *Journal of Biomechanics* 1991; **24**: 331–339.
21. Christie GW, Barratt-Boyes BG. Mechanical properties of porcine pulmonary valve leaflets: how do they differ from aortic leaflets? *The Annals of Thoracic Surgery* 1995; **60**: S195–199.
22. Stradins P, Lacis R, Ozolanta I, Purina B, Ose V, Feldmane L, et al. Comparison of biomechanical and structural properties between human aortic and pulmonary valve. *European Journal of Cardio-Thoracic Surgery* 2004; **26**: 634–639.
23. Robinson PS, Tranquillo RT. Planar biaxial behavior of fibrin-based tissue-engineered heart valve leaflets. *Tissue Engineering Part A* 2009; **15**: 2763–2772.
24. Matthews PB, Azadani AN, Jhun CS, Ge L, Guy TS, Guccione JM, et al. Comparison of porcine pulmonary and aortic root material properties. *Annals of Thoracic Surgery* 2010; **89**: 1981–1989.

25. Azadani AN, Chitsaz S, Matthews PB, Jaussaud N, Leung J, Wisneski A, et al. Biomechanical comparison of human pulmonary and aortic roots. *European Journal of Cardio-Thoracic Surgery* 2012; doi: 10.1093/ejcts/ezr163.
26. Butcher JT, Penrod AM, Garcia AJ, Nerem RM. Unique morphology and focal adhesion development of valvular endothelial cells in static and fluid flow environments. *Arteriosclerosis Thrombosis and Vascular Biology* 2004; **24**: 1429–1434.
27. Durbin AD, Gotlieb AI. Advances towards understanding heart valve response to in injury. *Cardiovascular Pathology* 2002; **11**: 69–77.
28. Butcher JT, Tressel S, Johnson T, Turner D, Sorescu G, Jo H, et al. Transcriptional profiles of valvular and vascular endothelial cells reveal phenotypic differences: influence of shear stress. *Arteriosclerosis Thrombosis and Vascular Biology* 2006; **26**: 69–77.
29. Butcher JT, Nerem RM. Valvular endothelial cells and the mechanoregulation of valvular pathology. *Philosophical Transactions of the Royal society B—Biological Sciences* 2007; **362**: 1445–1457.
30. Simmons CA, Grant GR, Manduchi E, Davies PF. Spatial heterogeneity of endothelial phenotypes correlates with side-specific vulnerability to calcification in normal porcine aortic valves. *Circulation Research* 2005; **96**: 792–799.
31. Holliday CJ, Ankeny RF, Jo H, Nerem RM. Discovery of shear- and side-specific mRNAs and miRNAs in human aortic valvular endothelial cells. *American Journal of Physiology—Heart and Circulatory Physiology* 2011; **301**: H856–H867.
32. Mohler ER, Gannon F, Reynolds C, Zimmerman R, Keane MG, Kaplan FS. Bone formation and inflammation in cardiac valves. *Circulation* 2001; **103**: 1522–1528.
33. Mohler ER. Mechanisms of aortic valve calcification. *American Journal of Cardiology* 2004; **94**: 1396–1402.
34. Simmons CA, Grant GR, Manduchi E, Davies PF. Spatial heterogeneity of endothelial phenotypes correlates with side-specific vulnerability to calcification in normal porcine aortic valves. *Circulation Research* 2005; **96**: 792–799.
35. Kilner PJ, Yang GZ, Wilkes AJ, Mohiaddin RH, Firmin DN, Yacoub MH. Asymmetric redirection of flow through the heart. *Nature* 2000; **404**: 759–761.

36. Liu AC, Joag VR, Gotlieb AI. The emerging role of valve interstitial cell phenotypes in regulating heart valve pathobiology. *American Journal of Pathology* 2007; **171**: 1407-1418.
37. Walker GA, Masters KS, Shah DN, Anseth KS, Leinwand LA. Valvular myofibroblast activation by transforming growth factor-beta: implications for pathological extracellular matrix remodeling in heart valve disease. *Circulation Research* 2004; **95**: 253-260.
38. Yip CYY, Chen JH, Zhao RG, Simmons CA. Calcification by valve interstitial cells is regulated by the stiffness of the extracellular matrix. *Arteriosclerosis Thrombosis and Vascular Biology* 2009; **29**: 936-U417.
39. Farrar EJ, Butcher JT. Valvular heart diseases in the developing world: developmental biology takes center stage. *Journal of Heart Valve Disease* 2012; **21**: 234-240.
40. Wyss K, Yip CYY, Mirzaei Z, Jin XF, Chen JH, Simmons CA. The elastic properties of valve interstitial cells undergoing pathological differentiation. *Journal of Biomechanics* 2012; **45**: 882-887.
41. Gould RA, Chin K, Santisakultarm TP, Dropkin A, Richards JM, Schaffer CB, et al. Cyclic strain anisotropy regulates valvular interstitial cell phenotype and tissue remodeling in three-dimensional culture. *Acta Biomaterialia* 2012; **8**: 1710-1719.
42. Dreger SA, Thomas P, Sachlos E, Chester AH, Czernuszka JT, Taylor PM, et al. Potential for synthesis and degradation of extracellular matrix proteins by valve interstitial cells seeded onto collagen scaffolds. *Tissue Engineering* 2006; **12**: 2533-2540.
43. Schoen F. Evolving concepts of cardiac valve dynamics the continuum of development, functional structure, pathobiology, and tissue. *Engineering Circulation* 2008; **118**: 1864-1880.
44. Liu AC, Gotlieb AI. Transforming growth factor-beta regulates in vitro heart valve repair by activated valve interstitial cells. *American Journal of Pathology* 2008; **173**: 1275-1285.
45. Li C, Xu SY, Gotlieb AI. The response to valve injury. A paradigm to understand the pathogenesis of heart valve disease. *Cardiovascular Pathology* 2011; **20**: 183-190.
46. Butcher JT, Nerem RM. Valvular endothelial cells regulate the phenotype of interstitial cells in co-culture: effects of steady shear stress. *Tissue Engineering* 2006; **12**: 905-915.
47. Mohler ER, Chawla MK, Chang AW, Vyavahare N, Levy RJ, Graham L, et al. Identification and characterization of calcifying valve cells

from human and canine aortic valves. *Journal of Heart Valve Disease* 1999; **8**: 254–260.

48. Blobe GC, Schiemann WP, Lodish HF. Mechanisms of disease: role of transforming growth factor beta in human disease. *New England Journal of Medicine* 2000; **342**: 1350–1358.

49. Cushing M, Liao J, Anseth K. Activation of valvular interstitial cells is mediated by transforming growth factor-beta 1 interactions with matrix molecules. *Matrix Biology* 2005; **24**: 428–437.

50. Li C, Gotlieb AI. Transforming growth factor-beta regulates the growth of valve interstitial cells in vitro. *American Journal of Pathology* 2011; **179**(4): 1746–1755.

51. Han L, Gotlieb AI. Fibroblast growth factor-2 promotes in vitro mitral valve interstitial cell repair through transforming growth factor-beta/smad signaling. *American Journal of Pathology* 2011; **178**: 119–127.

52. Gwanmesia P, Ziegler H, Eurich R, Barth M, Kamiya H, Karck M, et al. Opposite effects of transforming growth factor-beta 1 and vascular endothelial growth factor on the degeneration of aortic valvular interstitial cell are modified by the extracellular matrix protein fibronectin: implications for heart valve engineering. *Tissue Engineering Part A* 2010; **16**: 3737–3746.

53. Benton JA, Fairbanks BD, Anseth KS. Characterization of valvular interstitial cell function in three dimensional matrix metalloproteinase degradable PEG hydrogels. *Biomaterials* 2009; **30**: 6593–6603.

54. Benton JA, DeForest CA, Vivekanandan V, Anseth KS. Photocrosslinking of gelatin macromers to synthesize porous hydrogels that promote valvular interstitial cell function. *Tissue Engineering Part A* 2009; **15**: 3221–3230.

55. Schmittgraff A, Desmouliere A, Gabbiani G. Heterogeneity of myofibroblast phenotypic features-An example of fibroblastic cell plasticity. *Virchows Archiv—An International Journal of Pathology* 1994; **425**: 3–24.

56. Benton JA, Kern HB, Anseth KS. Substrate properties influence calcification in valvular interstitial cell culture. *Journal of Heart Valve Disease* 2008; **17**: 689–699.

57. Rodriguez KJ, Masters KS. Regulation of valvular interstitial cell calcification by components of the extracellular matrix. *Journal of Biomedical Materials Research Part A* 2009; **90A**: 1043–1053.

58. Rodriguez KJ, Piechura LM, Masters KS. Regulation of valvular interstitial cell phenotype and function by hyaluronic acid in 2-D and 3-D culture environments. *Matrix Biology* 2011; **30**: 70–82.
59. Kloxin A, Benton J, Anseth K. In situ elasticity modulation with dynamic substrates to direct cell phenotype. *Biomaterials* 2010; **31**: 1–8.
60. Quinlan AMT, Sierad LN, Capulli AK, Firstenberg LE, Billiar KL. Combining dynamic stretch and tunable stiffness to probe cell mechanobiology in vitro. *PloS One* 2011; **6**: e23272.
61. Butcher JT, Nerem RM. Porcine aortic valve interstitial cells in three-dimensional culture: comparison of phenotype with aortic smooth muscle cells. *Journal of Heart Valve Disease* 2004; **13**: 478–485.
62. Merryman WD, Lukoff HD, Long RA, Engelmayr GC, Hopkins RA, Sacks MS. Synergistic effects of cyclic tension and transforming growth factor-beta 1 on the aortic valve myofibroblast. *Cardiovascular Pathology* 2007; **16**: 268–276.
63. Stephens EH, Durst CA, West JL, Grande-Allen KJ. Mitral valvular interstitial cell responses to substrate stiffness depend on age and anatomic region. *Acta Biomaterialia* 2011; **7**: 75–82.
64. Ferdous Z, Jo H, Nerem RM. Differences in valvular and vascular cell responses to strain in osteogenic media. *Biomaterials* 2011; **32**: 2885–2893.
65. Hutmacher DW. Scaffold design and fabrication technologies for engineering tissues: state of the art and future perspectives. *Journal of Biomaterials Science—Polymer Edition* 2001; **12**: 107–124.
66. Goncalves AC, Griffiths LG, Anthony RV, Orton EC. Decellularization of bovine pericardium for tissue-engineering by targeted removal of xenoantigens. *Journal of Heart Valve Disease* 2005; **14**: 212–217.
67. Keane TJ, Londono R, Turner NJ, Badylak SF. Consequences of ineffective decellularization of biologic scaffolds on the host response. *Biomaterials* 2012; **33**: 1771–1781.
68. Kasimir MT, Rieder E, Seebacher G, Silberhumer G, Wolner E, Weigel G, et al. Comparison of different decellularization procedures of porcine heart valves. *International Journal of Artificial Organs* 2003; **26**: 421–427.
69. Akhyari P, Kamiya H, Gwanmesia P, Aubin H, Tschierschke R, Hoffmann S, et al. In vivo functional performance and structural maturation of decellularised allogenic aortic valves in the subcoronary position. *European Journal of Cardio-Thoracic Surgery* 2010; **38**: 539–546.

70. Crapo PM, Gilbert TW, Badylak SF. An overview of tissue and whole organ decellularization processes. *Biomaterials* 2011; **32**: 3233–3243.

71. Bader A, Schilling T, Teebken OE, Brandes G, Herden T, Steinhoff G, et al. Tissue engineering of heart valves: human endothelial cell seeding of detergent acellularized porcine valves. *European Journal of Cardio-Thoracic Surgery* 1998; **14**: 279–284.

72. Oswal D, Korossis S, Mirsadraee S, Wilcox H, Watterson K, Fisher J, et al. Biomechanical characterization of decellularized and cross-linked bovine pericardium. *Journal of Heart Valve Disease* 2007; **16**: 165–174.

73. Rieder E, Kasimir MT, Silberhumer G, Seebacher G, Wolner E, Simon P, et al. Decellularization protocols of porcine heart valves differ importantly in efficiency of cell removal and susceptibility of the matrix to recellularization with human vascular cells. *Journal of Thoracic Cardiovascular Surgery* 2004; **127**: 399–405.

74. Jiao T, Clifton RJ, Converse GL, Hopkins RA. Measurements of the effects of decellularization on viscoelastic properties of tissues in ovine, baboon, and human heart valves. *Tissue Engineering Part A* 2012; **18**: 423–431.

75. Liao J, Joyce EM, Sacks MS. Effects of decellularization on the mechanical and structural properties of the porcine aortic valve leaflet. *Biomaterials* 2008; **29**: 1065–1074.

76. da Costa FDA, Costa ACBA, Prestes R, Domanski AC, Balbi EM, Ferreira ADA, et al. The early and midterm function of decellularized aortic valve allografts. *Annals of Thoracic and Cardiovascular Surgery* 2010; **90**: 1854–1861.

77. Konuma T, Devaney EJ, Bove EL, Gelehrter S, Hirsch JC, Tavakkol Z, et al. Performance of cryovalve SG decellularized pulmonary allografts compared with standard cryopreserved allografts *Annals of Thoracic and Cardiovascular Surgery* 2009; **88**: 849–855.

78. Gerson CJ, Elkins RC, Goldstein S, Heacox AE. Structural integrity of collagen and elastin in SynerGraft (R) decellularized-cryopreserved human heart valves. *Cryobiology* 2012; **64**: 33–42.

79. Schenke-Layland K, Vasilevski O, Opitz F, Konig K, Riemann I, Halbhuber KJ, et al. Impact of decellularization of xenogeneic tissue on extracellular matrix integrity for tissue engineering of heart valves. *Journal of Structural Biology* 2003; **143**: 201–208.

80. Rieder E, Seebacher G, Kasimir MT, Eichmair E, Winter B, Dekan B, et al. Tissue engineering of heart valves: decellularized porcine and human valve scaffolds differ importantly in residual potential to attract monocytic cells. *Circulation* 2005; **111**: 2792–2797.

81. Simon P, Kasimir MT, Seebacher G, Weigel G, Ullrich R, Salzer-Muhar U, et al. Early failure of the tissue engineered porcine heart valve SYNERGRAFT (TM) in pediatric patients. *European Journal of Cardio-Thoracic Surgery* 2003; **23**: 1002–1006.

82. Flanagan TC, Cornelissen C, Koch S, Tschoeke B, Sachweh JS, Schmitz-Rode T, et al. The in vitro development of autologous fibrin-based tissue-engineered heart valves through optimised dynamic conditioning. *Biomaterials* 2007; **28**: 3388–3397.

83. Weber B, Scherman J, Emmert MY, Gruenenfelder J, Verbeek R, Bracher M, et al. Injectable living marrow stromal cell-based autologous tissue engineered heart valves: first experiences with a one-step intervention in primates. *European Heart Journal* 2011; **32**: 2830–2840.

84. Duan B, Hockaday LA, Kang KH, Butcher JT. 3D bioprinting of heterogeneous aortic valve conduits with alginate/gelatin hydrogels. *Journal of Biomedical Materials Research Part A* 2012; submitted.

85. Kasimir MT, Weigel G, Sharma J, Rieder E, Seebacher G, Wolner E, et al. The decellularized porcine heart valve matrix in tissue engineering: platelet adhesion and activation. *Thrombosis and Haemostasis* 2005; **94**: 562–567.

86. Lichtenberg A, Tudorache I, Cebotari S, Ringes-Lichtenberg S, Sturz G, Hoeffler K, et al. In vitro re-endothelialization of detergent decellularized heart valves under simulated physiological dynamic conditions. *Biomaterials* 2006; **27**: 4221–4229.

87. Ye XF, Zhao Q, Sun XN, Li HQ. Enhancement of mesenchymal stem cell attachment to decellularized porcine aortic valve scaffold by In vitro coating with antibody against CD90: a preliminary study on antibody-modified tissue-engineered heart valve. *Tissue Engineering Part A* 2009; **15**: 1–11.

88. Lee CH, Singla A, Lee Y. Biomedical applications of collagen. *International Journal of Pharmaceutics* 2001; **221**: 1–22.

89. Neidert MR, Tranquillo RT. Tissue-engineered valves with commissural alignment. *Tissue Engineering* 2006; **12**: 891–903.

90. Rothenburger M, Vischer P, Volker W, Glasmacher B, Berendes E, Scheld HH, et al. In vitro modelling of tissue using isolated vascular cells on a synthetic collagen matrix as a substitute for heart valves. *Thoracic and Cardiovascular Surgeon* 2001; **49**: 204–209.

91. Taylor PM, Allen SP, Dreger SA, Yacoub MH. Human cardiac valve interstitial cells in collagen sponge: a biological three-dimensional matrix for tissue engineering. *Journal of Heart Valve Disease* 2002; **11**: 298–306.

92. Parenteau-Bareil R, Gauvin R, Berthod F. Collagen-based biomaterials for tissue engineering applications. *Materials* 2010; **3**: 1863–1887.

93. Ahmed TAE, Dare EV, Hincke M. Fibrin: a versatile scaffold for tissue engineering applications. *Tissue Engineering Part B* 2008; **14**: 199–215.

94. Barsotti MC, Felice F, Balbarini A, Di Stefano R. Fibrin as a scaffold for cardiac tissue engineering. *Biotechnology and Applied Biochemistry* 2011; **58**: 301–310.

95. Ye Q, Zund G, Benedikt P, Jockenhoevel S, Hoerstrup SP, Sakyama S, et al. Fibrin gel as a three dimensional matrix in cardiovascular tissue engineering. *European Journal of Cardio-Thoracic Surgery* 2000; **17**: 587–591.

96. Williams C, Johnson SL, Robinson PS, Tranquillo RT. Cell sourcing and culture conditions for fibrin-based valve constructs. *Tissue Engineering* 2006; **12**: 1489–1502.

97. Syedain ZH, Tranquillo RT. Controlled cyclic stretch bioreactor for tissue-engineered heart valves. *Biomaterials* 2009; **30**: 4078–4084.

98. Flanagan TC, Sachweh JS, Frese J, Schnoring H, Gronloh N, Koch S, et al. In vivo remodeling and structural characterization of fibrin-based tissue-engineered heart valves in the adult sheep model. *Tissue Engineering Part A* 2009; **15**: 2965–2976.

99. Latif N, Sarathchandra P, Taylor PM, Antoniw J, Yacoub MH. Localization and pattern of expression of extracellular matrix components in human heart valves. *Journal of Heart Valve Disease* 2005; **14**: 218–227.

100. Stephens EH, Chu CK, Grande-Allen KJ. Valve proteoglycan content and glycosaminoglycan fine structure are unique to microstructure, mechanical load and age: relevance to an age-specific tissue-engineered heart valve. *Acta Biomaterialia* 2008; **4**: 1148–1160.

101. Johansson B, Holmgren A, Hedstrom M, Engstrom-Laurent A, Engstrom KG. Evaluation of hyaluronan and calcifications in stenotic and regurgitant aortic valves. *European Journal of Cardio-Thoracic Surgery* 2011; **39**: 27–32.

102. Camci-Unal G, Aubin H, Ahari AF, Bae H, Nichol JW, Khademhosseini A. Surface-modified hyaluronic acid hydrogels to capture endothelial progenitor cells. *Soft Matter* 2010; **6**: 5120–5126.

103. Ohri R, Hahn SK, Hoffman AS, Stayton PS. Hyaluronic acid grafting mitigates calcification of glutaraldehyde-fixed bovine pericardium *Journal of Biomedical Materials Research Part A* 2004; **70A**: 328-334.

104. Hahn SK, Ohri R, Giachelli CM. Anti-calcification of bovine pericardium for bioprosthetic heart valves after surface modification with hyaluronic acid derivatives. *Biotechnology and Bioengineering* 2005; **10**: 218-224.

105. Shinoka T, Breuer CK, Tanel RE, Zund G, Miura T, Ma PX, et al. Tissue engineering heart valves: valve leaflet replacement study in a lamb model. *Annals of Thoracic and Surgery* 1995; **60**: S513-S516.

106. Breuer CK, Shinoka T, Tane RE, Zund G, Mooney DJ, Ma PX, et al. Tissue engineering lamb heart valve leaflets. *Biotechnology and Bioengineering* 1996; **50**: 562-567.

107. Sodian R, Sperling JS, Martin DP, Stock U, Mayer JJ, Vacanti JP. Tissue engineering of a trileaflet heart valve-Early in vitro experiences with a combined polymer. *Tissue Engineering* 1999; **5**: 489-494.

108. Sodian R, Sperling JS, Martin DP, Egozy A, Stock U, Mayer JJ, et al. Fabrication of a trileaflet heart valve scaffold from a polyhydroxyalkanoate biopolyester for use in tissue engineering. *Tissue Engineering* 2000; **6**: 183-188.

109. Sodian R, Hoerstrup SP, Sperling JS, Daebritz SH, Martin DP, Schoen FJ, et al. Tissue engineering of heart valves: in vitro experiences. *Annals of Thoracic Surgery* 2000; **70**: 140-144.

110. Sodian R, Hoerstrup SP, Sperling JS, Daebritz S, Martin DP, Moran AM, et al. Early in vivo experience with tissue-engineered trileaflet heart valves. *Circulation* 2000; **102**: III-22-III-29.

111. Sodian R, Hoerstrup SP, Sperling JS, Daebritz SH, Martin DP, Schoen FJ, et al. Tissue engineering of heart valves: in vitro experiences. *Annals of Thoracic Surgery* 2000; **70**: 140-144.

112. Stock UA, Nagashima M, Khalil PN, Nollert GD, Herden T, Sperling JS, et al. Tissue-engineered valved conduits in the pulmonary circulation. *Journal of Thoracic Cardiovascular Surgery* 2000; **119**: 732-740.

113. Dvorin EL, Wylie-Sears J, Kaushal S, Martin DP, Bischoff J. Quantitative evaluation of endothelial progenitors and cardiac valve endothelial cells: proliferation and differentiation on poly-glycolic acid/poly-4-hydroxybutyrate scaffold in response to vascular endothelial growth factor and transforming growth factor beta(1). *Tissue Engineering* 2003; **9**: 487-493.

114. Schmidt D, Mol A, Odermatt B, Neuenschwander S, Breymann C, Gossi M, et al. Engineering of biologically active living heart valve leaflets using human umbilical cord-derived progenitor cells. *Tissue Engineering* 2006; **12**: 3223–3232.

115. Schmidt D, Dijkman PE, Driessen-Mol A, Stenger R, Mariani C, Puolakka A, et al. Minimally-invasive implantation of living tissue engineered heart valves. A comprehensive approach from autologous vascular cells to stem cells. *Journal of the American College of Cardiology* 2010; **56**: 510–520.

116. Weber B, Emmert MY, Behr L, Schoenauer R, Brokopp C, Drogemuller C, et al. Prenatally engineered autologous amniotic fluid stem cell-based heart valves in the fetal circulation. *Biomaterials* 2012; **33**: 4031–4043.

117. Ulery BD, Nair LS, Laurencin CT. Biomedical applications of biodegradable polymers. *Journal of Polymer Science Part B—Polymer Physics* 2011; **49**: 832–864.

118. Kloxin AM, Benton JA, Anseth KS. In situ elasticity modulation with dynamic substrates to direct cell phenotype. *Biomaterials* 2010; **31**: 1–8.

119. Schleicher M, Wendel HP, Fritze O, Stock UA. In vivo tissue engineering of heart valves: evolution of a novel concept. *Regenerative Medicine* 2009; **4**: 613–619.

120. Daly CD, Campbell GR, Walker PJ, Campbell JH. In vivo engineering of blood vessels. *Frontiers in Bioscience* 2004; **9**: 1915–1924.

121. Yamanami M, Yahata Y, Tajikawa T, Ohba K, Watanabe T, Kanda K, et al. Preparation of in-vivo tissue-engineered valved conduit with the sinus of Valsalva (type IV biovalve). *Journal of Artificial Organs* 2010; **13**: 106–112.

122. Hayashida K, Kanda K, Yaku H, Ando J, Nakayama Y. Development of an in vivo tissue-engineered, autologous heart valve (the biovalve): preparation of a prototype model. *Journal of Thoracic Cardiovascular Surgery* 2007; **134**: 152–159.

123. Jockenhoevel S, Chalabi K, Sachweh JS, Groesdonk HV, Demircan L, Grossmann M, et al. Tissue engineering: complete autologous valve conduit: a new moulding technique. *Thoracic and Cardiovascular Surgeon* 2001; **49**: 287–290.

124. Tedder ME, Simionescu A, Chen J, Liao J, Simionescu DT. Assembly and testing of stem cell-seeded layered collagen constructs for heart valve tissue engineering. *Tissue Engineering Part A* 2011; **17**: 25–36.

125. Sill TJ, von Recum HA. Electrospinning: applications in drug delivery and tissue engineering. *Biomaterials* 2008; **29**: 1989–2006.
126. Greiner A, Wendorff JH. Electrospinning: a fascinating method for the preparation of ultrathin fibres. *Angewandte Chemie—International Edition* 2007; **46**: 5670–5703.
127. Li WJ, Tuli R, Okafor C, Derfoul A, Danielson KG, Hall DJ, et al. A three-dimensional nanofibrous scaffold for cartilage tissue engineering using human mesenchymal stem cells. *Biomaterials* 2005; **26**: 599–609.
128. Wu SC, Chang WH, Dong GC. Cell adhesion and proliferation enhancement by gelatin nanofiber scaffolds. *Journal of Bioactive and Compatible Polymers* 2011; **26**: 565–577.
129. Li D, Xia YN. Electrospinning of nanofibers: reinventing the wheel? *Advanced Materials* 2004; **16**: 1151–1170.
130. Courtney T, Sacks MS, Stankus J, Guan J, Wagner WR. Design and analysis of tissue engineering scaffolds that mimic soft tissue mechanical anisotropy. *Biomaterials* 2006; **27**: 3631–3638.
131. Cynthia W, Shital P, Rui C, Owida A, Morsi Y. Biomimetic electrospun gelatin-chitosan polyurethane for heart valve leaflets. *Journal of Mechanics in Medicine and Biology* 2010; **10**: 563–576.
132. Peltola SM, Melchels FPW, Grijpma DW, Kellomaki M. A review of rapid prototyping techniques for tissue engineering purposes. *Annals of Medicine* 2008; **40**: 268–280.
133. Sodian R, Loebe M, Hein A, Martin DP, Hoerstrup SP, Potapov EV, et al. Application of stereolithography for scaffold fabrication for tissue engineered heart valves. *ASAIO Journal* 2002; **48**: 12–16.
134. Elomaa L, Teixeira S, Hakala R, Korhonen H, Grijpma DW, Seppala JV. Preparation of poly(epsilon-caprolactone)-based tissue engineering scaffolds by stereolithography. *Acta Biomaterialia* 2011; **7**: 3850–3856.
135. Ovsianikov A, Deiwick A, Van Vlierberghe S, Dubruel P, Moller L, Drager G, et al. Laser fabrication of three-dimensional CAD scaffolds from photosensitive gelatin for applications in tissue engineering. *Biomacromolecules* 2011; **12**: 851–858.
136. Hockaday LA, Kang KH, Colangelo NW, Cheung PYC, Malone E, Wu J, et al. Solid freeform fabrication of living aortic valve conduits. *Biofabrication* 2012; submitted.
137. Dijkman PE, Driessen-Mol A, Frese L, Hoerstrup SP, Baaijens FPT. Decellularized homologous tissue-engineered heart valves as off-the-shelf alternatives to xeno- and homografts. *Biomaterials* 2012; **33**: 4545–4554.

138. Taylor PA, Batten P, Brand NJ, Thomas PS, Yacoub MH. The cardiac valve interstitial cell. *International Journal of Biochemistry and Cell Biology* 2003; **35**: 113–118.

139. Messier RH, Bass BL, Aly HM, Jones JL, Domkowski PW, Walace RB, et al. Dual structural and functional phenotypes of the porcine aortic-valve interstitial population-Characteristics of the leaflet myofibroblast. *Journal of Surgical Research* 1994; **57**: 1–21.

140. Taylor PM, Allen SP, Yacoub MH. Phenotypic and functional characterization of interstitial cells from human heart valves, pericardium and skin. *Journal of Heart Valve Disease* 2000; **9**: 150–158.

141. Maish MS, Hoffman-Kim D, Krueger PM, Souza JM, Harper JJ, Hopkins RA. Tricuspid valve biopsy: a potential source of cardiac myofibroblast cells for tissue-engineered cardiac valves. *Journal of Heart Valve Disease* 2003; **12**: 264–269.

142. Hoffman-Kim D, Maish MS, Krueger PM, Lukoff H, Bert A, Hong T, et al. Comparison of three myofibroblast cell sources for the tissue engineering of cardiac valves. *Tissue Engineering* 2005; **11**: 288–301.

143. Shinoka T, ShumTim D, Ma PX, Tanel RE, Langer R, Vacanti JP, et al. Tissue-engineered heart valve leaflets: does cell origin affect outcome? *Circulation* 1997; **96**: 102–107.

144. Sutherland FWH, Perry TE, Yu Y, Sherwood MC, Rabkin E, Masuda Y, et al. From stem cells to viable autologous semilunar heart valve. *Circulation* 2005; **111**: 2783–2791.

145. Ramaswamy S, Gottlieb D, Engelmayr GC, Aikawa E, Schmidt DE, Gaitan-Leon DM, et al. The role of organ level conditioning on the promotion of engineered heart valve tissue development in-vitro using mesenchymal stem cells. *Biomaterials* 2010; **31**: 1114–1125.

146. Perry TE, Kaushal S, Sutherland FWH, Guleserian KJ, Bischoff J, Sacks M, et al. Bone marrow as a cell source for tissue engineering heart valves. *Annals of Thoracic Surgery* 2003; **75**: 761–767.

147. Sales VL, Mettler BA, Engelmayr GC, Aikawa E, Bischoff J, Martin DP, et al. Endothelial progenitor cells as a sole source for ex vivo seeding of tissue-engineered heart valves. *Tissue Engineering Part A* 2010; **16**: 257–267.

148. Colazzo F, Sarathchandra P, Smolenski RT, Chester AH, Tseng YT, Czernuszka JT, et al. Extracellular matrix production by adipose-derived stem cells: implications for heart valve tissue engineering. *Biomaterials* 2011; **32**: 119–127.

149. Colazzo F, Chester AH, Taylor PM, Yacoub MH. Induction of mesenchymal to endothelial transformation of adipose-derived stem cells. *Journal of Heart Valve Disease* 2010; **19**: 736–744.

150. Schmidt D, Achermann J, Odermatt B, Genoni M, Zund G, Hoerstrup SP. Cryopreserved amniotic fluid-derived cells: a life-long autologous fetal stem cell source for heart valve tissue engineering. *Journal of Heart Valve Disease* 2008; **17**: 446–455.

151. Schmidt D, Breymann C, Weber A, Guenter CI, Neuenschwander S, Zund G, et al. Umbilical cord blood derived endothelial progenitor cells for tissue engineering of vascular grafts. *Annals of Thoracic Surgery* 2004; **78**: 2094–2098.

152. Schmidt D, Mol A, Breymann C, Achermann J, Odermatt B, Gossi M, et al. Living autologous heart valves engineered from human prenatally harvested progenitors. *Circulation* 2006; **114**: I125–I131.

153. Weber B, Zeisberger SM, Hoerstrup SP. Prenatally harvested cells for cardiovascular tissue engineering: fabrication of autologous implants prior to birth. *Placenta* 2011; **32**: S316–S319.

154. Verter F. *Parent's Guide to Cord Blood Foundation: With Emphasis on How to Evaluate Bank Services.* Copyright 2000–2010 December 7, 2010 (cited; available from: http://parentsguidecordblood.org/content/usa/banklists/index.shtml?navid=14).

155. Emani S, Mayer JE, Emani SM. Gene regulation of extracellular matrix remodeling in human bone marrow stem cell-seeded tissue-engineered grafts. *Tissue Engineering Part A* 2011; **17**: 2379–2388.

156. Hoerstrup SP, Sodian R, Sperling JS, Vacanti JP, Mayer JE. New pulsatile bioreactor for in vitro formation of tissue engineered heart valves. *Tissue Engineering* 2000; **6**: 75–79.

157. Schmidt D, Dijkman P, Driessen-Mol A, Stenger R, Mariani C, Puolakka A, et al. Minimally-invasive implantation of living tissue engineered heart valves. A comprehensive approach from autologous vascular cells to stem cells. *Journal of the American College of Cardiology* 2010; **56**: 510–520.

158. Dagum P, Green GR, Nistal FJ, Daughters GT, Timek TA, Foppiano LE, et al. Deformational dynamics of the aortic root: modes and physiologic determinants. *Circulation* 1999; **100**: S54–S62.

159. Aikawa E, Whittaker P, Farber M, Mendelson K, Padera RF, Aikawa M, et al. Human semilunar cardiac valve remodeling by activated cells from fetus to adult: implications for postnatal adaptation, pathology, and tissue engineering. *Circulation* 2006; **113**: 1344–1352.

160. Brewer RJ, Mentzer RM, Deck JD, Ritter RC, Trefil JS, Nolan SP. In vivo study of the dimensional changes of the aortic valve leaflets during the cardiac cycle. *Journal of Thoracic and Cardiovascular Surgery* 1977; **74**: 645–650.

161. Kovacs G, Berghold A, Scheidl S, Olschewski H. Pulmonary arterial pressure during rest and exercise in healthy subjects: a systematic review. *European Respiratory Journal* 2009; **34**: 888–894.

162. Berry JL, Steen JA, Williams JK, Jordan JE, Atala A, Yoo JJ. Bioreactors for development of tissue engineered heart valves. *Annals of Biomedical Engineering* 2010; **38**: 3272–3279.

163. Jockenhoevel S, Zund G, Hoerstrup SP, Schnell A, Turina M. Cardiovascular tissue engineering: a new Laminar flow chamber for in vitro improvement of mechanical tissue properties. *ASAIO Journal* 2002; **48**: 8–11.

164. Ku CH, Johnson PH, Batten P, Sarathchandra P, Chambers RC, Taylor PM, et al. Collagen synthesis by mesenchymal stem cells and aortic valve interstitial cells in response to mechanical stretch. *Cardiovascular Research* 2006; **71**: 548–556.

165. Rubbens MP, Mol A, Boerboom RA, Bank RA, Baaijens FPT, Bouten CVC. Intermittent straining accelerates the development of tissue properties in engineered heart valve tissue. *Tissue Engineering Part A* 2009; **15**: 999–1008.

166. Balachandran K, Sucosky P, Jo H, Yoganathan AP. Elevated cyclic stretch alters matrix remodeling in aortic valve cusps: implications for degenerative aortic valve disease. *American Journal of Physiology— Heart and Circulatory Physiology* 2009; **296**: H756–H764.

167. Gupta V, Werdenberg JA, Lawrence BD, Mendez JS, Stephens EH, Grande-Allen KJ. Reversible secretion of glycosaminoglycans and proteoglycans by cyclically stretched valvular cells in 3D culture. *Annals of Biomedical Engineering* 2008; **36**: 1092–1103.

168. Engelmayr GC, Hildebrand DK, Sutherland FWH, Mayer JE, Sacks MS. A novel bioreactor for the dynamic flexural stimulation of tissue engineered heart valve biomaterials. *Biomaterials* 2003; **24**: 2523–2532.

169. Engelmayr GC, Rabkin E, Sutherland FW, Schoen FJ, Mayer JE, Sacks MS. The independent role of cyclic flexure in the early in vitro development of an engineered heart valve tissue. *Biomaterials* 2005; **26**: 175–187.

170. Engelmayr GC, Soletti L, Vigmostad SC, Budilarto SG, Federspiel WJ, Chandran KB, et al. A novel flex-stretch-flow bioreactor for the study of engineered heart valve tissue mechanobiology. *Annals of Biomedical Engineering* 2008; **36**: 700–712.

171. Engelmayr GC, Sales VL, Mayer JE, Sacks MS. Cyclic flexure and laminar flow synergistically accelerate mesenchymal stem cell-mediated engineered tissue formation: implications for engineered heart valve tissues. *Biomaterials* 2006; **27**: 6083–6095.

172. Deck JD, Thubrikar MJ, Schneider PJ, Nolan SP. Structure, stress, and tissue-repair in aortic valve leaflets. *Cardiovascular Research* 1988; **22**: 7–16.

173. Hildebrand DK, Wu ZJJ, Mayer JE, Sacks MS. Design and hydrodynamic evaluation of a novel pulsatile bioreactor for biologically active heart valves. *Annals of Biomedical Engineering* 2004; **32**: 1039–1049.

174. Schleicher M, Sammler G, Schmauder M, Fritze O, Huber AJ, Schenke-Layland K, et al. Simplified pulse reactor for real-time long-term in vitro testing of biological heart valves. *Annals of Biomedical Engineering* 2010; **38**: 1919–1927.

175. Durst CA, Grande-Allen KJ. Design and physical characterization of a synchronous multivalve aortic valve culture system. *Annals of Biomedical Engineering* 2010; **38**: 319–325.

176. Kortsmit J, Rutten MCM, Wijlaars MW, Baaijens FPT. Deformation controlled load application in heart valve tissue engineering. *Tissue Engineering Part C—Methods* 2009; **15**: 707–716.

177. Barzilla JE, McKenney AS, Cowan AE, Durst CA, Grande-Allen KJ. Design and validation of a novel splashing bioreactor system for use in mitral valve organ culture. *Annals of Biomedical Engineering* 2010; **38**: 3280–3294.

178. Sierad LN, Simionescu A, Albers C, Chen J, Maivelett J, Tedderm ME, et al. Design and testing of a pulsatile conditioning system for dynamic endothelialization of polyphenol-stabilized tissue engineered heart valves. *Cardiovascular Engineering and Technology* 2010; **1**: 138–153.

179. Hoerstrup SP, Sodian R, Daebritz S, Wang J, Bacha EA, Martin DP. Functional living trileaflet heart valves grown in vitro. *Circulation* 2000; **102**: III44–III49.

180. Sierad LN, Simionescu A, Albers C, Chen J, Maivelett J, Tedder ME, et al. Design and testing of a pulsatile conditioning system for dynamic endothelialization of polyphenol-stabilized tissue engineered heart valves. *Cardiovascular Engineering and Technology* 2010; **1**: 138–153.

181. Lichtenberg A, Tudorache I, Cebotari S, Suprunov M, Tudorache G, Goerler H, et al. Preclinical testing of tissue-engineered heart valves re-endothelialized under simulated physiological conditions. *Circulation* 2006; **114**: I559–I565.

182. Lichtenberg A, Cebotari S, Tudorache I, Sturz G, Winterhalter M, Hilfiker A, et al. Flow-dependent re-endothelialization of tissue-engineered heart valves. *Journal of Heart Valve Disease* 2006; **15**: 287–293.

183. Mol A, Driessen NJB, Rutten MCM, Hoerstrup SP, Bouten CVC, Baaijens FPT. Tissue engineering of human heart valve leaflets: a novel bioreactor for a strain-based conditioning approach. *Annals of Biomedical Engineering* 2005; **33**: 1778–1788.

184. Kloxin AM, Tibbitt MW, Anseth KS. Synthesis of photodegradable hydrogels as dynamically tunable cell culture platforms. *Nature Protocols* 2010; **5**: 1867–1887.

185. Pedron S, Kasko AM, Peinado C, Anseth KS. Effect of heparin oligomer chain length on the activation of valvular interstitial cells. *Biomacromolecules* 2010; **11**: 1692–1695.

186. Kloxin AM, Tibbitt MW, Kasko AM, Fairbairn JA, Anseth KS. Tunable hydrogels for external manipulation of cellular microenvironments through controlled photodegradation. *Advanced Materials* 2010; **22**: 61–66.

187. Benton JA, Kern HB, Leinwand LA, Mariner PD, Anseth KS. Statins block calcific nodule formation of valvular interstitial cells by inhibiting alpha-smooth muscle actin expression. *Arteriosclerosis Thrombosis and Vascular Biology* 2009; **29**: 1950–1957.

188. Zeltinger J, Landeen LK, Alexander HG, Kidd ID, Sibanda B. Development and characterization of tissue-engineered aortic valves. *Tissue Engineering* 2001; **7**: 9–22.

189. Schenke-Layland K, Opitz F, Gross M, Doring C, Halbhuber KJ, Schirrmeister F, et al. Complete dynamic repopulation of decellularized heart valves by application of defined physical signals-an in vitro study. *Cardiovascular Research* 2003; **60**: 497–509.

190. Dumont K, Yperman J, Verbeken E, Segers P, Meuris B, Vandenberghe S, et al. Design of a new pulsatile bioreactor for tissue engineered aortic heart valve formation. *Artificial Organs* 2002; **26**: 710–714.

191. Barzilla JE, Acevedo FE, Grande-Allen KJ. Organ culture as a tool to identify early mechanisms of serotonergic valve disease. *Journal of Heart Valve Disease* 2010; **19**: 626–635.

192. Wu S, Liu YL, Cui B, Qu XH, Chen GQ. Study on decellularized porcine aortic Valve/Poly (3-hydroxybutyrate-co-3-hydroxyhexanoate) hybrid heart valve in sheep model. *Artificial Organs* 2007; **31**: 689–697.

193. Honge JL, Funder JA, Jensen H, Dohmen PM, Konertz WF, Hasenkam JM. Recellularization of decellularized mitral heart valves in juvenile pigs. *Journal of Heart Valve Disease* 2010; **19**: 584–592.

194. Honge JL, Funder J, Hansen E, Dohmen PM, Konertz W, Hasenkam JM. Recellularization of aortic valves in pigs. *European Journal of Cardio—Thoracic Surgery* 2011; **39**: 829–834.

195. Ali ML, Kumar SP, Bjornstad K, Duran CM. The sheep as an animal model for heart valve research. *Cardiovascular Surgery* 1996; **4**: 543–549.

196. Rashid ST, Salacinski HJ, Hamilton G, Seifalian AM. The use of animal models in developing the discipline of cardiovascular tissue engineering: a review. *Biomaterials* 2004; **25**: 1627–1637.

197. Huysmans HA. Animal trials for heart valve substitutes. *Journal of Heart Valve Disease* 2004; **13**: S4–S6.

198. Wang N, Adams G, Buttery L, Falcone FH, Stolnik S. Alginate encapsulation technology supports embryonic stem cells differentiation into insulin-producing cells. *Journal of Biotechnology* 2009; **144**: 304–312.

199. Kallenbach K, Sorrentino S, Mertsching H, Kostin S, Pethig K, Haverich A, et al. A novel small-animal model for accelerated investigation of tissue-engineered aortic valve conduits. *Tissue Engineering Part C—Methods* 2010; **16**: 41–50.

200. Wang Q, McGoron AJ, Pinchuk L, Schoephoerster RT. A novel small animal model for biocompatibility assessment of polymeric materials for use in prosthetic heart valves. *Journal of Biomedical Materials Research Part A* 2010; **93A**: 442–453.

201. Gandaglia A, Bagno A, Naso F, Spina M, Gerosa G. Cells, scaffolds and bioreactors for tissue-engineered heart valves: a journey from basic concepts to contemporary developmental innovations. *European Journal of Cardio-Thoracic Surgery* 2011; **39**: 523–531.

202. Rippel RA, Ghanbari H, Seifalian AM. Tissue-engineered heart valve: future of cardiac surgery. *World Journal of Surgery* 2012; **36**: 1581–1591.

Chapter 20

Micro and Nanotechnology in Vascular Regeneration

Vivian Lee and Guohao Dai

Department of Biomedical Engineering, Rensselaer Polytechnic Institute, 110 8th Street, Troy, NY 12180, USA

daig@rpi.edu

While tissue engineering holds great potential to regenerate damaged tissues in the body, we have yet to realize much clinically relevant success [30,48]. As of today, only several tissue-engineered products are successful used in clinic, such as skin and cartilage replacement [35,62,108]. The lack of successful in vitro engineered tissues is due to multiple challenges that we are facing today in tissue engineering field [31,48]. One of the most significant challenges is the inability to create vascularized tissues [59,83,89]. Without vascular supplies, engineered tissues cannot grow more than a few hundred microns in size, which is also known as the diffusion limit [25]. There are reports of in vitro culture of large tissue-engineered constructs that can be sufficiently supplied with oxygen and nutrients by perfusion bioreactors [45,85]. However, after implanting these tissues, the diffusion processes are still limited due to the distance between capillaries and the center of the

---

Tissue and Organ Regeneration: Advances in Micro- and Nanotechnology
Edited by Lijie Grace Zhang, Ali Khademhosseini, and Thomas J. Webster
Copyright © 2014 Pan Stanford Publishing Pte. Ltd.
ISBN 978-981-4411-67-7 (Hardcover), 978-981-4411-68-4 (eBook)
www.panstanford.com

construct. In vivo, nearly all tissues are supplied with nutrients and oxygen by a highly branched network of blood vessels, which are then subdivided in the tissue into small capillaries. The maximum distance between these capillaries is 200 μm, which correlates with the diffusion limit of oxygen [10].

Over the past 10 years, there has been tremendous development in micro- and nanotechnologies, some of which are promising in promoting vascular regeneration in engineered tissues. The human vasculature spans a dramatically different length scale of more than 1000-fold, ranging from 10~20 mm in large vessels to 10 μm in smallest capillaries with more than 20 levels of branches and bifurcations. At the cellular level, the extracellular matrix (ECM) components and structure at the nanoscale level also have a great influence on the functions of vascular system. Because of these dramatic changes in length scale, micro- and nanotechnologies are especially useful to make an impact in vascular regeneration. In this chapter, we will review the current strategies to create vascularized tissues. In particular, we will emphasize the application of micro- and nanotechnologies in tissue revascularization at capillary level. We will not include technologies in fabricating tissue-engineered vascular graft, which is usually associated with large vessel and will be covered in other chapters.

20.1 Overview of Angiogenesis and Vasculogenesis

The formation of blood vessels in vivo is based on two underlying processes: angiogenesis and vasculogenesis. The basic concept of angiogenesis is the sprouting of capillaries from pre-existing blood vessels. Vasculogenesis describes a de novo assembly of undifferentiated ECs to capillaries in situ, such as the events during embryonic development. Initially, endothelial progenitor cells (EPCs) differentiate to mature ECs, these cells proliferate in former avascular areas and create first primitive vessel networks [10]. While it was once believed that vasculogenesis only appears during embryonic development, we now know that vasculogenesis also occurs in postnatal life [11]. For example, some of the current pre-vascularization strategies in tissue engineering recapitulate the postnatal vasculogenesis process [65,111]. The generation of more complex capillary networks occurs in the next step by the morphogenic process of angiogenesis with extensive ECM remodeling. Therefore, ECs release matrix metalloproteinases (MMPs) to degrade the surrounding ECM. The cells migrate into the newly developed gaps and sprout into novel blood vessels. This event is assisted by a complex interaction and crosstalk between adhesion proteins, growth factors, junctional molecules, oxygen sensors, endogenous inhibitors and many other molecules [44]. Furthermore, sequence of events between ECs and non-ECs of the surrounding tissue are involved in the formation of novel blood vessels from pre-existing vascular structures. Two important participants are differentiated pericytes (PCs) and smooth muscle cells (SMCs), which are critical for the stabilization and maturation of vessels [111]. In addition, mesenchymal progenitor cells from blood and bone marrow can also serve as the supporting cells to stabilize the blood vessel [58,65].

Understanding the fundamental principles of angiogenesis and vasculogenesis is important to vascular tissue engineering. The goal is to apply the basic principles of angiogenesis and vasculogenesis into practical solutions in vascularizing tissue-engineered constructs. In summary of various approaches, there are two main strategies utilized to engineer vascularized tissues. In the first approach, new vasculature is generated in free-form manner by ECs through angiogenesis or vasculogenesis when ECs are embedded in better designed biomaterials and growth factor environment. In the second approach, technologies are often used to precisely control the spatial localization of vascular cells and ECMs, such as Bio-MEMS, 3D cell printing, cell sheet engineering, hydrogel self-assembling, and many other microfabrication methods. Here we will review some of the most important strategies as illustrated below.

20.2 Biomaterial Scaffold to Promote Vascularization

20.2.1 Biomaterials for Controlled Release of Angiogenic Factors

To promote angiogenesis, biomaterial scaffolds are modified to incorporate or immobilize pro-angiogenic cytokines and growth factors [13,69,72,84]. The angiogenic growth factors are powerful initiators of neovascularization. They activate ECs from the surrounding tissues, and stimulate them to migrate toward the factor gradient. Afterwards, they also promote cell assembly, vessel formation and maturation. The main factors in up-regulating angiogenic processes are the vascular endothelial growth factor (VEGF), the basic fibroblast growth factor (bFGF) and the hepatocyte growth factor (HGF). Several other growth factors are also important such as insulin-like growth factor (IGF) and epidermal growth factor (EGF). In addition, a complex orchestra of cytokines such as platelet-derived growth factor (PDGF), transforming growth factor beta (TGFβ) and angiopoietin serve as indirect angiogenic factors and are involved in the regeneration of endothelial tubes through their action on ECs or the supporting mural cells around the vasculature [11].

While growth factors are powerful and promising for developing effective strategies in vascular regeneration, they also possess several potential drawbacks, such as high costs associated with recombinant proteins and susceptibility to degradation in vivo. Therefore, besides angiogenic growth factors, some small molecules have been discovered to stimulate angiogenesis. For example, medicinal chemistry and high throughput screening have been used to identify and synthesize non-peptide-based inducers of angiogenesis [113]. The identified small molecule compounds induce angiogenesis through increasing proliferative effects on vascular ECs. Another promising angiogenic molecule is sphingosine 1-phosphate (S1P). Sphingosine 1-phosphate is a bioactive phospholipid that impacts migration, proliferation, and survival in diverse cell types. Sphingosine 1-phosphate possesses significant ability to promote vascular stabilization by recruitment of pericytes and SMCs to newly formed vessels and stimulating SMC proliferation, migration and differentiation into a more contractile phenotype. Using biomaterials to deliver S1P, studies have shown that it dramatically promoted bone healing through arteriogenesis and microvessel diameter expansion [94].

To provide an effective angiogenic factor delivery, many challenges must be solved. In vivo, the angiogenic factors are typically unstable and large fluctuation in concentration often leads to undesired effects. Therefore, bolus injection of growth factors is increasingly replaced by local and sustained delivery strategy.

A promising approach to overcome the high degradation rate of the expensive growth factors is to design new biomaterial strategies. Therefore, various slow-release devices of natural, synthetic, and composite materials have been designed [106,119]. To provide better control of the local delivery concentration at the precise time, angiogenic factors can be encapsulated inside micro or nanoparticles, thus the rate and the amount of release can be tuned to satisfy particular applications [116]. Critical and important aspects, when designing an angiogenic therapy, are the dose and the composition of the delivered growth factors. For example high levels of PDGF induce vessel destabilization [1]. Enhancing the vascularization of 3D porous alginate scaffolds by an overexpression of angiopoietin-1 may result in endothelial hyperplasia and reduced vessel leakage [24]. The spatial pattern and concentration gradient of angiogenic factors are also important factors. To control the spatial pattern, VEGF were covalently bound through photopolymerization via laser scanning lithography to the surface of poly(ethylene glycol) (PEG) hydrogels in patterned micron-scale regions, and was found to accelerate endothelial tubulogenesis and increase cellular angiogenic responses [54].

Different control-releasing strategies can also be combined to achieve improved angiogenesis in tissue. For example, delivery of VEGF promotes neovascularization at early stages of ischemic tissue repair. However, its effects are very limited in longer term due to poorly organized, leaky, and/or hemorrhagic blood vessel formation after some period [106]. Additionally, nascent vascular networks formed in response to VEGF are often prone to regression if not adequately matured, or stabilized, by mural support cells [79]. This process of mural cell recruitment is a key component of arteriogenesis [44]. Therefore, strategies have been developed to deliver consecutive growth factors (e.g., VEGF, bFGF, PDGF, and angiopoietin-1) at the early, middle and late stages to induce capillary formation, to recruit mural cells and to stabilize the vessel for long-term functions [13,72,104,107]. A co-immobilization of two growth factors, PDGF-BB and FGF-2 resulted in a significantly increased EC migration compared to the presentation of each factor alone [55,90]. Promising results were achieved by combining the release of VEGF and angiopoietin-1, as well as the combination of VEGF, IGF-1, and SDF-1 from newly developed hydrogel matrices [104]. In this case, the induction of more and larger newly formed functional vessels in the surrounding host tissue could be observed. Because angiogenesis is a complex process involving spatial regulations of stimulatory and inhibitory mechanisms, biomimetic approaches have also been developed to co-delivery both angiogenic and anti-angiogenic factors from spatially restricted zones of a synthetic polymer to create temporally stable and spatially restricted angiogenic zones in vivo [123].

In some conditions, the delivery of angiogenic factors may still be not sufficient to grow large tissue implant. While neovascularization is being established, cells in the middle of the implant may already dead even before the complete vascularization has occurred. Therefore, oxygen generating scaffolds for enhancing tissue survival will be very useful [36]. To supply additional oxygen to the tissue, calcium peroxide-based oxygen generating particles were incorporated into 3D scaffolds of poly(D,L-lactide-co-glycolide) (PLGA). The scaffolds were designed to generate oxygen over the course of 10 days [74]. These biomaterials were able to extend cell viability and growth under hypoxic conditions. The use of oxygen generating biomaterials may allow for increased cell survivability while neovascularization is being established after implantation.

20.2.2 Immobilization of Bioactive Molecules to Enhance Angiogenesis

In addition to controlled release of angiogenic growth factors, various bioartificial matrices are also developed for therapeutic vascularization [84]. These bioartificial matrices mimic functionality and complexity of native tissues by incorporating the critical bioactive site of the ECM so that they can be sufficiently vascularized. For example, short peptide adhesion sequences derived from ECM-like fibronectin (e.g., RGD and REDV) or laminin (e.g., YIGSR) are well known to maintain cell adhesion through integrin binding [37,42,61,66,97,100,102,110]. They have been incorporated into biomimetic hydrogels to promote migration of ECs and enhance angiogenesis [34,71]. Besides adhesion peptides, another approach is to immobilize the glucosaminoglycane heparin on surfaces. Besides the antithrombotic effect of heparin, the polysaccharide contains growth factor–binding sites, so it can be used for a local and sustained release of angiogenic factors [121,122].

Another important feature of angiogenesis is the remodeling of the ECM by vascular cells. Degradation of the old matrix is necessary for the angiogenesis to happen. Therefore, synthetic matrix metalloproteinase (MMP)-sensitive hydrogels have been developed to promote angiogenesis [60]. West and Hubbell were the first to use protease-sensitive PEG-based biomaterials with degradation sites for proteases involved in cell migration [86]. By introducing MMP-sensitive peptide sequences into the backbone of PEG, the biodegradation rate and, therefore, the ability to increase angiogenesis performance, have been observed in vitro as well as in vivo [66].

20.2.3 Engineering Biomaterial Architecture to Promote Infiltration of Vascular Cells

The architecture of biomaterial scaffold has important effects on the angiogenesis process. The porosity is a main factor setting up suitable micro-architectures for supporting tissue neogenesis and blood vessel ingrowth. The topographic features at the micro- and nanoscales also influence the cell attachment, spreading, differentiation, and functions. Therefore, various strategies have been developed to create biomaterial scaffolds with desired special architectures.

Fabrication techniques, such as phase separation, freeze drying, particular leaching and gas foaming, have been used for different approaches in tissue engineering for years. The parameters associated with the fabrication process can be controlled to achieve desired porosity to facility vascular generation. However, those fabrication techniques hold some disadvantages concerning vascularized 3D scaffolds. Although it is possible to create hierarchical porous structures with variable shapes and sizes, the interconnectivity is not specified, which is important for successful vascularization. One way to obtain desired scaffold porosity with interconnected pores is the application of advanced electrospinning methods [82,99]. Recently, Leong and colleagues used ice crystals as templates to fabricate cryogenic electrospun scaffolds with large 3D and interconnected pores in a poly(D,L-lactide) matrix. They were able to show cells infiltration into the cryogenic electrospun scaffolds up to 50 μm in thickness in vitro, whereas cells did not infiltrate the conventional electrospun scaffolds [53]. Santos et al. fabricated by electrospun polycaprolactone based scaffold for bone tissue engineering, which contained a nano- and microfibrous network. The topography allowed ECs to stretch between single microfibers and guided the 3D distribution of ECs. For such structures an enhanced blood vessel formation after implantation was found [26]. Further investigations showed ECs on nano- and microfibers forming extensive networks of capillary-like structures, a clear indication of increased angiogenic potential [41,91].

In applications where a more complex tissue architecture with vasculature is desired, current fabrication technologies are still not sufficient to mimic the complete natural vascular architecture. Therefore, natural-derived scaffolds, which contain native vascular network, are often used. In this approach, the tissues or organs are decellularized while ECM and 3D vascular structure remain intact. This approach has proven to possess some advantages over the synthetic scaffold, especially naturally derived 3D structure supplying microvascular networks [3]. Using this approach, Doris Taylor's group created decellularized hearts by coronary perfusion with detergents. This resulted in a preserved underlying ECM, and produced an acellular perfusable vascular architecture. They reseeded these constructs with cardiac and ECs, and then subjected the construct under perfusion bioreactor. This procedure led to a functional heart with pump function. The re-established vascular system infiltrated with endothelial cells are thought to contribute to the successful of this approach [76]. Applying this approach, other tissues and organs have been generated for in vivo implantation, such as tissue-engineered lungs [81].

20.3 Micro- and Nanotechnologies to Create Precise Vascular Patterns

20.3.1 Microfabrication-Based Approaches

Recent development in microfabrication/Bio-MEMS enables the creation of various microscale features at the micron level [112]. This capability thus allows the fabricating of more complex branching networks at micron scale to mimic the native vascular geometries. First, micro features are fabricated using a molding process by soft lithography [6]. Using the microfabricated mold, artificial capillary networks are formed from biocompatible nondegradable materials such as silicone or polydimethyl siloxane (PDMS), or biodegradable elastomers, such as poly(glycerol sebacate) (PGS) [23]. This process resulted in mechanically robust devices with macroscopic fluidic connections. Afterwards, the devices were endothelialized under flow conditions [8,9,87]. In this approach, the vascular geometries and branches can be precisely controlled in the fabrication process. One problem associated with this approach is that the ECs are usually located on one side of the lumen and microchannels are typically rectangular cross section that do not recapitulate the circular cross section of the native vessels and result in nonuniform cell seeding and unnatural cellular responses. To overcome this limitation, ongoing efforts have developed method to construct microvascular networks with circular cross sections so that ECs can cover the entire lumen surface [8].

To mimic the exact pressure distribution, fluid flow and transport process, several biomimetic principles were established as the major design guidelines of branched vascular network. To implement these principles, computational fluid dynamic models have also been developed to optimize the design of the vascular pattern so that it resembles the in vivo physiological parameters [7]. These biomimetic design principles will provide a foundation for developing complex vascular networks for solid organ tissue engineering that can achieve physiologic blood flow in the future [39].

The microfabrication approaches can also be used to create physiologically relevant ex vivo model system for basic research in vascular biology. In one study, a 3D microfluidic device was used as a model system to study the molecular regulation of perivascular stem cell niches. ECs suspended within 3D fibrin gels were patterned in the device adjacent to stromal cells. It was found that the cells undergo a morphogenetic process similar to vasculogenesis, forming a primitive vascular plexus and maturing into a robust capillary network with hollow well-defined lumens [12]. Similarly, the differentiation of mesenchymal stem cells (MSC) within an EC-seeded modular construct in a microfluidic flow chamber can also be studied [49]. The advantages of these microfluidic approaches are the precise control of vascular geometries as well as physiological parameters such as pressure and flow. Using this system, the interstitial flow across hydrogel can be generated and precisely controlled, and its effects on the capillary morphogenesis can be monitored in real time [16,98,103,109].

In some of the microfluidic-based approaches, vascular patterns can be precisely controlled as designed. The limitation is associated with the limited selection of materials that are compatible with these processes. The limited biodegradability and biological activities (e.g., PDMS) of these materials forming the vascular channel often do not allow active remodeling between ECs and surrounding matrix. To overcome this problem, alternative approaches have been developed [14,29]. In this procedure, micromolded meshes of gelatin served as sacrificial materials following the microfabricated mold. Encapsulation of gelatin meshes in a hydrogel and subsequent melting and flushing of the gelatin left behind interconnected channels in the hydrogel. The channel was then seeded with ECs and perfused under flow condition. It was found that endothelial tubes displayed a strong barrier function over 5 days, resisted adhesion of leukocytes, and reacted quickly to inflammatory stimuli by breakdown of the barrier and support of leukocyte adhesion. These tubes resembled venules and "giant" capillaries in both their cellular organization and function. Therefore, this model can serve as useful in vitro models of inflammation under constant perfusion. The advantage of this approach is that the vascular channel is sitting directly on bioactive matrix in which the active remodeling between ECs and surround matrix can be achieved, as well as to recapitulate some important physiological parameters such as permeability, transmural pressure and fluid flow. Similarly, lithographic and microfluidic techniques have been used to form deterministic microstructures within hydrogels and thus enable rapid invasion and vascularization of soft tissue in vivo [15,125].

20.3.2 Multiphoton Polymerization of Hydrogels for Vascular Patterns

Multiphoton polymerization (MPP) of photosensitive materials is a 3D nanoscale manufacturing tool that offers great potential for rapid and flexible fabrication of fully 3D structures with sub-100 nm resolution [21]. This high-resolution technique thus enables the fabrication of engineered tissues with complex structures such as microvasculature. Currently, there are efforts to use MPP-technology for the fabrication of bioartificial small-lumen vessels from biocompatible synthetic materials [77]. Multiphoton polymerization is also used in tissue engineering approaches. West et al., for example, used the technology to micropattern cell adhesive ligands (RGDS) in hydrogels to guide cell migration along predefined 3D pathways. In this work, the two-photon laser scanning photolithographic technique was used to dictate the precise location of RGDS in collagenase-sensitive poly(ethylene glycol-co-peptide) diacrylate hydrogels. When human dermal fibroblasts cultured in fibrin clusters were encapsulated within the micropatterned collagenase-sensitive hydrogels, the cells underwent guided 3D migration only into the RGDS-patterned regions of the hydrogels. These results demonstrate the prospect of guiding tissue regeneration at the microscale in 3D scaffolds by providing appropriate bioactive cues in highly defined geometries. The advantage of this approach over many other approaches is that the two-photon polymerization is able to penetrate deeper into the gel thus enable generating complex 3D patterns to guide vascular regeneration [52,70]. This biomimetic hydrogel system can be readily modified with various biomolecules such as peptides, growth factors, and other signaling molecules and may lead to development of more native tissue-like constructs that can support and direct the complex processes of tissue regeneration.

20.3.3 Rapid Prototyping and Solid Free form Techniques

Recently, a manufacturing technique commonly used in industry, known as solid free-form fabrication (SFF), or rapid prototyping, has been successfully applied to tissue engineering by fabricating complex hierarchical biomaterial scaffolds [28,40,43,56,80,105,118,120]. Solid free-form fabrication systems build 3D structures by layering materials onto a moving platform. Commercially available systems (e.g., stereolithography, selective laser sintering, 3D inkjet, or laser printing) either photopolymerize liquid monomer, sinter powdered materials, process material either thermally or chemically as it passes through a nozzle, or print material, such as chemical binder onto powder. Solid free-form fabrication techniques can be easily automated and integrated with imaging techniques to produce scaffolds that are customized in size and shape for specific applications. Tissue engineering scaffolds, built by those layer-by-layer manufacturing processes, can match the in vivo paradigm of porosity and mechanical strength with the correct spatial positioning and morphology [40]. Unfortunately, toxic solvents and high temperatures are still widely used in most SFF techniques, making them not suitable to build live tissues and limiting their further applications in tissue engineering.

To engineer 3D live tissues, several groups around the world have begun to develop technology to simultaneously deposit hydrogels with live cells to form 3D tissue structures [51,57,67, 68,73,88,115]. This new concept, also called "organ printing," is an advanced form of SFF. The main features of this technology are using phase changing hydrogels without harsh chemicals as well as a dispensing technology that is gentle to the cells. Current strategies for inducing phase change (from liquid to solid form after printing) include UV, temperature, pH, and ion concentrations, which can be used on a variety of natural and synthetic hydrogels such as alginate, collagen, fibrin, agarose, gelatin and PEG based hydrogels. For instance, a pneumatic dispensing system has been utilized to build 3D structures by depositing a continuous stream of cell-laden photopolymerizable hydrogel before cross-linking via UV light excitation [22]. Commercial inkjet printers (e.g., piezoelectric and thermal) have been modified to print microdroplets of biological materials, including viable cells, with microscale precision [115] and a 10 kHz printing speed [92]. With the advances of cell printing, one may be able to build precise human microvasculature with suitable bio-ink. In one study, human microvascular ECs (HMVEC) and fibrin were studied as bio-ink for microvasculature construction. Micron-sized fibrin channel along with HMVECs was precisely fabricated using a drop-on-demand polymerization via thrombin solution [17]. It was found that the 3D tubular structure was formed in the printed patterns. Various approaches have used 3D printing technology to construct 3D tissue structures. However, a perfused vasculature has not been achieved. Toward this goal, a unique fabrication method was developed to construct a functional vascular perfusion channel within thick hydrogel scaffold [124]. Built on the success of this technique, a more complex thick viable tissue can be constructed in the future.

Although this technology is promising to build complex tissue structures with good cell viability, there are still considerable challenges, such as the low cell density associated with cell printing. This is in contrast to the cellular volume fraction observed in most live organs and cell aggregates [73]. This limitation comes from the need to use low cell concentrations (<5 × 10^6 cells/mL) in the bio-ink to avoid nozzle clogging from cell sedimentation and aggregation [78]. Therefore, alternative approaches must be developed in order to solve this problem.

One of them, based on the automated deposition of cell aggregates in 3D, has been reported [73]. Closely placed tissue spheroids undergo tissue fusion process that represents a fundamental biological and biophysical principle of developmental biology-inspired directed tissue self-assembly. In this approach, various vascular cell types, including SMCs and fibroblasts, were aggregated into discrete units, either multicellular spheroids or cylinders of controllable diameter (300–500 μm). These were printed layer-by-layer concomitantly with agarose rods, used here as a molding template. The postprinting fusion of the discrete units resulted in single- and double-layered small diameter vascular tubes (OD ranging from 0.9 to 2.5 mm). A unique aspect of the method is the ability to engineer vessels of distinct shapes and hierarchical trees that combine tubes of distinct diameters. Another approach used cell-laden hyaluronan (HA) hydrogel instead of cell aggregates, other tubular structures have been fabricated by means of an extrusion patterning system [101]. The composite material was deposited continuously as filaments (300–500 μm in diameter) on an agarose mold. These filaments then fused with each other as a tubular structure. In this study, a maximum cell density of 25 × 10^6 cells/mL was used without impeding hydrogel gelation [101].

Another printing technique is laser-assisted bio-printing (LAB) [33]. This technique is based on the principle of laser-induced forward transfer, also known as matrix-assisted pulse laser evaporation, laser induced direct writing, or biological laser printing [4,93]. A typical LAB setup comprises a pulsed laser beam, a focusing system, a "ribbon" (a transparent glass slide, possibly coated with a laser-absorbing layer of metal, onto which a thin layer of bio-ink is spread) and a receiving substrate facing the ribbon. The physical principle of LAB is based on the generation of a cavitation-like bubble, into the depth of the bio-ink film, whose expansion and collapse induces the formation of a jet and, thereby, the transfer of the bio-ink from the ribbon to the substrate. Previous studies have shown that LAB can print mammalian cells without affecting viability and function, and without causing DNA damage [32,93]. Laser-assisted bio-printing is a nozzle-free technology that prevents clogging issues and allows the printing of droplets from solutions of various viscosity (1–300 mPa/s) and with cell concentrations of the order of 1×10^8 cells/mL. Using LAB, cells can be individually aligned next to each other, and multiple cell types can be interfaced with micron-scale precision at a speed of 5 kHz [27]. A microvascular-like structure has been recently produced using LAB [114], and patterned human stem cells and ECs with laser printing was created for cardiac regeneration [27]. The principle of reconstructing a tissue in situ has also been demonstrated in vivo [47].

20.3.4 Bottom-Up Approach: Self-Assembling of Cell-Laden Hydrogels

Recently, modular approaches have emerged as attractive approaches in tissue engineering to achieve precisely controlled architectures by using micro-engineered components. In contrast to many "top-down" approaches, this molecular assembling is also called the "bottom-up" approach [19]. In some studies, the building blocks are often randomly assembled. For example, sub-millimeter-sized cylindrical modules of collagen have been seeded with cells and then randomly assembled inside a perfusion chamber to form a macroscopic tissue construct called an "organoid" [64]. To control the assembling process, a more detailed research on the interfacial phenomena between hydrogels and the liquid interface are needed, thus an improved assembling method can be developed [19]. In this approach, the shape and functional controlled microscale cell-laden microgels are self-assembled into desirable macro-scale tissue constructs. This assembly process is driven by the tendency of multiphase liquid–liquid systems to minimize the surface area and the resulting surface free energy between the phases. First, the shape-controlled cell-laden hydrogels (usually at the micron scale) were produced through micropatterned UV exposure on

PEG hydrogels and cells. Then the cell-laden hydrogels were spontaneously assembled within multiphase reactor systems into pre-determined geometric configurations. Finally, multicomponent cell-laden constructs could be generated by assembling microgel building blocks and performing a secondary cross-linking reaction.

Using this technology, Khademhosseini's group sequentially assembled microengineered hydrogels into hydrogel constructs with an embedded vascular-like microchannels [18]. First, arrays of microgels with predefined internal microchannels were fabricated by photolithography. Then, these microgels were assembled into 3D tubular construct with multilevel interconnected lumens. The sequential assembly of microgels occurred in a biphasic reactor and was initiated by swiping a needle to generate physical forces and fluidic shear. Finally, in an attempt to build a biomimetic 3D vasculature, they incorporated endothelial cells and SMCs into an assembled construct with a concentric microgel design. The sequential assembly is simple, rapid, cost-effective, and could be used for fabricating tissue constructs with biomimetic vasculature and other complex architectures. Other groups fabricated vascular-like tissues consisting of collagen gel rods seeded with ECs. The EC-covered modules were then assembled in a vascular shape to a macro-tissue, where the modules form a larger tube. The cell-covered interconnected channels provide an antithrombogenic surface that enables functional perfusion with medium or whole blood [46,64]. In comparison with conventional methods, this approach is simple and may provide a useful alternative for in vitro reconstruction of 3D vascular network for building vascularized tissue constructs.

20.3.5 Cell Sheet Technology

Cell sheet technology (CST) is a promising means for fabricating vascularized and complex tissues from the bottom up. Cell sheet technology is based on the thermo-responsive polymers, poly (*N*-isopropylacrylamide) (PIPAAm). The surface of PIPAAms is formulated in such a way as to make its typical thickness <100 nm. Cells are grown to confluency on the polymer substrate in culture conditions that favor ECM production. The cell sheet can be detached from the substrate below a crucial temperature (32°C) without the need for a proteinase treatment. This technique is beneficial to create 3D constructs containing EC networks, because it preserves normal and intrinsic cell-cell direct contact and various cell adhesive factors. Moreover, the thickness of these 3D constructs could be controlled by the number of layered cell sheets. Cell sheet technology has been very useful to create highly cellular sheets that can produce large amount of ECMs. For example, blood vessels have been created by rolling sheets of ECM produced by human skin fibroblasts [2,5,38,75,95,117].

Using CST, 3D stratified tissues were created by stacking cell sheets. The co-culture with ECs in the tissues was found to facilitate in vitro pre-vascular network formation and to promote in vivo neovascularization after their transplantation. In this study, HUVECs and human dermal fibroblasts (NHDFs), and their mixture were harvested as an intact cell sheet from temperature-responsive culture dish. Single mono-culture EC sheet was stacked with two NHDF-sheets in different orders, and 3 co-cultured cell sheets were layered by a cell sheet collecting device. Morphological analyses revealed that pre-vascular networks composing of HUVECs were formed in all the triple layer constructs. For this technique, the direct contact of ECs with fibroblasts contributed to the formation of a capillary-like network in vitro. It was also showed that the pre-vascular networks formed tube-like structures similar to native microvasculature [96].

Moreover, multiple cell types can be micropatterned in cells sheets. Cell sheet technology has found application in the regeneration of myocardial tissue, cornea and pancreas [20]. To construct hepatic-EC co-culture system, a monolayer cell sheet composed of EC was placed on top of a monolayer of hepatocytes (Hep). In this hybrid cell sheet format, histological examination revealed that bile canaliculi networks were formed and well developed among the hepatocytes in the layered Hep-EC sheet group. The albumin secretion level was highly preserved at least for 28 days in the hybrid Hep-EC sheet, whereas the monolayer of hepatocytes exhibited a markedly reduced time course of secretion. The expression levels of hepatocyte-specific genes were also significantly up-regulated. These results demonstrate that CST is a valuable technology to prolong hepatocyte functionality through vascularization of the construct [2,50]. Cell sheet technology can also improve in vivo vascular regeneration. Transplantation of the cardiac tissue sheet to a rat myocardial infarction model showed significant and sustained improvement of systolic function accompanied by neovascularization. Reduction of the infarct wall thinning and fibrotic length indicated the attenuation of LV remodeling [63].

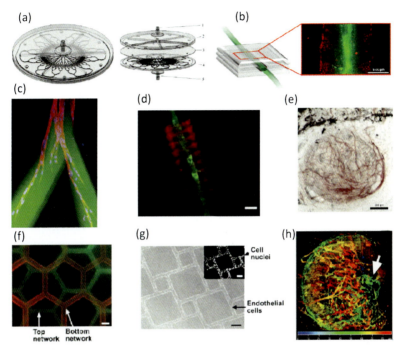

Figure 20.1 (a) Computational tools are implemented to guide the design of vascular network in hepatic tissue engineering. Shown here is isometric view of liver vascular network [39]. (b) Schematic diagram of the printed vascular channel construct, and fluorescence image of the printed vascular channel construct with fluid flow [126]. (c) Confocal microscope image of fibroblasts undergoing 3-D migration within RGDS-patterned region inside a collagenase-sensitive PEG hydrogel, scale bar 25 μm [52]. (d) Assembly of cell-laden hydrogel constructs to engineer vascular-like microchannels. Shown here is the perfusion of the stabilized tubular microgel assembly [18]. (e, h) Proteolytically degradable PEG hydrogels promote neovascularization in murine cornea [71]. (f, g) Microfabricated microvascular channels within collagen gels [29].

20.4 Summary

Vascularization remains one of the main obstacles that need to be overcome before large tissue-engineered constructs can be applied in clinical applications. Multiple strategies for improving vascularization in the field of tissue engineering have been developed. These strategies are based on our better understanding of the vascular development and vascular biology, as well as many enabling technology at the micro- and nanoscales.

Despite this progress in vascular bioengineering, at present it is still uncertain which will prove to be the best method for successful in vivo applications. There is no convincing evidence that any of the described strategies will be sufficient to sustain tissue-engineered constructs that are larger than several millimeters after implantation. To increase the chances of success, researchers should not focus solely on any one of these strategies but should instead investigate the integration of several strategies with the aim of combining their strong points and eliminating their weaknesses. Here we identify several critical challenges that need to be solved in order to move the field forward:

(1) Many of these technologies are functioning at certain length scale but there is not a single technology that can span across multiple length scales, which is necessary to mimic in vivo vasculature. The problem with microfabricated vascular network is how to anastomose these vessels at the micron level with the host blood vessel at the millimeter scale. Since the in vitro tissue is not microsurgically connected to the host vasculature, the diffusion limit still exists even after implant in vivo. The lack of microsurgical connections is a main issue in numerous in vitro approaches and needs to be addressed in future technology development.

(2) In some method, the 3D vascular structures are normally in two-dimensional manner with planar vascularized patterns starting from a single channel that branches out multiple times into thinner channels. Methods need to be developed so that a true 3D vascular pattern can be generated.

(3) Most researches focus on the formation of blood vessels by morphology, histology and immunostaining. But the functions of the newly generated vessels are largely unknown and it is difficult to compare different approaches to know which one

actually result in a functional vessel. Therefore, it is critical to study the functionality and maturation of the newly formed vessels. This means that a clear definition of functions needs to be justified accordingly based on its particular application.

(4) We now start to appreciate that vasculature exhibit huge diverse functions and heterogeneities depend on their tissue localization. For example, ECs from the artery, vein and microvasculature are different both functionally and genetically. ECs at different organ and tissue systems also have very different functions. The plasticity of vascular phenotype suggests that its surrounding cells have a major impact on its functions, such as neuron, hepatocyte, pancreatic islet cells, or SMCs in different organs. Therefore, it will be important to develop technologies and model systems to study their interactions and their impact on the functions of the tissue-engineered vascular system.

References

1. Andrae, J., Gallini, R., and Betsholtz, C. (2008). Role of platelet-derived growth factors in physiology and medicine. *Genes Dev,* **22**: 1276–1312.
2. Asakawa, N., Shimizu, T., Tsuda, Y., Sekiya, S., Sasagawa, T., Yamato, M., Fukai, F., and Okano, T. (2010). Pre-vascularization of in vitro three-dimensional tissues created by cell sheet engineering. *Biomaterials,* **31**: 3903–3909.
3. Badylak, S. F., Taylor, D., and Uygun, K. (2011). Whole-organ tissue engineering: decellularization and recellularization of three-dimensional matrix scaffolds. *Annu Rev Biomed Eng,* **13**: 27–53.
4. Barron, J. A., Wu, P., Ladouceur, H. D., and Ringeisen, B. R. (2004). Biological laser printing: a novel technique for creating heterogeneous 3-dimensional cell patterns. *Biomed Microdevices,* **6**: 139–147.
5. Bel, A., Planat-Bernard, V., Saito, A., Bonnevie, L., Bellamy, V., Sabbah, L., Bellabas, L., Brinon, B., Vanneaux, V., Pradeau, P., et al. (2010). Composite cell sheets: a further step toward safe and effective myocardial regeneration by cardiac progenitors derived from embryonic stem cells. *Circulation,* **122**: S118–S123.
6. Bettinger, C., Weinberg, E., Kulig, K., Vacanti, J., Wang, Y., Borenstein, J., and Langer, R. (2006). Three-dimensional microfluidic tissue-engineering scaffolds using a flexible biodegradable polymer. *Adv Mater,* **18**: 165–169.

7. Borenstein, J., Terai, H., King, K., Weinberg, E., Kaazempur-Mofrad, M., and Vacanti, J. (2002). Microfabrication technology for vascularized tissue engineering. *Biomed Microdevices,* **4**: 167–175.
8. Borenstein, J. T., Tupper, M. M., Mack, P. J., Weinberg, E. J., Khalil, A. S., Hsiao, J., and García-Cardeña, G. (2010). Functional endothelialized microvascular networks with circular cross-sections in a tissue culture substrate. *Biomed Microdevices,* **12**: 71–79.
9. Borenstein, J. T., Weinberg, E. J., Orrick, B. K., Sundback, C., Kaazempur-Mofrad, M. R., and Vacanti, J. P. (2007). Microfabrication of three-dimensional engineered scaffolds. *Tissue Eng,* **13**: 1837–1844.
10. Carmeliet, P. (2003). Angiogenesis in health and disease. *Nat Med,* **9**: 653–660.
11. Carmeliet, P., and Jain, R. K. (2011). Molecular mechanisms and clinical applications of angiogenesis. *Nature,* **473**: 298–307.
12. Carrion, B., Huang, C. P., Ghajar, C. M., Kachgal, S., Kniazeva, E., Jeon, N. L., and Putnam, A. J. (2010). Recreating the perivascular niche ex vivo using a microfluidic approach. *Biotechnol Bioeng,* **107**: 1020–1028.
13. Chiu, L. L., and Radisic, M. (2010). Scaffolds with covalently immobilized VEGF and Angiopoietin-1 for vascularization of engineered tissues. *Biomaterials,* **31**: 226–241.
14. Chrobak, K. M., Potter, D. R., and Tien, J. (2006). Formation of perfused, functional microvascular tubes in vitro. *Microvasc Res,* **71**: 185–196.
15. Chung, B. G., Lee, K. H., Khademhosseini, A., and Lee, S. H. (2012). Microfluidic fabrication of microengineered hydrogels and their application in tissue engineering. *Lab Chip,* **12**: 45–59.
16. Chung, S., Sudo, R., Mack, P. J., Wan, C.-R., Vickerman, V., and Kamm, R. D. (2009). Cell migration into scaffolds under co-culture conditions in a microfluidic platform. *Lab Chip,* **9**: 269–275.
17. Cui, X., and Boland, T. (2009). Human microvasculature fabrication using thermal inkjet printing technology. *Biomaterials,* **30**: 6221–6227.
18. Du, Y., Ghodousi, M., Qi, H., Haas, N., Xiao, W., and Khademhosseini, A. (2011). Sequential assembly of cell-laden hydrogel constructs to engineer vascular-like microchannels. *Biotechnol Bioeng,* **108**: 1693–1703.
19. Du, Y., Lo, E., Ali, S., and Khademhosseini, A. (2008). Directed assembly of cell-laden microgels for fabrication of 3D tissue constructs. *Proc Natl Acad Sci USA,* **105**: 9522–9527.

20. Elloumi-Hannachi, I., Yamato, M., and Okano, T. (2010). Cell sheet engineering: a unique nanotechnology for scaffold-free tissue reconstruction with clinical applications in regenerative medicine. *J Intern Med*, **267**: 54–70.
21. Farsari, M., and Chichkov, B. (2009). Materials processing: two-photon fabrication. *Nat. Photon*, **3**: 450.
22. Fedorovich, N. E., Swennen, I., Girones, J., Moroni, L., van Blitterswijk, C. A., Schacht, E., Alblas, J., and Dhert, W. J. (2009). Evaluation of photocrosslinked Lutrol hydrogel for tissue printing applications. *Biomacromolecules*, **10**: 1689–1696.
23. Fidkowski, C., Kaazempur-Mofrad, M. R., Borenstein, J., Vacanti, J. P., Langer, R., and Wang, Y. (2005). Endothelialized microvasculature based on a biodegradable elastomer. *Tissue Eng*, **11**: 302–309.
24. Fiedler, U., and Augustin, H. G. (2006). Angiopoietins: a link between angiogenesis and inflammation. *Trends Immunol*, **27**: 552–558.
25. Folkman, J., and Hochberg, M. (1973). Self-regulation of growth in three dimensions. *J Exp Med*, **138**: 745–753.
26. Fuchs, S., Ghanaati, S., Orth, C., Barbeck, M., Kolbe, M., Hofmann, A., Eblenkamp, M., Gomes, M., Reis, R. L., and Kirkpatrick, C. J. (2009). Contribution of outgrowth endothelial cells from human peripheral blood on in vivo vascularization of bone tissue engineered constructs based on starch polycaprolactone scaffolds. *Biomaterials*, **30**: 526–534.
27. Gaebel, R., Ma, N., Liu, J., Guan, J., Koch, L., Klopsch, C., Gruene, M., Toelk, A., Wang, W., Mark, P., et al. (2011). Patterning human stem cells and endothelial cells with laser printing for cardiac regeneration. *Biomaterials*, **32**: 9218–9230.
28. Giordano, R. A., Wu, B. M., Borland, S. W., Cima, L. G., Sachs, E. M., and Cima, M. J. (1996). Mechanical properties of dense polylactic acid structures fabricated by three dimensional printing. *J Biomater Sci Polym Ed*, **8**: 63–75.
29. Golden, A. P., and Tien, J. (2007). Fabrication of microfluidic hydrogels using molded gelatin as a sacrificial element. *Lab Chip*, **7**: 720–725.
30. Griffith, L. G., and Naughton, G. (2002). Tissue engineering–current challenges and expanding opportunities. *Science*, **295**: 1009–1014.
31. Griffith, L. G., and Swartz, M. A. (2006). Capturing complex 3D tissue physiology in vitro. *Nat Rev Mol Cell Biol*, **7**: 211–224.

32. Gruene, M., Deiwick, A., Koch, L., Schlie, S., Unger, C., Hofmann, N., Bernemann, I., Glasmacher, B., and Chichkov, B. (2010). Laser printing of stem cells for biofabrication of scaffold-free autologous grafts. *Tissue Eng Part C Methods,* **17**: 79–87.

33. Guillotin, B., Souquet, A., Catros, S., Duocastella, M., Pippenger, B., Bellance, S., Bareille, R., Rémy, M., Bordenave, L., Amédée, J., et al. (2010). Laser assisted bioprinting of engineered tissue with high cell density and microscale organization. *Biomaterials,* **31**: 7250–7256.

34. Hamada, Y., Nokihara, K., Okazaki, M., Fujitani, W., Matsumoto, T., Matsuo, M., Umakoshi, Y., Takahashi, J., and Matsuura, N. (2003). Angiogenic activity of osteopontin-derived peptide SVVYGLR. *Biochem Biophys Res Commun,* **310**: 153–157.

35. Harris, J. D., Siston, R. A., Pan, X., and Flanigan, D. C. (2010). Autologous chondrocyte implantation: a systematic review. *J Bone Joint Surg Am,* **92**: 2220–2233.

36. Harrison, B. S., Eberli, D., Lee, S. J., Atala, A., and Yoo, J. J. (2007). Oxygen producing biomaterials for tissue regeneration. *Biomaterials,* **28**: 4628–4634.

37. Hersel, U., Dahmen, C., and Kessler, H. (2003). RGD modified polymers: biomaterials for stimulated cell adhesion and beyond. *Biomaterials,* **24**: 4385–4415.

38. Hobo, K., Shimizu, T., Sekine, H., Shińoka, T., Okano, T., and Kurosawa, H. (2008). Therapeutic angiogenesis using tissue engineered human smooth muscle cell sheets. *Arterioscler Thromb Vasc Biol,* **28**: 637–643.

39. Hoganson, D. M., Pryor, H. I., Spool, I. D., Burns, O. H., Gilmore, J. R., and Vacanti, J. P. (2010). Principles of biomimetic vascular network design applied to a tissue-engineered liver scaffold. *Tissue Eng Part A,* **16**: 1469–1477.

40. Hollister, S. J. (2005). Porous scaffold design for tissue engineering. *Nat Mater,* **4**: 518–524.

41. Hu, J., Sun, X., Ma, H., Xie, C., Chen, Y. E., and Ma, P. X. (2010). Porous nanofibrous PLLA scaffolds for vascular tissue engineering. *Biomaterials,* **31**: 7971–7977.

42. Hubbell, J. A., Massia, S. P., Desai, N. P., and Drumheller, P. D. (1991). Endothelial cell-selective materials for tissue engineering in the vascular graft via a new receptor. *Biotechnology (NY),* **9**: 568–572.

43. Hutmacher, D. W., Sittinger, M., and Risbud, M. V. (2004). Scaffold-based tissue engineering: rationale for computer-aided design and solid free-form fabrication systems. *Trends Biotechnol,* **22**: 354–362.
44. Jain, R. K. (2003). Molecular regulation of vessel maturation. *Nat Med,* **9**: 685–693.
45. Janssen, F. W., Oostra, J., Oorschot, A., and van Blitterswijk, C. A. (2006). A perfusion bioreactor system capable of producing clinically relevant volumes of tissue-engineered bone: in vivo bone formation showing proof of concept. *Biomaterials,* **27**: 315–323.
46. Kelm, J. M., Lorber, V., Snedeker, J. G., Schmidt, D., Broggini-Tenzer, A., Weisstanner, M., Odermatt, B., Mol, A., Zünd, G., and Hoerstrup, S. P. (2010). A novel concept for scaffold-free vessel tissue engineering: self-assembly of microtissue building blocks. *J Biotechnol,* **148**: 46–55.
47. Keriquel, V., Guillemot, F., Arnault, I., Guillotin, B., Miraux, S., Amédée, J., Fricain, J.-C., and Catros, S. (2010). In vivo bioprinting for computer- and robotic-assisted medical intervention: preliminary study in mice. *Biofabrication,* **2**: 014101.
48. Khademhosseini, A., Vacanti, J. P., and Langer, R. (2009). Progress in tissue engineering. *Sci Am,* **300**: 64–71.
49. Khan, O. F., Chamberlain, M. D., and Sefton, M. V. (2012). Toward an in vitro vasculature: differentiation of mesenchymal stromal cells within an endothelial cell-seeded modular construct in a microfluidic flow chamber. *Tissue Eng Part A,* **18**: 744–756.
50. Kim, K., Ohashi, K., Utoh, R., Kano, K., and Okano, T. (2012). Preserved liver-specific functions of hepatocytes in 3D co-culture with endothelial cell sheets. *Biomaterials,* **33**: 1406–1413.
51. Landers, R., Hübner, U., Schmelzeisen, R., and Mülhaupt, R. (2002). Rapid prototyping of scaffolds derived from thermoreversible hydrogels and tailored for applications in tissue engineering. *Biomaterials,* **23**: 4437–4447.
52. Lee, S.-H., Moon, J. J., and West, J. L. (2008). Three-dimensional micropatterning of bioactive hydrogels via two-photon laser scanning photolithography for guided 3D cell migration. *Biomaterials,* **29**: 2962–2968.
53. Leong, M. F., Rasheed, M. Z., Lim, T. C., and Chian, K. S. (2009). In vitro cell infiltration and in vivo cell infiltration and vascularization

in a fibrous, highly porous poly(D,L-lactide) scaffold fabricated by cryogenic electrospinning technique. *J Biomed Mater Res A,* **91**: 231–240.

54. Leslie-Barbick, J. E., Shen, C., Chen, C., and West, J. L. (2011). Micron-scale spatially patterned, covalently immobilized vascular endothelial growth factor on hydrogels accelerates endothelial tubulogenesis and increases cellular angiogenic responses. *Tissue Eng Part A,* **17**: 221–229.

55. Li, J., Wei, Y., Liu, K., Yuan, C., Tang, Y., Quan, Q., Chen, P., Wang, W., Hu, H., and Yang, L. (2010). Synergistic effects of FGF-2 and PDGF-BB on angiogenesis and muscle regeneration in rabbit hindlimb ischemia model. *Microvasc Res,* **80**: 10–17.

56. Lin, C. Y., Kikuchi, N., and Hollister, S. J. (2004). A novel method for biomaterial scaffold internal architecture design to match bone elastic properties with desired porosity. *J Biomech,* **37**: 623–636.

57. Liu Tsang, V., Chen, A. A., Cho, L. M., Jadin, K. D., Sah, R. L., DeLong, S., West, J. L., and Bhatia, S. N. (2007). Fabrication of 3D hepatic tissues by additive photopatterning of cellular hydrogels. *FASEB J,* **21**: 790–801.

58. Loffredo, F., and Lee, R. T. (2008). Therapeutic vasculogenesis: it takes two. *Circ Res,* **103**: 128–130.

59. Lovett, M., Lee, K., Edwards, A., and Kaplan, D. L. (2009). Vascularization strategies for tissue engineering. *Tissue Eng Part B Rev,* **15**: 353–370.

60. Lutolf, M. P., Lauer-Fields, J. L., Schmoekel, H. G., Metters, A. T., Weber, F. E., Fields, G. B., and Hubbell, J. A. (2003). Synthetic matrix metalloproteinase-sensitive hydrogels for the conduction of tissue regeneration: engineering cell-invasion characteristics. *Proc Natl Acad Sci USA,* **100**: 5413–5418.

61. Ma, P. X. (2008). Biomimetic materials for tissue engineering. *Adv Drug Deliv Rev,* **60**: 184–198.

62. MacNeil, S. (2007). Progress and opportunities for tissue-engineered skin. *Nature,* **445**: 874–880.

63. Masumoto, H., Matsuo, T., Yamamizu, K., Uosaki, H., Narazaki, G., Katayama, S., Marui, A., Shimizu, T., Ikeda, T., Okano, T., et al. (2012). Pluripotent stem cell-engineered cell sheets reassembled with defined cardiovascular populations ameliorate reduction in infarct heart function through cardiomyocyte-mediated neovascularization. *Stem Cells,* **30**: 1196–1205.

64. McGuigan, A. P., and Sefton, M. V. (2006). Vascularized organoid engineered by modular assembly enables blood perfusion. *Proc Natl Acad Sci USA,* **103**: 11461–11466.
65. Melero-Martin, J. M., De Obaldia, M. E., Kang, S.-Y., Khan, Z. A., Yuan, L., Oettgen, P., and Bischoff, J. (2008). Engineering robust and functional vascular networks in vivo with human adult and cord blood-derived progenitor cells. *Circ Res,* **103**: 194–202.
66. Miller, J. S., Shen, C. J., Legant, W. R., Baranski, J. D., Blakely, B. L., and Chen, C. S. (2010). Bioactive hydrogels made from step-growth derived PEG-peptide macromers. *Biomaterials,* **31**: 3736–3743.
67. Mironov, V., Boland, T., Trusk, T., Forgacs, G., and Markwald, R. R. (2003). Organ printing: computer-aided jet-based 3D tissue engineering. *Trends Biotechnol,* **21**: 157–161.
68. Mironov, V., Visconti, R. P., Kasyanov, V., Forgacs, G., Drake, C. J., and Markwald, R. R. (2009). Organ printing: tissue spheroids as building blocks. *Biomaterials,* **30**: 2164–2174.
69. Miyagi, Y., Chiu, L. L., Cimini, M., Weisel, R. D., Radisic, M., and Li, R. K. (2011). Biodegradable collagen patch with covalently immobilized VEGF for myocardial repair. *Biomaterials,* **32**: 1280–1290.
70. Moon, J. J., Hahn, M. S., Kim, I., Nsiah, B. A., and West, J. L. (2009). Micropatterning of poly(ethylene glycol) diacrylate hydrogels with biomolecules to regulate and guide endothelial morphogenesis. *Tissue Eng Part A,* **15**: 579–585.
71. Moon, J. J., Saik, J. E., Poché, R. A., Leslie-Barbick, J. E., Lee, S.-H., Smith, A. A., Dickinson, M. E., and West, J. L. (2010). Biomimetic hydrogels with pro-angiogenic properties. *Biomaterials,* **31**: 3840–3847.
72. Nillesen, S. T., Geutjes, P. J., Wismans, R., Schalkwijk, J., Daamen, W. F., and van Kuppevelt, T. H. (2007). Increased angiogenesis and blood vessel maturation in acellular collagen-heparin scaffolds containing both FGF2 and VEGF. *Biomaterials,* **28**: 1123–1131.
73. Norotte, C., Marga, F. S., Niklason, L. E., and Forgacs, G. (2009). Scaffold-free vascular tissue engineering using bioprinting. *Biomaterials,* **30**: 5910–5917.
74. Oh, S. H., Ward, C. L., Atala, A., Yoo, J. J., and Harrison, B. S. (2009). Oxygen generating scaffolds for enhancing engineered tissue survival. *Biomaterials,* **30**: 757–762.
75. Ohashi, K., Yokoyama, T., Yamato, M., Kuge, H., Kanehiro, H., Tsutsumi, M., Amanuma, T., Iwata, H., Yang, J., Okano, T., et al. (2007). Engineering

functional two- and three-dimensional liver systems in vivo using hepatic tissue sheets. *Nat Med,* **13**: 880–885.

76. Ott, H. C., Matthiesen, T. S., Goh, S.-K., Black, L. D., Kren, S. M., Netoff, T. I., and Taylor, D. A. (2008). Perfusion-decellularized matrix: using nature's platform to engineer a bioartificial heart. *Nat Med,* **14**: 213–221.

77. Ovsianikov, A., Malinauskas, M., Schlie, S., Chichkov, B., Gittard, S., Narayan, R., Löbler, M., Sternberg, K., Schmitz, K.-P., and Haverich, A. (2011). Three-dimensional laser micro- and nano-structuring of acrylated poly(ethylene glycol) materials and evaluation of their cytoxicity for tissue engineering applications. *Acta Biomater,* **7**: 967–974.

78. Parzel, C. A., Pepper, M. E., Burg, T., Groff, R. E., and Burg, K. J. L. (2009). EDTA enhances high-throughput two-dimensional bioprinting by inhibiting salt scaling and cell aggregation at the nozzle surface. *J Tissue Eng Regen Med,* **3**: 260–268.

79. Peirce, S. M., Price, R. J., and Skalak, T. C. (2004). Spatial and temporal control of angiogenesis and arterialization using focal applications of VEGF164 and Ang-1. *Am J Physiol Heart Circ Physiol,* **286**: H918–H925.

80. Peltola, S. M., Melchels, F. P., Grijpma, D. W., and Kellomaki, M. (2008). A review of rapid prototyping techniques for tissue engineering purposes. *Ann Med,* **40**: 268–280.

81. Petersen, T. H., Calle, E. A., Zhao, L., Lee, E. J., Gui, L., Raredon, M. B., Gavrilov, K., Yi, T., Zhuang, Z. W., Breuer, C., et al. (2010). Tissue-engineered lungs for in vivo implantation. *Science,* **329**: 538–541.

82. Pham, Q. P., Sharma, U., and Mikos, A. G. (2006). Electrospinning of polymeric nanofibers for tissue engineering applications: a review. *Tissue Eng,* **12**: 1197–1211.

83. Phelps, E. A., and Garcia, A. J. (2010). Engineering more than a cell: vascularization strategies in tissue engineering. *Curr Opin Biotechnol,* **21**: 704–709.

84. Phelps, E. A., Landázuri, N., Thulé, P. M., Taylor, W. R., and García, A. J. (2010). Bioartificial matrices for therapeutic vascularization. *Proc Natl Acad Sci USA,* **107**: 3323–3328.

85. Portner, R., Nagel-Heyer, S., Goepfert, C., Adamietz, P., and Meenen, N. M. (2005). Bioreactor design for tissue engineering. *J Biosci Bioeng,* **100**: 235–245.

86. Raeber, G. P., Lutolf, M. P., and Hubbell, J. A. (2005). Molecularly engineered PEG hydrogels: a novel model system for proteolytically mediated cell migration. *Biophys J,* **89**: 1374–1388.
87. Raghavan, S., Nelson, C. M., Baranski, J. D., Lim, E., and Chen, C. S. (2010). Geometrically controlled endothelial tubulogenesis in micropatterned gels. *Tissue Eng Part A,* **16**: 2255–2263.
88. Roth, E. A., Xu, T., Das, M., Gregory, C., Hickman, J. J., and Boland, T. (2004). Inkjet printing for high-throughput cell patterning. *Biomaterials,* **25**: 3707–3715.
89. Rouwkema, J., Rivron, N. C., and van Blitterswijk, C. A. (2008). Vascularization in tissue engineering. *Trends Biotechnol,* **26**: 434–441.
90. Saik, J. E., Gould, D. J., Watkins, E. M., Dickinson, M. E., and West, J. L. (2011). Covalently immobilized platelet-derived growth factor-BB promotes angiogenesis in biomimetic poly(ethylene glycol) hydrogels. *Acta Biomater,* **7**: 133–143.
91. Santos, M. I., Tuzlakoglu, K., Fuchs, S., Gomes, M. E., Peters, K., Unger, R. E., Piskin, E., Reis, R. L., and Kirkpatrick, C. J. (2008). Endothelial cell colonization and angiogenic potential of combined nano- and micro-fibrous scaffolds for bone tissue engineering. *Biomaterials,* **29**: 4306–4313.
92. Saunders, R. E., Gough, J. E., and Derby, B. (2008). Delivery of human fibroblast cells by piezoelectric drop-on-demand inkjet printing. *Biomaterials,* **29**: 193–203.
93. Schiele, N. R., Corr, D. T., Huang, Y., Raof, N. A., Xie, Y., and Chrisey, D. B. (2010). Laser-based direct-write techniques for cell printing. *Biofabrication,* **2**: 032001.
94. Sefcik, L. S., Petrie Aronin, C. E., Wieghaus, K. A., and Botchwey, E. A. (2008). Sustained release of sphingosine 1-phosphate for therapeutic arteriogenesis and bone tissue engineering. *Biomaterials,* **29**: 2869–2877.
95. Sekine, H., Shimizu, T., Hobo, K., Sekiya, S., Yang, J., Yamato, M., Kurosawa, H., Kobayashi, E., and Okano, T. (2008). Endothelial cell coculture within tissue-engineered cardiomyocyte sheets enhances neovascularization and improves cardiac function of ischemic hearts. *Circulation,* **118**: S145–S152.
96. Sekiya, S., Muraoka, M., Sasagawa, T., Shimizu, T., Yamato, M., and Okano, T. (2010). Three-dimensional cell-dense constructs containing endothelial cell-networks are an effective tool for in vivo and in vitro vascular biology research. *Microvasc Res,* **80**: 549–551.

97. Shin, H., Jo, S., and Mikos, A. G. (2003). Biomimetic materials for tissue engineering. *Biomaterials,* **24**: 4353–4364.
98. Shin, Y., Jeon, J. S., Han, S., Jung, G.-S., Shin, S., Lee, S.-H., Sudo, R., Kamm, R. D., and Chung, S. (2011). In vitro 3D collective sprouting angiogenesis under orchestrated ANG-1 and VEGF gradients. *Lab Chip,* **11**: 2175–2181.
99. Sill, T. J., and von Recum, H. A. (2008). Electrospinning: applications in drug delivery and tissue engineering. *Biomaterials,* **29**: 1989–2006.
100. Singh, M., Berkland, C., and Detamore, M. S. (2008). Strategies and applications for incorporating physical and chemical signal gradients in tissue engineering. *Tissue Eng Part B Rev,* **14**: 341–366.
101. Skardal, A., Zhang, J., and Prestwich, G. D. (2010). Bioprinting vessel-like constructs using hyaluronan hydrogels crosslinked with tetrahedral polyethylene glycol tetracrylates. *Biomaterials,* **31**: 6173–6181.
102. Sreejalekshmi, K. G., and Nair, P. D. (2011). Biomimeticity in tissue engineering scaffolds through synthetic peptide modifications-altering chemistry for enhanced biological response. *J Biomed Mater Res A,* **96**: 477–491.
103. Sudo, R., Chung, S., Zervantonakis, I. K., Vickerman, V., Toshimitsu, Y., Griffith, L. G., and Kamm, R. D. (2009). Transport-mediated angiogenesis in 3D epithelial coculture. *FASEB J,* **23**: 2155–2164.
104. Sun, G., Shen, Y.-I., Kusuma, S., Fox-Talbot, K., Steenbergen, C. J., and Gerecht, S. (2011). Functional neovascularization of biodegradable dextran hydrogels with multiple angiogenic growth factors. *Biomaterials,* **32**: 95–106.
105. Sun, W., Darling, A., Starly, B., and Nam, J. (2004). Computer-aided tissue engineering: overview, scope and challenges. *Biotechnol Appl Biochem,* **39**: 29–47.
106. Tayalia, P., and Mooney, D. (2009). Controlled Growth Factor Delivery for Tissue Engineering. *Adv. Mater.,* **21**.
107. Tengood, J.E., Ridenour, R., Brodsky, R., Russell, A.J., and Little, S.R. (2011). Sequential delivery of basic fibroblast growth factor and platelet-derived growth factor for angiogenesis. *Tissue Eng Part A,* **17**: 1181–1189.
108. Vavken, P., and Samartzis, D. (2010). Effectiveness of autologous chondrocyte implantation in cartilage repair of the knee: a systematic review of controlled trials. *Osteoarthritis Cartilage,* **18**: 857–863.
109. Vickerman, V., Blundo, J., Chung, S., and Kamm, R. (2008). Design, fabrication and implementation of a novel multi-parameter control

microfluidic platform for three-dimensional cell culture and real-time imaging. *Lab Chip,* **8**: 1468–1477.

110. von der Mark, K., Park, J., Bauer, S., and Schmuki, P. (2010). Nanoscale engineering of biomimetic surfaces: cues from the extracellular matrix. *Cell Tissue Res,* **339**: 131–153.

111. Wang, Z.Z., Au, P., Chen, T., Shao, Y., Daheron, L.M., Bai, H., Arzigian, M., Fukumura, D., Jain, R.K., and Scadden, D.T. (2007). Endothelial cells derived from human embryonic stem cells form durable blood vessels in vivo. *Nat Biotechnol,* **25**: 317–318.

112. Whitesides, G.M., Ostuni, E., Takayama, S., Jiang, X., and Ingber, D.E. (2001). Soft lithography in biology and biochemistry. *Annu Rev Biomed Eng,* **3**: 335–373.

113. Wieghaus, K.A., Capitosti, S.M., Anderson, C.R., Price, R.J., Blackman, B.R., Brown, M.L., and Botchwey, E.A. (2006). Small molecule inducers of angiogenesis for tissue engineering. *Tissue Eng,* **12**: 1903–1913.

114. Wu, P.K., and Ringeisen, B.R. (2010). Development of human umbilical vein endothelial cell (HUVEC) and human umbilical vein smooth muscle cell (HUVSMC) branch/stem structures on hydrogel layers via biological laser printing (BioLP). *Biofabrication,* **2**: 014111.

115. Xu, T., Jin, J., Gregory, C., Hickman, J.J., and Boland, T. (2005). Inkjet printing of viable mammalian cells. *Biomaterials,* **26**: 93–99.

116. Yang, F., Cho, S., Son, S., Bogatyrev, S., Singh, D., Green, J., Mei, Y., Park, S., Bhang, S., Kim, B., et al. (2009). Regenerative Medicine Special Feature: Genetic engineering of human stem cells for enhanced angiogenesis using biodegradable polymeric nanoparticles. *Proc Natl Acad Sci USA.*

117. Yang, J., Yamato, M., Shimizu, T., Sekine, H., Ohashi, K., Kanzaki, M., Ohki, T., Nishida, K., and Okano, T. (2007). Reconstruction of functional tissues with cell sheet engineering. *Biomaterials,* **28**: 5033–5043.

118. Yang, S., Leong, K.F., Du, Z., and Chua, C.K. (2002). The design of scaffolds for use in tissue engineering. Part II. Rapid prototyping techniques. *Tissue Eng,* **8**: 1–11.

119. Yee, D., Hanjaya-Putra, D., Bose, V., Luong, E., and Gerecht, S. (2011). Hyaluronic Acid hydrogels support cord-like structures from endothelial colony-forming cells. *Tissue Eng Part A,* **17**: 1351–1361.

120. Yeong, W.-Y., Chua, C.-K., Leong, K.-F., and Chandrasekaran, M. (2004). Rapid prototyping in tissue engineering: challenges and potential. *Trends Biotechnol,* **22**: 643–652.

121. Yoon, J.J., Chung, H.J., Lee, H.J., and Park, T.G. (2006). Heparin-immobilized biodegradable scaffolds for local and sustained release of angiogenic growth factor. *J Biomed Mater Res A,* **79**: 934–942.

122. Yoon, J.J., Chung, H.J., and Park, T.G. (2007). Photo-crosslinkable and biodegradable Pluronic/heparin hydrogels for local and sustained delivery of angiogenic growth factor. *J Biomed Mater Res A*, **83**: 597–605.

123. Yuen, W.W., Du, N.R., Chan, C.H., Silva, E.A., and Mooney, D.J. (2010). Mimicking nature by codelivery of stimulant and inhibitor to create temporally stable and spatially restricted angiogenic zones. *Proc Natl Acad Sci USA*, **107**: 17933–17938.

124. Zhao, L., Lee, V.K., Yoo, S.-S., Dai, G., and Intes, X. (2012). The integration of 3-D cell printing and mesoscopic fluorescence molecular tomography of vascular constructs within thick hydrogel scaffolds. *Biomaterials*, **33**: 5325–5332.

125. Zheng, Y., Henderson, P.W., Choi, N.W., Bonassar, L.J., Spector, J.A., and Stroock, A.D. (2011). Microstructured templates for directed growth and vascularization of soft tissue in vivo. *Biomaterials*, **32**: 5391–5401.

Chapter 21

Micro- and Nanofabrication Approaches to Cardiac Tissue Engineering

Nicole Trosper,[a] Petra Kerscher,[b] Jesse Macadangdang,[a] Daniel Carson,[a] Elizabeth Lipke,[b] and Deok-Ho Kim[a,c,d]

[a]*Department of Bioengineering, University of Washington, 3720 15th Ave NE, Seattle, WA 98105, USA*
[b]*Department of Chemical Engineering, Auburn University, 212 Ross Hall, AL 36849, USA*
[c]*Center for Cardiovascular Biology, University of Washington, 850 Republican Street, Brotman Building 453, Seattle, WA 98195, USA*
[d]*Institute for Stem Cell and Regenerative Medicine, University of Washington, 850 Republican Street, Seattle, WA 98109, USA*

deokho@uw.edu, elipke@auburn.edu

In the effort to create cardiac tissue in vitro which closely mimics the structural and functional properties of native myocardium, cardiac tissue engineering needs to re-create the complex environment found in vivo; micro- and nanofabrication approaches are critical tools for accomplishing this objective. The cells of the heart, in vivo, are surrounded by an extracellular matrix that provides topographical cues on the micro- and nanoscale. Experimental studies have shown that topography influences cell organization, morphology, motility, and even proliferation. Understanding and recapitulating these influences is essential for guiding engineered cardiac tissue growth. This chapter reports on the fabrication techniques available for the creation of micro- and nanotopographically defined biomaterials, and examines the application of these biomimetic environments

---

Tissue and Organ Regeneration: Advances in Micro- and Nanotechnology
Edited by Lijie Grace Zhang, Ali Khademhosseini, and Thomas J. Webster
Copyright © 2014 Pan Stanford Publishing Pte. Ltd.
ISBN 978-981-4411-67-7 (Hardcover), 978-981-4411-68-4 (eBook)
www.panstanford.com

to produce organized and aligned cardiac constructs with function mimicking that of native tissue.

21.1 Introduction

The heart is a complex organ. Our efforts to understand and mimic it must span from the macroscale all the way down to the micro- and nanoscale (i.e., from synchronized muscle contraction to the fibers of the extracellular matrix (ECM)). The ECM proteins provide structural cues for heart cells and have major impact on cell and tissue function, acting to coordinate the various mechanical and biochemical factors within the cardiac microenvironment [10,11]. Soluble factors that are bound to the ECM provide molecular cues, which, in conjunction with its topographical cues, allow for the guidance of cellular structure and function. These micro- and nanoscale properties of cardiac tissue are the foundation on which macroscale functionality is built. In this chapter, we focus on the role of ECM as a type of scaffold to which cardiomyocytes, fibroblasts, and vasculature components attach in order to form aligned networks.

Cardiac ECM is made up of fibrillar collagens, basement membrane components, and proteoglycans, all of which are important for correct organ function. Collagens type I and III are the main constituents of fibrillar ECM and allow for the efficient propagation of cardiomyocyte force production and aid in the overall function of the ventricle as a pump [12]. The basement membrane is composed of a number of proteins including laminin, fibronectin, collagen type IV, and fibrillin [13]. These non-collagenous proteins of the basement membrane promote cell adhesion and cell–cell interaction. The role of proteoglycans in cardiac organ function is only beginning to be understood, but they are thought to be important both during cardiac development and in the progression of cardiac disease, such as heart failure [14,15].

Cells in the heart are connected to the ECM through integrins. Integrins bind to intracellular actin filaments through a plethora of linker proteins and aid in mechanically coupling intracellular and extracellular structures. Adjacent cardiomyocytes are connected through integrin-mediated insertion into the basal lamina of the cells [16]. Integrins also play a crucial role in cardiac mechanotransduction during development and in response to physiologic and pathologic signals [16].

Although the detailed physical structure (ECM components, integrins, tissue alignment, etc.) of the heart has been known for some time, in the past it was difficult to isolate these micro- and nanoscale features in vitro for investigation. Due to this, the biochemical influence of the cellular microenvironment dominated research efforts and the physical influence of this microenvironment was not widely investigated. Due to recent advances in micro- and nanofabrication techniques, scientists have been able to recapitulate and analyze the effect of the ECM's physical stimuli with a high degree of control.

The knowledge that the ECM provides direct structural guidance for overlying cardiomyocytes has led to the incorporation of anisotropically defined substrates for in vitro development of tissue constructs. It has provided the motivation to vary dimensions, shape, and mechanical stiffness of the underlying substrate to positively affect cultured heart tissue [17–22]. Within the heart, fibers have been shown to have feature sizes on the micron and nanometer scale in width while extending for much longer distances in length with a high level of fidelity. Thus, fabrication techniques intending to imitate the native ECM components must be robust and reproducible over a fairly large area. Micro- and nanotopographically defined substrates have produced tissue constructs demonstrating features and functional properties more similar to those of the in vivo cells and tissues [23–30]. This may provide a more physiologically relevant and cost-effective means of altering cell morphology, proliferation, and differentiation over traditional biochemical and chemical factors.

21.2 Multiscale Features of Cardiac Tissue Environments

The complex structure of the heart is organized on multiple scales and is present to help direct the collective movement of action potentials through this tissue, providing strong synchronous contractions. The alignment of tissue can be seen on all levels, from the three-dimensional ultra-structure down to the micron-scale sarcomeres (Fig. 21.1). The multilevel tissue organization of the heart is essential to proper function. The death of normal tissue following myocardial infarction leads to infiltration of fibrous scar tissue. Scar tissue not only lacks the contractile and electrical properties of native heart tissue, but the randomly oriented fibrous mesh also disrupts the high degree of alignment within the myocardium. Scar tissue patches cannot effectively participate in directional and synchronous contractions, giving rise to inhibited cardiac function. It is evident that the coupling of multiple scale organization directly influences the global function of the aligned, laminar tissue of the heart. Much work has been done to clearly characterize the anisotropic structure of the myocardium, and this understanding is vital to the efforts of cardiac tissue engineering.

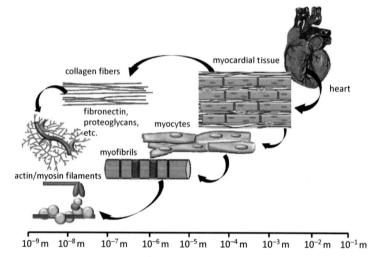

Figure 21.1 Schematic of various multiscale structures in the heart. The relative sizes need to be addressed in cardiac tissue engineering scale several orders of magnitude, from the 3D macro-scale structure to the sub-micron-sized actin-myosin motors and collagen fibers.

Investigation by Kim, Lipke et al. of the ultra-structure of the heart suggested that nanoscale ECM topography is present and that this topography is responsible for the structural orientation of native tissue [17]. By employing an ex vivo assessment of rat myocardium, their research revealed that the cellular alignment was strongly correlated with the alignment of the matrix fibers found directly underneath them (Fig. 21.2a). This result suggests that the nanoscale orientation and pattern of the underlying matrix could direct the alignment of cardiomyocytes and provide a means to attain anisotropic two-dimensional tissue. Cardiac tissue engineering aims to exploit this structural relationship for the purpose of improving in vitro mimicry.

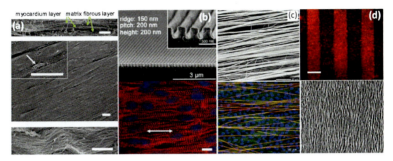

Figure 21.2 Many substrate fabrication approaches aim to mimic the structure of the native ECM, an image of which is shown in (a) revealing the fibrous matrix of the adult rat myocardium. (b) Capillary force lithography was used to create a ridge/groove array for stimulating cell alignment [58]. Cellular alignment is also shown with (c) electrospun fibers [8] and (d) micropatterned brush polymer [59].

21.3 Current Challenges in Cardiac Tissue Engineering

The primary goal of cardiac regeneration and tissue engineering is to repair damaged or diseased heart tissue. Success in accomplishing this goal can be evaluated by improved heart function, particularly by quantifying the ability of the heart to pump blood, which is measured by cardiac output. The major challenges facing cardiac tissue engineering today include (1) cardiomyocyte maturation, (2) electromechanical integration, (3) vascularization of the engineered and host tissues, and (4) cell delivery and survival. To this end, the use of micro- and nanofabricated biomaterials in cardiac tissue engineering has the potential to address and eventually overcome many of these obstacles.

In vitro responses, specifically those occurring from structural influences, have been widely characterized in literature for a number of cell types [31–34]. Cell morphology represents one of the most direct and easily identifiable characteristic responses of cells to structural guidance cues. It has been shown that cells are able to sense an underlying substrate by infiltrating grooves along the surface. The presence of anisotropic topographical cues promotes cell elongation, alignment, and increased cell area when compared to the responses observed from flat substrates. Either indirectly by dictating cell morphology or directly by other mechanisms, structural guidance cues are known to influence cellular function including migration, proliferation, and differentiation. Cell migration is influenced by different surface patterns and mechanical stiffness [35–37]. Although the proliferative capacity of mature cardiomyocytes is insignificant, it has been shown in some cases that the proliferative capacity of immature cell populations can be influenced by topography, as shown with the Notch1 signaling [38]. Studies examining the influence of topographical cues on cardiac differentiation are still limited [39,40], but as capabilities improve for the expansion and differentiation of human induced pluripotent stem cells stem cells (hiPSCs) into stem cell-derived cardiomyocytes (SC-CMs), substrate characteristics will likely play an increasing role in directing human stem cells to form functional engineered cardiac tissues.

Gene regulation is an important indicator of cellular function and can be used as one metric in quantifying cell maturation. Understanding the modulation of gene expression by tissue-engineered constructs, including the influence of structural guidance cues, is important in creating more accurate mimics of native cardiac tissue. Therefore, assessing gene expression of in vitro cardiac tissue constructs is an area of intensive research. Both structural and functional genes provide valuable information; specifically, the alpha-myosin heavy chain (a-MHC) to beta-myosin heavy chain (b-MHC) ratio and the slow-skeletal troponin I (ssTnI) to fast-skeletal troponin I (fsTnI) ratio are two key indicators of maturity [41–44]. Although the mature isoform of MHC varies between species, the ratio between the immature and mature isoform indicates the relative maturity of the construct. Other genes that are often observed in cardiac tissue constructs are atrial natriuretic peptide (ANP) and brain natriuretic peptide (BNP). Debate remains over these genes as to whether they are indicators of maturity or they are indicators of pathological hypertrophy [45,46]. Functional gene expression is also important including expression of genes for gap junctions, such as connexin 43, and ion channels, such as L-type Ca^{2+} channels, T-type Ca^{2+} channels, and HCN pacemaker channels, among others. While substantial fluctuations in gene expression can be seen in response to culture conditions, it is important to remember that the specific regulation observed is not necessarily the final indication of protein function. The presence of vast post-translation modifications may inhibit or further advance the function of resulting proteins. In addition, the localization of protein complexes impacts protein and tissue function. This makes cardiomyocyte maturation an intricate issue both as a matter of finding reliable means for quantification as well as understanding the numerous contributing factors.

Assessing the electrophysiological properties of in vitro cardiac tissues can give important information about tissue function. To use engineered cardiac tissue for in vitro drug screening, it is critical that these tissues can recapitulate the functional properties of the native heart. Electromechanical coupling of engineered cardiac tissue is equally important for clinical applications; inappropriate electromechanical properties could lead to the initiation of deadly cardiac arrhythmias. Characterization of action potential upstroke velocities, maximum diastolic potential, and specific ion channel functionality on the single cell level gives information about cardiomyocyte function, which is particularly important when cardiomyocytes are derived from pluripotent stem cells such as hiPSCs. To observe cellular interconnectivity, however, multicellular imaging is necessary. Optical mapping can be used to characterize action potential propagation through engineered cardiac tissues. Assessment of conduction velocity, action potential duration, maximum capture rate, conduction velocity heterogeneity, and anisotropic ratio provide a basis for comparison both between tissue-engineered constructs and native tissue. Structural guidance cues can influence these properties through modulation of functional protein expression and through directing cell and tissue alignment [17].

Just as biomimetic micro- and nanofabrication can be key to influencing myocytes within a cardiac construct, it can be equally critical in stimulating the population of endothelial cells responsible for developing vasculature [47]. Some engineered tissues such as skin and cartilage have been privileged with a much more rapid rise to human clinical applications due to the fact that they do not require extensive internal vasculature. Most tissues, however, will not be able to circumvent the need of a steady blood supply; this is especially true for functionally active tissues such as the heart. The diffusion limit for adequate delivery of oxygen and nutrients is a few hundred microns, meaning that tissue constructs that are too thick or have high metabolic demands will be prone to necrosis and cell death. This pressing need has led to a number of new engineering approaches within recent years aimed at facilitating rapid vasculogenesis.

Efforts have been made to stimulate growth of host vasculature into the implanted construct. Signaling from growth factors may facilitate this, but the process is quite slow and subjects the implanted tissue to a period of time without blood supply. Polysurgery is one means of overcoming this, but may be clinically undesirable in the context of the heart [48]. Ideally, engineered vasculature would align in parallel with the myocytes as seen naturally in the heart. This alignment helps optimize delivery of oxygen and other nutrients to the cells. For this reason, a pre-fabricated vasculature system that offers some degree of spatial control is desirable, with the understanding that angiogenic promotion will later be required to stimulate the connection between host and engineered vasculature.

The micropatterning of adhesion proteins onto a flat culture surface has been known to successfully influence endothelial cell organization and, under certain geometric configurations, can enhance the expression of von Willebrand factor in endothelial progenitor cells (EPCs) [49]. Gerecht et al. have demonstrated that EPCs, following 5 days of culture on a flat substrate with 50 µm wide fibronectin patterns, could be inverted onto a fibrin gel; three-dimensional tubular structures formed in this newly supportive microenvironment within only one day. [49]. Alternative approaches have suggested that interconnected, spherical pores 30–40 µm in diameter are capable of stimulating rapid vascularization [50].

Direct cell injection has long been pursued as a therapeutic approach for cardiac regeneration; however, its efficacy is often undermined by a low viability of the cells themselves. The post-infarct myocardium is a harsh environment with increased hypoxia and inflammation. This makes the transition from culture conditions to the site of injection a difficult for cell survival and results in poor cell retention and survival. Anoikis, programmed cell death due to a lack of attachment in anchorage-dependent cells, is thought to be the greatest perpetrator for initial clearance following injection. Engineered tissue constructs with topography enhanced cell–cell and cell–ECM contacts will provide a more substantial support system for the engrafted cell population and achieve higher degrees of cell survival [51].

In summary, micro- and nanofabrication techniques play an important role in overcoming the challenges facing cardiac tissue engineering. Structural guidance cues can influence cellular morphology as well as whole-tissue function, playing an important role in vascularization efforts, electromechanical maturation and integration, and cell survival upon engraftment.

21.4 Micro- and Nanofabrication Techniques

There are several different methods for fabricating nanotopographically defined substrates and each of these techniques produces different types of physical stimulation and presides over a limited range of feature resolution. For the purpose of this text, we can divide these methods into four categories: electron beam lithography, template molding, surface printing of ECM proteins, and methods for producing nanofibers. Here, we describe examples of these commonly used techniques, including their advantages and constraints [52–54].

21.4.1 Electron Beam Lithography

Electron beam lithography is a process by which a substrate is covered with an electron sensitive resist film and then selectively exposed to electron beam radiation. A positive resist becomes more soluble upon exposure as bonds are broken while a negative resist becomes less soluble due to cross-linking [55,56]. Therefore, the type of photoresist along with electron beam exposure pattern must be considered in order to yield the desired topography; this places some limitations on material choice. The pattern and duration of exposure is computer programmed, allowing for a high degree of control and reproducibility. Feature resolution down to a few nanometers has been achieved [57]. The effective beam broadening within the photoresist limits feature resolution while pitch resolution is determined by secondary electron travel within the photoresist. A key limitation of electron beam lithography is that the process has a very low throughput and high cost due to the fact that only the area of the electron beam is under exposure at any given time. Thus, master templates are often fabricated via electron beam and then replicated using other nanofabrication techniques such as hot embossing or capillary force lithography.

21.4.2 Template Molding

Hot embossing, also referred to as nano-imprint lithography, is a method of patterning where a rigid mold is pressed into a thermoplastic polymer that is heated above its glass transition temperature. By maintaining high temperature and pressure, material is transported into feature recesses in the mold and allowed to cool. The negative replicate of the master mold is then separated [60]. The temperature, pressure, and time at which they are maintained are important parameters for achieving ideal replication and should be selected with respect to the polymer being molded and the feature size. This is a relatively quick fabrication method that can be applied to large pattern areas. However, best pattern replication results are achieved with small, periodic feature sizes, and with positive molds as opposed to molds with recessed features. One drawback of this method is that it requires relatively high temperatures and pressures to transfer the nanopattern. This can cause deformation of the mold or result in the transfer of an inaccurate pattern. Another disadvantage of this method is that it requires a pre-existing mold with the nanotopography complementary to the desired pattern. However, this method is much quicker and does not require specialized equipment compared to electron beam lithography.

Capillary force lithography is a replication method quite similar to nano-imprint lithography, but it employs a softer master mold, typically made of polydimethylsiloxane (PDMS) or polyurethane acrylate (PUA). It also does not require high pressure conditions. A softer mold will make conformal contact with the substrate polymer and the pattern's recesses filled via capillary action [61]. The substrate polymer can be either thermoplastic or UV curable. UV curable polymers offer the most rapid means of replication (Figs. 21.2b and 21.3a). In addition, the entrapment of oxygen at the top of mold features results in incomplete curing in the upper regions of the replicate and can be utilized to create hierarchical structures. This technique has been demonstrated by Kwak et al. to fabricate monolithic bridge structures [62].

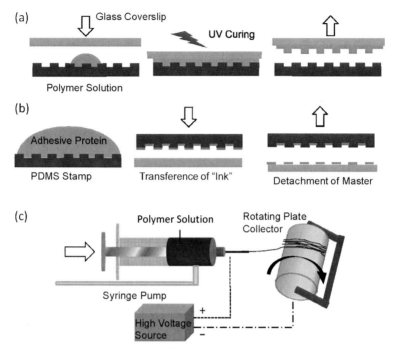

Figure 21.3 Schematics of fabrication techniques. (a) UV-assisted capillary force lithography, (b) microcontact printing, and (c) electrospinning.

21.4.3 Microcontact Printing

An alternative approach to controlling cellular organization at the microscale is to selectively deposit biologically relevant molecules which influence cell attachment. It should be noted that while this approach may achieve successful cell positioning and alignment, it does not contribute to topographical stimulation that has been found to profoundly influence cell morphology and function. Micro contact printing (µCP) is a method of direct stamping that typically employs a PDMS stamp that is "inked" with a thiol-terminated organic solution (Fig. 21.3b). Upon transfer to the substrate surface, the carbon chains of the thiol groups align to form a self-assembled monolayer within the restricted print region [63]. In addition to its simplicity and low cost, µCP is a fairly robust process that allows for relatively easy experimental manipulation. The feature resolution for µCP is limited by both the PDMS master (see hot-embossing) and the mobility of the biomolecule ink. In application, the selective deposition of adhesive proteins, such as lanes of fibronectin, can be used to direct cell attachment and achieve aligned and elongated cell morphology [1,64,65]. When a proliferating cell source is used, daughter cells will fill the protein- or biomolecule-free space between lanes to form an aligned, confluent monolayer. However, for non- or less proliferative lines (such as terminally differentiated cardiomyocytes), this may be a less viable method for creating aligned tissues.

Dip pen nanolithography is a deposition method similar to μCP wherein an atomic force microscope (AFM) tip is used in a positive printing fashion to write out patterns. Dip pen uses capillary transport to deliver the alkane thiolate ink via a water meniscus [66–68]. This method is far more time consuming and costly but can achieve nanometer scale line width resolution and can be directed by computer programming.

21.4.4 Electrospun Nanofibers

Polymeric nanofibers offer the distinct advantage of being most similar in geometry to the collagen fibers of the native ECM and are commonly produced via electrospinning, self-assembly of peptide-amphiphiles, or phase separation.

Electrospinning is the process of using electrostatic force to create nanoscale polymeric fibers (Fig. 21.3c). A viscous polymer solution is released from a syringe having a positively charged needle and attracted to a negatively charged collector some distance away [69]. The formation of a Taylor cone is seen and it is the inverted jet of solution that is transferred as fibrous deposition. The concentration of the polymer solution, the speed and relative direction of the emitter and collector, as well as the magnitude of the potential difference between the two all influence the fiber characteristics and allow for a high degree of manipulation. Unfortunately, control of fiber diameter is not exact and fiber density over the substrate area is not uniform. Electrospun fibers can be aligned in parallel by applying a magnetic or electric field across the collector, anisotropically stretching the scaffold after it has been fabricated, or by using a rotating plate as the collection surface.

Electrospinning is a relatively inexpensive method of making nanotopographically defined substrates [18,70–75]. Its use allows for a high degree of flexibility in material choice and results in a scaffold with high porosity when compared with the previously mentioned methods. This has significance for cell culture as it allows cells to receive both mechanical and chemical cues three-dimensionally.

Self-assembly techniques rely on the spontaneous aggregation of amphiphiles comprised of a peptide sequence at one end opposed by a relatively hydrophobic alkyl segment at the other end [76]. These peptide amphiphiles (PAs) self-assemble into cylindrical nanofibers, which can extend up to a few microns long, and are additionally capable of forming β-sheets at the collapse of the alkyl tail in the presence of a sequence of lysine and alanine peptide residues. Hydrogen bonding between the amino acid residues of adjacent PA molecules allows for the formation of fibrous strands, which entangle and create self-supporting networks, providing a scaffolding material for cell delivery [77,78].

One specific advantage of these SA-PAs is that they allow for the incorporation of epitopes, short polypeptide sequences, which can be used to influence cell-matrix interactions. For example, Supp et al., a leader in this particular field, displayed the fibronectin-derived EGDS epitope to promote cell adhesion within the scaffold [77]. SA-PAs have also been used to enhance endothelial cell growth through incorporation of YIGSR for endothelial cell adhesion, nitric oxide donating residues, and enzyme-degradable sites [79].

The methods reviewed here provide a sampling of the prominent approaches to fabricating biomimetic culture environments with micro- and nanoscale control. Table 21.1 provides a few key examples of fabricated substrates and the corresponding cellular response.

21.5 Applications of Micro- and Nanofabrication in Cardiac Tissue Engineering

Micro- and nanofabrication are being applied in cardiac tissue engineering and cardiac regeneration. Cell sheet engineering, nanoparticles for cardiac imaging and drug delivery, and cell-laden scaffolds all take advantage of these techniques.

Table 21.1 Fabricated substrates and the corresponding cellular response

	Material	Feature dimensions	Cell type	Relevant findings	Ref.
Capillary force lithography	Poly(ethylene glycol)-dimethacrylate (PEG-DMA)	Pillars 150 nm width, 250–300 nm height, 500 nm spacing; achieved robust patterning w/minimal defects	P19 EC cells, NRV fibroblasts	Nanofeatures increase hydrophobicity of surface; preferential cell adhesion to nanopatterned vs. unpatterned surfaces; attributed to increased protein adsorption	[2]
	Poly(ethylene glycol) (PEG)	Conical pillars, width tapering from 150 to 50 nm, 400 nm height, 500 nm spacing	Primary rat CMs	Nanopatterns stimulated self-assembled aggregates with globular morphology, spontaneous beating	[5]
	L-lactide/trimethylene carbonate copolymer (PLLA-TMC) films	10, 25, 50 µm width line patterns	C2C12	Fibronectin printing; alignment observed 24 h after seeding; 7D post confluence cells were fused, multinucleated, and exp. alpha-actinin	[1]
Microcontact printing	Poly(dimethyl siloxane) (PDMS) stamp onto poly (ethylene terephthalate) (PET)	5 µm spatial resolution, high reproducibility	None	Using the high-affinity streptavidin–biotin interaction, biological ligands were selectively patterned (MAPS)	[4]

Method	Material	Dimensions	Cell type	Results	Ref
	PDMS stamp onto polyacrylamide hydrogel surface	100 μm × 1 mm line patterns	NRVMs, C2C12, and primary myoblast satellite cells	Laminin printing achieved highly selective adhesion for both CMs and myoblasts; CMs formed aligned myofibers w/ synchronous contractions at 2D; myoblasts fuse, form aligned myotubes at 7D	[7]
	Non-cell adhesive chitosan surface	100 μm line patterns	Flk1+ angiogenic progenitors derived from mouse ESCs	VEGF linked to collagen surfaces; progenitors immobilized with VEGF yielded endothelial cells (53% CD31+, 17% SM actinin+); Col IV control favored vascular smooth muscle diff. (26% CD31+, 38% SM actinin+)	[9]
Electrospinning	Poly(L-lactide-c-ε-caprolactone)	Nanofibers 400–800 nm XS diameter	hSMCs and VEs	Successful cell attachment and proliferation	[3]
	Polymethylgluterarimide (PMGI)	Fibers 450 nm to 1.1 μm in XS diameter	NRVMs	CMs aligned along fiber orientation to form contractile tissue; higher nanofibre densities achieved better α-actinin alignment; anisotropy conduction velocity ratios of 1.8–2.4	[8]
	Copolymerization of 4% PEG—86% PCL—10% CPCL	0.5 μm XS diameter	Murine ECSs	Differentiation to CMs (viability, intracellular ROS, α-MHC, Ca^{2+} handling); reduced substrate elastic modulus led to inc. CM maturation	[9]

21.5.1 Cell Sheet Engineering

This chapter has focused strongly on fabrication methods for the incorporation of topography onto essentially flat substrates. This is motivated by the advantage that these platforms offer fine tuned control over the feature size, shape, and arrangement presented at the cell interface. Most of the known interplay between a cell and the topography of its surroundings has been elucidated using these controlled monolayer platforms. It is with recent advances in an application dubbed "cell sheet engineering" that these finely tuned monolayers can be use to create thick, implantable tissues of clinical relevance. Using a temperature responsive polymer, poly(N-isopropylacrylamide) (NIPAAm), to harvest intact cell sheets, the wealth of knowledge accumulated at the monolayer level and is being adapted for the use in advanced cell therapy [80].

NIPAAm grafted culture dishes present a slightly hydrophobic surface at 37°C to which adhesion proteins readily adsorb and cells will adhere. Once these cells have formed a confluent monolayer, the dish is cooled to below the polymer lower critical solution temperature (LCST), typically around 32°C, and the polymer undergoes a hydrophilic transition due to rapid hydration and swelling of the polymer chains [81]. Since no enzymatic degradation, such as the use of trypsin, is required for this cell detachment, cell–cell contacts are preserved and the deposited ECM remains intact and is released along with the cell sheet. Okano et al. employed NIPAAm culture surfaces to harvest intact cell sheets and developed a method for transferring and stacking these sheets using a gelatin-coated plunger. When cell sheets were combined in this manner they observed spontaneous electrical coupling between the layers (Fig. 21.4a) and in vivo survival of the grafts [80,82]. NIPAAm can be affixed to a growth surface via chemical grafting [83], electron beam irradiation [84], or initiated chemical vapor deposition [85]. Depending on the grafting method, the NIPAAm chain length and density can be adjusted to control the amount of protein adsorption and the release kinetics.

Microcontact printing of fibronectin onto these unique culture surfaces has allowed for 3D control of anisotropy as demonstrated by the alignment of human dermal fibroblasts [64]. Additionally, hot-embossing of polystyrene to produce micropatterned features of alternating grooves and ridges (50 μm wide, 5 μm deep) was shown to successfully align vascular smooth muscle cells on NIPAAm surfaces [86].

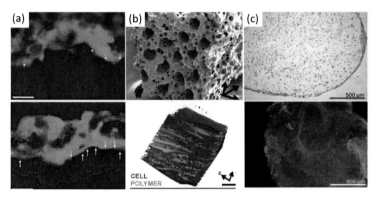

Figure 21.4 Engineered heart tissues have been formed using multiple materials and cell sources. Some examples of the systems used to create engineered heart tissues in vitro include: (a) layered cell sheets that support electrical propagation, (b) multidimensional poly(2-hydroxyethyl methacrylate-co-methacrylic acid) (pHEMA-co-MAA) scaffolds, which promote angiogenesis [91], and (c) PEGylated fibrinogen hydrogels [87].

Cell-seeded biomaterial–based approaches to tissue engineering face many limitations such as insufficient cell penetration into the construct and obstructed cell–cell contacts. Most importantly, the biodegradation of scaffolding materials following implantation commonly causes an inflammatory response, which can hinder the effectiveness of the therapy. Cell sheet engineering is rapidly rising as an advantageous approach that circumvents these issues by ultimately creating a scaffold-free thick tissue construct, which allows for a high degree of hierarchal control.

21.5.2 Cell-Laden Scaffolds

Even though the primary focus of this chapter is not on hydrogel scaffold approaches, it is important to note their presence in the field. Commonly referred to as the "cells in gels" approach, one such example may be seen in Fig. 21.4c wherein cardiomyocytes are imbedded within a photopolymerizable PEGylated fibrinogen (PF) hydrogel [87]. The benefits of implantable biomaterial scaffolds over cell sheet engineering include greater control over the mechanical properties of the construct as a whole and a more defined progression toward commercial implementation. The following research has been selected in part to highlight the diversity of the efforts to create organized and functionally relevant cardiac tissues and in part to discuss successful examples of mechanical and electrical preconditioning.

Zimmermann/Eschenhagen et al. have provided pioneering research in the field of cardiac regenerative medicine [88,89]. The group was able to establish a novel method for development of neonatal cardiac cells in three-dimensional collagen scaffolds. This technique was profound in the sense that the constructs demonstrated coordinated contractions and provided a means of measuring isometric force at the tissue level. Their original work was built upon to refine the casting mechanism for the circular engineered heart tissues while also improving the function of the resulting constructs [90]. It was shown that providing a phasic mechanical stimulus to cellularized constructs with a mixture of neonatal rat cardiomyocytes, collagen type I and matrix factors, showed extremely promising characteristics of mature myocardium including clear alignment of sarcomeres, gap junction formation, and basement membrane formation surrounding cardiac cells. Furthermore, the contractile properties achieved from their tissue constructs were highly representative of the native cardiac response. This indicates that preconditioning cell constructs with mechanical stress may be a critical means of attaining relevant cardiomyocyte force generation.

Madden et al. created a poly(2-hydroxyethyl methacrylate-co-methacrylic acid) (pHEMA-co-MAA) hydrogel scaffold using both polymer fiber and microsphere templating (Fig. 21.4b). The resulting construct contained parallel channels interconnected by smaller spherical pores, thereby successfully stimulating both cardiomyocyte development and angiogenesis [91]. This ingenuity uses microfabrication to not only provide topographical stimulation, but also to enforce organization within the tissue and to increase mass transport. Going forward, we will likely see increased efforts to take advantage of differences in topographical niches of cell populations to passively drive organization within engineered tissues.

Bursac et al. provide yet another important study into three-dimensional aligned scaffolds, which represents the next steps in cardiac tissue engineering. Three-dimensional anisotropic polymer (poly(lactic-co-glycolic acid)) (PLGA) scaffolds were made through leaching of aligned sucrose templates. Neonatal ventricular myocytes (NRVMs) were seeded and cultured in a rotating bioreactor for 6–14 days. The result was a successful attempt at creating a relatively large three-dimensional cardiac tissue construct. After two weeks of culture, the cells aligned and formed multiple bundles and showed anisotropic electrophysiological properties that closely mimicked the in vivo anisotropic ratio. The importance of this study is the transition from single monolayer constructs to three-dimensional tissue patches. The added dimensionality of in vitro constructs yields a more native-like tissue construct.

Radisic et al. investigated the effects of native-like electrical stimulation on the production of functional myocardium in vitro [92]. The goal of this study was to mimic the physiological electrical environment of the native heart during culturing of cardiomyocytes on scaffolds. The cell constructs were placed into a glass chamber containing 2.25 inch diameter carbon rods. Silicon spacers were used to separate wells. The chamber received electrical stimulation by a cardiac stimulator connected to platinum wires that were then connected to the carbon rods within the chamber. A constant pulsatile electrical stimulation was applied for 5 days to mimic physiological ranges of electrical activity (square wave, 2 ms, 5 V/cm, 1 Hz). Simultaneous culture of a cell construct without electric stimulation was also performed for comparison. The results of this study indicated that the presence of electrical stimulation resulted in a dramatic increase in the contractile properties of the cell constructs. The study displayed that the strength of contraction was seven times higher for the cell construct that had received electrical stimulation than non-stimulated tissue constructs, after 8 days of culture. The presence of electrical stimulation also resulted in increased levels of myosin heavy chain, connexin-43, creatine kinase-MM, cardiac troponin I, and other factors of cardiac maturation [93–95]. Another notable improvement of the myocardium subjected to electrical stimulation was the guided orientation and coupling of cells. The cells had increased alignment, elongation, and central positioning of nuclei. Electrical stimulation can also influence cardiac differentiation of pluripotent stem cells [96]. These findings suggest that electrical stimulation can be used to improve cardiomyocyte function. While the results from these groups as well as others provide a promising foundation for the field, it is important to remember that the ultimate goal of regenerating damaged or diseased tissue in the human heart remains elusive.

21.5.3 Nanoparticles

Beyond tissue engineering, cardiac regeneration can benefit from the use of nanoparticles to provide targeted drug delivery and to improve cardiac imaging. Targeted nanoparticles have been tested primarily for the use in delivering drugs to tumor specific sites for cancer therapy. However, this same approach of using nanoparticles as drug delivery devices has potential in cardiac regeneration as well. After myocardial infarction (MI), the left ventricle (LV) becomes leaky and allows increased penetration of targeted nanoparticles to the damaged tissue resulting in passive accumulation [97]. Additionally, active targeting is also possible. For example, the receptor for angiotensin (AT1) is overexpressed at sites of myocardial injury. It has been shown that the AT1 receptor can be targeted using a specific peptide sequence, which is comprised of four glycine residues that serve as a spacer and eight amino acids that mimic the angiotensin II sequence. To deliver a therapeutic drug to the site of cardiac tissue damage, this peptide sequence was attached to a PEGylated liposome to create a nanoparticle complex that was capable of carrying and releasing the therapeutic in a controlled manner at the infarct site following intravenous injection [98]. In vivo studies have shown that this nanoparticle complex binds to AT1 receptors over a 24 h circulation window and aids in regeneration of the infarcted heart [98]. Additional approaches for targeting nanoparticles to aid in cardiac regeneration have included coating with *N*-acetylglucosamine to increase uptake by cardiomyocytes [99], and using lipid nanoparticles that localize macrophages to deliver siRNA to reduce immune response and inflammation post-MI [100].

In addition to PEGylated liposomes, other nanoparticles have been tested for cardiac drug delivery including F-127/Capryol

90 hydrogel micelles [101] and chitosan-alginate nanoparticles [102]. The unique ability of F-127 when combined with Capryol 90 to form a micelle/hydrogel complex at 37°C enables extended release from this system. To form the F-127/Capryol 90 hydrogel, the engineered nanoparticle delivery system is injected into the epicardium next to the infarcted area. This system has been used to deliver vascular endothelial growth factor (VEGF). Upon injection the F-127/Capryol 90 hydrogel micelles formed a shell around a VEGF core, and the VEGF was released over a 42 day time period, resulting in improvement in overall heart function [101]. The chitosan-alginate nanoparticle system is biodegradable and biocompatible with low potential for toxicity, enables a slow release, and protects encapsulated protein from local enzymatic degradation [102]. Chitosan-alginate nanoparticles have been used to deliver placental growth factor (PIGF) via intramyocardial injections. PIGF has a positive effect on angiogenesis and cardiac function and, when delivered using the chitosan-alginate nanoparticles, decreased scar formation in the heart. One advantage of using PIGF over VEGF is the lack of undesired side effects such as edema, hypotension, and the formation of hemangiomas.

In summary, nanoparticles have high potential as drug delivery devices for cardiac regeneration. A number of materials can be chosen to obtain the desired release profile and targeting. Implementing a delivery system where the nanoparticles are targeted to a specific receptor which becomes overexpressed after MI further enhances the effectiveness of nanoparticle drug delivery. Targeted delivery will improve and ease the injection procedure and minimize non-specific binding.

In addition to being used for drug delivery, nanoparticles can also be used to improve cardiac imaging and the sensitivity of assays used to detect myocardial damage. The two most common nanoparticle types for imaging are iron oxide and manganese oxide nanoparticles. Superparamagnetic iron oxide (SPIO) nanoparticles are used as "negative contrast" agents due to the increase in R2 (45–84 1/s cellular relaxivities) to label cells for magnetic resonance imaging (MRI) [103,104]. In contrast, the use of manganese oxide (MnO) nanoparticles for cell labeling provides a "positive contrast" due to the increase in R1 (2.5–4.8 1/s cellular relaxivities). The use of nanoparticles can aid to visualize the myocardial infarct zone in a more accurate fashion than without the use of nanoparticles.

Nanoparticles can also be used to improve the sensitivity of assays used to detect proteins present when a person is having a MI [105], thereby facilitating earlier treatment, which is correlated with better outcomes.

Although the use of nanoparticles for drug delivery, imaging, and protein detection is, strictly speaking, not tissue engineering, it is important to recognize the scope to which nanoscale engineering efforts play a key role in advancing cardiac medicine.

21.6 Conclusion

The end goal of cardiac tissue engineering is not just to produce a complex of cells that can function well in a dish, but ultimately one that can survive successful engraftment into the host myocardium and achieve electrical, mechanical, and vascular integration. Going forward, we can see that the development of a multidimensional construct to improve heart function will require a greater understanding of the cardiac cellular micro- and nano-environment as well as greater collaboration between the fields of materials sciences and engineering and that of cell biology. This increased knowledge and appreciation of the importance of native micro- and nano-environment is motivating and informing the design and fabrication of advanced engineering platforms for cellular growth and implantable tissue therapies.

Acknowledgments

We gratefully acknowledge the support of the American Heart Association (AHA) Scientific Development Grant (AHA 13SDG 14560076) and the Wallace H. Coulter Foundation Translational Research Partnership Award for the work in this chapter.

References

1. Altomare, L., R. M., Gadegaard, N., Tanzi, M., and Fare, S., Microcontact printing of fibronectin on a biodegradable polymeric surface fo skeletal muscle cell orientation. *Intl J Artif Organs*, 2010. **33**(8): 535–543.

2. Kim, P., et al., Fabrication of nanostructures of polyethylene glycol for applications to protein adsorption and cell adhesion. *Nanotechnology*, 2005. **16**(10): 2420.
3. Chen, V. J., and P. X. Ma, Nano-fibrous poly(L-lactic acid) scaffolds with interconnected spherical macropores. *Biomaterials*, 2004. **25**(11): 2065–2073.
4. Yang, Z., et al., Molecular imaging of a micropatterned biological ligand on an activated polymer surface. *Langmuir*, 2000. **16**(19): 7482–7492.
5. Kim, D.-H., et al., Guided three-dimensional growth of functional cardiomyocytes on polyethylene glycol nanostructures. *Langmuir*, 2006. **22**(12): 5419–5426.
6. Anokye-Danso, F., et al., Highly efficient miRNA-mediated reprogramming of mouse and human somatic cells to pluripotency. *Cell Stem Cell*, 2011. **8**(4): 376–388.
7. Cimetta, E., et al., Production of arrays of cardiac and skeletal muscle myofibers by micropatterning techniques on a soft substrate. *Biomed Microdevices*, 2009. **11**(2): 389–400.
8. Orlova, Y., et al., Electrospun nanofibers as a tool for architecture control in engineered cardiac tissue. *Biomaterials*, 2011. **32**(24): 5615–5624.
9. Chiang, C. K., et al., Engineering surfaces for site-specific vascular differentiation of mouse embryonic stem cells. *Acta Biomater*, 2010. **6**(6): 1904–1916.
10. Bowers, S. L. K., I. Banerjee, and T. A. Baudino, The extracellular matrix: at the center of it all. *J Mol Cell Cardiol*, 2010. **48**(3): 474–482.
11. Hinds, S., et al., The role of extracellular matrix composition in structure and function of bioengineered skeletal muscle. *Biomaterials*, 2011. **32**(14): 3575–3583.
12. Zile, M. R., New concepts in diastolic dysfunction and diastolic heart failure: Part II: causal mechanisms and treatment. *Circulation*, 2002. **105**(12): 1503–1508.
13. Bosman, F. T., and I. Stamenkovic, Functional structure and composition of the extracellular matrix. *J Pathol*, 2003. **200**(4): 423–428.
14. Fomovsky, G. M., S. Thomopoulos, and J. W. Holmes, Contribution of extracellular matrix to the mechanical properties of the heart. *J Mol Cell Cardiol*, 2010. **48**(3): 490–496.

15. Hatano, S., et al., Versican/PG-M is essential for ventricular septal formation subsequent to cardiac atrioventricular cushion development. *Glycobiology*, 2012. **22**(9): 1268–1277.
16. Kassiri, Z., and R. Khokha, *Myocardial Extra-Cellular Matrix and Its Regulation by Metalloproteinases and their Inhibitors.* Thrombosis and Haemostasis, 2005.
17. Kim, D. H., et al., Nanoscale cues regulate the structure and function of macroscopic cardiac tissue constructs. *Proc Natl Acad Sci USA*, 2010. **107**(2): 565–570.
18. Orlova, Y., et al., Electrospun nanofibers as a tool for architecture control in engineered cardiac tissue. *Biomaterials*, 2011. **32**(24): 5615–5624.
19. Venugopal, J. R., et al., Biomaterial strategies for alleviation of myocardial infarction. *J R Soc Interface*, 2012. **9**(66): 1–19.
20. Ishii, O., et al., In vitro tissue engineering of a cardiac graft using a degradable scaffold with an extracellular matrix-like topography. *J Thoracic Cardiovasc Surg*, 2005. **130**(5): 1358–1363.
21. Luna, J. I., et al., Multi-scale biomimetic topography for the alignment of neonatal and embryonic stem cell-derived heart cells. *Tissue Eng Part C: Methods*, 2011. **17**(5) 579–588.
22. Shah, U., H. Bien, and E. Entcheva, Microtopographical effects of natural scaffolding on cardiomyocyte function and arrhythmogenesis. *Acta Biomater*, 2010. **6**(8): 3029–3034.
23. Andersson, A.-S., et al., Nanoscale features influence epithelial cell morphology and cytokine production. *Biomaterials*, 2003. **24**(20): 3427–3436.
24. Deok-Ho, K., et al. *Modulation of Adhesion and Growth of Cardiac Myocytes by Surface Nanotopography.* in *Engineering in Medicine and Biology Society, 2005. IEEE-EMBS 2005. 27th Annual International Conference of the* 2005.
25. Kim, D. H., et al., Matrix nanotopography as a regulator of cell function. *J Cell Biol*, 2012. **197**(3): 351–360.
26. Salvi, J. D., J. Yul Lim, and H. J. Donahue, Increased mechanosensitivity of cells cultured on nanotopographies. *J Biomechan*, 2010. **43**(15): 3058–3062.
27. Tajima, S., et al., Differential regulation of endothelial cell adhesion, spreading, and cytoskeleton on low-density polyethylene by nanotopography and surface chemistry modification induced by

argon plasma treatment. *J Biomed Mater Res Part A*, 2008. **84A**(3): 828–836.

28. Wang, P., et al., Modulation of alignment, elongation and contraction of cardiomyocytes through a combination of nanotopography and rigidity of substrates. *Acta Biomater*, 2011. **7**(9): 3285–3293.
29. Yim, E. K. F., and K. W., Leong, Significance of synthetic nanostructures in dictating cellular response. *Nanomed Nanotechnol, Biol, Med*, 2005. **1**(1): 10–21.
30. Yim, E. K. F., et al., Nanopattern-induced changes in morphology and motility of smooth muscle cells. *Biomaterials*, 2005. **26**(26): 5405–5413.
31. Boyan, B. D., et al., Role of material surfaces in regulating bone and cartilage cell response. *Biomaterials*, 1996. **17**(2): 137–146.
32. Deng, M., et al., Nanostructured polymeric scaffolds for orthopaedic regenerative engineering. *IEEE Trans Nanobiosci*, 2012. **11**(1): 3–14.
33. Li, D., et al., Role of mechanical factors in fate decisions of stem cells. *Regen Med*, 2011. **6**(2): 229–240.
34. Khan, S., and G. Newaz, A comprehensive review of surface modification for neural cell adhesion and patterning. *J Biomed Mater Res A*, 2010. **93**(3): 1209–1224.
35. Charest, J. M., et al., Fabrication of substrates with defined mechanical properties and topographical features for the study of cell migration. *Macromol Biosci*, 2012. **12**(1): 12–20.
36. Davis, M. E., et al., Custom design of the cardiac microenvironment with biomaterials. *Circ Res*, 2005. **97**(1): 8–15.
37. Kim, D., et al., Guided cell migration on microtextured substrates with variable local density and anisotropy. *Adv Funct Mater*, 2009. **19**(10): 1579–1586.
38. Collesi, C., et al., Notch-1 signaling stimulates proliferation of immature cardiomyocytes. *J Cell Biol*, 2008. **183**(1): 117–128.
39. Charest, J. L., A. J. García, and W. P. King, Myoblast alignment and differentiation on cell culture substrates with microscale topography and model chemistries. *Biomaterials*, 2007. **28**(13): 2202–2210.
40. Kim, D. H., et al., Matrix nanotopography as a regulator of cell function. *J Cell Biol*, 2012. **197**(3): 351–360.
41. Chan, S. S.-K., et al., Salvianolic acid B–vitamin C synergy in cardiac differentiation from embryonic stem cells. *Biochem Biophys Res Commun*, 2009. **387**(4): 723–728.

42. Murphy, A. M., et al., Molecular cloning of rat cardiac troponin I and analysis of troponin I isoform expression in developing rat heart. *Biochemistry*, 1991. **30**(3): 707–712.
43. Swynghedauw, B., Developmental and functional adaptation of contractile proteins in cardiac and skeletal muscles. *Physiol Rev*, 1986. **66**(3): 710–771.
44. Morkin, E., Control of cardiac myosin heavy chain gene expression. *Micros Res Techniq*, 2000. **50**(6): 522–531.
45. Rockwood, D. N., et al., Culture on electrospun polyurethane scaffolds decreases atrial natriuretic peptide expression by cardiomyocytes in vitro. *Biomaterials*, 2008. **29**(36): 4783–4791.
46. Schellings, M. W. M., Y. M. Pinto, and S. Heymans, Matricellular proteins in the heart: possible role during stress and remodeling. *Cardiovas Res*, 2004. **64**(1): 24–31.
47. Kshitiz, et al., Matrix rigidity controls endothelial differentiation and morphogenesis of cardiac precursors. *Sci Signal*, 2012. **5**(227): ra41.
48. Shimizu, T., et al., Polysurgery of cell sheet grafts overcomes diffusion limits to produce thick, vascularized myocardial tissues. *FASEB J*, 2006. **20**(6): 708–710.
49. Dickinson, L. E., M. E. Moura, and S. Gerecht, Guiding endothelial progenitor cell tube formation using patterned fibronectin surfaces. *Soft Matter*, 2010. **6**(20): 5109–5119.
50. Marshall, et al., *Biomaterials with Tightly Controlled Pore Size that Promote Vascular in-Growth*, vol. 45. 2004, Boston, MA, ETATS-UNIS: American Chemical Society. 2.
51. Kim, D. H., et al., Nanopatterned cardiac cell patches promote stem cell niche formation and myocardial regeneration. *Integr Biol* (Camb), 2012. **4**(9): 1019–1033.
52. Dehne, T., et al., Regenerative potential of human adult precursor cells: cell therapy: an option for treating cartilage defects?. *Z Rheumatol*, 2009. **68**(3): 234–238.
53. Bratton, D., et al., Recent progress in high resolution lithography. *Polymers Adv Technol*, 2006. **17**(2): 94–103.
54. Kim, H., et al., Patterning methods for polymers in cell and tissue engineering. *Ann Biomed Eng*, 2012. **40**(6): 1339–1355.
55. Cheung, H. S., Biologic effects of calcium-containing crystals. *Curr Opin Rheumatol*, 2005. **17**(3): 336–340.
56. Joseph, R. M., Osteoarthritis of the ankle: bridging concepts in basic science with clinical care. *Clin Podiatr Med Surg*, 2009. **26**(2): 169–184.

57. Broers, A. N., A. C. F. Hoole, and J. M. Ryan, Electron beam lithography–Resolution limits. *Microelectron Eng*, 1996. **32**(1–4): 131–142.
58. Kim, D.-H., et al., Nanoscale cues regulate the structure and function of macroscopic cardiac tissue constructs. *Proc Natl Acad Sci*, 2010. **107**(2): 565–570.
59. Takahashi, H., et al., Anisotropic cell sheets for constructing three-dimensional tissue with well-organized cell orientation. *Biomaterials*, 2011. **32**(34): 8830–8838.
60. Guo, L. J., Nanoimprint lithography: methods and material requirements. *Adv Mater*, 2007. **19**(4): 495–513.
61. Suh, K.-Y., M. C. Park, and P. Kim, Capillary force lithography: a versatile tool for structured biomaterials interface towards cell and tissue engineering. *Adv Funct Mater*, 2009. **19**(17): 2699–2712.
62. Kwak, R., H. E. Jeong, and K. Y. Suh, Fabrication of monolithic bridge structures by vacuum-assisted capillary-force lithography. *Small*, 2009. **5**(7): 790–794.
63. Burns, K., C. Yao, and T. J. Webster, Increased chondrocyte adhesion on nanotubular anodized titanium. *J Biomed Mater Res A*, 2009. **88**(3): 561–568.
64. Takahashi, H., et al., Anisotropic cell sheets for constructing three-dimensional tissue with well-organized cell orientation. *Biomaterials*, 2011. **32**(34): 8830–8838.
65. Kim, D., et al., Biomimetic nanopatterns as enabling tools for analysis and control of live cells. *Adv Mater*, 2010. **22**(41): 4551–4566.
66. Ginger, D. S., H. Zhang, and C. A. Mirkin, The evolution of dip-pen nanolithography. *Angew Chem Int Ed Engl*, 2004. **43**(1): 30–45.
67. Piner, R. D., "Dip-Pen" Nanolithography. *Science*, 1999. **283**(5402): 661–663.
68. Lee, K. B., et al., Protein nanoarrays generated by dip-pen nanolithography. *Science*, 2002. **295**(5560): 1702–1705.
69. Ikeda, T., et al., Distinct roles of Sox5, Sox6, and Sox9 in different stages of chondrogenic differentiation. *J Bone Miner Metab*, 2005. **23**(5): 337–340.
70. Yim, E. K. F., and K. W. Leong, Significance of synthetic nanostructures in dictating cellular response. *Nanomed Nanotechnol, Biol Med*, 2005. **1**(1): 10–21.
71. Gupta, M. K., et al., Combinatorial polymer electrospun matrices promote physiologically-relevant cardiomyogenic stem cell differentiation. *PLoS One*, 2011. **6**(12): e28935.

72. Kai, D., et al., Polypyrrole-contained electrospun conductive nanofibrous membranes for cardiac tissue engineering. *J Biomed Mater Res Part A*, 2011. **99A**(3): 376–385.
73. Kumbar, S. G. et al., Electrospun nanofiber scaffolds: engineering soft tissues. *Biomed Mater*, 2008. **3**(3): 034002.
74. Martins, A., et al., Electrospun nanostructured scaffolds for tissue engineering applications. *Nanomedicine*, 2007. **2**(6): 929–942.
75. Zong, X., et al., Electrospun fine-textured scaffolds for heart tissue constructs. *Biomaterials*, 2005. **26**(26): 5330–5338.
76. Berndt, P., G. B. Fields, and M. Tirrell, Synthetic lipidation of peptides and amino acids: monolayer structure and properties. *J Am Chem Soc*, 1995. **117**(37): 9515–9522.
77. Webber, M. J., et al., Development of bioactive peptide amphiphiles for therapeutic cell delivery. *Acta Biomater*, 2010. **6**(1): 3–11.
78. Zhang, S., F. Gelain, and X. Zhao, Designer self-assembling peptide nanofiber scaffolds for 3D tissue cell cultures. *Semin Cancer Biol*, 2005. **15**(5): 413–420.
79. Kushwaha, M., et al., A nitric oxide releasing, self assembled peptide amphiphile matrix that mimics native endothelium for coating implantable cardiovascular devices. *Biomaterials*. **31**(7): 1502–1508.
80. Shimizu, T., et al., Electrically communicating three-dimensional cardiac tissue mimic fabricated by layered cultured cardiomyocyte sheets. *J Biomed Mater Res*, 2002. **60**(1): 110–117.
81. Heskins, M., and J. E. Guillet, Solution properties of poly(N-isopropylacrylamide). *J Macromol Sci Part A—Chem*, 1968. **2**(8): 1441–1455.
82. Shimizu, T., Fabrication of pulsatile cardiac tissue grafts using a novel 3-dimensional cell sheet manipulation technique and temperature-responsive cell culture surfaces. *Circ Res*, 2002. **90**(3): 40e–48e.
83. Virtanen, J., C. Baron, and H. Tenhu, Grafting of poly(N-isopropylacrylamide) with poly(ethylene oxide) under various reaction conditions. *Macromolecules*, 1999. **33**(2): 336–341.
84. Akiyama, Y., et al., Surface characterization of Poly(N-isopropylacrylamide) grafted tissue culture polystyrene by electron beam irradiation, using atomic force microscopy, and X-ray photoelectron spectroscopy. *J Nanosci Nanotechnol*, 2007. **7**(3): 796–802.
85. Jones, C. W., et al., Confocal laser scanning microscopy in orthopaedic research. *Prog Histochem Cytochem*, 2005. **40**(1): 1–71.

86. Isenberg, B. C., et al., A thermoresponsive, microtextured substrate for cell sheet engineering with defined structural organization. *Biomaterials*, 2008. **29**(17): 2565–2572.
87. Shapira-Schweitzer, K., et al., A photopolymerizable hydrogel for 3-D culture of human embryonic stem cell-derived cardiomyocytes and rat neonatal cardiac cells. *J Mol Cell Cardiol*, 2009. **46**(2): 213–224.
88. Eschenhagen, T., et al., Three-dimensional reconstitution of embryonic cardiomyocytes in a collagen matrix: a new heart muscle model system. *FASEB J*, 1997. **11**(8): 683–694.
89. Zimmermann, W. H., Tissue engineering of a differentiated cardiac muscle construct. *Circ Res*, 2001. **90**(2): 223–230.
90. Zimmermann, W.-H., et al., Engineered heart tissue grafts improve systolic and diastolic function in infarcted rat hearts. *Nat Med*, 2006. **12**(4): 452–458.
91. Madden, L. R., et al., Proangiogenic scaffolds as functional templates for cardiac tissue engineering. *Proc Natl Acad Sci*, 2010. **107**(34): 15211–15216.
92. Radisic, M., et al., Functional assembly of engineered myocardium by electrical stimulation of cardiac myocytes cultured on scaffolds. *Proc Natl Acad Sci*, 2004. **101**(52): 18129–18134.
93. Au, H. T. H., et al., Interactive effects of surface topography and pulsatile electrical field stimulation on orientation and elongation of fibroblasts and cardiomyocytes. *Biomaterials*, 2007. **28**(29): 4277–4293.
94. Tandon, N., et al., Electrical stimulation systems for cardiac tissue engineering. *Nat. Protocols*, 2009. **4**(2): 155–173.
95. Huang, G., et al., The role of cardiac electrophysiology in myocardial regenerative stem cell therapy. *J Cardiovasc Translational Res*, 2011. **4**(1): 61–65.
96. Limpitikul, W., et al., Influence of electromechanical activity on cardiac differentiation of mouse embryonic stem cells. *Cardiovasc Eng Technol*, 2010. **1**(3): 179–193.
97. Weis, S. M., Vascular permeability in cardiovascular disease and cancer. *Curr Opin Hematol*, 2008. **15**(3): 243–249 10.1097/MOH.0b013e3282f97d86.
98. Dvir, T., et al., Nanoparticles targeting the infarcted heart. *Nano Lett*, 2011. **11**(10): 4411–4414.

99. Gray, W., et al., *N*-acetylglucosamine conjugated to nanoparticles enhances myocyte uptake and improves delivery of a small molecule p38 inhibitor for post-infarct healing. *J Cardiovasc Translational Res*, 2011. **4**(5): 631–643.

100. Leuschner, F., et al., Therapeutic siRNA silencing in inflammatory monocytes in mice. *Nat Biotech*, 2011. **29**(11): 1005–1010.

101. Oh, K. S., et al., Temperature-induced gel formation of core/shell nanoparticles for the regeneration of ischemic heart. *J Control Release*, 2010. **146**(2): 207–211.

102. Binsalamah, Z. M., et al., Intramyocardial sustained delivery of placental growth factor using nanoparticles as a vehicle for delivery in the rat infarct model. *Intl J Nanomed*, 2011. **6**: 2667–2678.

103. Gilad, A. A., et al., MR tracking of transplanted cells with "positive contrast" using manganese oxide nanoparticles. *Magn Reson Med*, 2008. **60**(1): 1–7.

104. Yilmaz, A., et al., Magnetic resonance imaging (MRI) of inflamed myocardium using iron oxide nanoparticles in patients with acute myocardial infarction–Preliminary results. *Intl J Cardiol*, 2011. **163**(2): 175–182.

105. Goluch, E. D., et al., A bio-barcode assay for on-chip attomolar-sensitivity protein detection. *Lab Chip*, 2006. **6**(10): 1293–1299.

Chapter 22

Engineering of Skeletal Muscle Regeneration: Principles, Current State, and Challenges

Weining Bian,[a] Mark Juhas,[b] and Nenad Bursac[b]

[a]*Department of Anesthesia and Cardiovascular Division, Brigham and Women's Hospital, 75 Francis St, Boston, MA 02115, USA*
[b]*Department of Biomedical Engineering, Duke University, 3000 Science Dr, Durham, NC 27705, USA*

wbian1@partners.org, mark.juhas@duke.edu, nbursac@duke.edu

This chapter discusses the biological processes involved in skeletal muscle repair and regeneration, the use of tissue engineering technologies to reconstitute bioengineered muscle tissues in vitro and in vivo, and challenges and future directions in the field of regenerative muscle therapy.

22.1 Biology of Skeletal Muscle Regeneration

Skeletal muscle is the most abundant tissue in our body comprising nearly 45% of the total body weight. The main characteristic of muscle tissue is its ability to contract by coordinated activity of aligned bundles of multinucleated and striated muscle cells called myofibers. The contractile function of muscle is supported by a

---

Tissue and Organ Regeneration: Advances in Micro- and Nanotechnology
Edited by Lijie Grace Zhang, Ali Khademhosseini, and Thomas J. Webster
Copyright © 2014 Pan Stanford Publishing Pte. Ltd.
ISBN 978-981-4411-67-7 (Hardcover), 978-981-4411-68-4 (eBook)
www.panstanford.com

network of nerves, blood vessels, and extracellular matrix. When functioning properly, skeletal muscle has the capacity to mount a robust regenerative response to exercise or injury by sequentially preparing, and then repairing, the area of tissue damage; a process that involves a pool of endogenous progenitors, termed "satellite cells." In this section of the chapter, we will discuss important biological aspects of skeletal muscle development and repair, including skeletal myogenesis, muscle regeneration in acute trauma and chronic degenerative disease, and the roles that satellite cells, non-myogenic cell types, extracellular matrix, and mechanical loading play in muscle regeneration.

22.1.1 Overview of Skeletal Myogenesis

Skeletal myogenesis (Fig. 22.1), i.e., the formation of skeletal muscle, is a fundamental and complex process that occurs during both muscle development and repair. During early development, a major portion of skeletal muscle in the body of vertebrates, including the trunk and limbs, is derived from the paraxial mesodome of the somite [25]. This process is driven by primary progenitor cells that co-express two paired-box transcription factors, Pax3 and Pax7 [61], which control expression of a family of myogenic regulatory factors (MRF), including myoblast determination protein (MyoD), myogenic factor 5 (Myf5), muscle-specific regulatory factor 4 (MRF4), and myogenin, all of which coordinately initiate and regulate the myogenic program [17]. Pax3 and Pax7 are also expressed in satellite cells, a group of small mononuclear progenitor cells located between the basal lamina and sarcolemma of individual myofibers in postnatal skeletal muscle [22]. Satellite cells are responsible for maintenance, growth and regeneration of adult skeletal muscle [19]. Upon activation by exercise or injury, satellite cells proliferate and either commit to myogenic differentiation, yielding a pool of mononucleated myoblasts, or forestall differentiation and self-renew, ultimately returning to quiescence. Similar to their embryonic ancestors, myogenic differentiation of satellite cells relies on the coordinated expression of the four MRFs [22].

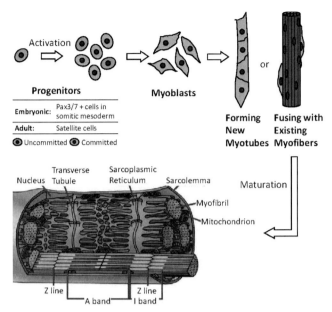

Figure 22.1 Stages of skeletal myogenesis in embryonic development and adult regeneration. Distinct populations of skeletal muscle progenitors drive myogenesis during embryonic development and adult regeneration. Activated progenitors proliferate and either become muscle committed myoblasts or self-renew and replenish the progenitor pool. Myoblasts then fuse with each other to form nascent myotubes, or with existing mature muscle fibers to augment muscle mass and capacity. As myotubes mature, highly specialized excitation-contraction apparatus emerges, including specific sarcolemmal ion channels, extensive transverse tubular (T-tubular) network, fully-developed sarcoplasmic reticulum for calcium storage, mature sarcommeric structures, and numerous mitochondria for cellular respiration. Nuclei also undergo peripheral translocation. Histological drawing adapted from Gartner et. al., *Color Textbook of Histology*, 2nd edition, 2001.

Myoblast fusion into multinucleated myofibers is a crucial step in skeletal myogenesis. During embryonic development, myoblasts first fuse with each other to generate primary myofibers, thereby defining the overall organization of the skeletal muscle tissue. This is followed by the formation of secondary myofibers to augment the muscle mass by fusion between myoblasts and the primary myofibers [94]. Similarly, myoblasts derived from satellite cells fuse with one another or existing muscle fibers during postnatal muscle growth and regeneration [19,26]. The process of myoblast fusion begins with cell migration, recognition, and adhesion and is followed by membrane fusion and the formation of a multinucleated syncytium. Myoblasts migrate in response to a plethora of chemokines [51] and growth factors [93] secreted by differentiated muscle cells [51] or supporting non-myocytes [93]. Various regulatory factors have also been discovered that either facilitate migration, bringing cells closer to each other [57], or inhibit migration to promote cell-cell contacts and adhesion [13]. Differentiating myoblasts form long membrane protrusions (i.e., filopodia and lamellipodia) in order to recognize and contact adjacent myoblasts and muscle cells [129]. A number of adhesion molecules such as cadherins [26], integrins [103], and associated proteins such as beta-catenin [121] then accumulate at cell contact sites and activate intracellular signaling pathways that initiate membrane fusion [121].

Nascent myofibers formed via myoblast fusion subsequently undergo structural and functional maturation, including the development of a specialized contractile apparatus consisting of parallel myofibrils made of repeating sarcomeres [100]. As myofibrils start to occupy the majority of the intracellular space, myonuclei become translocated from the center to the periphery of the myofiber [50]. Concurrently, the expression of myosin, the major protein constituent of the thick filament in a myofibril, gradually shifts from the embryonic and neonatal to the adult isoform types. This isoform switch alters the filament sliding kinetics in myofibrils leading to more forceful contraction [101]. Furthermore, specialized excitation-contraction (E-C) coupling structures called "triads" form as transverse (T)-tubules (deep invaginations of the sarcolemma) become coupled on both sides with the terminal cisternae of the sarcoplasmic reticulum (SR). Within T-tubules, concentrated L-type Ca^{2+} channels (dihydropyridine receptors, DHPR) activate by membrane depolarization during action potential generation. Muscle action potentials are triggered by the transmembrane inflow of Na^+ ions through nicotinic receptors upon their activation by acetylcholine release from motor neurons at neuromuscular junctions. DHPR activation yields calcium influx, which activates the ryanodine receptors (RyRs) on the adjacent SR membrane yielding the release of calcium ions from the SR into the cytoplasm. The generated excess intracellular calcium binds to troponin-C on the thin filaments of the myofibrils and causes muscle contraction by initiating the sliding movement of thick filaments along the thin filaments. Mitochondria, the major metabolic organelle that generates the sufficient amount of ATP required for muscle contraction, also become increasingly associated with triads during muscle maturation [12].

22.1.2 Muscle Regeneration in Acute Trauma and Chronic Degenerative Diseases

Skeletal muscle has a remarkable capacity for regeneration, which allows the tissue to undergo daily renewal even in a matured state, a process lacking in other tissues such as cardiac muscle. Skeletal muscle regeneration involves synchronization of numerous responses at the cellular and molecular level which are coordinated with the inflammatory response [22] (Fig. 22.2). Following common acute injuries, such as exercise-induced tears or lacerations, muscle is regenerated in a robust and efficient manner, restoring contractile function [115]. However, in cases of trauma resulting in significant loss of muscle (i.e., volumetric muscle loss) or chronic degenerative diseases, such as muscular dystrophies, inadequate regenerative process can yield the formation of scar tissue, denervation, and loss of contractile function [115].

The generation of new muscle following injury can be separated into a *degenerative* and a *regenerative* phase. The degenerative phase is responsible for both clearing necrotic myofibers, as well as activating the subsequent regenerative phase. Following injury, the myofiber sarcolemma is disrupted and intracellular components, such as creatine kinase, leak into the extracellular space [30]. Inflammatory cells, primarily neutrophils, begin to infiltrate the site of injury within 1–6 h [73]. By 48 h, pro-inflammatory M1 phenotype macrophages are the predominant inflammatory cell type at the site of injury. The cells act to clear necrotic debris through phagocytosis, further amplify the inflammatory response, and activate satellite cells for regeneration through release of soluble factors [111].

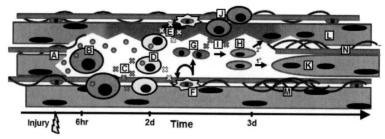

Figure 22.2 Sequence of events during muscle regeneration. Upon injury, myofiber intracellular components are released to extracellular environment (A). Neutrophils (B) arrive first at the site of injury to clear debris and release proinflammatory cytokines (C). They are followed by M1-macrophages (D) that further clear debris and release pro-myogenic factors (E) to activate local satellite cells. Satellite cells (F) asymmetrically divide, creating a pool of myogenic cells (G) which differentiate into myoblasts (H) upon exposure to interleukins (I) released from M2-macrophages (J). Terminally differentiated myoblasts undergo either primary (1°) fusion to each other to form new myofibers (K) or secondary (2°) fusion to rebuild injured myofibers (L). Throughout the regeneration process, excess secreted ECM (M) provides a temporary support for cell migration, proliferation, and restoration of the vascular network (N).

The regenerative phase involves the fundamental process of skeletal myogenesis occurring simultaneously with extracellular matrix (ECM) deposition and angiogenesis. Myogenesis is initiated by the local activation of satellite cells that enter the cell cycle, proliferate, and differentiate into myoblasts. Myoblasts will continue to proliferate, activated by M2 phenotype macrophages [111], and fuse with one another or with existing myofibers. Concurrent with myogenesis, a temporary ECM is produced as fibroblasts proliferate and migrate to the injury site due to the release of profibrotic factors, namely transforming growth factor-β (TGF-β), in the degenerative phase [133]. The temporary fibrous matrix stabilizes the damaged site, preserves transduction of force within the muscle, serves as a scaffold for regenerating myofibers, and guides proper innervations [70]. Maintaining blood supply through revascularization is also essential, with new capillaries and myofibers being formed simultaneously [102] and high levels of angiogenic factors being seen as early as day 3 post injury [125]. All three mechanisms of the regenerative phase (i.e., myogenesis,

ECM synthesis, and angiogenesis) provide a proper environment for regrowth and maturation of skeletal muscle to restore muscle function following common acute injuries.

In the case of significant muscle loss (greater than 20% of total muscle), the regeneration phase is unable to fully restore muscle function. As reviewed in [115], in these severe injuries, fibrotic response to stabilize the tissue proceeds more rapidly than myogenesis. Accelerated ECM deposition results in a dense cap of scar tissue, inhibiting myofibers from bridging the damaged site. As a result, the distal tissue, lacking any neuromuscular junctions, becomes denervated.

In the case of chronic degenerative diseases, such as muscular dystrophy, repetitive muscle injuries elicit continuous cycles of degeneration and regeneration, eventually leading to severe fibrosis and fat accumulation as well as exhaustion of the myogenic capacity associated with loss of satellite cell pool. In Duchenne muscular dystrophy (DMD), the most severe form of muscular dystrophy, muscle lacks the membrane-bound protein dystrophin, a critical force-bearing link between the myofiber cytoskeleton and the ECM [40]. In the absence of dystrophin, the cellular membrane becomes vulnerable to contraction-induced injury and the sarcolemma undergoes repeated tearing [76]. The regenerative process, although present, is inefficient since regenerating myofibers also contain the dystrophin mutation and remain prone to further degeneration. The persistent cycles of degeneration result in chronic activation of the inflammatory response leading to fibrosis [88]. The fibrotic environment and disarrayed ECM further hinder the ability to fully restore healthy muscle structure, innervation, and function.

22.1.3 Role of Satellite Cells in Muscle Regeneration

Muscle satellite cells, first described over 50 years ago, are named for their proximity to the myofiber periphery where they reside surrounded by the basement membrane [22]. In adult muscle, satellite cells are quiescent but able to proliferate, differentiate, and self-renew in response to injury, allowing for myofiber repair as well as the continued maintenance of the muscle stem cell pool [19]. At birth, satellite cells account for a large portion of myonuclei (~30%); however, as skeletal muscle matures and reaches homeostasis, this percentage drops to under 5% [22]. Satellite cells are observed with increased density in specific locations within muscle; primarily at neuromuscular junctions and adjacent to capillaries [22]. They are identified by molecular markers such as Pax7, α7β1-integrin, CD34, syndecan 3 and 4, caveolin 1, M-cadherin, and CXCR4 [22].

Regulation of satellite cell quiescence is attributed to Notch signaling [10] and the involvement of microRNAs [23]. Once activated, satellite cells exit the quiescent state, enter the cell cycle, and begin to proliferate. In the proliferating satellite cells, the Notch-inhibiting protein Numb is localized asymmetrically in the two daughter cells [28]. Activation of Notch-1 in a fraction of cells promotes their proliferation and self-renewal, while its inhibition leads to myogenic commitment and differentiation toward more mature myoblasts. The differentiation process is associated with upregulation of MyoD and Myf5, loss of Pax7 expression, and subsequent upregulation of more mature MRFs, such as myogenin [17]. The self-renewal of Notch-1–activated cells appears essential to prevent the depletion of the satellite cell pool [10].

22.1.4 Role of Non-Myogenic Cells in Muscle Regeneration

Two major populations of non-myogenic cells that are present in regenerating skeletal muscle are immune or inflammatory cells, and tissue resident mesenchymal stromal cells (MSCs). Emerging evidence shows that these non-myogenic cells are crucial modulators of regenerative myogenesis that act through both the secretion of paracrine factors and direct contact with myogenic cells [83].

Specifically, inflammatory response to muscle injury starts with infiltration of special leukocytes, mostly neutrophils and macrophages, into the damage site. Neutrophils release free radicals and proteases to degrade tissue debris, as well as proinflammatory cytokines to chemoattract macrophages and stimulate their proliferation [126]. M1 macrophages are activated mostly in the early stage of regeneration and function similar to neutrophils to remove tissue debris. These cells also protect muscle progenitors and differentiating myofibers from apoptosis [108]. M2 macrophages appear later in the regenerative process to attenuate inflammation [111]. Importantly, M1 macrophages have been shown to stimulate myoblast proliferation, while M2 macrophages enhance myoblast fusion and myogenic differentiation [111], suggesting that time course of myogenic repair may be determined by changes in macrophage types.

Muscle-resident MSCs, as another non-myogenic cell type involved in muscle regeneration, exhibit the same key defining characteristics of MSCs originally discovered in bone marrow, including clone-forming capacity [43] and tri-potency to differentiate into adipocytes, chondrocytes and osteoblasts [44]. Resident MSCs of hematopoietic origin are able to generate myogenic progeny along with progenies of mesenchymal, hematopoietic and vascular lineages [90,131]. By contrast, the other subsets of muscle-resident MSCs are limited in their myogenic potential, but play a supportive role in muscle regeneration by secreting paracrine factors to stimulate proliferation and migration of myogenic progenitors and myoblasts [59].

22.1.5 Role of Extracellular Matrix in Muscle Regeneration

Extracellular matrix (ECM) in adult skeletal muscle consists of two major components, interstitial connective tissue, and basement membrane. Hierarchically, interstitial ECM comprises the endomysium ensheathing individual myofibers, the perimysium surrounding each fascicle (i.e., bundle) of myofibers, and the outermost collagen I-rich epimysium surrounding the bundles of fascicles (i.e., the entire muscle) [49]. The basement membrane, or basal lamina, is a thin ECM sheet, rich in type IV collagen and laminin, in close contact with muscle sarcolemma [99]. Both interstitial connective tissue and basement membrane are known to play significant roles in the muscle force transmission [78]. Recently, a growing body of evidence has shown that these ECM components are also critically involved in different phases of muscle regeneration, including inflammation, revascularization, and myogenesis.

In particular, cell-ECM binding via integrins is known to mediate outside-in signaling that ultimately leads to changes in cellular processes such as survival, activation, proliferation and differentiation. Specifically, binding of $\alpha 7\beta 1$ integrins in satellite cells to laminin in basement membrane is required to enhance the motility of satellite cells facilitating their migration out of the resident niches [106]. In the later stages of myogenesis, adhesion to laminin-based ECM through integrins or the dystrophin glycoprotein complex (DGC) is required for the differentiation of myoblasts into striated muscle fibers [53]. Conversely, the absence of instructive ECM cues has been shown to hamper myoblast fusion and myofibril assembly without interfering with expression and nuclear localization of differentiation-associated MRFs such as MyoD and myogenin [81].

In addition to ECM proteins, both the interstitial and basement membrane of skeletal muscle contain abundant glycosaminoglycans (GAGs) capable of binding a wide variety of growth factors and cytokines secreted by myogenic and ancillary cells. Other ECM components, including interstitial collagens, can also entrap different growth factors, including transforming growth factor-β (TGF-β) and insulin-like growth factor (IGF) [47]. The spatiotemporal changes in the distribution and presence of specific GAGs during ECM remodeling enable localized and concentrated paracrine actions of their binding growth factors and cytokines that regulate the process of muscle regeneration. For example, binding of fibroblast growth factor 2 (FGF2) to syndecan-1 has been shown to enhance its affinity to tyrosine kinase receptors in myoblasts and stimulate their proliferation. In contrast, sequestration of FGF2 by glypican promotes myofiber formation by attenuating the inhibitory effect of FGF2 on myoblast differentiation [122].

In addition to ECM components, various proteases have been shown to regulate inflammation, angiogenesis and myogenesis, all of which are known to significantly impact regeneration of injured muscle [54]. Specifically, matrix metalloproteinases and their tissue inhibitors (MMPs/TIMPs) [20] and plasmin/plasminogen activation systems (PAs) [109] are shown to play key roles in the degradation of ECM proteins (e.g., collagen, laminin, fibronectin) during the early stages of muscle regeneration [109]. The ECM proteolytic fragments can in turn serve as chemotactic signals to promote the infiltration of inflammatory cells into the sites of injury [52]. Proteolytic degradation of ECM also allows invasion of endothelial cells that initiates neovascularization in regenerating muscle [20]. Moreover, certain proteases can bind to ECM and interact with ECM-bound growth factors (e.g., IGFs) to modulate their downstream roles in the regenerative process [71].

22.2 Current Advances toward Therapeutic Muscle Regeneration

Over the last few decades, various approaches to augment the regenerative capacity of severely injured or chronically diseased muscle have been explored in clinical and animal studies.

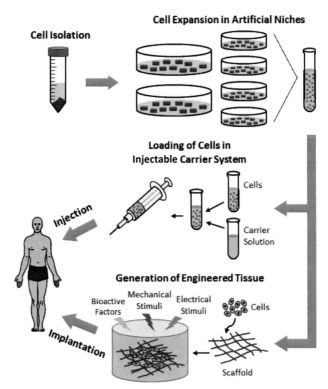

Figure 22.3 Cell transplantation strategies for skeletal muscle repair. Following tissue dissociation, isolated muscle progenitor cells or multipotent stem cells are expanded in well-controlled in vitro conditions designed to mimic microenvironment of native niches where these cells normally reside. Cells can be subsequently loaded in an injectable carrier with tunable bioactivity and stiffness, capable of promoting cell survival, growth, and differentiation upon injection. Alternatively, cells are seeded onto scaffolds and exposed to biophysical and biochemical stimuli to form functional muscle tissue constructs in vitro. The obtained engineered tissue is then surgically implanted into the injured muscle to aid regeneration.

One of the widely pursued strategies has been the transplantation of exogenous adult stem cells into the muscle tissue to synergistically restore muscle structure and function and augment the resident progenitor cell pools. In general, the use of adult stem cells for myogenic repair is a practical option. The cells are relatively easy to isolate and expand in vitro. However, ensuring the sustained proliferation, self-renewal, and myogenic differentiation of implanted cells in vivo remains challenging and limits the potential for clinical application. This section will describe recent progress in stem cell–based muscle repair, including the methods to expand stem cells in vitro, induce or support muscle repair in situ by use of different biomaterials, and engineer living skeletal muscle tissues in vitro to enable rapid restoration of impaired muscle function (Fig. 22.3).

22.2.1 Artificial Stem Cell Niches for Cell Expansion

Adult stem cells, including those from skeletal muscle, reside in specialized tissue "niches" where their quiescence, self-renewal, and differentiation are regulated by different biophysical cues, cell–cell, cell-ECM, paracrine and autocrine interactions present within the niche [72]. Exposure of isolated muscle-, adipose- or bone marrow–derived stem cells to an in vitro or in vivo microenvironment resembling that of the muscle stem cell niche has shown promise in controlling cell self-renewal and acquisition of a myogenic fate.

For example, mechanical stiffness of cell adhesion substrate has been suggested to play a pivotal role in the preservation of the self-renewal and regenerative capacity of muscle progenitor cells. Specifically, in vitro expansion of myogenic cells on stiff substrates, such as tissue culture plastic, increased differentiation and limited the ability of cells to engraft, survive, and retain regenerative capacity upon implantation [77,90]. On the other hand, culture of CD34+/integrin-α7+/Pax7+ muscle stem cells (MuSCs) on a polyethylene glycol (PEG) hydrogel with a stiffness similar to that of skeletal muscle (i.e., 12 kPa) yielded enhanced cell survival and reduced differentiation (myogenin expression) compared to culture on stiffer substrates. Upon implantation, the cells that were expanded on the soft substrate homed to native satellite cell niches and retained self-renewal and regenerative potential comparable to those of freshly isolated MuSCs. This work emphasizes the importance of the proper in vitro expansion conditions to enable efficient and sustained repair of injured muscle by implanted myogenic cells [18,27,41,48,77,96].

Substrate stiffness can also guide differentiation of stem cells toward unwanted cell fates. By virtue of their myogenic potency, adult human stem cells, such as those derived from bone marrow (BMSCs) and adipose tissue (ASCs), represent potential cell sources for muscle repair. However, the damaged site in the muscle, whether resulting from degenerative disease or a large defect, is often fibrous and stiffer than the healthy surrounding muscle. This can lead to osteogenic differentiation of implanted, undifferentiated stem cells [18]. To generate myogenically primed cells expressing myoD and myogenin, BMSCs and ASCs were cultured on substrates mimicking the stiffness of skeletal muscle [24]. This environment allowed differentiating stem cells to efficiently assemble focal adhesions and muscle contractile proteins. Furthermore, upon subsequent exposure to a stiff substrate, the derived myogenic cells were able to maintain their muscle lineage and function [24]. These studies suggest that appropriate in vitro conditions can also allow expansion of myogenic cells obtained from relatively abundant and accessible sources such as bone marrow or adipose tissue.

22.2.2 In situ Tissue Regeneration

Successful muscle repair by implanted cells will depend on their ability to replenish resident stem cell population and repeatedly undergo self-renewal and myogenic commitment to aid in future muscle regeneration. As both a load-bearing and load-generating tissue, injured muscle may also require temporary structural support that would mechanically stabilize tissue during the repair process [95]. Implantation of biocompatible scaffolds, alone or together with cells, may help form or maintain the native muscle structure, concentrate and retain implanted cells at the injury site, protect cells from the initial inflammatory or immune response, promote cell migration and proliferation, stimulate angiogenesis and synaptogenesis, and progressively degrade away to allow regenerated myofibers to reconstitute lost muscle tissue [16,95].

Various bioresorbable synthetic and natural scaffolds, including micro-patterned poly(glycolic acid) [11], collagen hydrogels [105], and hyaluronic acid hydrogels [96] have been utilized to deliver cells in the injured muscle. Rossi et al. injected freshly isolated satellite cells together with in situ polymerizable hydrogel to yield functional recovery of the injured muscle and replenishment of the satellite cell pool [96]. As satellite cells are limited in their number and potentially impractical for human use, Borselli et al. have combined satellite cell-derived myoblasts with a porous alginate scaffold able to provide sustained and local release of the angiogenic growth factor VEGF and the myogenic growth factor IGF-1 [16]. Delivery of the two growth factors dramatically enhanced participation of myoblasts in muscle regeneration, reduced muscle inflammation and fibrosis, improved formation of vasculature, and increased contractile function compared to implantation of the scaffold with only growth factors or the scaffold alone. It is, however, unlikely that the myoblasts implanted in this study could restore the satellite cell pool and support future muscle regeneration. In addition to use of myogenic cells, treatment of significant muscle loss or ischemia may be further aided by addition of angiogenic stem cells [128].

In addition to injectable hydrogels, muscle repair in situ has been attempted using two types of biological scaffolds: (1) small intestinal submucosa (SIS) [114,127] and (2) decellularized skeletal muscle ECM [127]. A few weeks after implantation, both matrices yielded a robust remodeling response marked by scaffold degradation, vasculature formation, and myogenesis [114,127]. However, in a complex injury setting, the SIS proved unable to restore muscle function and yielded dense areas of collagenous tissue [114]. Thus, although promising, biological scaffolds in cases of severe muscle damage could promote strong wound healing response and, instead of myogenesis, ultimately generate harmful tissue fibrosis.

22.2.3 In vitro Generation of Functional Skeletal Muscle Tissues

Compared to in situ muscle regeneration by implantation of exogenous, undifferentiated muscle progenitor cells and/or temporary scaffolds, the transplantation of fully differentiated tissue-engineered muscle may offer several unique benefits for muscle repair [6], including (1) the precise and instant structural repair at the injured site using muscle constructs engineered with patient-specific tissue architecture, (2) prompt relief of the mechanical overload that would prevent the adverse, compensatory tissue remodeling after injury, and (3) the ability to precondition muscle constructs prior to transplantation to match specific mechanical or metabolic demands of the host tissue. In addition, engineered muscle could be designed to promote effective communication among different cell types within the construct leading to successful reparative myogenesis, innervation, and vascularization.

In vitro generation of muscle constructs with native-like architecture (i.e., made of dense and aligned myofibers) was initially achieved by constraining muscle cell growth within thin and long muscle bundles by (1) centrifugal packing in cylindrically shaped collagen gels [80], (2) casting a mixture of muscle cells, collagen and Matrigel in cylindrical tissue molds [89], and (3) self-assembly of muscle cells into scaffold-free "myooids" under the influence of passive tension [58]. The diameter of such engineered muscle bundles has thus far been limited to a few hundred microns. Thicker engineered muscle bundles with diameters exceeding 1 mm were generated by casting cells and hydrogel; however, the limited oxygen and nutrient transport to the bundle center caused outward migration of muscle cells to bundle periphery, yielding the formation of an acellular core [92]. Advanced fabrication techniques were recently applied to create porous collagen scaffolds in an attempt to uniformly distribute and orient muscle cells throughout a large tissue volume [64]. However, collagen scaffolds have been shown to limit cellular migration [95] and may hinder myofiber hypertrophy and secondary fusion.

To address the above limitations, our group has recently developed a novel biofabrication method to generate large, relatively thick, and contractile muscle tissues composed of dense, uniformly distributed and aligned cells [7,8]. Specifically, an optimized mixture of muscle cells and fibrin-based hydrogel was cultured in photolithographically fabricated elastomeric molds containing an array of uniformly spaced posts. The posts were shaped as 1–2 mm-tall, 0.2 mm-wide, and 0.6–2 mm-long hexagonal prisms that were staggered and oriented in one direction. Through cell-mediated gel compaction, the posts generated elliptical pores in the tissue construct that facilitated oxygen and nutrient transport and guided cell alignment in the direction of the posts. The size and thickness of the muscle constructs were directly controlled by the dimensions of the tissue molds, while local and global directions and degrees of cell alignment were controlled by the orientation and length-to-width ratio of the posts [7–9]. Fibrin remodeling and compaction during culture enabled a large increase in final cell density and alignment and, along with high fibrin compliance that supported macroscopic tissue contractions, greatly facilitated myotube fusion and structural and functional maturation of formed muscle constructs.

In addition to stimulation of myofiber alignment and fusion by structural or topographical cues, different biophysical and biochemical factors have been studied for their capacity to augment the differentiation and function of engineered muscle tissues. For example, static mechanical stretch has been shown to enhance 3D cell spreading in collagen-based matrices [120], and when uniaxially applied, promote alignment and fusion of myoblasts [119]. Specific regimens of cyclic stretch also increased the myofiber diameter and density in human engineered muscle [89]. Moreover, muscle cells in hydrogel-based constructs subject to mechanical stress secreted VEGF that stimulated co-cultured endothelial cells to form vascular structures [117]. Similar to mechanical stimulation, electrical stimulation has been shown to have multiple beneficial effects on 3D cultured muscle cells [85,105]. Furthermore, addition of soluble factors (IGF-1, TGF-β, FGF-2) to culture media or release from bioactive scaffolds have been shown to promote the differentiation, hypertrophy, and contractile function of engineered muscle [16,68,118]. Combining the biochemical and biophysical stimulation (to engage their distinct and shared downstream signaling pathways) may further enhance the structure, maturation, and function of 3D engineered muscle, and remains to be explored in the future. In addition, we have shown that cell-matrix interactions play an important role in the force production of engineered muscle [56]. Optimizing the hydrogel composition to enhance the cell-ECM interactions significantly increased the myofiber diameter, Ca^{2+} transient duration, and contractile output of engineered muscle bundles.

22.3 Existing Challenges and Future Work

Although significant progress has been made toward the development of different strategies for skeletal muscle repair, a number of critical issues remain to be resolved. These challenges and potential directions for their resolution will be discussed in this section.

22.3.1 Optimal Cell Source

A variety of possible cell source candidates have been explored for use in skeletal muscle cell therapy (Table 22.1). An optimal cell source for human transplantation would be: (1) *easily accessible,* (2) *readily expandable* in vitro, (3) *self-renewing,* (4) *non-immunogenic and non-tumorigenic,* and (5) *able to engraft and continually regenerate muscle* in vivo.

Table 22.1 Potential cell sources for muscle regeneration

Cell type	Advantages	Disadvantages	References
Muscle Satellite Cells	– Fill Satellite Cell Niche (SCN) – Engraft in vivo	– Loss of myogenic capacity during expansion	[21,27, 95,96]
Muscle-derived Stem Cells/ Myoendothelial Cells	– Fill SCN – Expandable in vitro – Systemic delivery – Engraft in vivo	– Unestablished ability to aid in functional recovery	[36,79, 90,112]
Muscle Side Population Cells	– Fill SCN	– Non-myogenic in vitro	[2,110]
Blood/Muscle-derived CD133+ Cells	– Fill SCN – Easily accessible – Systemic delivery	– Difficult to expand in vitro	[4,42,113]
Mesoangioblasts / Human pericytes	– Fill SCN – Expandable in vitro – Systemic delivery	– Mesoangioblasts: derivedfrom embryo – Reproducibility of results	[37,98]
Bone marrow-derived Stem Cells	– Fill SCN – Engraft in vivo – Expandable in vitro	– Difficulties engrafting in fibrotic conditions	[18,38]
Adipose-derived Stem Cells	– Easily accessible – Engraft in vivo	– Potential inability to fill SCN	[69,84]

(Continued)

Table 22.1 (Continued)

Cell type	Advantages	Disadvantages	References
Embryonic Stem Cells (Pax7-driven)	– Fill SCN – Engraft in vivo – Expandable in vitro	– Ethical concerns – Need for immunosuppression	[32–34]
Induced Pluripotent Stem Cells (Pax7-driven)	– Fill SCN – Engraft in vivo – Expandable in vitro – Easily accessible	– Differentiation using integrative genetic methods	[34]

Specifically, muscle satellite cells (SCs) are the local resident muscle stem cells that can be isolated from single muscle fibers and expanded in vitro. However, following extended passage, these cells lose myogenic potential and ability for self-renewal. Freshly isolated satellite cells do maintain their regenerative capacity following transplantation and are able to engraft, proliferate, and add to the satellite cell niche [21,27,95,96]. The inability to proliferate and preserve "stemness" of SCs in vitro is currently the main obstacle to their use in muscle repair or treatment of different genetic disorders, including muscular dystrophies.

Vessel-associated stem cells, termed mesoangioblasts, have been shown by Cossu's group to differentiate toward myogenic lineage when exposed to certain cytokines or differentiating myoblasts, [29]. Mesoangioblasts grow extensively in vitro (over 50 passages) and are not tumorigenic [97]. Following injection into the femoral artery of a mouse, they homed in all hindlimb muscles and contributed satellite cells and regenerating myofibers as well as smooth muscle and endothelial cells [97]. Pretreatment of the cells with certain cytokines (SDF-1 and TNF-α) and transient expression of $\alpha 4$ integrin further increased homing of these cells [45]. The use of mesoangioblasts for muscle repair has since been applied to a dog model of DMD, in which dystrophin expression and muscle morphology and function were rescued [45]. Furthermore, Cossu's group has identified a pericyte cell population similar to that of embryonic mesangioblasts that can contribute to regeneration during postnatal life and populate the satellite cell niche [37]. While these vessel-associated stem cells may represent a highly promising source for muscle therapy, the results await confirmation by other groups [32].

Peripheral blood- or skeletal muscle-derived cells expressing human antigen CD133 can also undergo myogenic differentiation in co-culture with C2C12 mouse myoblasts or Wnt-producing fibroblasts, as evidenced by their de novo expression of M-cadherin, Pax7, CD34, and Myf5 [113]. Upon intra-muscular or intra-arterial injection, they have been shown to contribute to myofibers and satellite cells within muscle [113]. In addition, CD133$^+$ cells isolated from human DMD patients were genetically corrected (exon skipping) to express a shorter, yet functional, form of the dystrophin protein [4]. The corrected cells fused to host fibers, expressed functional human dystrophin, and appeared to fill the SC niche when injected systemically or locally in the muscle [4]. While relatively easy to isolate, CD133$^+$ cells may be difficult to expand in vitro [42,113] which may eventually limit their therapeutic potential.

Multi-potent stem cells from mouse muscle, termed muscle-derived stem cells (MDSCs) can self-renew, differentiate to various mesodermal cell types, and preserve their myogenic potential in vitro [98] for up to 200 population doublings [36,90]. Following in vivo injection, both locally [35,36] and systemically [112], MDSCs show ability to participate in muscle regeneration and self-renewal. Furthermore, a human analog to MDSCs has been identified based on co-expression of both myogenic and endothelial markers (CD56, CD34, CD144), termed myoendothelial cells [131]. These cells can undergo long term expansion without loss of myogenic potential and regenerate myofibers in vivo [131]. While potentially promising, these cells remain to be characterized for their potential to aid in functional recovery of diseased muscle [79].

Mouse muscle side population cells (SPs) and PW1-interstitial cells (PICs) are two additional resident cell types able to aid in muscle repair. SPs are Sca-1$^+$/Lin-1$^-$ cells [2,55] which are unable to undergo myogenesis in vitro [2], but can participate in muscle regeneration in vivo [2,55]. A SP subset expressing the ATP-binding transporter ABCG2, Syndecan-4, and Pax7, can engraft into the regenerating muscle with remarkable efficiency to contribute 75% of the SCs and 30% of myonuclei [110]. PICs are muscle interstitial cells positive for the stress mediator PW1 and negative for SC marker Pax7 [75]. PICs can undergo myogenesis to express both MyoD and Pax7 in vitro and efficiently replenish both the SC and PIC pools in regenerating muscle in vivo [75].

Human bone marrow-derived (BMSCs) and adipose-derived (ASCs) stem cells are also able to undergo myogenic differentiation.

Pittenger et al. demonstrated that a fraction of adult human BMSCs, when exposed to myogenic growth factors can be converted to myoblasts that express functional dystrophin [87]. Dezawa et al. generated a myogenic population containing Pax7+ cells from BMSCs at 89% efficiency through Notch1 intracellular domain gene transfer and exposure to various cytokines [38]. BMSCs, however, face difficulties engrafting into diseased, fibrotic muscle [18,46], a problem that may not be shared by ASCs [69]. When co-cultured with human DMD myoblasts, ASCs partially restored dystrophin expression in vitro [123] and when transplanted into dystrophic mice, they led to muscle regeneration and expression of human dystrophin protein in host myofibers [69,124]. The potential for long-term therapeutic effects remains to be established since the benefits from cell transplantation have been shown to disappear after few weeks due to the disappearance of injected cells [84].

Embryonic stem cells (ESCs) have remarkable potential for regeneration and self-renewal. In co-cultures with myogenic cells [5] or upon treatment with IGF2 [60], mouse ESCs have been shown to acquire myogenic phenotype. Darabi et al. demonstrated that overexpression of Pax3 during embryoid body differentiation increased myogenic potential of mouse ESCs and that Pax3$^+$/PDGFRα^+/Flk-1$^-$ progenitors engrafted and improved contractile function upon injection without causing tumors [31]. Inducible Pax7 overexpression yielded similar results, including the ability of derived progenitors to self-renew and respond to injury in vivo [33]. More recently, by applying the similar approach to inducible pluripotent stem cells (iPSCs), the same group reported the derivation of human muscle progenitors [34]. When transplanted into dystrophic mice, these cells successfully engrafted, improved muscle contractility, populated the SC compartment (for at least 11 months), and yielded expression of human dystrophin in host muscle [34]. While highly promising, the derivation of muscle progenitors from pluripotent stem cells should be ideally achieved through non-integrating genetic methods to reduce the mutagenic risks.

22.3.2 Optimal Biomaterial

Various bioactive materials have been explored as means to regulate cell fate and function and control different phases of tissue repair

[86]. Ideally, these scaffolds should be independently tunable for their: (1) physical, biochemical and topographical properties and (2) the ability to deliver multiple biofactors (including chemical drugs, proteins and nucleic acids) with individually controlled timing and dose. In addition, smart multifunctional scaffolds could bes designed to alter properties in response to externally applied stimuli such as electrical current, light, magnetic force, temperature, pH, or enzymatic reaction.

Synthetic polymers such as poly(acrylamide) (PAA) [24,41] and poly(ethylene glycol) (PEG) [48] have been used to create 2-D substrates with tunable stiffness supportive of myogenic cell growth. The 3D PAA or PEG scaffolds are, however, bioinert and unable to support high cell density and spreading needed for the engineering of functional muscle. Therefore, the composite biomaterials containing both natural and synthetic building blocks have been utilized to generate scaffolds with the optimal stiffness and abundant cell attachment sites. For example, conjugation of acrylated PEG with fibrinogen monomers yielded a hybrid PEG-fibrin hydrogel with the stiffness that could be modulated by varying the molecular weight of PEG and its fraction relative to fibrin, while the presence of fibrin still supported 3D spreading and growth of smooth muscle cells [1]. Similarly, PEG-collagen hybrid scaffolds have been generated in the form of modular hydrogels by assembling collagen I and functionalized PEG microgels [104]. The addition of collagen did not significantly alter the stiffness of PEG gels, enabling the decoupling of physical and biochemical cues in these 3D scaffolds, while it also enhanced the survival and proliferation of encapsulated neural cells.

A growing body of evidence suggests important regulatory roles of nanotopographical cues in the control of cellular behavior and function [62]. For example, electrospun nanofibrous scaffolds made of collagen [3] or polyurethane [67,107] were used to align skeletal myoblasts and demonstrate that the nanofiber diameter can influence the efficiency of myoblast fusion [107]. In addition, electrically conductive carbon nanotubes were incorporated into the nanofibers to enhance the beneficial effect of electrical stimulation on muscle differentiation and maturation [107]. Nevertheless, limited cell penetration inside the electrospun scaffolds remains the major drawback of this fabrication method. Another class of nanomaterials with potential use in muscle regeneration are self-assembled peptide amphiphile (PA) nanofibers. The PA-based 3D scaffolds can be designed to contain a specific set of functional motifs to modulate 3D adhesion, proliferation and differentiation of encapsulated cells [66,132]. These scaffolds have been used to enhance angiogenesis [91] and promote endogenous nerve regeneration in injured spinal cord [116]. PAs can be also made in injectable form in which they were applied to deliver exogenous cells and/or therapeutic proteins for in situ myocardial regeneration [82].

Recently, macroporous alginate scaffolds able to release both VEGF and IGF-1 have been implanted in injured or ischemic muscle [15,16] and shown to induce multiple beneficial effects, including reduction of inflammatory response and cell apoptosis, increase in satellite cell proliferation and differentiation, and enhancement of innervation and vascularization [15]. These scaffolds also supported in vivo retention and engraftment of implanted exogenous myoblasts in a model of severe muscle injury [16]. While promising, this and similar approaches for muscle regeneration need to be optimized with respect to a combination of growth factors and their release profiles. In addition, several studies have focused on design of scaffolds that can incorporate and release non-viral gene delivery vehicles, such as nanoparticles and nanocapsules containing plasmid DNA, mitochondrial RNA and small interfering RNAs (siRNA) [86]. Development of multifunctional scaffolding systems that can simultaneously deliver growth factors and genetic materials and possess stimulus-responsive features [86] is expected to provide improved control of various aspects of muscle regeneration and significantly promote future therapies for muscle injury and disease.

22.3.3 Neurovascular Integration

Rapid vascularization and innervation of implanted or regenerated muscle are critical for its survival and the ability to function within the native neouromuscular system. Major approaches currently employed to promote vascularization of implanted muscle grafts include (1) genetic modification of donor cells to express angiogenic factors [128] or controlled release of these factors from polymer scaffolds [15] and (2) prevascularization of engineered tissue constructs prior to transplantation by co-culturing muscle cells with endothelial cells or vascular progenitors in vitro [63], or growth of muscle cells around blood vessels (e.g., arterio-venous loop or femoral artery) in vivo [14,74]. Importantly, the increased organization of vascular structures obtained by an extended co-culture of myoblasts, fibroblasts, and endothelial cells has been shown to yield faster inosculation, perfusion, and functional maturation of engineered muscle post-implantation [63]. While promising, the above approaches need to be validated and likely specifically tailored to address complex and highly variable conditions encountered in different types of muscle injury and disease. Regarding that speed of vascular integration will be crucial for the graft survival, approaches combining a shorter co-culture to induce a degree of prevascularization with angiogenic gene or protein delivery may yield the optimal cell transplantation strategies for efficient muscle repair.

Although somewhat underappreciated in tissue engineering studies, the successful innervation of implanted engineered muscle will be crucial for the maintenance of its tone and the ability to efficiently support the function of the host muscle. Recent studies have shown functional innervation of engineered muscle constructs in co-cultures with neuronal cells in vitro [65] or after implantation adjacent to the transected nerves in vivo [39]. In these conditions, differentiated muscle fibers in tissue constructs exhibited enhanced assembly of acetylcholine-sensitive postsynaptic structures, which are an essential constituent of the neuromuscular junction (NMJ). These postsynaptic structures could facilitate the integration of engrafted muscle into the host neuromuscular system. Enhanced myogenic differentiation and force production have also been observed in these conditions, likely due to the trophic effect of nerve-derived factors on muscle cells. Neural agrin, a critical synaptogenic factor involved in NMJ development, has recently been identified by our group as one of those neurotrophic factors that can directly improve sarcolemmal clustering of achetylcholine receptors and enhance the contractile force production of engineered muscle [9]. In addition, several molecular pathways are known to be shared in vascular and neuronal development [130]. Delivery of specific effector molecules to selectively target these common pathways may simultaneously promote vascularization and innervation of the implanted engineered muscle, and remains to be explored in the future.

22.4 Concluding Remarks

Extensive trauma or chronic degenerative disease of skeletal muscle can yield persistent inflammatory response and significant depletion of progenitor cells, and eventually diminish the muscle capacity for self-repair. Over the last few decades, continued progress in our understanding of the biology of muscle development and repair has set the grounds for the pursuit of more effective therapies for muscle injury and disease. In particular, transplantation of exogenous myogenic cells and tissues has been regarded as a promising therapeutic strategy to enhance compromised muscle function and efficiently rebuild lost muscle tissue. The combined use of biological, biomaterial, and bioengineering techniques in the past decade have led to marked progress in the areas of (1) in vitro reconstruction of stem cell niche-like environments to preserve or enhance the self-renewing and differentiation capacity of muscle progenitor cells, (2) bioactive scaffold design to promote in situ muscle repair through anti-apoptotic, angiogenic and myogenic stimulation of implanted or host cells, and (3) engineering of functional muscle tissue substitutes to support rapid structural and functional repair of the injured muscle. However, a number of critical issues related to the lack of adequate source of human muscle progenitor cells, inefficient methods for their expansion and delivery, unknown biological roles of different non-muscle cells, and the inability to engineer highly functional human muscle tissues in vitro, remain to be resolved to allow the development of clinically applicable cell therapies for muscle repair. Future progress in the areas of micro- and nanotechnology will be a key to success in this important endeavor.

Acknowledgments

This work was supported in part by the grant AR055226 from National Institute of Arthritis and Musculoskeletal and Skin Diseases.

References

1. Almany, L., and Seliktar, D. (2005). Biosynthetic hydrogel scaffolds made from fibrinogen and polyethylene glycol for 3D cell cultures. *Biomaterials*, **26**, 2467–2477.

2. Asakura, A., Seale, P., Girgis-Gabardo, A., and Rudnicki, M. A. (2002). Myogenic specification of side population cells in skeletal muscle. *J Cell Biol,* **159**, 123–134.
3. Beier, J. P., Klumpp, D., Rudisile, M., Dersch, R., Wendorff, J. H., Bleiziffer, O., Arkudas, A., Polykandriotis, E., Horch, R. E., and Kneser, U. (2009). Collagen matrices from sponge to nano: new perspectives for tissue engineering of skeletal muscle. *BMC Biotechnol,* **9**, 34.
4. Benchaouir, R., Meregalli, M., Farini, A., D'Antona, G., Belicchi, M., Goyenvalle, A., Battistelli, M., Bresolin, N., Bottinelli, R., Garcia, L., and Torrente, Y. (2007). Restoration of human dystrophin following transplantation of exon-skipping-engineered DMD patient stem cells into dystrophic mice. *Cell Stem Cell,* **1**, 646–657.
5. Bhagavati, S., and Xu, W. (2005). Generation of skeletal muscle from transplanted embryonic stem cells in dystrophic mice. *Biochem Biophys Res Commun,* **333**, 644–649.
6. Bian, W., and Bursac, N. (2008). Tissue engineering of functional skeletal muscle: challenges and recent advances. *IEEE Eng Med Biol Mag,* **27**, 109–113.
7. Bian, W., and Bursac, N. (2009). Engineered skeletal muscle tissue networks with controllable architecture. *Biomaterials,* **30**, 1401–1412.
8. Bian, W., Liau, B., Badie, N., and Bursac, N. (2009). Mesoscopic hydrogel molding to control the 3D geometry of bioartificial muscle tissues. *Nat Protoc,* **4**, 1522–1534.
9. Bian, W., and Bursac, N. (2012). Soluble miniagrin enhances contractile function of engineered skeletal muscle. *FASEB J,* **26**, 955–965.
10. Bjornson, C. R., Cheung, T. H., Liu, L., Tripathi, P. V., Steeper, K. M., and Rando, T. A. (2012). Notch signaling is necessary to maintain quiescence in adult muscle stem cells. *Stem Cells,* **30**, 232–242.
11. Boldrin, L., Elvassore, N., Malerba, A., Flaibani, M., Cimetta, E., Piccoli, M., Baroni, M. D., Gazzola, M. V., Messina, C., Gamba, P., Vitiello, L., and De Coppi, P. (2007). Satellite cells delivered by micro-patterned scaffolds: a new strategy for cell transplantation in muscle diseases. *Tissue Eng,* **13**, 253–262.
12. Boncompagni, S., Rossi, A. E., Micaroni, M., Beznoussenko, G. V., Polishchuk, R. S., Dirksen, R. T., and Protasi, F. (2009). Mitochondria are linked to calcium stores in striated muscle by developmentally regulated tethering structures. *Mol Biol Cell,* **20**, 1058–1067.
13. Bondesen, B. A., Jones, K. A., Glasgow, W. C., and Pavlath, G. K. (2007). Inhibition of myoblast migration by prostacyclin is associated with enhanced cell fusion. *FASEB J,* **21**, 3338–3345.

14. Borschel, G. H., Dow, D. E., Dennis, R. G., and Brown, D. L. (2006). Tissue-engineered axially vascularized contractile skeletal muscle. *Plast Reconstr Surg,* **117**, 2235–2242.

15. Borselli, C., Storrie, H., Benesch-Lee, F., Shvartsman, D., Cezar, C., Lichtman, J. W., Vandenburgh, H. H., and Mooney, D. J. (2010). Functional muscle regeneration with combined delivery of angiogenesis and myogenesis factors. *Proc Natl Acad Sci USA,* **107**, 3287–3292.

16. Borselli, C., Cezar, C. A., Shvartsman, D., Vandenburgh, H. H., and Mooney, D. J. (2011). The role of multifunctional delivery scaffold in the ability of cultured myoblasts to promote muscle regeneration. *Biomaterials,* **32**, 8905–8914.

17. Braun, T., and Gautel, M. (2011). Transcriptional mechanisms regulating skeletal muscle differentiation, growth and homeostasis. *Nat Rev Mol Cell Biol,* **12**, 349–361.

18. Breitbach, M., Bostani, T., Roell, W., Xia, Y., Dewald, O., Nygren, J. M., Fries, J. W., Tiemann, K., Bohlen, H., Hescheler, J., Welz, A., Bloch, W., Jacobsen, S. E., and Fleischmann, B. K. (2007). Potential risks of bone marrow cell transplantation into infarcted hearts. *Blood,* **110**, 1362–1369.

19. Campion, D. R. (1984). The muscle satellite cell: a review. *Int Rev Cytol,* **87**, 225–251.

20. Carmeli, E., Moas, M., Reznick, A. Z., and Coleman, R. (2004). Matrix metalloproteinases and skeletal muscle: a brief review. *Muscle Nerve,* **29**, 191–197.

21. Cerletti, M., Jurga, S., Witczak, C. A., Hirshman, M. F., Shadrach, J. L., Goodyear, L. J., and Wagers, A. J. (2008). Highly efficient, functional engraftment of skeletal muscle stem cells in dystrophic muscles. *Cell* **134**, 37–47.

22. Charge, S. B., and Rudnicki, M. A. (2004). Cellular and molecular regulation of muscle regeneration. *Physiol Rev,* **84**, 209–238.

23. Cheung, T. H., Quach, N. L., Charville, G. W., Liu, L., Park, L., Edalati, A., Yoo, B., Hoang, P., and Rando, T. A. (2012). Maintenance of muscle stem-cell quiescence by microRNA-489. *Nature,* **482**, 524–528.

24. Choi, Y. S., Vincent, L. G., Lee, A. R., Dobke, M. K., and Engler, A. J. (2012). Mechanical derivation of functional myotubes from adipose-derived stem cells. *Biomaterials,* **33**, 2482–2491.

25. Christ, B., Huang, R., and Scaal, M. (2007). Amniote somite derivatives. *Dev Dyn,* **236**, 2382–2396.

26. Cifuentes-Diaz, C., Nicolet, M., Alameddine, H., Goudou, D., Dehaupas, M., Rieger, F., and Mege, R. M. (1995). M-cadherin localization in developing adult and regenerating mouse skeletal muscle: possible involvement in secondary myogenesis. *Mech Dev,* **50**, 85–97.
27. Collins, C. A., and Partridge, T. A. (2005). Self-renewal of the adult skeletal muscle satellite cell. *Cell Cycle,* **4**, 1338–1341.
28. Conboy, I. M., and Rando, T. A. (2002). The regulation of Notch signaling controls satellite cell activation and cell fate determination in postnatal myogenesis. *Dev Cell,* **3**, 397–409.
29. Cossu, G., and Bianco, P. (2003). Mesoangioblasts–vascular progenitors for extravascular mesodermal tissues. *Curr Opin Genet Dev,* **13**, 537–542.
30. Coulton, G. R., Morgan, J. E., Partridge, T. A., and Sloper, J. C. (1988) The mdx mouse skeletal muscle myopathy: I. A histological, morphometric and biochemical investigation. *Neuropathol Appl Neurobiol,* **14**, 53–70.
31. Darabi, R., Gehlbach, K., Bachoo, R. M., Kamath, S., Osawa, M., Kamm, K. E., Kyba, M., and Perlingeiro, R. C. (2008). Functional skeletal muscle regeneration from differentiating embryonic stem cells. *Nat Med,* **14**, 134–143.
32. Darabi, R., Santos, F. N., and Perlingeiro, R. C. (2008). The therapeutic potential of embryonic and adult stem cells for skeletal muscle regeneration. *Stem Cell Rev,* **4**, 217–225.
33. Darabi, R., Santos, F. N., Filareto, A., Pan, W., Koene, R., Rudnicki, M. A., Kyba, M., and Perlingeiro, R. C. (2011). Assessment of the myogenic stem cell compartment following transplantation of Pax3/Pax7-induced embryonic stem cell-derived progenitors. *Stem Cells,* **29**, 777–790.
34. Darabi, R., Arpke, R. W., Irion, S., Dimos, J. T., Grskovic, M., Kyba, M., and Perlingeiro, R. C. (2012). Human ES- and iPS-derived myogenic progenitors restore DYSTROPHIN and improve contractility upon transplantation in dystrophic mice. *Cell Stem Cell,* **10**, 610–619.
35. Deasy, B. M., Jankowski, R. J., and Huard, J. (2001). Muscle-derived stem cells: characterization and potential for cell-mediated therapy. *Blood Cells Mol Dis,* **27**, 924–933.
36. Deasy, B. M., Gharaibeh, B. M., Pollett, J. B., Jones, M. M., Lucas, M. A., Kanda, Y., and Huard, J. (2005). Long-term self-renewal of postnatal muscle-derived stem cells. *Mol Biol Cell,* **16**, 3323–3333.

37. Dellavalle, A., Maroli, G., Covarello, D., Azzoni, E., Innocenzi, A., Perani, L., Antonini, S., Sambasivan, R., Brunelli, S., Tajbakhsh, S., and Cossu, G. (2011). Pericytes resident in postnatal skeletal muscle differentiate into muscle fibres and generate satellite cells. *Nat Commun,* **2**, 499.

38. Dezawa, M., Ishikawa, H., Itokazu, Y., Yoshihara, T., Hoshino, M., Takeda, S., Ide, C., and Nabeshima, Y. (2005). Bone marrow stromal cells generate muscle cells and repair muscle degeneration. *Science,* **309**, 314–317.

39. Dhawan, V., Lytle, I. F., Dow, D. E., Huang, Y. C. and Brown, D. L. (2007). Neurotization improves contractile forces of tissue-engineered skeletal muscle. *Tissue Eng,* **13**, 2813–2821.

40. Emery, A. E. (2002). The muscular dystrophies. *Lancet,* **359**, 687–695.

41. Engler, A. J., Sen, S., Sweeney, H. L., Discher, D. E. (2006). Matrix elasticity directs stem cell lineage specification. *Cell,* **126**, 677–689.

42. Farini, A., Razini, P., Erratico, S., Torrente, Y., and Meregalli, M. (2009). Cell based therapy for Duchenne muscular dystrophy. *J Cell Physiol,* **221**, 526–534.

43. Friedenstein, A. J., Deriglasova, U. F., Kulagina, N. N., Panasuk, A. F., Rudakowa, S. F., Luria, E. A., and Ruadkow, I. A. (1974). Precursors for fibroblasts in different populations of hematopoietic cells as detected by the in vitro colony assay method. *Exp Hematol,* **2**, 83–92.

44. Friedenstein, A. J., Gorskaja, J. F., and Kulagina, N. N. (1976). Fibroblast precursors in normal and irradiated mouse hematopoietic organs. *Exp Hematol,* **4**, 267–274.

45. Galvez, B. G., Sampaolesi, M., Brunelli, S., Covarello, D., Gavina, M., Rossi, B., Constantin, G., Torrente, Y., and Cossu, G. (2006). Complete repair of dystrophic skeletal muscle by mesoangioblasts with enhanced migration ability. *J Cell Biol,* **174**, 231–243.

46. Gang, E. J., Darabi, R., Bosnakovski, D., Xu, Z., Kamm, K. E., Kyba, M., and Perlingeiro, R. C. (2009). Engraftment of mesenchymal stem cells into dystrophin-deficient mice is not accompanied by functional recovery. *Exp Cell Res,* **315**, 2624–2636.

47. Gelse, K., Poschl, E., and Aigner, T. (2003). Collagens--structure, function, and biosynthesis. *Adv Drug Deliv Rev,* **55**, 1531–1546.

48. Gilbert, P. M., Havenstrite, K. L., Magnusson, K. E., Sacco, A., Leonardi, N. A., Kraft, P., Nguyen, N. K., Thrun, S., Lutolf, M. P., and Blau, H. M. (2010). Substrate elasticity regulates skeletal muscle stem cell self-renewal in culture. *Science,* **329**, 1078–1081.

49. Gillies, A. R., and Lieber, R. L. (2011). Structure and function of the skeletal muscle extracellular matrix. *Muscle Nerve,* **44**, 318–331.
50. Grefte, S., Kuijpers-Jagtman, A. M., Torensma, R., and Von den Hoff, J. W. (2007). Skeletal muscle development and regeneration. *Stem Cells Dev,* **16**, 857–868.
51. Griffin, C. A., Apponi, L. H., Long, K. K., and Pavlath, G. K. (2010). Chemokine expression and control of muscle cell migration during myogenesis. *J Cell Sci,* **123**, 3052–3060.
52. Grounds, M. D., and Davies, M. J. (1996). Chemotaxis in myogenesis. *Basic Appl Myol,* **6**, 469–483.
53. Grounds, M. D., Sorokin, L., and White, J. (2005). Strength at the extracellular matrix-muscle interface. *Scand J Med Sci Sports,* **15**, 381–391.
54. Grounds, M. D. (2008). Complexity of extracellular matrix and skeletal muscle regeneration, in *Skeletal Muscle Repair and Regeneration* (Schiaffino, S., and Partridge, T. eds.) pp. 269–301, Springer, The Netherlands.
55. Gussoni, E., Soneoka, Y., Strickland, C. D., Buzney, E. A., Khan, M. K., Flint, A. F., Kunkel, L. M., and Mulligan, R. C. (1999). Dystrophin expression in the mdx mouse restored by stem cell transplantation. *Nature,* **401**, 390–394.
56. Hinds, S., Bian, W., Dennis, R. G., and Bursac, N. (2011). The role of extracellular matrix composition in structure and function of bioengineered skeletal muscle. *Biomaterials,* **32**, 3575–3583.
57. Horsley, V., Jansen, K. M., Mills, S. T., and Pavlath, G. K. (2003). IL-4 acts as a myoblast recruitment factor during mammalian muscle growth. *Cell,* **113**, 483–494.
58. Huang, Y. C., Dennis, R. G., Larkin, L., and Baar, K. (2005). Rapid formation of functional muscle in vitro using fibrin gels. *J Appl Physiol,* **98**, 706–713. Epub 2004 Oct 2008.
59. Joe, A. W., Yi, L., Natarajan, A., Le Grand, F., So, L., Wang, J., Rudnicki, M. A., and Rossi, F. M. (2010). Muscle injury activates resident fibro/adipogenic progenitors that facilitate myogenesis. *Nat Cell Biol,* **12**, 153–163.
60. Kamochi, H., Kurokawa, M. S., Yoshikawa, H., Ueda, Y., Masuda, C., Takada, E., Watanabe, K., Sakakibara, M., Natuki, Y., Kimura, K., Beppu, M., Aoki, H., and Suzuki, N. (2006). Transplantation of myocyte precursors derived from embryonic stem cells transfected with IGFII gene in a mouse model of muscle injury. *Transplantation,* **82**, 516–526.

61. Kassar-Duchossoy, L., Giacone, E., Gayraud-Morel, B., Jory, A., Gomes, D., and Tajbakhsh, S. (2005). Pax3/Pax7 mark a novel population of primitive myogenic cells during development. *Genes Dev*, **19**, 1426–1431.

62. Kim, D. H., Provenzano, P. P., Smith, C. L., and Levchenko, A. (2012). Matrix nanotopography as a regulator of cell function. *J Cell Biol*, **197**, 351–360.

63. Koffler, J., Kaufman-Francis, K., Shandalov, Y., Egozi, D., Pavlov, D. A., Landesberg, A., and Levenberg, S. (2011). Improved vascular organization enhances functional integration of engineered skeletal muscle grafts. *Proc Natl Acad Sci USA*, **108**, 14789–14794.

64. Kroehne, V., Heschel, I., Schugner, F., Lasrich, D., Bartsch, J. W., and Jockusch, H. (2008). Use of a novel collagen matrix with oriented pore structure for muscle cell differentiation in cell culture and in grafts. *J Cell Mol Med.*, **12**, 1582–1838.

65. Larkin, L. M., Van der Meulen, J. H., Dennis, R. G., and Kennedy, J. B. (2006). Functional evaluation of nerve-skeletal muscle constructs engineered in vitro. *In vitro Cell Dev Biol Anim*, **42**, 75–82.

66. Li, Q., and Chau, Y. (2010). Neural differentiation directed by self-assembling peptide scaffolds presenting laminin-derived epitopes. *J Biomed Mater Res A*, **94**, 688–699.

67. Liao, I. C., Liu, J. B., Bursac, N., and Leong, K. W. (2008). Effect of electromechanical stimulation on the maturation of myotubes on aligned electrospun fibers. *Cell Mol Bioeng*, **1**, 133–145.

68. Liao, I. C., and Leong, K. W. (2011). Efficacy of engineered FVIII-producing skeletal muscle enhanced by growth factor-releasing co-axial electrospun fibers. *Biomaterials*, **32**, 1669–1677.

69. Liu, Y., Yan, X., Sun, Z., Chen, B., Han, Q., Li, J., and Zhao, R. C. (2007) Flk-1+ adipose-derived mesenchymal stem cells differentiate into skeletal muscle satellite cells and ameliorate muscular dystrophy in mdx mice. *Stem Cells Dev*, **16**, 695–706.

70. Lluri, G., Langlois, G. D., McClellan, B., Soloway, P. D., and Jaworski, D. M. (2006). Tissue inhibitor of metalloproteinase-2 (TIMP-2) regulates neuromuscular junction development via a beta1 integrin-mediated mechanism. *J Neurobiol*, **66**, 1365–1377.

71. Loechel, F., Fox, J. W., Murphy, G., Albrechtsen, R., and Wewer, U. M. (2000). ADAM 12-S cleaves IGFBP-3 and IGFBP-5 and is inhibited by TIMP-3. *Biochem Biophys Res Commun*, **278**, 511–515.

72. Lutolf, M. P., and Blau, H. M. (2009). Artificial stem cell niches. *Adv Mater,* **21**, 3255–3268.
73. McClung, J. M., Davis, J. M., and Carson, J. A. (2007). Ovarian hormone status and skeletal muscle inflammation during recovery from disuse in rats. *Exp Physiol,* **92**, 219–232.
74. Messina, A., Bortolotto, S. K., Cassell, O. C., Kelly, J., Abberton, K. M., and Morrison, W. A. (2005). Generation of a vascularized organoid using skeletal muscle as the inductive source. *FASEB J,* **19**, 1570–1572.
75. Mitchell, K. J., Pannerec, A., Cadot, B., Parlakian, A., Besson, V., Gomes, E. R., Marazzi, G., and Sassoon, D. A. (2010). Identification and characterization of a non-satellite cell muscle resident progenitor during postnatal development. *Nat Cell Biol,* **12**, 257–266.
76. Mokri, B., and Engel, A. G. (1975). Duchenne dystrophy: electron microscopic findings pointing to a basic or early abnormality in the plasma membrane of the muscle fiber. *Neurology,* **25**, 1111–1120.
77. Montarras, D., Morgan, J., Collins, C., Relaix, F., Zaffran, S., Cumano, A., Partridge, T., and Buckingham, M. (2005). Direct isolation of satellite cells for skeletal muscle regeneration. *Science,* **309**, 2064–2067.
78. Monti, R. J., Roy, R. R., Hodgson, J. A., and Edgerton, V. R. (1999). Transmission of forces within mammalian skeletal muscles. *J Biomech,* **32**, 371–380.
79. Mueller, G. M., O'Day, T., Watchko, J. F., and Ontell, M. (2002). Effect of injecting primary myoblasts versus putative muscle-derived stem cells on mass and force generation in mdx mice. *Hum Gene Ther,* **13**, 1081–1090.
80. Okano, T., and Matsuda, T. (1998). Tissue engineered skeletal muscle: preparation of highly dense, highly oriented hybrid muscular tissues. *Cell Transplant,* **7**, 71–82.
81. Osses, N., and Brandan, E. (2002). ECM is required for skeletal muscle differentiation independently of muscle regulatory factor expression. *Am J Physiol Cell Physiol,* **282**, C383–C394.
82. Padin-Iruegas, M. E., Misao, Y., Davis, M. E., Segers, V. F., Esposito, G., Tokunou, T., Urbanek, K., Hosoda, T., Rota, M., Anversa, P., Leri, A., Lee, R. T., and Kajstura, J. (2009). Cardiac progenitor cells and biotinylated insulin-like growth factor-1 nanofibers improve endogenous and exogenous myocardial regeneration after infarction. *Circulation,* **120**, 876–887.

83. Paylor, B., Natarajan, A., Zhang, R. H., and Rossi, F. (2011). Nonmyogenic cells in skeletal muscle regeneration. *Curr Top Dev Biol,* **96**, 139–165.
84. Pecanha, R., Bagno, L. L., Ribeiro, M. B., Robottom Ferreira, A. B., Moraes, M. O., Zapata-Sudo, G., Kasai-Brunswick, T. H., Campos-de-Carvalho, A. C., Goldenberg, R. C., and Saar Werneck-de-Castro, J. P. (2012). Adipose-derived stem-cell treatment of skeletal muscle injury. *J Bone Joint Surg Am,* **94**, 609–617.
85. Pedrotty, D. M., Koh, J., Davis, B. H., Taylor, D. A., Wolf, P., and Niklason, L. E. (2005). Engineering skeletal myoblasts: roles of three-dimensional culture and electrical stimulation. *Am J Physiol Heart Circ Physiol,* **288**, H1620–H1626.
86. Perez, R. A., Won, J. E., Knowles, J. C., and Kim, H. W. (2012). Naturally and synthetic smart composite biomaterials for tissue regeneration. *Adv Drug Deliv Rev,* **65**, 471–496.
87. Pittenger, M. F., Mackay, A. M., Beck, S. C., Jaiswal, R. K., Douglas, R., Mosca, J. D., Moorman, M. A., Simonetti, D. W., Craig, S., and Marshak, D. R. (1999). Multilineage potential of adult human mesenchymal stem cells. *Science,* **284**, 143–147.
88. Porter, J. D., Khanna, S., Kaminski, H. J., Rao, J. S., Merriam, A. P., Richmonds, C. R., Leahy, P., Li, J., Guo, W., and Andrade, F. H. (2002). A chronic inflammatory response dominates the skeletal muscle molecular signature in dystrophin-deficient mdx mice. *Hum Mol Genet,* **11**, 263–272.
89. Powell, C. A., Smiley, B. L., Mills, J., and Vandenburgh, H. H. (2002). Mechanical stimulation improves tissue-engineered human skeletal muscle. *Am J Physiol Cell Physiol,* **283**, C1557–1565.
90. Qu-Petersen, Z., Deasy, B., Jankowski, R., Ikezawa, M., Cummins, J., Pruchnic, R., Mytinger, J., Cao, B., Gates, C., Wernig, A., and Huard, J. (2002). Identification of a novel population of muscle stem cells in mice: potential for muscle regeneration. *J Cell Biol,* **157**, 851–864.
91. Rajangam, K., Behanna, H. A., Hui, M. J., Han, X., Hulvat, J. F., Lomasney, J. W., and Stupp, S. I. (2006). Heparin binding nanostructures to promote growth of blood vessels. *Nano Lett,* **6**, 2086–2090.
92. Rhim, C., Lowell, D. A., Reedy, M. C., Slentz, D. H., Zhang, S. J., Kraus, W. E., and Truskey, G. A. (2007). Morphology and ultrastructure of differentiating three-dimensional mammalian skeletal muscle in a collagen gel. *Muscle Nerve,* **36**, 71–80.
93. Robertson, T. A., Maley, M. A., Grounds, M. D., and Papadimitriou, J. M. (1993). The role of macrophages in skeletal muscle regeneration with particular reference to chemotaxis. *Exp Cell Res,* **207**, 321–331.

94. Ross, J. J., Duxson, M. J., and Harris, A. J. (1987). Formation of primary and secondary myotubes in rat lumbrical muscles. *Development,* **100**, 383–394.
95. Rossi, C. A., Pozzobon, M., and De Coppi, P. (2010). Advances in musculoskeletal tissue engineering: moving towards therapy. *Organogenesis,* **6**, 167–172.
96. Rossi, C. A., Flaibani, M., Blaauw, B., Pozzobon, M., Figallo, E., Reggiani, C., Vitiello, L., Elvassore, N., and De Coppi, P. (2011). In vivo tissue engineering of functional skeletal muscle by freshly isolated satellite cells embedded in a photopolymerizable hydrogel. *FASEB J,* **25**, 2296–2304.
97. Sampaolesi, M., Torrente, Y., Innocenzi, A., Tonlorenzi, R., D'Antona, G., Pellegrino, M. A., Barresi, R., Bresolin, N., De Angelis, M. G., Campbell, K. P., Bottinelli, R., and Cossu, G. (2003). Cell therapy of alpha-sarcoglycan null dystrophic mice through intra-arterial delivery of mesoangioblasts. *Science,* **301**, 487–492.
98. Sampaolesi, M., Blot, S., D'Antona, G., Granger, N., Tonlorenzi, R., Innocenzi, A., Mognol, P., Thibaud, J. L., Galvez, B. G., Barthelemy, I., Perani, L., Mantero, S., Guttinger, M., Pansarasa, O., Rinaldi, C., Cusella De Angelis, M. G., Torrente, Y., Bordignon, C., Bottinelli, R., and Cossu, G. (2006). Mesoangioblast stem cells ameliorate muscle function in dystrophic dogs. *Nature,* **444**, 574–579.
99. Sanes, J. R. (2003). The basement membrane/basal lamina of skeletal muscle. *J Biol Chem,* **278**, 12601–12604.
100. Sanger, J. W., Chowrashi, P., Shaner, N. C., Spalthoff, S., Wang, J., Freeman, N. L., and Sanger, J. M. (2002). Myofibrillogenesis in skeletal muscle cells. *Clin Orthop Relat Res,* S153–S162.
101. Schiaffino, S., and Reggiani, C. (1994). Myosin isoforms in mammalian skeletal muscle. *J Appl Physiol,* **77**, 493–501.
102. Scholz, D., Thomas, S., Sass, S., and Podzuweit, T. (2003). Angiogenesis and myogenesis as two facets of inflammatory post-ischemic tissue regeneration. *Mol Cell Biochem,* **246**, 57–67.
103. Schwander, M., Leu, M., Stumm, M., Dorchies, O. M., Ruegg, U. T., Schittny, J., and Muller, U. (2003). Beta1 integrins regulate myoblast fusion and sarcomere assembly. *Dev Cell,* **4**, 673–685.
104. Scott, R. A., Elbert, D. L., and Willits, R. K. (2011). Modular poly(ethylene glycol). scaffolds provide the ability to decouple the effects of stiffness and protein concentration on PC12 cells. *Acta Biomater,* **7**, 3841–3849.

105. Serena, E., Flaibani, M., Carnio, S., Boldrin, L., Vitiello, L., De Coppi, P., and Elvassore, N. (2008). Electrophysiologic stimulation improves myogenic potential of muscle precursor cells grown in a 3D collagen scaffold. *Neurol Res,* **30,** 207–214.

106. Siegel, A. L., Atchison, K., Fisher, K. E., Davis, G. E., and Cornelison, D. D. (2009). 3D timelapse analysis of muscle satellite cell motility. *Stem Cells,* **27,** 2527–2538.

107. Sirivisoot, S., and Harrison, B. S. (2011). Skeletal myotube formation enhanced by electrospun polyurethane carbon nanotube scaffolds. *Int J Nanomedicine,* **6,** 2483–2497.

108. Sonnet, C., Lafuste, P., Arnold, L., Brigitte, M., Poron, F., Authier, F. J., Chretien, F., Gherardi, R. K., and Chazaud, B. (2006). Human macrophages rescue myoblasts and myotubes from apoptosis through a set of adhesion molecular systems. *J Cell Sci,* **119,** 2497–2507.

109. Suelves, M., Vidal, B., Ruiz, V., Baeza-Raja, B., Diaz-Ramos, A., Cuartas, I., Lluis, F., Parra, M., Jardi, M., Lopez-Alemany, R., Serrano, A. L., and Munoz-Canoves, P. (2005). The plasminogen activation system in skeletal muscle regeneration: antagonistic roles of urokinase-type plasminogen activator (uPA) and its inhibitor (PAI-1). *Front Biosci,* **10,** 2978–2985.

110. Tanaka, K. K., Hall, J. K., Troy, A. A., Cornelison, D. D., Majka, S. M., and Olwin, B. B. (2009). Syndecan-4-expressing muscle progenitor cells in the SP engraft as satellite cells during muscle regeneration. *Cell Stem Cell,* **4,** 217–225.

111. Tidball, J. G., and Villalta, S. A. (2010). Regulatory interactions between muscle and the immune system during muscle regeneration. *Am J Physiol Regul Integr Comp Physiol,* **298,** R1173–R1187.

112. Torrente, Y., Tremblay, J. P., Pisati, F., Belicchi, M., Rossi, B., Sironi, M., Fortunato, F., El Fahime, M., D'Angelo, M. G., Caron, N. J., Constantin, G., Paulin, D., Scarlato, G., and Bresolin, N. (2001). Intraarterial injection of muscle-derived CD34(+)Sca-1(+) stem cells restores dystrophin in mdx mice. *J Cell Biol,* **152,** 335–348.

113. Torrente, Y., Belicchi, M., Sampaolesi, M., Pisati, F., Meregalli, M., D'Antona, G., Tonlorenzi, R., Porretti, L., Gavina, M., Mamchaoui, K., Pellegrino, M. A., Furling, D., Mouly, V., Butler-Browne, G. S., Bottinelli, R., Cossu, G., and Bresolin, N. (2004). Human circulating AC133(+) stem cells restore dystrophin expression and ameliorate function in dystrophic skeletal muscle. *J Clin Invest,* **114,** 182–195.

114. Turner, N. J., Badylak, J. S., Weber, D. J., and Badylak, S. F. (2011). Biologic scaffold remodeling in a dog model of complex musculoskeletal injury. *J Surg Res,* **176**, 490–502.
115. Turner, N. J., and Badylak, S. F. (2012). Regeneration of skeletal muscle. *Cell Tissue Res,* **347**, 759–774.
116. Tysseling-Mattiace, V. M., Sahni, V., Niece, K. L., Birch, D., Czeisler, C., Fehlings, M. G., Stupp, S. I., and Kessler, J. A. (2008). Self-assembling nanofibers inhibit glial scar formation and promote axon elongation after spinal cord injury. *J Neurosci,* **28**, 3814–3823.
117. van der Schaft, D. W., van Spreeuwel, A. C., van Assen, H. C., and Baaijens, F. P. (2011). Mechanoregulation of vascularization in aligned tissue-engineered muscle: a role for vascular endothelial growth factor. *Tissue Eng Part A,* **17**, 2857–2865.
118. Vandenburgh, H., Shansky, J., Benesch-Lee, F., Barbata, V., Reid, J., Thorrez, L., Valentini, R., and Crawford, G. (2008). Drug-screening platform based on the contractility of tissue-engineered muscle. *Muscle Nerve,* **37**, 438–447.
119. Vandenburgh, H. H., Hatfaludy, S., Karlisch, P., and Shansky, J. (1989). Skeletal muscle growth is stimulated by intermittent stretch-relaxation in tissue culture. *Am J Physiol,* **256**, C674–C682.
120. Vandenburgh, H. H., and Karlisch, P. (1989). Longitudinal growth of skeletal myotubes in vitro in a new horizontal mechanical cell stimulator. *In vitro Cell Dev Biol,* **25**, 607–616.
121. Vasyutina, E., Martarelli, B., Brakebusch, C., Wende, H., and Birchmeier, C. (2009). The small G-proteins Rac1 and Cdc42 are essential for myoblast fusion in the mouse. *Proc Natl Acad Sci USA,* **106**, 8935–8940.
122. Velleman, S. G., Liu, X., Coy, C. S., and McFarland, D. C. (2004). Effects of syndecan-1 and glypican on muscle cell proliferation and differentiation: implications for possible functions during myogenesis. *Poult Sci,* **83**, 1020–1027.
123. Vieira, N. M., Brandalise, V., Zucconi, E., Jazedje, T., Secco, M., Nunes, V. A., Strauss, B. E., Vainzof, M., and Zatz, M. (2008). Human multipotent adipose-derived stem cells restore dystrophin expression of Duchenne skeletal-muscle cells in vitro. *Biol Cell,* **100**, 231–241.
124. Vieira, N. M., Bueno, C. R., Jr., Brandalise, V., Moraes, L. V., Zucconi, E., Secco, M., Suzuki, M. F., Camargo, M. M., Bartolini, P., Brum, P. C., Vainzof, M., and Zatz, M. (2008). SJL dystrophic mice express a significant

amount of human muscle proteins following systemic delivery of human adipose-derived stromal cells without immunosuppression. *Stem Cells,* **26**, 2391–2398.

125. Wagatsuma, A. (2007). Endogenous expression of angiogenesis-related factors in response to muscle injury. *Mol Cell Biochem,* **298**, 151–159.

126. Wiedow, O., and Meyer-Hoffert, U. (2005). Neutrophil serine proteases: potential key regulators of cell signalling during inflammation. *J Intern Med,* **257**, 319–328.

127. Wolf, M. T., Daly, K. A., Reing, J. E., and Badylak, S. F. (2012). Biologic scaffold composed of skeletal muscle extracellular matrix. *Biomaterials,* **33**, 2916–2925.

128. Yang, F., Cho, S. W., Son, S. M., Bogatyrev, S. R., Singh, D., Green, J. J., Mei, Y., Park, S., Bhang, S. H., Kim, B. S., Langer, R., and Anderson, D. G. (2010). Genetic engineering of human stem cells for enhanced angiogenesis using biodegradable polymeric nanoparticles. *Proc Natl Acad Sci USA,* **107**, 3317–3322.

129. Yoon, S., Molloy, M. J., Wu, M. P., Cowan, D. B., and Gussoni, E. (2007). C6ORF32 is upregulated during muscle cell differentiation and induces the formation of cellular filopodia. *Dev Biol,* **301**, 70–81.

130. Zacchigna, S., Ruiz de Almodovar, C., and Carmeliet, P. (2008). Similarities between angiogenesis and neural development: what small animal models can tell us. *Curr Top Dev Biol,* **80**, 1–55

131. Zheng, B., Cao, B., Crisan, M., Sun, B., Li, G., Logar, A., Yap, S., Pollett, J. B., Drowley, L., Cassino, T., Gharaibeh, B., Deasy, B. M., Huard, J., and Peault, B. (2007). Prospective identification of myogenic endothelial cells in human skeletal muscle. *Nat Biotechnol,* **25**, 1025–1034.

132. Zhou, M., Smith, A. M., Das, A. K., Hodson, N. W., Collins, R. F., Ulijn, R. V., and Gough, J. E. (2009). Self-assembled peptide-based hydrogels as scaffolds for anchorage-dependent cells. *Biomaterials,* **30**, 2523–2530.

133. Zhou, X. D., Xiong, M. M., Tan, F. K., Guo, X. J., and Arnett, F. C. (2006). SPARC, an upstream regulator of connective tissue growth factor in response to transforming growth factor beta stimulation. *Arthritis Rheum,* **54**, 3885–3889.

Index

adipose stem/progenitor cells (ASCs) 575–76, 767, 773–74
adipose tissues 431, 542, 590, 594, 767
alveolar bone 549, 566, 568, 573, 575, 593–94
angiogenesis 90, 118, 120, 501–2, 518, 572, 602, 696–98, 700–1, 741–42, 745, 760–61, 764, 767, 776
angiogenic growth factors 698, 700
aortic heart valve tissue regeneration 645–46, 648, 650, 652, 654, 656, 658, 660, 662, 664, 666, 668, 670, 672, 674
aortic valves 645–50, 654, 672
articular cartilage, self-assembling of 370, 372, 374, 376, 378, 380, 382, 384, 386, 388, 390, 392, 394
ASCs, see adipose stem/progenitor cells

biodegradable polyurethanes 243, 254
biomaterial scaffolds 37–40, 42, 44, 46, 48, 50, 52, 54, 56–58, 60, 62, 64, 66, 507, 701
  three-dimensional micropatterning of 37–38, 40, 42, 44, 46, 48, 50, 52, 54, 56, 58, 60, 62, 64, 66

biomaterials
  elastomeric 241, 245, 250, 253–54
  functional 79, 266–68, 270
  hydrogel 40, 42, 46
  Notch ligand–modified 548–49, 551
  peptide 283–84
  scaffold 320, 590, 595–96
  smart 342, 355, 413
  synthetic 255
biomimetic design principles 298, 309, 312, 314, 316, 703
biomimetic microvascular architecture 295–96, 298, 300, 302, 304, 306, 308, 310, 312, 314, 316, 318, 320, 322
biomimetic vascular design principles 298–99, 301, 303, 305, 307, 309, 311
bioreactor culture systems 412, 515–16
bladder reconstruction 250–51, 336, 350
bladder regeneration 348–50
bladder replacement 336, 339, 348–53
bladder tissue 158, 250, 335–36, 338, 340–42, 344, 346, 348, 350, 352, 354–55
  engineered 352–53, 355
blend electrospinning 84–86
BMA, see bone marrow aspirates
BMPs, see bone morphogenetic proteins
BMSCs, see bone marrow stromal cells

bone
  cortical 458–60, 467
  lamellar 458, 469
  native 131, 206, 381, 469,
    471–73, 606
  subchondral 141, 622–23,
    625–26, 632
  tissue engineering of 456, 471,
    590
  trabecular 458, 460, 470, 475
bone defects 517–18, 520, 593,
  595
bone formation 13, 118–19, 134,
  462, 497, 500, 502, 506–7,
  511, 515, 517–19, 591, 597
bone graft substitutes 463–66
bone grafts 381, 463–65, 496, 600
bone marrow 116, 344–45, 381,
  431, 475–76, 479, 500, 503,
  592, 594, 659, 661, 666, 763,
  767
bone marrow aspirates (BMA)
  466, 574
bone marrow MSCs 435, 592, 595,
  599, 668
bone marrow stromal cells (BMSCs)
  110, 132, 548, 575–76, 598,
  666, 767, 773–74
bone morphogenetic protein-2
  127, 496, 633–34
bone morphogenetic proteins
  (BMPs) 84, 160, 170, 211,
  283, 432, 466, 504, 519, 545,
  549, 574, 601–2
bone regeneration 10, 495–502,
  504, 506, 508, 510–14, 516,
  518–20, 548–49, 593,
  595–97, 601, 603–4, 607, 609
  calvarial 548, 575–76
  enhanced 602, 604
bone regenerative engineering
  455, 458, 460, 462, 464, 466,
  468, 470, 472, 474, 476, 478,
  480, 482

bone repair 25, 463, 471, 497,
  500–3, 506–7, 512, 515,
  517–19, 602
bone substitutes 463, 591–92
bone tissue 10, 24, 208, 210, 220,
  381–82, 460–61, 467–69,
  496, 498, 500–1, 507, 509,
  512, 514–15
bone tissue engineering (BTE) 10,
  24, 140, 208, 210, 498, 501,
  507, 516, 590–93, 595, 597,
  604, 607–8, 630
bone tissue formation 131, 503,
  520
bone tissue regeneration 19, 495,
  514–15, 549
bone tissue repair 503, 520
BTE, see bone tissue engineering

CAD, see computer-aided design
cardiac regeneration 550–51, 708,
  729, 732, 737, 744–45
cardiac tissue 246, 251, 253,
  725–26, 728–29, 733, 737,
  743, 746
  engineered 731
cardiac tissue engineering 251,
  725–26, 728–32, 734, 736,
  738, 740, 742, 744, 746
cartilage 116, 125–26, 131, 141,
  158–59, 169, 176, 373–74,
  387, 391–92, 410–11, 418,
  621–22, 626, 628
  engineered 158, 412, 417–18,
    420, 423, 425–26, 428–30,
    626
  tissue-engineered 412, 417–20,
    425, 427–28
cartilage repair 412–13, 424, 432,
  437
cartilage tissue 14, 159–60, 215,
  410, 413, 415–16, 418, 432,
  437, 599, 634

cell differentiation   157, 176, 188, 456, 468, 498, 503, 541, 548
cell homing   78, 566, 570–73, 577–79
cell printing   140, 697, 706–7
cell transplantation   78, 336, 566, 571–73, 576–79, 774
cell–biomaterial interactions   466, 609
cells
  autologous   342–44, 351, 574, 592
  bone-lining   461–62
  bone marrow   569, 574–75, 595
  dental follicle   568–69, 594, 604
  fibroblast   42, 56, 58
  glial   113, 206
  implanted   162–63, 766–67
  inflammatory   759, 762, 764
  interstitial   645, 647, 649, 671
  mesenchymal   461, 475, 548, 569, 571, 659
  muscle   249, 343, 350–51, 666, 758, 769–70, 777
  myogenic   760, 762, 766–68, 774
  osteoblast   467, 471
  osteoprogenitor   456, 461, 463, 508, 590, 602
  periodontal   544
  precursor   697
  primary   394, 435, 594
  renal tubular   300
  seeded   656, 658
  somatic   164, 346–47, 476
  stem/progenitor   566, 568, 571–72
  stromal   548, 595, 703
  transplanted   78, 337–38, 572
  urothelial   250, 342
  valve endothelial   663–64
  vascular   697, 701
cementum   549, 566, 568, 570, 573, 575, 594
chondrocytes   109–10, 116, 118, 124, 159–60, 163, 389, 410–13, 415, 418, 423, 426, 430–31, 434, 623–24
chondrogenesis   373, 422–24, 431–33
chondrogenic differentiation   15, 433, 628
co-culture systems   107–9, 111, 113–19, 141
collagen fibers   107, 201, 211, 458–61, 507, 549, 608, 623, 665, 728, 736
collagen fibrils   410, 420, 460, 507, 624–25
collagen gels   57, 273, 317, 510, 652, 656, 665, 711
collagen molecules   340, 459–60
composite nanofibers   15, 206
computer-aided design (CAD)   17, 22, 139–40, 600, 636
craniofacial graft design principles   591, 593, 595, 597, 599, 601, 603, 605
craniofacial tissue   575
craniofacial tissue engineering   565–66, 568, 570, 572, 574, 576, 578

DBD, *see* DNA-binding domain
degradable elastomers for tissue regeneration   231–32, 234, 236, 238, 240, 242, 244, 246, 248, 250, 252, 254
dental pulp   543, 566, 568–69, 571–72, 578
dental pulp stem cells (DPSCs)   543, 571, 594
dentin regeneration   543, 571
direct-write bioprinting   40, 42–43, 66
DNA-binding domain (DBD)   172, 182–83
DPSCs, *see* dental pulp stem cells

ECM-like substrate for tissue regeneration 200, 202, 204, 206, 208, 210, 212, 214, 216, 218, 220
ECs, see endothelial cells
elastomeric materials 241–42, 248, 251
elastomeric proteins 241
elastomers 232–40, 248, 255
  biodegradable 234–35, 237, 239, 241–43, 245, 247–49, 251, 253–55, 316, 703
  degradable 232, 235, 237–39, 248, 250, 252, 254
  electrospinning 11–13, 15–16, 28, 83–84, 135–36, 142, 199, 201–3, 215–16, 218, 220–21, 472–73, 607, 659, 735–36
  coaxial 85–86, 203, 208–10
  wet 13, 205
electrospun fibers 201–4, 209, 729, 736
electrospun nanofibers 199, 201, 205, 218, 221, 659, 736
embryonic stem cells (ESCs) 90, 114, 121, 241, 252, 335, 344–47, 350, 382, 498–99, 569, 592, 772, 774
  human 95, 241, 252, 345
endothelial cells (ECs) 47–52, 60–61, 109–12, 118–20, 321–22, 513, 566–67, 656–57, 668–69, 671, 697–98, 702–4, 708–10, 713, 777
endothelial progenitor cells (EPCs) 43, 696, 732
EPCs, see endothelial progenitor cells
epithelial cells 200, 254, 550–51, 567
  differentiation of 544, 550–51
ESCs, see embryonic stem cells
exogenous growth factors 422–25

FGFs, see fibroblast growth factor
fibers, spatial arrangement of 211, 213
fibroblast growth factor (FGFs) 85–86, 110, 127, 160, 173–74, 209, 211, 422, 504, 545, 601–2, 651, 698, 764
fibrocartilage 112, 124, 369, 387, 389–92
functional bone grafts for craniofacial regeneration 589–90, 592, 594, 596, 598, 600, 602, 604, 606, 608, 610
fusion proteins 55, 167, 172–74, 176, 182, 184

gene expression 111–12, 158, 161, 163, 165, 168, 170, 177–78, 186–88, 371, 373, 504, 506, 511, 730–31
gene regulation 157–58, 164–65, 167, 169, 171, 173, 175, 730
genes 76, 79, 84–85, 89–90, 158, 162–65, 169, 171, 175, 178, 181–82, 186–87, 504, 514, 730
  endogenous 164–65, 175
GFP, see green fluorescent protein
green fluorescent protein (GFP) 88, 176, 178–80, 182, 186–87, 514, 576, 592
GTR, see guided tissue regeneration
guided tissue regeneration (GTR) 550, 573, 634

heart valve disease 645–46
heart valve function 647, 649, 651
heart valve tissue 656
  engineered 667

heart valves 214, 647, 650, 657, 659, 667, 673, 675
hematopoietic stem cells (HSCs) 344, 462, 500, 541, 548, 571
hepatocyte growth factor (HGF) 244, 253, 698
hepatocytes 111, 120–21, 170, 299, 301, 318, 323, 375, 379–80, 710, 713
HGF, *see* hepatocyte growth factor
HSCs, *see* hematopoietic stem cells
human umbilical vein endothelial cells (HUVECs) 22, 90, 272–73, 281, 322–23, 656, 710
HUVECs, *see* human umbilical vein endothelial cells
hydrogel systems 53, 79–80, 277, 281, 283
hydrogels 38, 50–51, 54–63, 80–81, 115–17, 125, 137–38, 245–47, 267–71, 273–75, 278–81, 319–20, 322, 413–14, 704–5
  agarose 44, 54–56, 116, 430
  alginate 508
  bioactive 268–69, 271, 278, 280
  cell-laden 18, 62, 708–9
  multi-functional 268, 280, 283
  PEG-based 51–53, 55, 57, 60, 63–64, 137
  preformed 50, 58
  protein 269, 278–79, 281
  protein-based 270

inkjet bioprinting 40, 43–45, 66
inkjet printing 23, 44, 67, 139–40, 635
interface tissue engineering (ITE) 105–8, 115, 119–29, 131–32, 138, 141–44, 625

ITE, *see* interface tissue engineering

laser printing, biological 40, 46–48, 66–67, 707
liver tissue 379–80, 392

MDSCs, *see* muscle-derived stem cells
mesenchymal stem cells (MSCs) 90–91, 160, 246, 431–35, 475, 478–79, 500–3, 505–6, 508–9, 511–14, 516, 519, 551, 590–92, 659–60
  adipose-derived 542, 661
  human 57, 95, 247, 273, 477, 481
  multipotent 431, 433, 435, 592
microenvironments 53–54, 57, 96–97, 218, 232, 338, 414, 433, 476–77, 509, 650–51, 658, 660, 676, 727
microfluidic system 63–64
micromolding 81, 314, 318
microspheres 107, 122, 130
microstructures 18–19, 38, 46, 57, 67, 310, 339, 459–60, 467, 659, 671
mineralized tissue 107, 568, 598
MITCH, *see* mixing-induced, two component hydrogels
mixing-induced, two component hydrogels (MITCH) 271–73
MSC chondrogenic differentiation 432, 434–36
MSCs, *see* mesenchymal stem cells
multiwalled carbon nanotubes (MWCNTs) 15, 630–31
muscle-derived stem cells (MDSCs) 127, 160, 771, 773

muscle regeneration 756, 760–64, 767–68, 773–76
muscle repair 767–68, 772–73, 778
muscle satellite cells 761, 771–72
MWCNTs *see* multiwalled carbon nanotubes
myoblasts 165, 475, 739, 757–58, 760, 763–64, 768, 770, 772, 774, 777
myofibers 755–56, 758, 760, 762–63, 773
myogenesis 757, 760–61, 763–64, 768, 773
myogenic differentiation 127, 756, 763, 766, 773

nanobiomaterials 627, 631, 633–34, 636–37
  carbon-based 630–31
nanofabrication 627, 731, 737, 739, 741, 743, 745
nanofibers 15, 84, 129, 135, 199, 201, 203–20, 472–74, 607–8, 739, 775–76
  PCL/collagen 206, 212, 218–19
nanoparticles 77, 89–91, 163, 604, 699, 737, 744–46, 776
native bone tissue 206, 465, 507, 510, 515
native tissue morphogenesis 383, 388, 394
neovascularization 514, 572, 698–700, 711, 764
nerve growth factor (NGF) 86, 127, 211, 572
neural stem cells (NSCs) 60, 95, 127–28, 273, 475, 569
NGF, *see* nerve growth factor
Notch ligands 536–39, 542, 544–47, 549–51
Notch receptors 537–39, 546

Notch signaling 535–36, 538, 540–45, 547–51, 762
Notch signaling biomaterials 535–36, 538, 540, 542, 544–52
Notch signaling pathway 536–37, 539–41, 550
Notch signaling pathway, canonical 539–40
NSCs, *see* neural stem cells

odontoblast differentiation 543, 569
orofacial structures 565–66, 578
osteoblast differentiation 38, 479, 548–49
osteochondral regeneration 116, 123, 126, 621–22, 624–28, 630, 632, 634, 636
osteochondral tissue 621, 623, 626
osteochondral tissue regeneration 625, 627, 629–33, 635
osteogenic differentiation 127, 498, 502, 505, 507–11, 513–14, 516, 549, 575, 605, 767
oxygen 37, 158, 177, 252, 296–97, 299, 419, 458, 465, 515, 517, 605, 695–96, 700, 734

PDGF, *see* platelet-derived growth factor
pellet culture 373
peptide amphiphile 133, 272, 278–79, 281, 312, 516, 598–99, 606, 608, 627, 652, 737, 776
peptide fibers 280, 282
peptide ligands 274–75, 281
peptides 57, 60, 77, 243, 265–67, 269, 274–75, 277–78, 280, 282, 520, 608, 627–28, 705

self-assembling   280–81, 414, 416
periodontal defects   550, 573–74, 592, 594, 604
periodontal ligament stem cells   550, 594
periodontal regeneration   549, 573–75, 594–95
periodontal tissues   544, 594
PGS, *see* poly-glycerol-sebacate
photolithography   24, 39, 49, 51, 53, 55, 57, 59, 61, 65, 81, 315, 317–18, 608, 709
platelet-derived growth factor (PDGF)   86, 162, 211, 283, 428, 572–74, 601–3, 698–99
PLLA, *see* poly-L-lactic acid
pluripotent stem cells (PSCs)   78, 164, 346–47, 475, 497–99, 512, 514, 519, 731, 744, 772, 774
poly-glycerol-sebacate (PGS)   235–37, 250–52, 254, 316, 703
poly-L-lactic acid (PLLA)   13, 129, 134, 202, 205, 245, 414, 474, 628–29
polyamides   240–41, 598–99
polyesters   234–35, 239, 241, 244, 341, 507
polymeric nanofibers   206, 473, 736
polymers
  elastomeric   81, 232, 250, 254
  natural   79–80, 83, 115, 199, 205, 231, 241, 247, 596, 626
  synthetic   79–80, 83, 95, 205–6, 231–32, 234, 240–41, 245, 339, 341, 507, 573, 599, 626, 657–58
polypeptides   266, 271
polyurethanes   81, 241–44, 253–54, 336, 775
post-gelation photopatterning   50–51, 54, 61, 64

progenitor cells   79, 342–43, 354, 566–67, 591, 595, 778
  adult   78, 345
protein fibers   269–70, 278
proteins, non-collagenous   459, 461–62, 726
PSCs, *see* pluripotent stem cells

rapid prototyping   16–17, 80, 139, 200, 318, 600–1, 659, 705
regenerative medicine   75–80, 82–84, 86, 88, 90–94, 96–97, 254–55, 335–36, 338, 341–42, 350, 354, 376, 535–36, 542
regenerative therapies   255, 345, 509, 574, 577–78

scaffold-based tissue   372
scaffold design   19, 76, 97, 144, 199–200, 217, 220, 626, 776
scaffold fabrication   16, 19, 25–26, 28, 76, 133, 135, 137, 139, 205
scaffold materials   23, 118, 241, 314, 317–19, 340, 352–53, 372, 596, 656–57, 667–68, 675
scaffold types   121–23, 125, 127, 129, 131, 142, 430
scaffoldless approaches   43, 132, 370, 375, 377
scaffolds
  anisotropic   128
  biodegradable   413, 456, 467, 591
  braided   122, 129–30, 142
  cartilage   126, 626
  collagen   40–41, 117, 138, 170, 317, 352, 572, 575, 596, 769

composite nanofiber/microsphere 474–75
electrospun 10, 14–15, 83–84, 87, 135–36, 414, 701, 775
exogenous 372, 377
fibrous 129, 136, 236, 243
gradiated 107, 122–24, 127–28, 133–34, 136, 142–43
microsphere-based 122
nanofiber 472, 507
nanofibrous 85–86, 125–26, 133, 135, 142, 201, 205, 414, 607
nanostructured 15, 25, 608
natural 119, 131, 200, 767
osteochondral 141, 635–37
polymer 350, 776
porous 13, 27, 322, 341, 604
printed 23–24, 43
tissue-engineered 26, 298, 314
valve 657, 659, 661
scanning electron microscopy (SEM) 84, 90, 134, 202, 631
SCs, see stem cells
selective laser sintering (SLS) 19–21, 139, 318, 598, 600–1, 635, 705
self-assembling tissues 370, 376–77, 385, 390–91, 393–94
self-organization 370, 372, 374–79, 382, 394
SEM, see scanning electron microscopy
SFF, see solid freeform fabrication
skeletal muscle 173, 431, 755–56, 759, 761–62, 764, 766–67, 778
skeletal muscle regeneration 755–64, 766, 768, 770, 772, 774, 776, 778
skeletal myogenesis 756–57, 760
SLS, see selective laser sintering
SMCs, see smooth muscle cells
smooth muscle cells (SMCs) 117, 127, 162, 218–19, 243, 249–50, 335, 338, 342–43, 354, 661, 666, 697–98, 709, 713
solid freeform fabrication (SFF) 18, 139, 660, 705–6
spatiotemporal gene regulation systems 177, 179, 181, 183, 185, 187
stem cell differentiation 51, 91, 409, 463, 477–79, 481, 497, 503, 515, 520
stem cell phenotype 508, 512, 514, 516
stem cell proliferation 475, 477, 551
stem cell sources 476, 497, 499, 501, 661
stem cells (SCs) 246–47, 344–47, 475–79, 495–520, 535–36, 540–44, 550–51, 566–67, 569–71, 578–79, 590–94, 658–61, 730–31, 765–68, 771–74
  adipose-derived 382, 771
  adult 250, 344–46, 475, 497, 499, 766
  human 344, 730
  human-induced pluripotent 91
  marrow-derived 350, 771
  marrow-derived mesenchymal 208, 218
  osteogenic differentiation of 505–6, 509, 512
  osteogenic induction of 503, 505, 507, 509, 511, 513
  tissue-derived mesenchymal 542
  undifferentiated 345, 500, 767
stimuli, biochemical 142, 425, 427, 429, 765

TEHV, see tissue-engineered heart valve

TGF, *see* transforming growth factor
therapeutic muscle regeneration 765, 767, 769
time-independent gene regulation systems 158–59, 161, 163
tissue
 adult 344–46, 476, 497–98, 503
 connective 549, 566, 578, 763
 diseased 343, 353–54, 744
 fetal 503
 normal 126, 200, 338, 343–44, 354, 727
 orofacial 571, 578
 scaffoldless 369–72, 374–76
 scar 173, 566, 728, 759, 761
 self-organizing 370, 375, 377, 380
 vascularized 17, 695–97
tissue alignment 727, 731
tissue culture 112
tissue-engineered heart valve (TEHV) 645, 647, 653, 655, 657, 659, 661–62, 667, 673–76
tissue engineers 39, 369, 371, 381, 592
tissue fusion 378, 383
tissue growth 124, 430
tissue ingrowth 124, 129, 204, 339
tissue regeneration 78–81, 83, 199–202, 231–32, 234–36, 244–54, 348, 456–57, 498–99, 535–36, 550–52, 566, 578–79, 630, 634
 functional 209, 249, 337
 guided 573, 634
 periodontal 549–50
tissue repair 75, 78, 176, 495–97, 501, 519, 774
 ischemic 280, 699

tissues, engineered 158, 165, 296–98, 304, 338–39, 352–53, 377, 380, 415–16, 419, 422–23, 425, 427–28, 695–96, 704
tooth regeneration 569–70
transforming growth factor (TGF) 110, 160, 411, 496, 574, 601, 628, 651, 698, 760, 764
transgene expression 169, 183–84
transwell systems 109–10, 114

valvular endothelial cells (VEC) 650–51, 661, 664
valvular interstitial cells (VICs) 648, 664–65
vascular endothelial growth factor (VEGF) 55, 90, 118, 209–11, 274–75, 502, 572, 576, 601–2, 651, 698–99, 739, 745, 776
vascular regeneration 695–96, 698, 700, 702, 704, 706, 708, 710, 712
vascular structures 119, 317, 319, 321, 543, 702, 712, 777
vasculogenesis 602, 696–97, 703
VEC, *see* valvular endothelial cells
VEGF, *see* vascular endothelial growth factor
vessel diameter 301, 303, 307
VICs, *see* valvular interstitial cells

wavy-walled bioreactor (WWB) 420–21, 425, 427–28
WWB, *see* wavy-walled bioreactor

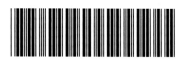